# Palliative care nursing
## Second edition

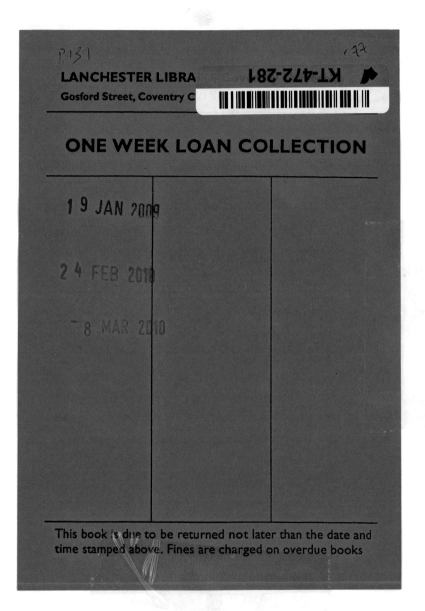

# Palliative care nursing

## Principles and evidence for practice

## Second edition

*Edited by Sheila Payne, Jane Seymour and Christine Ingleton*

(Payne, 2008)

Open University Press

Open University Press
McGraw-Hill Education
McGraw-Hill House
Shoppenhangers Road
Maidenhead
Berkshire
England
SL6 2QL

email: enquiries@openup.co.uk
world wide web: www.openup.co.uk

and
Two Penn Plaza, New York, NY 10121-2289, USA

First published 2004
Second edition published 2008

A catalogue record of this book is available from the British Library

ISBN13: 978 0 335 22181 3 (pb)
ISBN10: 0 335 22181 5 (pb)

Library of Congress Cataloging-in-Publication Data
CIP data has been applied for

Typeset by RefineCatch Limited, Bungay, Suffolk
Printed in Great Britain by Bell and Bain Ltd., Glasgow

Fictitious name of companies, products, people, characters and/or data
that may be used herein (in case studies or in examples) are not intended
to represent any real individual, company, product or event.

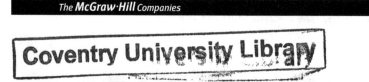

# Contents

# Contributors

**Julia Addington-Hall**, Professor in End of Life Care, Co-Director of the NCRI-funded Cancer Experiences Supportive and Palliative Care Research Collaborative (CECo), School of Nursing and Midwifery, University of Southampton, Southampton, UK

**Kendra Albright**, Lecturer and Deputy Director, Centre for Health Information Management Research, University of Sheffield, Sheffield, UK

**Sanchia Aranda**, Professor of Nursing and Head, School of Nursing and Social Work, The University of Melbourne and Director of Cancer Nursing Research, Peter MacCallum Cancer Centre, Melbourne, Australia

**Christopher Bailey**, Senior Research Fellow and Academic Co-ordinator, Cancer Experiences Research Collaborative, School of Nursing and Midwifery, University of Southampton, Southampton, UK

**Peter Bath**, Senior Lecturer in Health Informatics and Director, Centre for Health Information Management Research (CHIMR), University of Sheffield, Sheffield, UK

**Michael Bennett**, Professor of Palliative Medicine, International Observatory on End of Life Care, Lancaster University, Lancaster, UK

**Bert Broeckaert**, Professor, Interdisciplinary Centre for the Study of Religion and Worldview, University of Leuven, Leuven, Belgium

**Margaret Camps**, Palliative Care Macmillan Nurse, Cancer Centre Mount Vernon Hospital, East and North Herts NHS Trust, Middlesex, UK

**Ann Carter**, Complementary Therapy Co-ordinator, St Ann's Hospice, Manchester, UK

**David Clark**, Professor of Medical Sociology, International Observatory on End of Life Care, Lancaster University, Lancaster, UK

**José Closs**, Professor of Nursing, School of Health Care, University of Leeds, Leeds, UK

**Reverend Mark Cobb**, Clinical Director and Senior Chaplain at Sheffield Teaching Hospitals NHS Foundation Trust, Directorate of Professional Services, Royal Hallamshire Hospital, Sheffield, UK

**Jessica Corner**, Professor, Director of Improving Cancer Services, Macmillan Cancer Support, London, UK

**Karen Cox**, Professor of Cancer and Palliative Care, Faculty of Medicine and Health Sciences, University of Nottingham, Nottingham, UK

**Sue Duke**, Consultant Practitioner/Senior Lecturer in Cancer and Palliative Care, School of Nursing and Midwifery, University of Southampton, Southampton, UK

**Katherine Froggatt**, Senior Lecturer, International Observatory on End of Life Care, Lancaster University, Lancaster, UK

**Gunn Grande**, Senior Lecturer Palliative Care, School of Nursing, Midwifery and Social Work, University of Manchester, Manchester, UK

**Jenny Hockey**, Professor of Sociology, Department of Sociological Studies, University of Sheffield, Sheffield, UK

**Jo Hockley**, Research Fellow/Clinical Nurse Specialist, School of Community Health Sciences, University of Edinburgh, Edinburgh, UK

**Matthew Hotopf**, Professor of General Hospital Psychiatry, Department of Psychological Medicine, King's College London, London, UK

**John Hughes**, Research Fellow, Academic Palliative and Supportive Care Studies Group (APSCSG), University of Liverpool, Liverpool, UK

**Jennifer Hunt**, Independent Consultant, Harare, Zimbabwe

**Christine Ingleton**, Reader in Palliative Care, Centre for Health and Social Care, University of Sheffield, Sheffield, UK

**Veronica James**, Professor of Nursing Studies, School of Nursing, Nottingham University, Nottingham, UK

**Jeanne Samson Katz**, Senior Lecturer and Director of Postgraduate Studies, Faculty of Health and Social Care, The Open University, Milton Keynes, UK

**David Kissane**, Professor of Psychiatry, Department of Psychiatry and Behavioural Sciences, Weill Medical College of Cornell University, New York, USA

**Jonathan Koffman**, Lecturer in Palliative Care, Department on Palliative Care, Policy and Rehabilitation, King's College London, London, UK

**Carol Komaromy**, Director (Health and Social Care), Faculty of Health and Social Care, The Open University, Milton Keynes, UK

**Philip Larkin**, Senior Lecturer in Nursing (Palliative Care), School of Nursing and Midwifery Studies, The National University of Ireland, Galway, Ireland

**William Lee**, Clinical Lecturer in General Hospital Psychiatry, Department of Psychological Medicine, King's College London, London, UK

**Mari Lloyd-Williams**, Professor/Honorary Consultant in Palliative Medicine, Academic Palliative and Supportive Care Studies Group (APSCSG), University of Liverpool, Liverpool, UK

**Peter Mackereth**, Clinical Lead and Senior Lecturer University of Derby, Rehabilitation Unit, Christie Hospital NHS Foundation Trust, Manchester, UK

**Margaret O'Connor**, Professor of Palliative Care Nursing, Monash University, Melbourne, Australia

**Sheila Payne**, Help the Hospices Chair in Hospice Studies, Co-Director of the NCRI-funded Cancer Experiences Supportive and Palliative Care Research Collaborative (CECo), International Observatory on End of Life Care, Lancaster University, Lancaster, UK

**Silvia Paz**, Palliative Care Physician, Palliative Care Unit, Institut Catalá d'Oncologia, L'Hospitalet de Llobregat, Barcelona, Spain

**Marilyn Relf**, Head of Education, Sir Michael Sobell House, Oxford, UK

**Liz Rolls**, Clara Burgess Charity Senior Research Fellow, Department of Natural and Social Sciences, University of Gloucestershire, Cheltenham, UK

**Barbara Sen**, Lecturer in Information and Library Management, Department of Information Studies, University of Sheffield, Sheffield, UK

**Jane Seymour**, Sue Ryder Care Professor in Palliative and End of Life Studies, School of Nursing, Faculty of Medicine and Health Sciences, University of Nottingham, Nottingham, UK

**Julie Skilbeck**, Senior Lecturer in Nursing, Faculty of Health and Wellbeing, Sheffield Hallam University, Sheffield, UK

**Paula Smith**, Lecturer, Faculty of Health and Wellbeing, Sheffield Hallam University, Sheffield, UK

**Tony Stevens**, Research Fellow, International Observatory on End of Life Care, Lancaster University, Lancaster, UK

**Carol Thomas**, Professor of Sociology, Institute for Health Research, Lancaster University, Lancaster, UK

**Mary Turner**, Research Fellow, International Observatory on End of Life Care, Lancaster University, Lancaster, UK

**Reverend Michael Wright**, Senior Research Fellow, International Observatory on End of Life Care, Lancaster University, Lancaster, UK

# Foreword

Nurse academics are an interesting if somewhat capricious breed. We tend to want a foot in both camps. Not content with expecting students to inwardly digest a wealth of knowledge from the weighty volumes of literature put before them, we also demand that they seek ways of blending this knowledge with the reality of the clinical world they live in. The ultimate aim of this arduous process is to enable the practitioners of the future to articulate their unique contribution to their chosen field of practice. In this second edition, we are fortunate in having a thoughtful and scholarly resource which clearly articulates that unique contribution for palliative care nursing. The fact that Sheila Payne, Jane Seymour and Christine Ingleton have chosen to offer a new revised edition since the book was first published in 2004, demonstrates the pace of change facing palliative care today. It may seem that palliative care is at a crossroads and that decisions need to be made as to its place within mainstream health care and where it is going. Even the language which shaped the thinking of many early pioneers in the field may no longer fit comfortably with a technologically driven model of practice based on an interventionist process and outcome mentality. In bringing together a group of internationally renowned experts to provide a critical review of where palliative nursing fits within this shifting paradigm, the editors offer a body of evidence by which nurses can validate their real worth and contribution to palliative care practice.

Most importantly, the second edition does not try to 're-invent the wheel'. Readers familiar with the framework of the first edition will find similarity in layout and in some of the chapters which follow. Such a framework, which embraces a life-limiting illness approach, not only acknowledges the breadth of palliative care beyond malignant disease, but strengthens the call for a legitimate palliative care agenda based on a public health approach. Today, this is an important consideration in challenging the status quo of clinically led models of care for those facing the end of life. Equally, this new edition is neither complacent nor in anyway indulgent of its success to date. It is aware of the need to set palliative care in a global context and, in particular, a chapter on palliative care in resource poor countries offers a platform from which the success and failures of some of the arguments which have shaped palliative care to date (such as the need for specialization) may be judged. The second edition also includes new chapters which provide a comprehensive and reflective balance between the political nature of palliative care and interpreting the true essence of end-of-life care – a fundamental respect for the personhood of the other.

In using this book as a resource for teaching, learning and practice, the reader will find clear evidence that palliative care based within humanity frames the beliefs and views of the many experts who have contributed to this edition. Neither should it be forgotten that this book is edited by nurses who, by virtue of their clinical and academic experiences over many years, are able to examine the critical issues of palliative care from a variety of perspectives and to reach considered and sound conclusions about that unique contribution of nursing to the wider dimension of practice.

There are clearly going to be challenges for nurses involved in palliative care in the future. To meet those challenges, it will be imperative that we, as nurses, are clearly able to articulate who we are and what we do, so that others, particularly the patient, family and carer, will also understand our contribution to their care. Each of the chapters in this book enables nurses to reflect on those challenges, so that the roles and responsibilities in light of the changing dynamic of palliative care can be appraised. I am particularly indebted to the authors for their revisioning of the traditional model of palliative care (which they term 'the wedge') into a more fluid and realistic model for chronic disease, 'the wave'. I have no doubt that this will prove to be one of the most important innovations within this second edition and demonstrates the leadership which this book will bring to the field of palliative care in general. I make this final point because this book should not just be read and used by nurses but has a message for the wider multidisciplinary community which is involved in end-of-life. We owe a debt of gratitude to the authors for helping to articulate the voice of nursing within palliative care. It is now for nurses to take the foundations offered in this book and share the vision which has been so ably presented here.

**Philip J. Larkin**
Former Vice President of the European Association for Palliative Care

# Introduction
*Sheila Payne, Jane Seymour and Christine Ingleton*

Fifty-six million people die in the world each year and, according to the World Health Organization (WHO), approximately 60 per cent could benefit from palliative care (Davies and Higginson 2004a). Some infants may die shortly after life has begun but, increasingly, people are surviving longer into adulthood, with growing numbers dying in late old age. Death may come in many different ways such as after an acute illness, a sudden violent road accident, on the battlefield, following a chronic illness or after a prolonged decline in physical fitness in late old age. While all of us will die; most of us cannot determine the manner of our dying. Patterns of dying vary over time and in different contexts but current global public health challenges are related to ten risk factors which are implicated in over 40 per cent of all deaths including; being underweight (especially for women and children), unsafe sexual behaviour, hypertension, tobacco use, alcohol consumption, unsafe water, lack of sanitation, high cholesterol, indoor smoke from cooking and heating fires, iron deficiency anaemia and obesity (World Health Organization 2002). There are stark contrasts between causes of death in different parts of the world, and in overall life expectancy and in healthy life expectancy. In the resource-rich regions of the world, death is most frequently associated with chronic illness and occurs in later life (Davis and Higginson 2004b). In resource-poor regions, acute infectious illness such as malaria and tuberculosis continue to cause death, while globally HIV/AIDS is now rated as the fourth leading cause of death. Cancer is a major cause of death globally. Estimates from the WHO (2007) indicate that 7.6 million people died of cancer in 2005 and 84 million people may die of the disease in the next decade. Over 70 per cent of all cancer deaths occur in countries where health care resources are limited.

Health care agendas, the organization and funding of health care services and resources for health and social care are remarkably variable throughout the world (Sepulveda *et al.* 2002). So, the majority of dying people do not benefit from supportive and palliative care or even have sufficient access to medication to relieve suffering. Five years after the preparation of the first edition of this book, there is now much more evidence about the distribution and nature of palliative care services worldwide. In 2007, 115 of the world's 234 countries had established one or more hospice or palliative care services (Clark and Wright 2007), but only in 35 countries had these services become sufficiently well established to become part of national health care policies and be integrated with other health care providers. More detailed mapping of services has been undertaken for certain areas including Eastern Europe and Central Asia (Clark and Wright 2003), Africa (Wright and Clark 2006), the 52 countries of Europe (Centeno *et al.* 2007) and the Middle East (Bingley and Clark in press). This information, along with reports on individual countries, helps both to demonstrate what has been achieved in the global development of palliative care but also to show how much still needs to be done.

This book is about the care of people facing death, both those who will die and those who accompany them – families, friends, community supporters, volunteer workers, health and social care workers. In particular, the book focuses on the role of nurses in providing care throughout the trajectory of advanced illness, the process of dying and in the respectful care of the dead person. Nurses generally work closely with family members, if they are available, supporting them through the process of illness and bereavement. We have focused attention on those who die as adults rather than those who die as babies and young children. Paediatric palliative nursing care is an important topic but requires the attention of a different book. However, dying adults are often in close relationships with children as parents, grandparents or guardians, so to ensure the needs of children are not overlooked a chapter about the impact of death on children and services for bereaved children has been included.

The palliation of distressing symptoms, the care of patients approaching death, the laying out of the body and the care of newly bereaved relatives have long formed an important part of nursing work. In the latter part of the twentieth century, the emergence of the modern hospice movement has provided an impetus to reconceptualizing the delivery of some aspects of this care (Clark and Seymour 1999). Nursing has been central to a new style of end-of-life care, both in specialist contexts such as in hospices, hospital teams and community teams, and more broadly in delivering care to terminally ill people in a range of settings. There has been an increasing recognition of the importance of nursing care provided in patients' homes. Specialist education for nurses in 'Care of the Dying' has been available in post-qualifying courses in the UK since the 1980s. In 2004, the European Association for Palliative Care endorsed an educational curriculum for nurses at three levels of expertise (Vliegner _et al._ 2004) and curriculum developments for nurses have been progressed in the United States of America through the End of Life Nursing Education Consortium and The Education on Palliative and End-of-Life Care Project. Across the world, nursing roles have been extended to develop advanced practice and specialist expertise, such as Clinical Nurse Specialists and Nurse Consultants, but in most regions they are a limited resource.

Current debates in health care recognize a number of tensions which are likely to impact upon specialist palliative care services. They include: concerns about the medicalization of dying; issues around equity of access; appropriateness of service models; cost effectiveness; and problems with funding sources. In some parts of the world, such as the Indian subcontinent, palliative care services remain virtually non-existent or overwhelmingly stretched and in these situations nurses are required to be resourceful in using community support (Graham and Clark 2005a). In these situations, there is relatively little choice for patients. In other countries such as the USA, Canada, Australia and the UK, political and economic agendas are encouraging patients to participate more actively in expressing preferences about place of care; often with the implicit assumption that home care is 'best'. This raises important questions and roles for nurses in facilitating advance care planning, comparability of care options and reasons of choices. The relationship of specialist palliative care services and central health care planning and policy remains controversial in some countries because most hospices have arisen independently of central control (Clark and Wright 2003). This means these services do not form part of the main health care agenda and therefore do not secure necessary resources. However, they have offered opportunities for innovation in care and pioneering new ways of working.

## What is palliative care?

The use and evaluation of specialist palliative care services is based on an assumption that people share a common understanding of the terminology and purpose of palliative care. However, most of the evidence indicates that definitions and terminology are poorly understood and not agreed (Praill 2000; Payne *et al.* 2002). Terminology is influenced by the historical development and the nature of end-of-life health care services in different countries and changes over time (see Box 1). In the UK, terminology relating to end-of-life care has undergone a number of transitions from hospice care and terminal care in the early period of the hospice movement (1960s and 1970s) to palliative care towards the turn of the last century (1980–2000). Clark and Seymour (1999) provide an account of these transitions in terminology in relation to the UK context. They have noted how terminology has changed as tensions in the boundaries between generalist and specialist skills, activities and services have become more contentious.

Recently, supportive care has emerged as an accepted term within the context of services that are provided in addition to curative treatments for cancer patients (Department of Health 2000). While the term end-of-life care was first applied to care of dying patients in Canada, this term is now widely used in North America.

---

**Box 1**  Terms associated with caring for dying people

- Hospice care
- Terminal care
- Continuing care
- Care of the dying
- Palliative care
- End-of-life care
- Supportive care

There may be a number of reasons for the increasing number of terms used to describe health and social care services provided for those near the end of life. While the early hospice movement in the UK was unambiguously concerned with terminal care, predominantly for those with cancer, subsequent developments have sought to extend the range of services in terms of both client groups (non-cancer) and types and timing of interventions during the illness trajectory. Current policies in the UK have sought to introduce palliative or supportive care much earlier in the illness trajectory (Department of Health 2000; National Institute for Clinical Excellence (NICE) 2003). Most discussion of supportive care and the definition offered by the National Council for Hospices and Specialist Palliative Care Services (2002) are located in the context of cancer care but there is no good reason why supportive care could not be applicable to those with other chronic illnesses (Addington Hall and Higginson 2001; National Council for Hospices and Specialist Palliative Care Services 2003). Praill (2000) has argued that the transition in terminology from 'terminal care' to 'palliative care' reflects a 'death denying' tendency. These changes in terminology have paralleled the growth in medical involvement in end-of-life care services more generally. McNamara (2001), writing from an Australian perspective, has observed how the medical component has gradually come to frame and dominate definitions of palliative care. It is therefore hardly surprising that most major medical and nursing textbooks in palliative care prioritize symptom control as a key function (e.g. Doyle *et al.* 1998; Ferrell and Coyle 2001).

In an attempt to establish greater clarity, predominantly directed at an audience within specialist palliative care, the National Council for Hospices and Specialist Palliative Care Services (2002) published a briefing paper which offers a series of definitions of common terms. Many other organizations and countries have sought to establish working definitions and standards to guide service provision, for example in Australia and New Zealand. There has yet to be a consensus view. For the purposes of this book, we will draw upon the working definitions proposed by the National Council for Hospices and Specialist Palliative Care Services (2002) and the World Health Organization's recently revised definitions (Sepulveda *et al.* 2002). However, we do not agree with the abrupt demarcation between supportive/palliative care and bereavement depicted in the National Council for Hospices and Specialist Palliative Care Services (2002) model, instead, we regard it as a transition, in that preparation for bereavement care for families may start prior to the death of the patient, as will be explained in greater detail in Part Three of this book.

Definition of palliative care (Sepulveda *et al.* 2002: 94)

> Palliative care is an approach that improves the quality of life of patients and their families facing the problems associated with life-threatening illness, through the prevention and relief of suffering by means of early identification and impeccable assessment and treatment of pain and other problems, physical, psychosocial and spiritual.

Palliative care:

- provides relief from pain and other distressing symptoms;
- affirms life and regards dying as a normal process;
- intends neither to hasten nor postpone death;
- integrates the psychological and spiritual aspects of patient care;
- offers a support system to help patients live as actively as possible until death;
- offers a support system to help the family cope during the patient's illness and in their own bereavement;
- uses a team approach to address the needs of patients and their families, including bereavement counselling, if indicated;
- will enhance quality of life, and may also positively influence the course of illness;
- is applicable early in the course of illness, in conjunction with other therapies that are intended to prolong life, such as chemotherapy or radiation therapy, and include those investigations needed to better understand and manage distressing clinical complications.

The National Council for Hospices and Specialist Palliative Care Services (2002: 2) differentiate between:

- *general palliative care*, which 'is provided by the usual professional carers of the patient and family with low to moderate complexity of palliative care need', and
- *specialist palliative care services*, which 'are provided for patients and their families with moderate to high complexity of palliative care need. They are defined in terms of their core service components, their functions and the composition of the multi-professional teams that are required to deliver them.'

In the following sections, a number of key debates and questions in contemporary palliative care will be highlighted. Many of these topics will be discussed in greater depth in the ensuing chapters.

## What is the remit of palliative care?

The twentieth century was remarkable in the successful development of a large range of new health technologies (such as blood transfusion, radiotherapy), pharmaceutical agents (such as antibiotics, insulin, antiretroviral agents) and preventive health care procedures (such as immunization and various types of screening). Combined with improved nutrition, better housing, sanitation and clean water, many of the citizens of resource-rich regions of the world have opportunities for healthy living, unrivalled in history. The profession of medicine has been seen as pivotal in contributing to these developments and arguably a culture of 'cure' was seen to marginalize the dying. However, the rise in medical power did not go unchallenged (Illich 1976) and throughout the century (see Winslow and Clark 2005 history of St Joseph's Hospice in Hackney, London), but particularly from the 1950s onwards, there was a growing interest in improving the care of dying people (Clark's chapter provides a fuller account of the history of hospice development).

Figure 1 demonstrates two possible models of palliative care: the 'wedge' was the traditional model where curative treatment input declined as palliative input increased, and bereavement support was only provided after the death. In comparison, the 'wave' model indicates the concurrent provision of supportive and palliative care with curative treatment. This model is particularly appropriate for chronic diseases with an uncertain and remitting nature, like heart failure. In some countries palliative care may be used concurrently with active treatment, while in others palliative care services are restricted only to those who have completed all available curative treatment. For example, with HIV the treatment of opportunistic infections need active treatment but the underlying disease cannot be cured; this would be the same for end-stage heart failure, chronic obstructive airways disease (COPD) and renal failure. This presents considerable dilemmas for when referral to supportive and palliative care services should be initiated. It is often the case in resource-poor settings that patients do not access care early enough, which means that potentially curable treatments are ineffective because they are delivered too late.

Contemporary debates focus on whether palliative care services should concentrate attention on terminal care or extend its remit to those at earlier stages of the illness. Arguably, the success of the early 'hospice' period was because it had a clear goal in improving the quality of dying, especially for

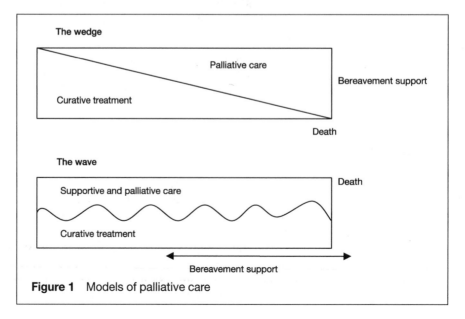

**Figure 1**   Models of palliative care

those dying of cancer. The advantage of this approach is that it makes good use of limited resources and practitioners develop specific skills in controlling difficult symptoms associated with the dying phase. Moreover, professionals can also concentrate their efforts on addressing the psychosocial and spiritual concerns of patients and the supporting of family members. The disadvantage of offering services just to those who are imminently dying is the difficulty in accurate prognostication. Therefore, people, especially those who have precipitous deaths, may miss out and, alternatively, those whose final illness is very protracted may exhaust the resources of some charitable services. In the UK, palliative care services generally have a great deal of expertise in caring for people with cancer but rather less expertise in caring for patients dying of other conditions. There have been concerns raised about the arbitrary definitions of 'dying' applied to different groups of people. In the US access to insurance funded hospice care programmes has been dependent upon people agreeing to no longer seek curative treatment. This has created great dilemmas and conflict within families as different members may or may not wish to continue to seek active interventions. The consequence is that many people are admitted to palliative care programmes when it is almost too late for them or their families to benefit from care (Shockett *et al.* 2005).

An emerging model of palliative care emphasizes the supportive role of health and social care practitioners throughout the trajectory of illness. This model, which arguably is driven by a medical agenda, suggests that symptom control is the major priority. There are now many more well-established medical interventions than were available in the early days of hospice care. For example, the syringe driver has revolutionized the way medication may be delivered subcutaneously in those with advanced illness (Graham and Clark 2005b). It offers many benefits for people who are unable to take oral medication. Its use has become pervasive in many palliative care contexts in the UK but is not commonly used in all countries. The advantage of a supportive care model is that skilled medical and nursing symptom control interventions are not limited to one period of a patient's life (the final stage), so that suffering can be relieved at all stages of their illness. In the UK the primary reason for admission to inpatient palliative care is for treatment of complex symptoms. Once there is resolution of symptoms or acceptable management, patients are discharged home or to other types of care. The use of skilled specialist palliative care resources can be targeted at those with severe and/or complex needs, rather than diagnostic category (Skilbeck and Payne 2005). The disadvantage of this model of palliative care is the lack of clarity in its implementation. In particular, there are concerns about territorial disputes between generalists (such as general practitioners and community nurses, or hospital based practitioners) and specialist palliative care providers. This model has the potential to deskill other health and social care providers because they come to believe that only specialist palliative care professionals are competent to work with dying people. Caring for patients with advanced disease and those who are dying is an important aspect of many health care professionals workload, especially for those working in care homes for older people (Froggatt *et al.* 2006). It is therefore important not to disempower them but instead to work in collaboration while acknowledging the skills that each practitioner may bring. This model of care also raises concerns about boundaries between the areas of expertise in specialist workers. Since many older patients have a number of co-morbidities which may be treated by different specialists such as a cardiologist, a neurologist and an oncologist, there are real dangers of overtreatment. By extending the remit of specialist palliative care to patients who are at earlier stages of their disease, this raises issues about availability of funding and resources, and their optimal use.

# Who gets palliative care? Who should get palliative care?

Access to palliative care typically relates to the availability of services, the funding models of health care, and the nature of disease. For example, access to hospice programmes (generally home care) in the USA is generally a balance between people with cancer and other conditions, while in many African countries hospices predominantly care for people with HIV/AIDS (Wright and Clark 2006). One contemporary debate has focused on whether access to palliative care should be needs based or based on diagnostic categories (Skilbeck and Payne 2005). In the UK, despite repeated calls to widen access to patients whatever their diagnosis who are nearing the end of life, approximately 95 per cent of those referred to hospices have cancer. About 50 per cent of cancer patients receive some care from hospices. The preponderance of patients with cancer accessing palliative care in the UK is probably related to the historical development of early hospices and funding from key cancer charities. The only other medical condition with a history of specialist hospices is HIV/AIDS. In the UK during the 1990s a number of reports and other documents explored what came to be known as the cancer–non-cancer debate (Field and Addington-Hall 1991). These publications rehearsed arguments for and against extending specialist palliative care to non-cancer patients. One of the chief concerns being that if access was widened to those with other conditions, there would be insufficient resources (the 'flood-gates' argument) and current services would be overwhelmed. This prediction has proven not to be convincing as, despite repeated calls to widen access, little has changed, indicating that either patients without cancer may be reluctant to be admitted to institutions so closely associated with cancer or that practitioners remain unwilling to refer them. These debates have largely been superseded by a public health agenda that calls for access to specialist palliative care based on levels of distress and disease burden rather than diagnostic category (Foley 2003). In this book, we make no assumption that palliative care is restricted to people with cancer.

# Where is palliative care delivered?

Palliative care is a philosophy of care and therefore it can be delivered in a variety of settings, including institutions such as hospitals, inpatient hospices and care homes for older people as well as in people's own homes. What constitutes specialist palliative care and hospice care varies both within and across countries. In the UK, the early development was marked by the construction of dedicated separate buildings as inpatient hospices. In the USA, a hospice programme tends to refer to community based support. As we have reiterated before, most patients receive palliative care from their usual health care providers. In the UK this means that most patients with advanced illness are in the care of the primary health care team, consisting of general practitioners, community nurses and associated health and social care professionals. Care is therefore delivered in patients' homes where they spend the majority of their time during the final year of life. Moreover, home is overwhelmingly the preferred place of care for the majority of people. General practitioners and community nurses may make referrals to specialist palliative care providers. Specialist palliative care services themselves offer a range of provision, from a single specialist nurse to a comprehensive multidisciplinary team. Specialist palliative care services have developed an array of different types of provision including: inpatient units, hospices, hospital teams, community teams, outpatient clinics, day care, respite services, bereavement support services, complementary therapies, counselling and psychological support, spiritual and religious support.

# Who provides palliative care?

There is a danger that in providing a list of who provides palliative care that some people may be overlooked. With this proviso in mind, Box 2 offers a broad overview of the types of individuals who may be engaged in providing both paid and unpaid palliative care.

Corner (2003) discriminates between two types of nurses working in specialist palliative care; those who have additional post-basic qualifications in palliative care and provide direct patient care in various contexts including inpatient hospices and in the patient's home, and the clinical nurse specialist. The latter nursing role has been developed in the UK largely through the funding made available from a cancer charity now called Macmillan Cancer Relief. These specialist nurses tend to use the title 'Macmillan' nurse. Research evidence demonstrates that a large proportion of their role involves direct face-to-face contact with patients (89 per cent) and that the most common reason for referral was for emotional support (Corner *et al.* 2002; Skilbeck *et al.* 2002). Most of the nurses did not provide 'hands-on' physical care but did offer support and information to patients. They also

---

**Box 2**   Palliative care work force

| | |
|---|---|
| Patient's carers: | families, friends and neighbours |
| Nursing care: | general nurses and specialist nurses |
| Medical care: | general practitioners |
| | specialists in palliative medicine |
| | specialists in other areas of medicine |
| Social care: | social worker |
| Spiritual care: | chaplaincy, faith advisors |
| Therapists: | occupational therapists, physiotherapists |
| | (physical therapists), speech and language |
| | therapists, art, drama, music therapists |
| Psychological care: | counsellors, clinical and health psychologists, |
| | psychotherapists, liaison psychiatrists |
| Specialist staff: | nutritionists, dieticians |
| | pharmacists |
| Support staff: | care assistants, administrative, domestic, |
| | gardeners, transport, and other workers |
| Volunteer staff | |

---

worked behind the scenes in coordinating care and offering specialist advice to generalists including general practitioners and community nurses. Their work served to promote better standards of palliative care by disseminating good practice and current evidence. They were therefore an important resource in trying to improve palliative care provision. There remains much that is not known about how clinical nurse specialists develop and sustain their role, what attributes are required and how they may be supported. Skilbeck and Payne (2003) have drawn attention to the ambivalence in these nurses about taking on emotional labour and emotional support functions when they are often poorly prepared and inadequately supported in this aspect of their role. Many of the subsequent chapters in this book will explore how nurses work to provide palliative care and the challenges this may create for them.

---

## Overview of the book

In this final part of the Introduction we will introduce ourselves as editors and say how we have revised the structure and content of the book in the second edition. The second edition has been a pleasure and a challenge to produce. We were heartened and encouraged to produce a second edition by supportive and some constructive feedback from reviewers, colleagues and our publishers.

### The editors

We are academics, nurses and researchers in palliative care. We share attributes as well as contributing our unique perspectives. We have drawn upon our academic disciplines of health psychology and medical sociology and many years of research in the field of palliative care. In addition, we have expertise in education for health and social care professionals in higher and continuing education. The experience of designing, coordinating and teaching on Masters level courses in palliative care has been very influential in developing this book. The many students on these courses have taught us much, and we are grateful to them. We are indebted to Jeni Hulme, who has helped us manage the clerical work involved in this book.

*Sheila Payne* has a background in nursing and health psychology. For over 20 years she has conducted numerous research studies in palliative care and worked with colleagues in developing palliative care and bereavement services. She co-directs the Cancer Experiences Collaborative (with Professor Julia Addington-Hall) which brings together five leading universities to improve the quantity and quality of research in supportive and palliative care. She has published widely in academic and professional journals and authored or edited ten books.

*Jane Seymour* is a nurse and medical sociologist. She leads a team of researchers working closely with a charity, Sue Ryder Care. Her research focuses primarily on older people's knowledge, attitudes and experiences of end-of-life care, and issues in advance care planning.

*Christine Ingleton* is a nurse and has worked as a clinician, manager, educationalist and researcher. Over the past 15 years she has been involved in a variety of funded research projects in the area of end-of-life care, including service evaluation, needs assessment, satisfaction with bereavement care, the provision and quality of respite services, and the role of non-specialist providers of palliative care. She has published widely in academic and professional journals.

### The authors

In preparing the second edition, we carefully reviewed the content and accessibility of all the chapters. We have commissioned 13 new chapters from international authors who are leading experts in palliative care. The authors represent a range of expertise and are drawn from different professional and academic backgrounds. They include: academics, researchers, professional practitioners, managers, policy makers and educators. We believe that the diversity of backgrounds and perspectives enhance the depth of coverage. However, it does mean that the writing styles vary and while some editorial work has been undertaken, we are keen that the chapters reflect the views and attitudes of our authors rather than conform to our perspectives. We have urged authors to take an international perspective when possible, but each person is likely to know their own country's health care systems and issues best. We realize there are some important omissions; namely we have decided not to include a chapter written by a patient or carer presenting the 'user' perspective. While this has become fashionable, we are concerned about tokenism and we also acknowledge that people hold multiple roles – in that some of our chapter authors may also be a patient and/or a carer. Most of the authors work in resource-rich countries, but we have added a chapter which considers palliative care in resource-poor contexts.

### Aims of the book

This second edition, like the first edition, aims to present the principles and evidence in palliative care nursing that underpin practice in order to support both nurses and other health professionals working in specialist palliative care settings and those whose work involves general end-of-life care. The book will focus on palliative care for adults. The first edition introduced a novel organizing framework – the trajectory of life-limiting illness – and we have retained this. Namely, the book is structured around important transitions in the trajectory of illness and dying (e.g. suspecting illness, confirmation of diagnosis, living with dying, and bereavement). Organizing the book in this way enables the examination of complex issues in a longitudinal way and from a variety of perspectives. We have rejected the old four-part framework of physical, psychological, social and spiritual care because it tends to prevent an acknowledgement of the integration of patient experience, and there is a tendency to privilege physical aspects of care. The book has dedicated sections on research issues as well as integrating research findings throughout. The book draws extensively from literature in fields related to, and informing, nursing – history, psychology, sociology, social policy, anthropology and ethics. The book emphasizes the phenomenology or experience of care-giving and care-receiving throughout. It offers an agenda for change and future research. We are mindful that people experiencing these transitions in their lives are often connected with families and friends, and a wider social network, and we will attempt to suggest how nursing interventions may encompass a socially embedded approach to care. We make no assumptions that end-of-life care is concerned merely with those who have cancer, but much of current specialist palliative care is provided for those with cancer and therefore the research literature reflects this reality.

### Who is this book for?

This book is aimed at practitioners following basic professional qualifications. The first edition was widely used as a core text for students undertaking Master's level courses in palliative care and related courses in health and social care. The book also contributes to courses aimed at developing a conceptual understanding of the theories and evidence that underpin clinical skills. In addition, the book aims to be a resource for Clinical Nurse Specialists and Nurse Consultants, and those working in nurse education and management. The book is aimed predominantly at those working in the UK and other resource-rich countries such as Australia, New Zealand,

Canada, and for those working in Europe. While aimed primarily at nurses, we hope that this book will be read widely by a range of health and social care practitioners, helping them to think more critically about palliative care. This book is not primarily a 'how to do' book or a practical guide to delivering care; instead, it seeks to intellectually challenge the reader and promote debate and discussion about the nature and purpose of palliative care.

### *Overview of Parts One to Four*

This book is structured around a framework of four major parts based on a trajectory of illness model (in the first three parts) and a final part addressing contemporary issues in nursing and interprofessional working. Each part is introduced by an overview chapter dealing with the principles and theoretical issues underpinning practice, which is authored by one or more of the editors. This is followed by shorter and more focused chapters written by experts in the area, which deal with specific contexts, conditions and practical issues. These are meant to be illustrative of the issues raised in the overview chapter. All chapters start with a summary of key points to assist readers identify their contents.

## | References

Addington-Hall, J.M. and Higginson, I.J. (eds) (2001) *Palliative care for non-cancer patients*. Oxford: Oxford University Press.

Bingley, A.F. and Clark, D. (in press) *Palliative care developments in the region represented by the Middle East Cancer Consortium: review and comparative analysis*. Bethesda, MD: National Cancer Institute. NIH Publications.

Centeno, C., Clark, D., Lynch, T., Rocafort, J., Flores, L.A, Greenwood, A., Brasch, S., Praill, D., Giordano, A. and de Lima, L. (2007) *EAPC Atlas of Palliative Care in Europe*. Milano: European Association for Palliative Care.

Clark, D. and Seymour, J. (1999) *Reflection on Palliative Care*. Buckingham: Open University Press.

Clark, D. and Wright, M. (2003) *Transition in end of life care: Hospice and related developments in Eastern Europe and Central Asia*. Buckingham: Open University Press.

Clark, D. and Wright, M. (2007) The International Observatory on End of Life Care: a global view of palliative care development. *Journal of Pain and Symptom Management*, 33(5): 542–46.

Corner, J. (2003) Nursing management in palliative care. *European Journal of Oncology Nursing*, 7(2): 83–90.

Corner, J., Clark, D. and Normand, C. (2002) Evaluating the work of clinical nurse specialists in palliative care. *Palliative Medicine*, 16: 275–7.

Davies, E. and Higginson, I.J. (2004a) *The solid facts: Palliative Care*. Copenhagen: World Health Organization.

Davies, E. and Higginson, I.J. (2004b) *Better Palliative Care for Older People*. Copenhagen: World Health Organization.

Department of Health (2000) *The NHS Cancer Plan: a plan for investment, a plan for reform*. London: HMSO.

Doyle, D., Hanks, W.C. and MacDonald, N. (eds) (1998) *Oxford Textbook of Palliative Medicine* 2nd edn. Oxford: Oxford University Press.

Ferrell, B.R. and Coyle, N. (eds) (2001) *Textbook of Palliative Nursing*. Oxford: Oxford University Press.

Field, D. and Addington-Hall, J. (1991) Extending specialist palliative care to all? *Social Science and Medicine*, 48: 1271–80.

Foley, K.M. (2003) How much palliative care do we need? *European Journal of Palliative Care*, 10(2): 5–7.

Froggatt, K.A., Wilson, D., Justice, C., MacAdam, M., Leibovici, K., Kinch, J., Thomas, R. and Choi, J. (2006). End-of-life care in long-term care settings for older people: a literature review. *International Journal of Older People Nursing*, 1: 45–50.

Graham, F. and Clark, D. (2005a) Addressing the basics of palliative care. *International Journal of Palliative Nursing*, 11(1): 36–9.

Graham, F. and Clark, D. (2005b) The Syringe Driver and the Subcutaneous Route in Palliative Care: The Inventor, the History and the Implications. *Journal of Pain and Symptom Management*, 29(1): 32–40.

Illich, I. (1976) *Limits to Medicine*. Harmondsworth: Penguin.

McNamara, B. (2001) *Fragile Lives: Death Dying and Care*. Buckingham: Open University Press.

National Council for Hospices and Specialist Palliative Care Services (2002) *Definitions of Supportive and Palliative Care*. London: National Council for Hospices and Specialist Palliative Care Services.

National Council for Hospices and Specialist Palliative Care Services (2003) *Palliative Care for Adults with Non-malignant Diseases*. London: National Council for Hospices and Specialist Palliative Care Services.

National Institute for Clinical Excellence (2003) *Supportive and Palliative Care Guidance for Cancer*. London: National Institute for Clinical Excellence.

Payne, S., Sheldon, F., Jarrett, N., Large, S., Smith, P., Davis, C., Turner, P. and George, S. (2002) Differences in understandings of Specialist Palliative Care amongst service providers and commissioners in South London. *Palliative Medicine*, 16: 395–402.

Praill, D. (2000) Who are we here for? (editoral). *Palliative Medicine*, 14: 91–2.

Sepulveda, C., Marlin, A., Yoshida, T. and Ullrich, A. (2002) Palliative care: The World Health Organization's global perspective. *Journal of Pain and Symptom Management*, 24(2): 91–6.

Shockett, E.R., Teno, J., Miller, S.C. and Stuart, B. (2005) Late referral to hospice and bereaved family member perception of quality of end-of-life care. *Journal of Pain and Symptom Management*, 30(5): 400–7.

Skilbeck, J., Corner, J., Bath, P., Beech, N., Clark, D., Douglas, H-R., Halliday, D., Haviland, J., Hughes, P., Marples, R., Normand, C., Seymour, J. and Webb, T. (2002) Clinical Nurse Specialists in Palliative Care (1): a description of the Macmillan Nurse caseload. *Palliative Medicine*, 16: 285–96.

Skilbeck, J. and Payne, S. (2003) Emotional support and the role of Clinical Nurse Specialists in palliative care. *Journal of Advanced Nursing*, 43(5): 521–30.

Skilbeck, J. and Payne, S. (2005) End-of-Life care: a discursive analysis of specialist palliative care nursing, *Journal of Advanced Nursing*, 51(4): 325–34.

Vliegner, M., Gorchs, N., Larkin, P. and Porchet, F. (2004) Palliative nurse education: towards a common language (editorial). *Palliative Medicine*, 18: 401–3.

Winslow, M. and Clark, C. (2005) *St Joseph's Hospice, Hackney*. Lancaster: Observatory Publications.

World Health Organization (2002) Report on 'Preventing Risks, Promoting Healthy Life' (http://who.int/mediacentre/releases/pr84/en/), accessed March 2003.

World Health Organization (2007) *Cancer Control: Knowledge into Action. WHO Guide for Effective Programmes. Palliative Care*. Geneva, Switzerland: World Health Organization.

Wright, M. and Clark, D. (2006) *Hospice and Palliative Care in Africa: a review of developments and challenges*. Oxford: Oxford University Press.

# PART ONE

**Encountering illness**

# 1

# Overview

*Sheila Payne and Jane Seymour*

Over the last century, public health programmes and improvements in living conditions have delivered some remarkable benefits to humanity (Payne 2007). This means that more people live with chronic illness, and they survive longer with advanced disease and probably live with more co-morbidities. Arguably some will live with a potential awareness that they are dying, and perhaps a greater number do not regard themselves as 'dying'. Therefore there is considerable ambivalence in how people construct the social position of a 'dying' person and whether they identify with that social category. In our view, this has transformed the nature of what it means to be dying and the status of a 'dying person'. For example, medical treatments and technologies have enabled some people to live much longer with formerly fatal conditions such as end-stage renal disease where haemodialysis may enable people to survive for many years. Societal expectations that medical interventions will prolong life place great pressures on nurses and medical staff, and it may have become difficult in some cultures when to recognize that a person is really dying, until almost the final stages of life.

This chapter explores what it means for people who become ill to take up the social role of 'patient' and the implications this has for family members and friends who will be designated as 'carers' or 'care-givers'. We also examine how and when they start to realize that they are approaching the end of life. We examine various perspectives on the self and introduce models of illness drawn from the social sciences, considering how they inform our understandings of palliative care nursing and how they have influenced the development of palliative care both over time and across geographical boundaries. In addition, we draw upon current conceptualizations of palliative care to consider how very ill and dying people are perceived by different societies, how the 'good death' has been constructed and reshaped over time, and what is considered to be 'normal' care for those with end-stage disease. For example, in developed societies, people with diseases such as heart failure are more likely to be treated with intensive medical and nursing interventions like artificial ventilation in intensive care units right to the end of their lives (Seymour 2001), whereas others with conditions such as dementia are less likely to receive such treatments (Small *et al.* 2007).

In the latter part of this chapter, we discuss the impact of disease and illness upon those in close relationships with the ill person. These are usually assumed to be family members or relatives, but the changes wrought by divorce, geographical mobility, increased longevity and declining birth rates may mean that friends or employed care workers provide more significant and meaningful relationships, for example for older people living in care homes. Human beings are embedded within social systems, kinship networks and cultural groups: the lack of such networks is potentially problematic for those reaching the end of their life, particularly the socially excluded, such as refugees and asylum seekers, and those living in regions where war, famine, migration, poverty and social upheaval have destroyed normal family patterns of care and support (Wright and Clark 2006). We therefore introduce basic concepts about social support, social networks and social relationships. Finally, this overview chapter aims to provide a clear framework to guide the reader through the ensuing chapters in Part One.

## What does it mean to become a patient?

The sociological and anthropological literature has long emphasized the impact of illness and subsequent contact with health care services on personal identity and feelings of personhood (Kleinman 1980; Helman 2000). While early functionalist accounts of the 'patient's role' (in which patient-hood was conceptualized as a 'social role' with its own set of expectations, responsibilities and constraints) are now largely discounted, there remain a few elements that are highly salient for consideration when thinking about palliative care. The use of the label 'patient' continues to be dominant in the language of health care workers, health care managers and policy makers, and is widely used by the public. It serves to differentiate the 'well' from the 'ill', the 'cared for' from the 'care workers'.

Typically, life-threatening illness changes the outlook of the person it affects and alters the possibilities available to them. One's taken-for-granted life and the expectation of an almost limitless future diminish, and with increasing physical and/or mental decline imposed by illness comes creeping social isolation as treasured roles are modified and eventually relinquished. For example, employment provides many opportunities, including financial security, social relationships with work colleagues, social status, power and enhanced self-esteem. Of course, not all work-related experiences are life-enhancing, but to be forced to leave work because of ill health is particularly symbolic of the way in which life-threatening illness eventually leads to a transition from activity to passivity. At this point, there may also be an incremental dismantling of essential features of personhood, such as the appearance of the physical body, as in cachexia, the destruction of cognitive and emotional capacity, as in end-stage dementia, and a transformation and eventual withdrawal of social relationships, described by Sudnow (1967) as 'social death'.

## Concepts of the self and identity

Nurses have traditionally engaged with the physical body of the patient by providing comfort care, observing and recording physiological changes, assisting with activities of living and administering medical treatments. These complex skills are often referred to as 'basic' nursing care. However, research by Lawler (1991) has shown how nursing work also involves a detailed *social* understanding of the body. Her research has demonstrated that nurses are skilled at managing intimate bodily care while engaging in strategies to minimize embarrassment and discomfort for the patient. Changes in nursing education, knowledge and concepts of the professional role in the latter part of the twentieth century opened up new possibilities for how nurses engage with and 'know' patients. May (1992) argues that nurses now seek to 'know' patients in terms of 'foreground' and 'background' knowledge. 'Foreground' knowledge relates to the clinical definition of the body: this allows nurses to establish what nursing work needs to be under-taken. 'Background' knowledge concerns the person as an individual, and it is this engagement of nurses with a person who is a complex social being with an unique identity that is arguably new. Although there are evident benefits for nurses and patients in moving beyond stereotypical portrayals of patients (such as 'the lung cancer in bed 6'), this can represent a challenge to nurses because it requires sensitive communication and an openness to the full extent of each person's experience of suffering. It is also potentially more invasive for patients because they are expected to reveal to nurses not only their physical bodies, but also their thoughts, feelings and existential concerns. Claims to 'know' the whole person and to deliver 'holistic' care have been made particularly loudly in palliative care (e.g. Buckley 2002).

If 'knowing the person' is regarded as fundamental to palliative care nursing, what theories of the self and identity influence our understanding? In this section, we consider how concepts of the self and identity are described from various perspectives. Psychological approaches to questions of self and identity fall into four major groups: psychoanalytic and psycho-dynamic therapists have drawn upon their clinical work (e.g. Freud 1923), humanistic psychologists have drawn upon insights from psychotherapeutic work (e.g. Kelly 1955; Rogers 1961; Maslow 1970), social psychologists have used experimental methods (e.g. Bem 1972) and, more recently, social constructivist theorists have drawn upon narrative methods (e.g. Crossley 2000). Sociologists tend to emphasize the influence of socialization or 'cultural programming' (Giddens 1998) on self-identity. Critically important here are the accidents of birth that tend to give individuals differential educational and employment opportunities and thus ensure that they occupy

**Box 1.1** An example of a study of people with lung cancer from the Netherlands (The 2002)

A social science researcher, Anne-Mei The (2002), conducted an ethnographic study in a cancer centre focusing on the experience of a group of patients with advanced small-cell lung cancer. Anne-Mei The spent a great deal of time in the clinics listening to the doctors and nurses and sharing the experiences of the patients and their families as they underwent diagnosis, initial treatment, recurrence and through to their final days and deaths. Readers are introduced to the key people: Mr van der Ploeg, Mr Dekker, Mr Henvel, Mr Wiersema, Mr Wessels and other patients early in their illness, their spouses and families. We also learn about medical and nursing staff not as stereotypical consultant oncologists, junior doctors and ward nurses, but as complex individuals who vary both between each other and also between their handling of each patient. The research sought to address the questions about why and how patients remain so optimistic throughout their illness when the outcome is known (by medical staff) to be almost invariably fatal. This research offers an antidote to simplistic communication research in cancer care that focuses solely on 'the bad news' interview as though it were a single event. It demonstrates the complex interactions between patients, families, medical and nursing professionals in constructing what is 'known', and when and how it is 'known'. Anne-Mei The argues that both patients and their doctors collude in minimizing the significance of the disease in the early stages by concentrating their attention on short-term outcomes such as planning and starting treatment. In her view, this serves to deflect attention away from the more unpleasant long-term outcome that will be the patient's inevitable death. This analysis confirms other research such as that by Christakis (1999), which indicates that doctors are less likely to offer a prognosis than a diagnosis.

Patients and their families come to understand the implications of their disease through processes of social comparison with other patients. Once again, this is rarely acknowledged in the communication literature, where health professionals are often portrayed as virtually the only sources of information. By comparison, in this research we are shown how patients hear about the recurrences and deaths of their peers, and how they both learn from, and distance themselves from, these events. Anne-Mei The also describes how nurses are placed in the difficult position of having to 'fish' for information about the level of awareness of patients because they are not party to the communication that has occurred between medical consultants and patients. The picture of fluctuating awareness is akin to that described by Field and Copp (1999) as 'conditional awareness'. The research paints a complex picture of the tangled web of truths, half-truths and deceptions that are, in our view, the pattern of communication that most patients, families and health care workers participate in creating.

This research study is a very good example of ethnography. Ethnographic methodology has a long tradition in social research about end-of-life care, from the influential work of Glaser and Strauss (1965) in which 'awareness contexts' were described in acute care hospitals in the USA, to more recent UK examples in a cancer hospital (Costain Schou and Hewison 1999), in a hospice (Lawton 2000) and in intensive care (Seymour 2001). It is a powerful research methodology that enables rich analytical accounts to be developed. One of the markers of a good ethnographic account is an acknowledgement of the role of the researcher in the collection of the data and the construction of the analysis. In the epilogue, Anne-Mei The demonstrates how she coped with the emotional involvement in the participants' lives and deaths. She addresses the dilemma between over-involvement and academic detachment which is faced by all researchers who see themselves as part of the process of research.

particular positions in society. Traditional sociological approaches have emphasized: the influence of historical, cultural and economic circumstances (for example, the theories of Karl Marx about the way in which social conditions shape human existence); the influence of ethical or 'normative' standards on identity (for example, Talcott Parson's idea of a 'sick role' as a set of normative expectations that shape the identity of patients); and how self-perception is fashioned through the way in which others respond to us during social interaction. This latter idea has emerged in different ways in the work of symbolic interactionists who have followed George Herbert Mead and in the work of those who follow Erving Goffman. Goffman showed how the small rituals of everyday life constrain our behaviour and shape our sense of self as we learn to 'play the game' (May 1996). Contemporary sociologists have used these traditional perspectives in new ways. Most notable among these is Giddens' theory of 'structuration', in which he draws together a range of perspectives to argue that social structures (of which culture is pre-eminent) do not merely *influence* a person's sense of self, but are manifest *through* individuals' engagement with the practices that make up social life (Giddens 1976).

Identity has been posited to be derived predominantly from one's social position at birth (e.g. being born to wealthy or poor parents), acquired through education and employment, or derived from performance of social roles like being a parent, a widower or widow, which determine to some extent what are regarded as appropriate behaviours and ways of interacting with others. More recently, identity has been presented as a more flexible and negotiated construct, and it has been suggested that people living in contemporary Western societies take a more reflexive and internalized position to identity in which traditional belief systems play little part. Thus Taylor (1989) argues that in some countries people now spend more time pondering existential questions about the meaning of life and their role in it, because there is less acceptance of broad frameworks like religion.

Rumsey and Harcourt (2005) have highlighted the psychological importance of physical appearance in defining identity and individuality, and how the body is used to convey powerful messages about culture. For example, our choice of clothing and accessories can signify wealth, culture, social class, age and gender. Similarly, body art (e.g. tattoos, ear rings and nose studs) is closely linked with the way we wish to convey both our identity as cultural group members and as individuals. Wearing make-up and styling hair in certain ways are gender markers in most cultures. Thus, difficulty in maintaining one's usual standards of personal dress and grooming may be profoundly challenging for people with advanced disease (Lawler 1997). For example, the thinness associated with cachexia or the swelling arising from ascites may be difficult to mask by clothing and may lead people and their families to feel depersonalized by the experience of illness. At St Christopher's Hospice, in London, fashion students worked with patients to create special clothing designed to their taste to cover the effects of physical changes resulting from advanced disease and treatment (Tasker 2005).

Narratives, or stories, have become a powerful and popular way to construct identity, with increasing interest over the last decade from sociologists and others in the use of narrative research methods (e.g. Riessman 1993). Sociologists highlight how serious and chronic illness disrupts individuals' sense of identity and the taken-for-grantedness of continuity that characterizes most people's lives (see, for example, Bury 1982; Charmaz 1991). Most of us optimistically assume that we will live to a happy and healthy old age and we plan and live our lives based on these assumptions. Therefore, when illness occurs, especially if this is sudden like a stroke, there are major psychological and social adjustments to be made, as well as the challenges of managing the physical and functional changes associated with illness. Written accounts produced as biographies, autobiographies and more recently as Internet 'blogs' have been used by people to convey their experiences of dying (Bingley *et al.* 2006). Crossley (2000) argues that people use stories to create accounts of themselves that are flexible over time. Written narratives also provide an opportunity for professionals to make sense of experiences of caring for dying cancer patients (McDermott *et al.* 2006) and analysis of their accounts revealed how they constructed the 'good' death.

'Narrative medicine' is a comparatively new development that seeks to take account of how people understand their identity and how illness impacts on their sense of self and the meaning that illness has at each stage in their life (Greenhalgh and Hurwitz 1998; Launer 2003). It also seeks to redefine the role of medicine by emphasizing the more fundamental and humanitarian aspects of care. It is argued that by using narrative (stories) patients can be encouraged to share their experiences, which provides an insight into their predicaments. There is evidence from psychological research that writing stories is potentially therapeutic and helps people to manage loss (e.g. Pennebaker and Seagal 1999). Arguably, one of the functions of counselling is to provide the opportunity for people to tell their story, from which they may gain insights into themselves and they may even find the storytelling healing (Frank 1995). Many bereavement counsellors report that being available to listen to the story of the death is an important aspect of their role (Payne *et al.* 2002) (for more about narrative in bereavement see Overview chapter to Part Three). Crossley (2000) suggests that the way the story is told and the language used serve to shape people's understanding of their own identity. Thus, some people with cancer object strongly to the term 'cancer victim' because it positions them as passive, helpless and deserving of pity. They prefer to use language which indicates a more active and positive stance, such as 'cancer survivor' (Feuerstein 2007).

---

**Box 1.2**   An example of a study of a person with oral cancer (Crossley 2003)

John Diamond, a British broadcaster and journalist, wrote an account of his experience of oral cancer in a series of articles in *The Times* newspaper over a period of four years, from diagnosis to one week before his death. His account provided a narrative of one man's experience of living with cancer. Through writing the articles in the form of a diary, he attempted to find meaning in his experiences and, according to his brother-in-law, the writing was his method of coping with illness. Crossley (2003), a health psychologist, undertook a narrative analysis of Diamond's articles, which she interpreted in the context of Del Vecchio Good *et al.*'s (1994) notion of 'therapeutic emplotment'. Del Vecchio Good *et al.* (1994) have argued that oncologists and patients creatively manage time and the patients' experience of illness as part of 'a larger therapeutic story' (p. 855). This serves to highlight particular events and episodes that appear to maintain the possibility of hope. Crossley examined Diamond's articles for evidence of his unfolding story. She categorized them into six sequential stages.

1   *Pre-cancer: touch wood.* In the first article on 14 September 1996, he reported the possibility that his mouth swelling *might be* cancer but distanced himself.
2   *Learning to live in 'therapeutic emplotment'.* Over the next six months, Diamond's articles were full of accounts of various medical and surgical treatments and their associated side effects. His language appeared to be optimistic, with an emphasis on the future expectation that after six weeks of daily radiotherapy and surgery, he would achieve full recovery. He was encouraged by health professionals to live in the 'immediacy of treatment' while the future held the promise of a certainty of outcome (cure).
3   *In limbo: holding one's breath.* Following treatment, he came to realize that 'the truth is . . . I still don't know whether I'm cured. Nor will I know for weeks, or months, or possibly years'. This period is sometimes described as 'watchful waiting' and can be even more stressful than undergoing active medical treatment (Jones and Payne 2000).
4   *Recurrence: 'therapeutic emplotment' continued.* Ten months after what appeared to be the 'end' of treatment, his cancer recurred. Diamond tried to be optimistic in the face of further radical head and neck surgery. He wrote, 'if the surgeons slash and burn in the right way, then I have a reasonable chance of a cure'.
5   *Through the mirror: the 'unspoken narrative'.* Following surgery, there was evidence that Diamond started to abandon his previous expectations of cure and gave up his 'almost childish belief in the power of modern medicine'. However, he consented to chemotherapy, which he described as 'stale hell' and some four months later another swelling in his neck was confirmed as cancer recurrence.
6   *Endings or the end?* The final period of writing was characterized by a lethargy and resignation. Further recurrence and spread to his lungs were responded to by his agreement to a further three courses of chemotherapy but with no optimistic expectations. One week later, he died in hospital.

This is a tale of one person's experience of oral cancer. As readers we know the outcome, but as Crossley points out in her analysis, Diamond did not. How he engaged with this uncertainty is powerfully revealed in his writing.

# The distinction between *illness* and *disease*

In this book, we make the distinction between *illness*, which refers to the subjective experience of being unwell and may or may not be linked to an organic disease, and *disease*, which refers to a recognized pathological state. It is therefore possible for a person to have a life-threatening disease and to describe themselves as 'well'. Similarly, it is also possible for a person to feel ill but not have a disease. The recognition and labelling of disease states (i.e. diagnosis) has traditionally been the role of medicine, but a diagnostic label takes no account of the meaning a person places on the set of symptoms. There are worldwide agreed systems of classification of diseases, for example DSM-IV-R (American Psychiatric Association 1994) for psychiatric conditions. The fact that disease classification systems are revised and modified indicates that notions of disease change over time and across cultures. Research indicates that nurses find diagnostic labels highly salient. In a study of information transfer between nurses working in wards for older people, most nurses reported that the essential information they required during handovers (reports between nursing shifts) included patient's name, age, diagnosis and resuscitation status (Payne *et al.* 2000).

Patterns of disease have traditionally been categorized as chronic or acute. Palliative care services have predominantly been concerned with providing care for people with chronic rather than acute diseases. This distinction has, arguably, become blurred by changes in diseases themselves, in medical technology and in treatment. For example, a century ago childhood leukaemias were regarded as acute and rapidly fatal diseases but now most children with leukaemia survive. Similarly, antiretroviral agents have transformed AIDS into a chronic disease, or at least for those who have access to appropriate medication. Many cancers are now also experienced as an intermittent chronic condition, as patients encounter repeated episodes of recurrence and further treatment. However, many people continue to perceive of cancer as a rapidly fatal disease. Heart failure predominantly affects older people and, in Scotland, hospitalization rates are higher than for any other condition, and it is among the top five reasons for GP consultations among men over 75 years and women over 85 years (Murphy *et al.* 2004) and a major cause of death. For example, the introduction of ACE inhibitors have prolonged the lives of those with heart failure (British Heart Foundation 2001) but research has revealed the poor quality of general palliative care delivered to patients with heart failure (Barnes *et al.* 2006). While attention is beginning to be focused on the need to improve end-of-life care in a range of chronic physical diseases, those with mental health conditions and dementia remain largely neglected (Small *et al.* 2007).

Underpinning much of the palliative care literature is an assumption that people have a single identifiable disease. Yet evidence from Western countries suggests that the majority of older people and an increasing proportion of younger people are living with at least one chronic disease and a range of co-morbidities (Williams and Botti 2002). As life expectancy has increased in the majority of countries, most people can anticipate dying in old age with a number of chronic co-morbidities (Seymour *et al.* 2005). For example, an 88-year-old person may live with pain from osteoarthritis, asthma that results in acute episodes of breathlessness and is complicated by recurrent chest infections, and osteoporosis that has resulted in hip fractures. This person has, therefore, several chronic diseases that result in chronic pain and also a number of acute problems requiring a complex range of health and social care interventions. The outcome of experiencing a number of chronic diseases may include reduced quality of life, repeated and sometimes unpredictable requirements for health and social care services, and increased health care costs. Unfortunately, the organization of medical services generally focuses on specific types of pathology (e.g. oncology or orthopaedics) with little integration between services, which necessitates visits to different physicians at different clinics and possibly in different hospitals.

There is evidence that the end-of-life care needs of older people have been relatively neglected by palliative care services (Seymour *et al.* 2005). In a review of the policy and practice literature, Seymour *et al.* argued that many older people approaching the last phase of their lives, and their carers, experience systematic and structurally related disadvantage and discrimination, partly because the course of their deterioration and dying may be less clear-cut than in younger people. For many older people, physical and mental decline, which is often combined with social withdrawal, may be drawn out over many years, and it is more difficult to recognize a clearly terminal phase (Lynn and Adamson 2003). In recognition that care homes are a major provider of end-of-life care for older people it has been highlighted that there is a need to build collaboratively upon the skills and expertise of care workers located in care home environments rather than assume that specialist palliative care workers are expert in all types of dying (Froggatt *et al.* 2006).

There has been growing pressure from palliative care services to better understand 'typical' trajectories of dying to determine when and how interventions may be best delivered. Arguably early hospice development, especially in the UK (see chapter by Clark) was based on the 'typical' trajectory of cancer. The assumption was that patients were largely cognitively intact until almost the end of life and wished to engage in social and psychological processes such as 'leave taking' with family and friends. Clark (1999) argued that these elements of end-of-life care became possible because hospices pioneered and delivered improved pain control. Also Saunder's notion of 'total pain' encouraged hospice workers to engage with psychological, spiritual and social aspects of pain, in addition to providing exemplary attention to physical care. As palliative care services have spread to those with a range of diseases, the limitations of assumptions of homogeneity in dying experiences have been revealed.

Based upon analysis of US data, Lunney *et al.* (2002: 1108) have proposed four distinct 'ideal' trajectories each differing in length and slope of functional decline (that) appear to account for most persons' last phase of life. They described them as: 1) sudden death with little prior warning and minimal interaction with health services before death; 2) death following a distinct terminal phase of illness occurring after a long period of high functioning and rapid decline, most characteristic of cancer patients; 3) death from organ failure (including COPD and heart failure) where a gradual decline in functional status occurs interspersed with acute periods of deterioration which could cause death; and 4) death following progressive deterioration accompanying frailty, stroke or dementia. While these trajectories are intuitively appealing, evidence from heart failure patients in the UK fails to confirm the commonality implied by this model (Gott *et al.* 2007). However, it is perhaps not surprising that the experiences of a relatively small group of patients may not 'map' well to 'ideal' types of trajectory. Further research is required to explore the robustness of this model in larger samples of people dying from a diversity of diseases.

So far, we have differentiated between illness and disease and highlighted how important these are for understanding the experience of patients. But we have not yet mentioned or sought to define 'health' in the context of palliative care. Readers may be surprised to consider this as an outcome of palliative care. Yet Kellehear (1999) has argued for a 'health promoting palliative care', and enhanced quality of life is widely regarded as a successful outcome for palliative and supportive care. Another way to construe this is that the outcome of palliative care interventions and nursing care is to foster and enhance remaining opportunities for healthy living. This does not just mean eating more fruit and vegetables or stopping smoking, but enhancing perceived well-being and health. Of course, 'health' is a notoriously difficult concept to define. However, it is possible to identify a number of differing perspectives on health and illness to provide a foundation to thinking about health in advanced disease. Within each perspective there are numerous debates and we do not claim to do justice to the complexity of the positions introduced here. The following is merely an introduction to these and readers are encouraged to seek more information from specialist texts.

## Models of health and illness

Anthropologists have emphasized that Western notions of biomedicine are just one of a number of ways to understand health, illness and the body (Kleinman 1980). Moreover, Western medicine should not be thought of as a static or uniformly agreed set of ideas, as caricatured in the 'medical model'. Biomedicine is constantly evolving; for example, recent research on genetics and the human genome project bring new ways to conceive of the body and to think about the genetic and foetal origins of disease. As well as Western biomedicine, there are other well-accepted medical systems such as that used in traditional Chinese medicine. And, of course, people also have access to their own culturally defined folk beliefs that may incorporate aspects of other health beliefs, such as those derived from biomedicine. These health and illness beliefs may be complex and influence health-seeking behaviours, especially in relation to common ailments and normal life transitions. Thus, as we will see in Part Three, folk beliefs about what are 'normal' bereavement experiences incorporate psychological models of phases and beliefs that bereavement represents a 'process' (Payne *et al.* 1999).

In the UK and in North America, a heterogeneous group of therapies, dietary practices and types of healing have been labelled as 'complementary medicine' (see chapter by Carter and Mackereth). The use of this term to describe a diverse range of therapeutic and diagnostic interventions positions them as adjuncts to biomedicine, although this relationship is ambivalent. The critics of complementary medicine highlight the lack of scientific evidence to support the use of many of the therapies, while their supporters emphasize the popularity of these interventions with the general public and how some therapies have gained acceptance as supportive treatments in hospice and palliative care contexts. In many areas, nurses have been active in including complementary therapies – especially 'touch therapies' like aromatherapy and massage – in the repertoire of interventions available to palliative care patients.

Evidence from major surveys in the UK (e.g. Blaxter 1990) has been used by sociologists to demonstrate that health and illness are regarded in different ways by different groups of people. Field (1993) reminds us that social factors such as gender, age, social class, economic and educational abilities, all influence what people regard as normal health and how they define themselves as ill. For example, in some communities where smoking is common, older people have described a cough as 'normal'. The apparent paradox in contemporary societies is that there appears to be greater mistrust and disillusionment with medical practitioners and health care institutions than in the past but, at the same time, greater attention is devoted to risk management and seeking health care (Lupton 1994). There are a plethora of health information sources but access to them, especially via electronic computer-based media, are known to be related to socio-demographic factors such as age and economic resources, which may exacerbate health inequalities.

## The impact of the illness on the family

So far, we have concentrated on people facing the end of their lives and not the people who populate their lives and social worlds. Field (2000) has argued that while specialist palliative care workers acknowledge the psychosocial impact of illness and the need to recognize psychosocial care needs, the emphasis has tended to be on the psychological care of patients with much less attention being directed to social aspects. Whatever your views are about this criticism, in this book we intend to consider explicitly the social relationships and social contexts in which people live. The remainder of this chapter is therefore devoted to considering the impact of illness and approaching death upon families and friends. These people are often labelled by health care workers as carers or care-givers. We also provide a brief account of how 'social support' and 'social network' are conceptualized in the literature. In many nursing textbooks, patients' families and friends remain marginal in the text and therefore, by implication, in the lives and deaths of patients. In community or institutional contexts, nurses are constantly interacting with the families and friends in their dealings with patients.

## Definitions of family

Internationally, 'family' is a contested notion, and may comprise anything from a couple or dyad (for example, a mother and child) to an extended multigenerational network. In many families there is a network of support and care from people who may or may not be co-located. One definition of family is: 'those related through committed heterosexual or same sex partnerships, birth and adoption, and others who have strong emotional and social bonds with a patient' (NICE 2004: 155). This broad definition of family encapsulates people who share biological, economic, social or legal ties. It also includes wider culturally recognized groups such as the New Zealand Maori *whanau* and other extended families through birth, adoption or legal contract (marriage). Nurses should be aware that notions of what constitute a 'family' may vary between cultures. Families are dynamic social structures which change over time as members are added through marriage, birth and adoption or lost through death and, in some cultures, following marriage. There are role expectations, responsibilities and commitments that are often related to economic provision, child-bearing and child-raising activities and in some cultures the roles may be defined by gender, birth order or economic position. Theories tend to describe family relationships in terms of complex systems of reciprocal demands and support.

Social changes in many countries have influenced family structures and the availability of family members to fulfill caring roles. These changes include increasing divorce and separation, with some individuals experiencing a series of marital relationships. Their children thus experience a series of family relationships with step-parenting and step siblings becoming more common. In many countries there is a declining birth rate, with some people remaining childless either through choice or enforced national policies (e.g. in China). In many resource-rich countries family size has declined to one or two children per partnership. This reduces the potential number of people related by kinship who may be available to offer care near the end of life. Economic pressures for two incomes combined with other factors has increased female employment rates, while male employment patterns have become less stable with greater geographical mobility and more part-time working in multiple jobs. Economic migration in parts of Eastern Europe and Asia mean that younger generations are not available to provide care to older or dying family members (Kellerhear forthcoming). One of the most dramatic changes of recent years relates to the high incidence of AIDS in

Africa that has massively increased the numbers of children orphaned and growing up in unprotected or institutional environments (Wright and Clark 2006).

Certain groups in society are less likely to have close family ties. Socially disadvantaged or socially excluded people such as refugees, homeless people and prisoners are less likely to have access to families or friends to support them during times of crisis. Other people may reject, or have been rejected by, their families. It is important to remember that not all families are mutually supportive or beneficial to their members. Rather, some may experience abusive, exploitative or threatening relationships that undermine or threaten an individual's welfare. Increased longevity may result in greater numbers of people enjoying being grandparents or great grandparents, but also an increased possibility of experiencing the loss of, or distancing from, family members in late old age. Older people, especially those in later old age (more than 85 years), are an increasing proportion of the population in many resource-rich countries, and are vulnerable to social isolation as their families disperse and their friends die. Approximately one-fifth of all people over 85 years in the UK die in care homes (Froggatt *et al.* 2006). For many, close emotional and social relationships with their peers and with staff members assume a special importance.

## Definitions of carers

> Carers, who may or may not be family members, are lay people in a close supportive role who share in the illness experience of the patient and who undertake vital care work and emotion management.
>
> (National Institute of Clinical Excellence 2004: p.155)

The terminology of care-giving is potentially confusing with a number of terms being used in various situations, countries and in the research literature (Payne 2007). The following terms are widely used to describe people who provide unpaid care in existing relationships including: carer, care-giver, informal carer, care-taker, relative, family, companion and significant other. They may be family members, friends or neighbours, although it should not be assumed that all family members are able to, or wish to, take on a caring role. Evidence suggests that more women than men take on a caring role (Hudson and Payne in press), and that in palliative care there is more within-generational than cross-generational care-giving. Being a carer is a social relationship that can only be undertaken in the context of another person, even if that person rejects the carer or is reluctant to be cared for. Research undertaken with older people indicates that many people, including those from minority ethnic groups, are fearful of becoming dependent upon family members and do not wish to 'burden' their adult children (Gott *et al.* 2004; Seymour *et al.* 2007). So becoming a 'carer' and becoming a 'cared for' person are roles that many people approach with some ambivalence. It should not be assumed that family members or patients are necessarily comfortable with the term 'carer' or attribute it to themselves.

# Social support and social network

Here, we briefly introduce the concepts of 'social support' and 'social network' to provide a wider theoretical context within which to situate the subsequent chapters about carers. Social support has been defined as information leading individuals to believe they are cared for and loved, esteemed and valued, and belong to a network of communication and mutual obligation (Cobb 1976). Several different types of social support have been identified. They function in different ways and may involve 'doing for' the cared-for person, encouraging activity in others, taking responsibility or just 'being there' for others. The following list defines key types of social support:

- *Informational support* refers to the provision of knowledge relevant to the situation the individual is experiencing.
- *Tangible support* refers to specific activities that others provide which are perceived to be helpful.
- *Emotional support* is the perceived availability of thoughtful, caring individuals who can share thoughts and feelings.
- *Affirmatory or validatory support* is given when others acknowledge the appropriateness of a person's beliefs and feelings.
- *Social affiliation* refers to an individual's system of mutual obligations and reciprocal help with other individuals and institutions.

Social support can be differentiated from 'social network', which is a system of social ties such as those formed between family, relatives and friends. Simmons (1994) suggested that there are seven functions of a social network: intimacy, social integration, nurturing others, reassurance of worth, assistance, guidance and access to new contacts. Social networks are generally defined in terms of their structural properties, including:

- *Size*: the number of people within the network.
- *Network density*: the amount of contact between members.
- *Accessibility*: the ease with which members can be contacted.
- *Stability over time*: the duration of the relationship.
- *Reciprocity*: the amount of give and take in the relationship.
- *Content*: the nature of the involvement in the relationship.
- *Intensity*: the degree of closeness within the relationship.

The mechanism by which social support mediates the effects of stress upon health remains controversial. Two main hypotheses have been postulated: the main effects hypothesis, which suggests that social support is beneficial whether or not the individual is experiencing stress, and the stress-buffering hypothesis, which suggests that social support influences individual appraisals of stressful stimuli. No one model adequately explains all the variance found in the literature. However, it is generally accepted that the extent of the social network is not sufficient to account for the health-enhancing effects; rather, it is the perception of the availability of appropriate support and the social skills needed to elicit them that are the key determinants.

## Overview of chapters in Part One

In the remainder of this chapter, we introduce the other eight chapters in Part One. Our aim is to guide the reader by providing a framework to understand the content and purpose of this part. Many factors influence the experience of dying including structural features such as culture, economic resources, health care system, and individual characteristics such as ethnicity, social position and time in the life span of the person. Paradoxically, while it is an experience which all of us will undergo, it is arguably highly individual and is shaped by our social position, culture and location in the world (Field *et al.* 1997).

In Chapter 2, David Clark presents an updated analysis of the care provided for dying people drawing upon a global perspective. He traces back the roots of modern palliative care to before the mid-twentieth-century developments led by Cicely Saunders in the UK. Many of the early pioneers trying to improve the care of dying people were inspired and motivated by religion, especially Christian teaching. He highlights the important role of women, some of whom were nurses, in responding to the needs of dying people. He emphasizes how people are shaped by the understanding of death and dying in their culture and the resources available to them.

In Chapter 3, Tony Stevens presents a new chapter on the engagement of patients and others in shaping palliative care services and research, referred to as 'user involvement'. He argues that service users contribute different types of knowledge drawn from a distillation of their experiences. The policy of involving people other than professionals in influencing health and social care services has been growing in popularity since the early 1990s in many European, North American and other countries. It has arisen from social changes that have challenged medical hegemony and paternalism, and involves a broader recognition of rights of citizens in health care services and in medical research. Stevens highlights both the advantages and challenges of implementing user involvement activities, especially the dangers of tokenism. He discusses practical strategies to facilitate the involvement of frail, ill and tired patients near the end of life such as greater use of information technology. He argues that careful consideration of potential costs or benefits for users and for organizations is required to ensure that initiatives are sustainable and effective.

In Chapter 4, Julia Addington-Hall has extensively revised and updated her original chapter to reflect more critically on the factors that determine referral and access to specialist palliative care services. This chapter draws predominantly upon comparisons between the organization and funding of services in the UK and the USA. She highlights how services have evolved in each country in rather different ways, which she largely attributes to different funding mechanisms and the extent to which there is public and professional support for palliative care. Addington-Hall goes on to consider two groups of people: those with diseases other than cancer and older people. They are not mutually exclusive groups, as older people are more likely to die of chronic diseases other than cancer. She argues that while there is evidence to indicate bias in current referrals and the uptake of specialist palliative care services in the UK (this is less evident in the USA), it cannot be concluded that older people and those without cancer would necessarily benefit from additional services. She challenges readers to think critically about the essential elements of services that define them as 'palliative care'.

In a new Chapter 5, Carol Thomas examines the relationship between the quality of dying experience and the place of death. She reviews the extensive and emerging literature on place of death and illustrates the key issues with examples from a study conducted in the north of England. Her analysis goes beyond simplistic notions to question the meaning of home, hospice and hospitals as environments of dying.

In a revised Chapter 6, Margaret O'Connor attends first to the experience of the person with a life-threatening condition and then to the response of health care policies and services. Her main focus is on the experience of *living with* illness. She argues that life transitions can be regarded as normal. While it is well recognized that illness causes biological disruption, it is also compounded by complex psychological, social and cultural changes. O'Connor draws attention to the differing ways in which illness is understood and experienced. She presents stages of transition through illness and wellness, with differing outcomes including survival, which has been mainly researched in relation to those with cancer, and terminal decline (Feuerstein 2007). She explores some of the tensions in access to palliative care policy in Australia where assumptions are made about the stage of illness (end-stage versus throughout the illness trajectory), the types of diseases (cancer versus non-cancer) and the special needs of older people. These themes resonate with issues introduced by Addington-Hall in Chapter 4 on access to palliative care. They are themes that will recur throughout this book.

In a new Chapter 7, Sue Duke and Chris Bailey argue that communication is fundamental to good palliative care. Drawing upon their insights as practitioners and researchers, they discuss the challenges of effective communication in the context of life-threatening illness. Their methodical examination of the topic highlights the role of information provision, emotional support and therapeutic listening in effective communication.

In a further new Chapter, 8, Mike Bennett and Jose Closs combine their medical and nursing perspectives to offer a comprehensive account of assessment and measurement issues in clinical practice. They argue that accurate, regular and meticulous assessment is the foundation of effective palliative care. They caution against simple tick box approaches which fail to grasp the complexity and holistic nature of human experience. They wisely highlight the difference between measuring what is important to patients and families, and using measures just because they are available. The chapter clearly describes the principles of reliability and validity which should help readers in selecting appropriate assessment procedures.

In Chapter 9, Ann Carter and Peter Mackereth introduce a new topic in the second edition, that of using complementary therapies in palliative care contexts. They start by clarifying the terminology and indicating the main types of therapy that may safely be provided to dying patients. In the UK and similar resource-rich countries there has been a remarkable increase in the acceptability and utilization of complementary therapies in cancer care and in palliative care, such that most hospices provide a range of therapies generally for patients and, in some cases, for their carers. Nurses have been enthusiastic supporters of the introduction of these therapies and may have undergone additional training in order to deliver these interventions. However, in some quarters there remain concerns about the lack of scientific evidence to demonstrate the safety and efficacy of these therapies, and they largely remain supplementary to the 'core' functions of many palliative care services. Carter and Mackereth call for more rigorous investigation of these therapies, using appropriate and sensitive methods, to establish and justify their use with patients and carers, and as a means to reduce staff stress.

# References

American Psychiatric Association (1994) *Diagnostic and Statistical Manual of Mental Disorders*, 4th edn. Washington, DC: APA.

Barnes, S., Gott, M., Payne, S., Seamark, D., Parker, C., Gariballa, S. and Small, N. (2006) Prevalence of symptoms in a community-based sample of heart failure patients. *Journal of Pain and Symptom Management*, 33(3): 208–16.

Bem, D. (1972) Self perception theory. In: L. Berkowitz (ed.) *Advances in Experimental Social Psychology*, Vol. 6. New York: Academic Press.

Bingley, A.F., McDermott, E., Thomas, C., Payne, S., Seymour, J.E. and Clark, D. (2006) Making sense of dying: a review of narratives written since 1950 by people facing death from cancer and other diseases. *Palliative Medicine*, 20(3): 183–95.

Blaxter, M. (1990) *Health and Lifestyle*. London: Heinemann.

British Heart Foundation (2001) *Palliative care of heart failure, Factfile No. 5.* London: BHF.

Buckley, J. (2002) Holism and a health-promoting approach to palliative care. *International Journal of Palliative Nursing*, 8(10): 505–8.

Bury, M. (1982) Chronic illness as biographical disruption. *Sociology of Health and Illness*, 4(2): 167–82.

Charmaz, K. (1991) *Good Days, Bad Days: The Self in Chronic Illness and Time.* New Brunswick, NJ: Rutger University Press.

Christakis, C.A. (1999) *Death, Foretold Prophecy and Prognosis in Medical Care.* London: University of Chicago Press.

Clark, D. (1999) 'Total pain', disciplinary power and the body in the work of Cicely Saunders 1958–67. *Social Science and Medicine,* 49(6): 727–36.

Cobb, S. (1976) Social support as a moderator of life stress. *Psychosomatic Medicine,* 38(5): 300–14.

Costain Schou, K. and Hewison, J. (1999) *Experiencing Cancer: Quality of Life in Treatment.* Buckingham: Open University Press.

Crossley, M. (2000) *Introducing Narrative Psychology: Self, Trauma and the Construction of Meaning.* Buckingham: Open University Press.

Crossley, M. (2003) 'Let me explain': narrative emplotment and one patient's experience of oral cancer. *Social Science and Medicine,* 56: 439–48.

Del Vecchio Good, M., Munakata, T., Kobayashi, Y., Mattingly, C. and Good, B. (1994) Oncology and narrative time. *Social Science and Medicine,* 38: 855–62.

Feuerstein, M. (ed.) (2007) *Handbook of Cancer Survivorship.* New York: Springer.

Field, D. (1993) Social definitions of health and illness. In: S. Taylor and D. Field (eds) *Sociology of Health and Health Care,* 2nd edn. Oxford: Blackwell Science.

Field, D. (2000) *What Do We Mean by 'Psychosocial'? Briefing 4.* London: National Council for Hospice and Specialist Palliative Care Services.

Field, D. and Copp, G. (1999) Communication and awareness about dying in the 1990s. *Palliative Medicine,* 13: 459–68.

Field, D., Hockey, J. and Small, N. (1997) *Death, Gender and Ethnicity.* London: Routledge.

Frank, A. (1995) *The Wounded Storyteller: Body, Illness and Ethics.* Chicago, IL: University of Chicago Press.

Freud, S. (1923) *The Ego and the Id.* Standard edition. London: Howarth Press.

Froggatt, K.A., Davies, S., Atkinson, L., Aveyard, B., Binney, S., Kent, Y., McCaffrey, S. and Townend, C. (2006) The joys and tribulations of partnership working in care homes for older people. *Quality in Ageing,* 7(3): 26–32.

Froggatt, K.A., Wilson, D., Justice, C., MacAdam, M., Leibovici, K., Kinch, J., Thomas, R. and Choi, J. (2006). End-of-life care in long-term care settings for older people: a literature review. *International Journal of Older People Nursing,* 1: 45–50.

Giddens, A. (1976) *New Rules of Sociological Method: A Positive Critique of Interpretive Sociologies.* London: Hutchinson.

Giddens, A. (1998) *Sociology.* Cambridge: Polity Press.

Glaser, B.G. and Strauss, A.L. (1965) *Awareness of Dying.* New York: Aldine.

Gott, M., Seymour, J.E., Bellamy, G., Clark, D. and Ahmedzai, S. (2004) How important is dying at home to the 'good death'? Findings from a qualitative study with older people. *Palliative Medicine,* 18: 460–7.

Gott, M., Barnes, S., Payne, S., Seamark, D., Parker, C., Gariballa, S. and Small, N. (2007) Dying trajectories in heart failure. *Palliative Medicine,* 21: 95–9.

Greenhalgh, T. and Hurwitz, B. (1998) *Narrative Based Medicine.* London: British Medical Journal Books.

Helman, C.G. (2000) *Culture, Health and Illness,* 4th edn. Oxford: Butterworth Heinemann.

Hudson, P. and Payne, S. (eds) *Family Caregivers and Palliative Care.* Oxford University Press: Oxford (in press).

Jones, G.Y. and Payne, S. (2000) Searching for safety signals: the experience of medical surveillance amongst men with testicular teratomas. *Psycho-Oncology*, 9: 385–95.

Kellehear, A. (1999) *Health Promoting Palliative Care*. Oxford: Oxford University Press.

Kellehear, A. (forthcoming) Care giving social and cultural aspects. In: P. Hudson and S. Payne (eds) *Family Caregivers and Palliative Care*. Oxford: Oxford University Press.

Kelly, G. (1955) *A Theory of Personality – The Psychology of Personal Constructs*. New York: W.W. Norton.

Kleinman, A. (1980) *Patients and Healers in the Context of Culture*. Berkeley, CA: University of California Press.

Launer, J. (2003) Narrative-based medicine: a passing fad or a giant leap for general practice? (editorial) *British Journal of General Practice*, 53(2): 91–2.

Lawler, J. (1991) *Behind the Screens: Somology and the Problem of the Body*. London: Churchill Livingstone.

Lawler, J. (1997) *The Body in Nursing*. Melbourne, VIC: Churchill Livingstone.

Lawton, J. (2000) *The Dying Process: Patients' Experiences of Palliative Care*. London: Routledge.

Lunney, J.R, Lynn, J. and Hogan, C. (2002) Profiles of older Medicare decedents. *Journal of the American Geriatrics Society*, 50(6): 1008–12.

Lupton, D. (1994) *Medicine as Culture: Illness, Disease and the Body in Western Societies*. London: Sage.

Lynn, J. and Adamson, D.M. (2003) *Living well at the end of life. Adapting health care to serious chronic illness in old age*. Washington: Rand Health.

Maslow, A.H. (1970) *Motivation and Personality*, 2nd edn. New York: Harper & Row.

May, C. (1992) Nursing work, nurses' knowledge and subjectification of the patient. *Sociology of Health and Illness*, 14: 472–87.

May, T. (1996) *Situating Social Theory*. Buckingham: Open University Press.

McCarthy, M., Lay, M. and Addington-Hall, J.M. (1996) Dying from heart disease. *Journal of the Royal College of Physicians*, 30: 325–8.

McDermott, E., Bingley, A.F., Thomas, C., Payne, S., Seymour, J. and Clark, D. (2006) Viewing patient need through professional writings: a systematic 'ethnographic' review of palliative care professionals' experiences of caring for people with cancer at the end of life. *Progress in Palliative Care*, 14(1): 9–18.

Murphy, N.F., Simpson, C.R., McAlister, F.A., Stewart, S., MacIntyre, K., Kirkpatrick, M., Chalmers, J., Redpath, A., Capewell, S. and McMurray, J.J.V. (2004) National survey of the prevalence, incidence, primary care burden, and treatment of heart failure in Scotland. *Heart*, 90: 1129–36.

National Institute for Clinical Excellence (NICE) (2004) *Guidance on cancer services. Improving supportive and palliative care in adults with cancer*. London: National Institute of Clinical Excellence.

Payne, S. (2007) Public health and palliative care (editorial) *Progress in Palliative Care*, 15(3): 101–2.

Payne, S. (2007) Resilient carers. In: B. Monroe and D. Oliviere (eds) *Resilience in Palliative Care – Achievement in Adversity*. Oxford: Oxford University Press.

Payne, S., Horn, S. and Relf, M. (1999) *Loss and Bereavement*. Buckingham: Open University Press.

Payne, S., Hardey, M. and Coleman, P. (2000) Interactions between nurses during handovers in elderly care. *Journal of Advanced Nursing*, 32(2): 277–85.

Payne, S., Jarrett, N., Wiles, R. and Field, D. (2002) Counselling strategies for bereaved people offered in primary care. *Counselling Psychology Quarterly*, 15(2): 161–77.

Pennebaker, J.W. and Seagal, J.D. (1999) Forming a story: the health benefits of narrative. *Journal of Clinical Psychology*, 55(10): 1243–54.

Riessman, C. (1993). *Narrative Analysis*. London: Sage.

Rogers, C. (1961) *On Becoming a Person: A Therapist's View of Psychotherapy*. London: Constable.

Rumsey, N. and Harcourt, D. (2005) *The Psychology of Appearance*, Maidenhead: McGraw-Hill Press.

Seymour, J. (2001) *Critical Moments: Death and Dying in Intensive Care*. Buckingham: Open University Press.

Seymour, J.E., Gott, M., Bellamy, G., Clark, D. and Ahmedzai, S. (in press) Planning for the end of the life: the views of older people about advance statements. *Social Science and Medicine*.

Seymour, J., Witherspoon, R., Gott, M., Ross, H. and Payne, S. (2005) *Dying in Older Age: End-of-Life Care*, Bristol: Policy Press.

Seymour, J.E., Payne, S., Chapman, A. and Holloway, M. (2007) Hospice or Home? Expectations about end of life care among older white and Chinese people living in the UK. *Sociology of Health and Illness, Special Edition on Ethnicity & Health*, 29(6): 872–890.

Simmons, S. (1994) Social networks: their relevance to mental health nursing. *Journal of Advanced Nursing*, 19: 281–9.

Small, N., Froggatt, K., and Down, M. (2007) *Living and Dying with Dementia: Dialogues about Palliative Care*. Oxford: Oxford University Press.

Sudnow, D. (1967) *Passing On*. Englewood Cliffs, NJ: Prentice-Hall.

Tasker, M. (2005) Something inside so strong . . . *Hospice Information Bulletin*, 4(3): 1–2.

Taylor, C. (1989) *Sources of the Self: The Making of Modern Identity*. Cambridge: Cambridge University Press.

The, A-M. (2002) *Palliative Care and Communication: Experiences in the Clinic*. Buckingham: Open University Press.

Williams, A. and Botti, M. (2002) Issues concerning the on-going care of patients with comorbidities in acute care and post-discharge in Australia: a literature review. *Journal of Advanced Nursing*, 40(2): 131–40.

Wright, M. and Clark, D. (2006) *Hospice and Palliative Care in Africa: a review of developments and challenges*. Oxford: Oxford University Press.

# 2

# History and culture in the rise of palliative care

*David Clark*

---

**Key points**

- Presents a history of palliative care in the global context.
- Highlights the particular contribution of Cicely Saunders.
- Shows how palliative care emerged as a field of specialization.
- Describes patterns of global development.
- Presents an overview of current hospice palliative care provision around the world.

---

As the work of palliative care expands around the world, there is a growing interest in understanding how this field of activity first began to develop in its modern form and how that history is shaping its current development. This chapter draws on an established programme of research at the International Observatory on End of Life Care at Lancaster University, which is now recognized as a key source of information about the history of modern hospice and palliative care and the global analysis of current developments.[1] Acknowledging some important nineteenth-century influences and the new interest in the care of the dying that began to emerge at that time, the chapter analyses key developments taking place in the twentieth century that began to establish the care of the dying not just as the interest of religiously and philanthropically motivated individuals and groups, but as something that might be capable of finding a place within wider systems of health and social care delivery. The history of modern hospice palliative care is a short one, and many of those who have shaped it are still alive to tell their stories and to reflect on their experience. Learning from that history is a crucial way in which an increasingly specialized field can better understand its current dilemmas and also develop effective strategies for the future.

# A summary view

In many parts of Europe, North America and Australia, as the nineteenth century advanced, an epidemiological transition got underway which saw the beginnings of a shift in the dominant causes of death: from fatal infectious diseases of rapid progression, to chronic and life-threatening diseases of longer duration. As this transition became more marked, the departure from life for many people became an extended and sometimes uneven process. Consequently, people called 'the dying' began to emerge more clearly as a social category; and over time, the most common place for life to end began to shift from the domestic home to some form of institution. For the first time in history, special institutions were formed, often the work of religious orders or religiously-motivated philanthropists, that were uniquely concerned with the care of dying people. At first the influence of these 'hospices' and 'homes for the dying' was quite limited, scarcely capable of changing attitudes and practices more generally. They appeared in several countries through the later nineteenth and into the early decades of the twentieth centuries, but seemed to make little impact on the wider environment of care for dying people (Humphreys 2001).

In the second half of the twentieth century however, major innovations did begin to take place, building on and developing some of the ideas which prevailed in the original religious and philanthropic homes. By this time a modern 'movement' was emerging: reformist in character, advocating new approaches to old experiences, and above all opening up a space in which the 'the process of dying' could be newly problematized, shaped and moulded. Hospice care came to be defined in quite specific terms, emphasizing 'quality of life', 'pain and symptom management', and 'psychosocial care'. In several countries, palliative medicine gained recognition as a specialty and advanced programmes of training developed, not only for physicians, but also for nurses, social workers and others involved in what came to be seen as the multi-disciplinary activity of modern palliative care. During the last quarter of the twentieth century, and particularly in the 1990s, there was a steady growth in the number of services operating in this way, across countries and continents. By the start of the twenty-first century, palliative care had reached a stage of relative maturation, gaining a measure of recognition on the part of the public, the professions and the policy makers. Yet, in most resource-poor regions of the world, hospice and palliative care were still struggling to gain a foothold, seen as a low priority in settings where overall health care expenditure remained limited and where other social problems appeared more pressing. Over a relatively short period of time, the achievements made by palliative care protagonists, as well as the definition of the challenges that remained, reveal a line of development which could be traced back to nineteenth-century foundations. These were laid by nursing orders, philanthropic associations and voluntary medical practitioners. Now transformed into the guise of modern palliative care, the achievements and challenges took on a new character. They were accompanied by different ways of thinking and behaving towards dying members of society. Indeed, they seemed capable of generating previously unimagined ways of experiencing illness, suffering, and even mortality itself.

## Key developments in the twentieth century

We know that the nineteenth-century hospice founders were a key source of inspiration to Cicely Saunders (1918–2005) as in the late 1950s she set about her life's work to improve the care of dying people. Indeed, they influenced her clinical activities, her research and teaching, and the formation of St Christopher's Hospice in 1967. They were also a source of inspiration for her continuing leadership and inspiration to palliative care workers in many places (Clark 2001a). We also know that Cicely Saunders was acting as part of an international network of like-minded people, even from as early as 1958 when she published her first paper in *The St Thomas' Hospital Gazette*. This network covered North America, India and Ceylon, Australia, France, Switzerland, the Netherlands and communist Poland, and is revealed in her remarkable and extensive correspondence of the time (Clark 2002a). Indeed it can be argued that the foundation of St Christopher's Hospice in London in 1967 by Cicely Saunders and her colleagues should be seen, not as the beginning of the modern hospice movement; but rather, as the conclusion to the first stage of its international development – a process that had already been underway for a decade or more when the hospice opened (Clark 1998).

By the late 1950s the British National Health Service had been in existence for more than a decade; it formed part of a welfare state pledged to provide care 'from the cradle to the grave'. Yet, the new health service had done nothing to promote the care of its dying patients. Instead, the thrust of policy was moving towards acute medicine and rehabilitation. Yes, there was

---

**Box 2.1**

I am a doctor of medicine, having read this rather late in life after training first as a nurse and then as an almoner. I read medicine because I was so interested and challenged by the problems of patients dying of cancer, and have for the past twelve years had in mind the hope that I might be led to found a new Home for these patients . . . I am enclosing a reprint of some articles which I wrote for the 'Nursing Times' at their request last year, and which contain something of what I have learnt so far. I am also enclosing a scheme for a Home which I am trying to plan for at the moment.

Cicely Saunders to Olive Wyon, 4 March 1969.

(Clark 2002a: 23)

increasing awareness of the demographic changes which would lead to far more elderly people in the population, but the consequences for their care, and in particular for those affected by malignant disease, received scant attention. Cicely Saunders was one of a handful of clinicians on both sides of the Atlantic who began to take a special interest in the care of the dying in this context. There were others working towards similar goals elsewhere. In the mid-1960s the Swiss-born psychiatrist Dr Elisabeth Kubler Ross was running a weekly seminar talking to dying patients at the Billings Hospital in Chicago. Her first book, published in the autumn of 1969, became a worldwide bestseller, though her ideas on the stages of dying and how to communicate with dying patients did much to polarize medical opinion (Kubler Ross 1969). In New Haven, Florence Wald, Dean of Nursing at Yale, and her associates were also making plans for a hospice service and working in close dialogue with colleagues in London, Chicago and elsewhere (Buck 2007).

It is important to note that the most immediate audience for Cicely Saunders's writings was among nurses. While she struggled to get *medical* interest in her work (Clark 1998; Faull and Nicholson 2003), nursing colleagues encouraged her, became involved in her plans and fostered the publication of her ideas. A series of six articles she wrote for *Nursing Times* in the autumn of 1959 provoked a huge written response from the readership, as well as an editorial in the *Daily Telegraph* (Clark 1997). The articles were among the first to elucidate a set of principles for the care of the dying that could be used as a guide to practice. Rooted in strong personal, religious and moral convictions they also made compelling, if controversial, reading. The following year they were reproduced in a *Nursing Times* pamphlet entitled *Care of the Dying* (Saunders 1960a) and Cicely Saunders continued to write for the journal throughout the early 1960s. Likewise, in 1964, she was invited to contribute a piece to the *American Journal of Nursing* (Clark 2001b). When it appeared, the article used case illustrations from St Joseph's Hospice to focus on nursing aspects of care, giving particular prominence to a major point of discussion at that time: the question of whether or not to reveal the patient's prognosis. Once again, the article produced a considerable postbag, and every nurse who wrote in from across the United States received a personal reply from the author.

Why were nurses so eager to read such material and how was it that these writings on terminal care found such resonances within nursing audiences? By the mid-twentieth century important changes were occurring in Western medicine and health care. Specialization was advancing rapidly; new treatments were proliferating; and there was an increasing emphasis upon cure and rehabilitation. At the same time, death in the hospital, rather than at home, was becoming the norm; and the dying patient or 'hopeless case' was often viewed as a failure of medical practice. In a series of famous lectures in the 1930s, the American physician and champion of nursing revisionism, Alfred Worcester had noted: '. . . many doctors nowadays, when the death of their patients becomes imminent, seem to believe that it is quite proper to leave the dying in the care of the nurses and the sorrowing relatives. This shifting of responsibility is unpardonable. And one of its results is that as less professional interest is taken in such service less is known about it' (1935: 33). It seems that nurses bridled at such trends and observations. If Worcester thought it unpardonable that patients should be left in this way, nurses considered that they and their dying patients had been abandoned by their medical colleagues and, indeed, ignored by society. Nurses who had remained with the task of staying with their dying patients therefore found some endorsement and succour in the early writings of Cicely Saunders and indeed showed a willingness to contribute to the new thinking, even when doctors remained sceptical and doubting. It was as if in reading this new writing on a traditional aspect of nursing care, in some way the notion of nursing as a 'calling' was being rekindled: 'you have been a guiding light in helping me to discover what I have been searching for as a student nurse', observed one American correspondent (Clark 1998: 54).

## An emerging specialization

Despite these concerns, some initiatives for improving care at the end of life did begin to gain a wider hearing from the early 1960s. In Britain attention focused on the medical 'neglect' of the terminally ill; whereas in the United States a reaction to the medicalization of death began to take root. Four particular innovations can be identified (Clark 1999a). First, a shift took place within the professional literature of care of the dying, from idiosyncratic anecdote to systematic observation. New studies, by nurses, doctors, social workers and social scientists provided evidence about the social and clinical aspects of dying in contemporary society. By the early 1960s, leading articles in *The Lancet* and *British Medical Journal* were drawing on the evidence of research to suggest ways in which terminal care could be promoted and how arguments in favour of euthanasia might be countered. Second, a new view of dying began to emerge which sought to foster concepts of dignity and meaning. Enormous scope was opened up here for refining ideas about the dying process and exploring the extent to which patients should and did know about their terminal condition. Third, an active rather than a passive approach to the care of the dying was promoted with increasing vigour. Within this, the fatalistic resignation of the doctor was supplanted by a determination to find new and imaginative ways to continue caring up to the end of life, and indeed beyond it, in the care of the bereaved. Fourth, a growing recognition of the interdependency of mental and physical distress created the potential for a more embodied notion of suffering, thus constituting a profound challenge to the body–mind dualism upon which so much medical practice of the period was predicated.

As we have already observed, it was the work of Cicely Saunders, first developed in St Joseph's Hospice in Hackney, East London that was to prove most consequential, for it was she that began to forge a peculiarly modern philosophy of terminal care (Winslow and Clark 2005). Through

---

**Box 2.2**

Key innovations in care of the dying in the 1950s and 1960s

● Emergence of the first research studies
● A new approach to dignity and meaning in dying
● Active solutions to clinical problems
● Recognition of the interdependency of mental and physical suffering

---

systematic attention to patient narratives, listening carefully to stories of illness, disease and suffering, she evolved the concept of 'total pain' (Clark 1999b). This view of pain moved beyond the physical to encompass the social, emotional, even spiritual aspects of suffering – captured so comprehensively by the patient who told her: 'All of me is wrong' (Saunders 1964: viii). But it was also linked to a hard-headed approach to pain management. Her message was simple: 'constant pain needs constant control' (1964: 17). Analgesics should be employed in a method of regular giving which would ensure that pain was prevented in advance, rather than alleviated once it had become established; and they should be used progressively, from mild, to moderate to strong.

Even before the opening of St Christopher's Hospice, in South London, in 1967, it had become a source of inspiration to others and was also firmly established in an international network. The correspondence of Cicely Saunders shows clearly how it attracted the interests of senior academics and managers in American nursing, as well as those from many countries who were eager to develop their practical skills through work on the wards of the hospice (Clark 2002a). As the first 'modern' hospice, it sought to combine three key principles: excellent clinical care, education and research. It therefore differed significantly from the other homes for the dying which had preceded it and sought to establish itself as a centre of excellence in a new field of care. Its success was phenomenal and it soon became the stimulus for an expansive phase of hospice development, not only in Britain, but also around the world.

An extensive 'oral history' of the hospice movement in Britain (Clark *et al.* 2005) shows how the development of hospices can be seen as a force shaped by the commitment and imagination of many individuals, found in varied settings and circumstances and at different times. Hospices and the hospice movement attracted charismatic leaders who found ways to integrate a particular vision into a whole programme of activity, wherein the person and the cause were sometimes difficult to distinguish. For some the hospice represented a welcome institutional home, separate from but working alongside the National Health Service (NHS). Others felt a commitment both to hospice care and to the NHS and were pleased to bring the two together in their work. This exposed some limitations to the model, however – it was often based on a costly inpatient care unit that served as a hub reaching out to relatively small numbers of patients; it was predominantly a model for cancer care (although some interest was shown in patients with neurological conditions); and it was delivered from non-profit charitable organizations, situated outside the formal health care system. Despite this, it served as a useful platform upon which other ideas could be built and adapted and quite quickly some NHS hospice services did begin to appear in the UK. Elsewhere patterns of development took different forms and the balance between voluntary and public sector provision varied enormously between different countries.

## Growth and diversification in the later twentieth century: the global perspective

From the outset, ideas developed in the voluntary hospices and elsewhere were applied differently in other places and contexts. Within a decade after St Christopher's opened in the UK it was accepted that the principles of hospice care could be practised in many settings: in specialist inpatient units, but also in home care and day care services; likewise, hospital units and support teams were established that brought the new thinking about dying into the very heartlands of acute medicine. By the mid-1990s there were over 1,000 specialist Macmillan nurses working in palliative care in the UK, as well as some 5,000 Marie Curie nurses providing care in the home. In 2005 there were 63 NHS inpatient units in the UK and 158 voluntary hospices, comprising a total of 3,180 beds. There was also a large array of other services: day care (257); hospital based (305); home care teams (356) (Centeno *et al.* 2007).

Modern hospice developments took place first in affluent countries but, in time, they also gained a hold in poorer countries, often supported by mentoring and 'twinning' arrangements with more established hospices in the West. Pioneers of first-wave hospice development and some of their second generation successors worked to promote palliative care in many countries of the world, building increasingly on international networks of support and collaboration. Table 2.1 lists a timeline of organizational developments among pan-national associations and initiatives to promote palliative care around the world.

Globally, however, palliative care development appears patchy and until recently comparative data about the distribution of services has been difficult to obtain. Clark and Wright (2007) have categorized hospice-palliative care development, country by country, throughout the world and depicted this development in a series of world and regional maps. Adopting a multi-method approach, which involves the synthesis of evidence from published and grey literature as well as information from regional experts, has enabled the creation of a four-part typology at the country level: 1) no identified hospice-palliative care activity, 2) capacity building activity, but no service, 3) localized palliative care provision and 4) countries where palliative care

**Table 2.1**   Pan-national associations and initiatives in hospice and palliative care

| | |
|---|---|
| **1973** | International Association for the Study of Pain, founded Issaquah, Washington, USA |
| **1976** | 1st International Congress on the Care of the Terminally Ill, Montreal, Canada |
| **1977** | Hospice Information Service, founded at St Christopher's Hospice, London, UK. |
| **1980** | International Hospice Institute, became International Hospice Institute and College (1995) and International Association for Hospice and Palliative Care (1999) |
| **1982** | World Health Organization Cancer Pain Programme initiated |
| **1988** | European Association of Palliative Care founded in Milan, Italy |
| **1998** | Poznan Declaration leads to the foundation of the Eastern and Central European Palliative Task Force (1999) |
| **1999** | Foundation for Hospices in sub-Saharan Africa founded in USA |
| **2000** | Latin American Association of Palliative care founded |
| **2001** | Asia Pacific Hospice Palliative Care Network founded |
| **2002** | UK Forum for Hospice and Palliative Care Worldwide founded by Help the Hospices<br>Hospice Information Service re-launched as Hospice Information – a joint venture between Help the Hospices and St Christopher's Hospice |
| **2004** | African Palliative Care Association founded |
| **2005** | First World Hospice and Palliative Care Day |

**Sources:** Swerdlow and Stjernswärd 1982; Saunders 2000; Luczak and Kluziak 2001; Woodruff *et al.* 2001; Blumhuber, Kaasa and de Conno 2002; Bruera, de Lima and Woodruff 2002; FHSSA 2002; Goh 2002; Richardson, Praill and Jackson 2002.

activities are approaching integration with mainstream service providers. Overall, they found palliative care services in 115 out of 234 countries and the following distribution within the categories: no identified activity, 78 (33 per cent); capacity building, 41 (18 per cent); localized provision, 80 (34 per cent); approaching integration, 35 (15 per cent). The typology differentiates levels of palliative care development across hemispheres and in rich and poor settings and highlights both where successes have been achieved and where challenges remain.

Such a picture must be set against the stark realities of global need for palliative care at the beginning of the twenty-first century: 56 million deaths per year, with an estimated 60 per cent who could benefit from some form of palliative care (Stjernswärd and Clark 2003). A substantial literature on national developments in hospice and palliative care records important achievements and many developments in the face of adversity, together with a large agenda of 'unfinished business'.

### North and South America

Hospice services in the USA grew dramatically from the founding organization in New Haven in 1974, to some 3,000 providers by the end of the twentieth century. These services evolved in the USA had much less contact with oncology than their UK counterparts and have a much greater involvement of non-cancer patients. American hospices focus primarily on home care and the concept of hospital teams and inpatient hospice beds is much less developed. In 1982, a major milestone was the achievement of funding recognition for hospices under the Medicare programme. Several key developments occurred in the 1990s. National representative bodies appeared to take a more professionalized approach to their activities, giving greater emphasis to palliative care as a specialized field of activity (the National Hospice Association became the National Hospice and Palliative Care Association; the American Academy of Hospice Physicians became the American Academy of Hospice and Palliative Medicine). At the same time two major foundations developed extensive programmes concerned with improving the culture of end-of-life care in American society (the Robert Wood Johnson Foundation created the Last Acts initiative; and the Open Society Institute established the Project on Death in America). An influential report by the Institute of Medicine (IoM), published in 1997, sought to strengthen popular and professional understanding of the need for good care at the end of life (Field and Cassel 1997). This was followed in 2001 by a further report from the IoM listing ten recommendations addressing the role of the National Cancer Institute (NCI) in promoting palliative care (Foley and Gelband 2001). In 2004 the National Institutes of Health held a 'State-of-the-Science' meeting on Improving End-of-Life Care, which brought together prominent clinicians and researchers to focus on defining and understanding major considerations related to end-of-life care, and developing interventions for symptom management, social and spiritual care and care-giver support (Grady 2005). Meanwhile, in neighbouring Canada, where Balfour Mount first coined the term 'palliative care' in 1974 (Mount 1997), a Senate report in 2000 stated that no extension of palliative care provision had occurred in the previous five years, and set out recommendations for further development among the country's 600 services (Carstairs and Chochinov 2001). In Latin America, there was evidence of faltering progress, with palliative care services existing in seven countries, and the greatest amount of development in Argentina (de Lima 2001). A chief problem here, as in other developing regions, was the problem of poor opioid availability, an issue highlighted in the 1994 Declaration of Florianopolis (Stjernswärd *et al.* 1995).

### Asia Pacific

The first evidence of hospice developments in the Asia Pacific region came with a service for dying patients in Korea, at the Calvary Hospice of Kangung, established by the Catholic Sisters of the Little Company of

Mary, in 1965; services had increased to 60 by 1999 (Chung 1999). In Japan, the first hospice was also Christian, established in the Yodogwa Christian Hospital in 1973; by the end of the century, the country had 80 inpatient units (Maruyama 1999). In Australia, the country that established the world's first chair in palliative care, commonwealth and state funds for palliative care increased steadily from 1980 and palliative medicine was recognized as a specialty in 2000; by 2002 there were 250 designated palliative care services (Hunt *et al.* 2002). Protocols for the WHO three-step analgesic ladder were first introduced into China in 1991 and there were said to be hundreds of palliative care services in urban areas by 2002 (Wang *et al.* 2002).

An extensive review of hospice and palliative care developments in India has mapped the existence of services state by state and explored the perspectives and experiences of those involved, with a view to stimulating new development (McDermott *et al.* in press). The study found that 135 hospice and palliative care services exist in 16 states. These are usually concentrated in large cities, with the exception of the state of Kerala, where services are much more widespread. Non-government organizations and public and private hospitals and hospices are the predominant sources of provision. Palliative care provision could not be identified in 19 states or union territories. Nevertheless, successful models exist in Kerala for the development of affordable, sustainable community-based hospice and palliative care services (Shabeer and Kumar 2005) and these may have potential for replication elsewhere.

### Africa

About one million Africans will develop cancer every year, but for most, treatment remains unattainable (Morris 2003). The need for palliative care is now hugely increased by the epidemic of HIV/AIDS. Wright and Clark (2006), in a review of hospice and palliative care developments in Africa, have mapped the existence of services country by country and explored the perspectives and experiences of those involved. The 47 countries studied were grouped into the four categories of palliative care development adopted by the International Observatory on End of Life Care: no identified hospice or palliative care activity, 21; capacity building activity underway to promote hospice and palliative care delivery, 11; localized provision of hospice and palliative care in place, 11; hospice and palliative care services achieving some measure of integration with mainstream service providers and gaining wider policy recognition, 4. Major difficulties included: opioid availability; workforce development; achieving sustainable critical mass; absorption capacity in relation to major external funding initiatives; coping with the scale of HIV/AIDS-related suffering. The authors concluded that models exist in Uganda, Kenya, South Africa and Zimbabwe for the development of affordable, sustainable community-based hospice and palliative care services and that the newly formed African Palliative Care Association has huge potential to promote innovation, in a context where interest in the development of hospice and palliative care in Africa has never been greater. A small number of further studies have also appraised the development of palliative care in sub-Saharan Africa and stimulated interest in the evaluation of services (Harding *et al.* 2003; Sepulveda *et al.* 2003; Harding and Higginson 2005).

### Europe

In the former communist countries of Eastern Europe and Central Asia, there were few palliative care developments in the years of Soviet domination. Most initiatives can be traced to the early 1990s, after which many projects got underway. These have been documented in detail (Clark and Wright 2003) and show evidence of some service provision in 23 out of 28 countries in the region. Poland and Russia have the most advanced programmes of palliative care, with considerable achievements also made in Romania and Hungary. Nevertheless, in a region of over 400 million people there were just 467 palliative care services in 2002, more than half of which were found in a single country, Poland.

Palliative care in Western Europe made rapid progress from the early 1980s, but by the late 1990s there were still striking differences in provision across different states (ten Have and Clark 2002). After the foundation of St Christopher's in England, in 1967, it was ten years until the first services began to appear elsewhere: in Sweden (1977), Italy (1980), Germany (1983), Spain (1984), Belgium (1985), France (1986) and the Netherlands (1991). In all of these countries the provision of palliative care has moved beyond isolated examples of pioneering services run by enthusiastic founders. Palliative care is being delivered in a variety of settings (domiciliary; quasi-domiciliary; and institutional), though these are not given uniform priority everywhere.

The Council of Europe published a set of European guidelines on palliative care in 2003 and described palliative care as an essential and basic service for the whole population. Its recommendations appear to have been used quite actively in some countries with less-developed palliative care systems, particularly in Eastern Europe, where they have served as a tool for advocacy and lobbying. Policy issues relating to end-of-life care in Europe have also been raised by other non-governmental and inter-governmental organizations. At palliative care conferences in 1995 (Barcelona) and 1998 (Poznan) exhortatory declarations were made, calling for government action on palliative care at the national level and drawing attention to key problems and issues facing palliative care as it develops internationally. By 2003 the European Society for Medical Oncology was giving greater recognition to palliative care (Cherny *et al.* 2003). In 2004 the European Federation of Older Persons launched a campaign to make palliative care a priority topic on the European health agenda.[2] The same year, WHO Europe produced an important document on *Better Palliative Care for Older People*. Its aim is 'to incorporate palliative care for serious chronic progressive illnesses within ageing policies, and to promote better care towards the end of life' (Davies and Higginson 2004a). Its companion volume, *Palliative Care: The solid facts*, is a resource for policy makers in a context where 'the evidence available on palliative care is not complete and . . . there are differences in what can be offered across the European region' (Davies and Higginson 2004b). In 2007, a set of 'commitments' for palliative care improvement was entered into by palliative care associations at the Budapest congress of the European Association for Palliative Care (Radbruch *et al.* 2007). Despite the powerful symbolic language of these and other documents, however, evidence of their impact remains unclear (Clark and Centeno 2006).

## Conclusion

In the early period of development, modern hospice and palliative care in the West had many of the qualities of a social movement. This movement may well have contributed to a new openness about death and bereavement that was in evidence in the late twentieth century (one of the first persons ever to be seen to die on television, for example, was in the care of an Irish 'hospice at home service'). Inspired by charismatic leadership, it was a movement which condemned the neglect of the dying in society; called for high quality pain and symptom management for all who needed it; sought to reconstruct death as a natural phenomenon, rather than a clinical failure; and marshalled practical and moral argument to oppose those in favour of euthanasia. For Cicely Saunders and her followers, such work served as a measure of the very worth of a culture: 'A society which shuns the dying must have an incomplete philosophy' (Saunders 1961: 3).

At the same time, other interests were at work. In several countries (Britain, Australia, Canada, United States) professional recognition of this emerging area of expertise seemed desirable. Specialty recognition occurred first in Britain, in 1987, and was seen by some as a turning point in hospice history (James and Field 1992). It was part of a wider shift away from 'terminal' and 'hospice' care towards the concept of palliative care. Today, 'modernizers' claim that specialization, the integration of palliative care into the mainstream health system, and the development of an 'evidence-based' model of practice and organization are crucial to long-term viability. Yet others mourn the loss of early ideals and regret what they perceive to be an emphasis upon physical symptoms at the expense of psychosocial and spiritual concerns. In short, there have been assertions that forces of 'medicalization' and 'routinization' are at work, or even that the putative 'holism' of palliative care philosophy masks a new, more subtle form of surveillance of the dying and bereaved in modern society (Clark and Seymour 1999). Perhaps it is more helpful to see the rise of modern palliative care as creating and then colonizing a space somewhere between the hope of cure and the acceptance of death – a view of the response to life-threatening illness which is more consistent with the concerns and perspectives of patients in late modern culture (Clark 2002b).

By the end of the twentieth century two forces for expansion were also clearly visible in the new specialty. First was the impetus to move palliative care further upstream in the disease progression, thereby seeking integration with curative and rehabilitation therapies and shifting the focus beyond terminal care and the final stages of life. Second, there was a growing interest in extending the benefits of palliative care to those with diseases other than cancer, in order to make 'palliative care for all' a reality. The new specialty was therefore delicately poised. For some, such integration with the wider system was a *sine qua non* for success; for others, it marked the entry into a risky phase of new development in which early ideals might be compromised.

Hospice care and palliative care have a shared and brief history. The evolution of one into the other marks a transition which, if successful, could ensure that the benefits of a model of care previously available to just a few people at the end of life, and will in time be extended to all who need it, regardless of diagnosis, stage of disease, social situation or means. As the field of palliative care matures, so too our knowledge of its history is deepening and widening. What emerges is a rich field of innovation, taking place in different forms in many varied settings. Out of this has emerged the potential not only to relieve individual suffering at the end of life, but also to transform the social dimensions of dying, death and bereavement in the modern world.

## Notes

1   See: http://www.eolc-observatory.net
2   See: http://www.eurag-europe.org/palliativ-en.htm

## References

Barcelona Declaration on Palliative Care (1995) *European Journal of Palliative Care*. 3(1): 15.

Buck, J. (2007) Reweaving a tapestry of care: religion, nursing and the meaning of hospice, 1945–1978. *Nursing History Review*, 15: 113–45.

Blumhuber, H., Kaasa, S. and de Conno, F. (2002) The European Association for Palliative Care. *Journal of Pain and Symptom Management*, 24(2): 124–7.

Bruera, E., de Lima, L. and Woodruff, R. (2002) The International Association for Hospice and Palliative Care. *Journal of Pain and Symptom Management*, 24(2): 102–5.

Carstairs, S. and Chochinov, H. (2001) Politics, palliation and Canadian progress in end-of-life care. *Journal of Palliative Medicine*, 4(3): 396–9.

Centeno, C., Clark, D., Lynch, T., Rocafort, J., Greenwood, A., Flores, L.A., de Lima, L., Giordano, A., Brasch, S. and Praill, D. (2007) *EAPC Atlas of Palliative Care in Europe*. Houston: IAHPC Press.

Cherny, N.I., Catane, R. and Kosmidis, P. (2003) ESMO takes a stand on supportive and palliative care. *Annals of Oncology*. 14(9): 1335–7.

Chung, Y. (1999) Palliative care in Korea: a nursing point of view. *Progress in Palliative Care*, 8(1): 12–16.

Clark, D. (1997) Someone to watch over me: Cicely Saunders and St Christopher's Hospice, *Nursing Times*, 26 August: 50–1.

Clark, D. (1998) Originating a movement: Cicely Saunders and the development of St Christopher's Hospice, 1957–67. *Mortality*, 3(1): 43–63.

Clark, D. (1999a) Cradle to the grave? Preconditions for the hospice movement in the UK, 1948–67. *Mortality*, 4(3): 225–47.

Clark, D. (1999b) 'Total pain', disciplinary power and the body in the work of Cicely Saunders 1958–67. *Social Science and Medicine*, 49(6): 727–36.

Clark, D. (2001a) Religion, medicine and community in the early origins of St Christopher's Hospice, *Journal of Palliative Medicine*, 4(3): 353–60.

Clark, D. (2001b) A special relationship: Cicely Saunders, the United States and the early foundations of the modern hospice movement. *Illness, Crisis and Loss*, 9(1): 15–30.

Clark, D. (2002a) *Cicely Saunders Founder of the Hospice Movement, Selected letters 1959–1999*. Oxford: Oxford University Press.

Clark, D. (2002b) Between hope and acceptance: the medicalisation of dying. *British Medical Journal*, 324: 905–7.

Clark, D. and Seymour, J. (1999) *Reflections on Palliative Care*. Buckingham: Open University Press.

Clark, D. and Wright, M. (2003) *Transitions in End of Life Care. Hospice and Related Developments in Eastern Europe and Central Asia*. Buckingham: Open University Press.

Clark, D., Small, N., Wright, M., Winslow, M. and Hughes, N. (2005) *A Bit of Heaven for the Few? An oral history of the modern hospice movement in the United Kingdom*. Lancaster: Observatory Publications.

Clark, D. and Centeno, C. (2006) Palliative care in Europe: an emerging approach to comparative analysis. *Clinical Medicine*, 6(2): 197–201.

Clark, D. and Wright, M. (2007) The International Observatory on End of Life Care: a global view of palliative care development. *Journal of Pain and Symptom Management*, 33(5): 542–6.

Davies, E. and Higginson, I.J. (eds) (2004a) *Better Palliative Care for Older People*. Copenhagen: World Health Organization.

Davies, E. and Higginson, I.J. (eds) (2004b) *Palliative Care: The solid facts*. Copenhagen: World Health Organization.

de Lima, L. (2001) Advances in palliative care in Latin America and the Caribbean: ongoing projects of the Pan American Health Association (PAHO). *Journal of Palliative Medicine*, 4(2): 228–31.

Faull, C. and Nicholson, A. (2003) Taking the myths out of the magic: Establishing the use of opioids in the management of cancer pain. In: C. Bushnell and M. Meldrum (eds) *Opioids, the Janus Drugs, and the Relief of Pain*. Seattle: IASP Press.

Field, M.J. and Cassel, C.K. (eds) (1997) *Approaching Death. Improving care at the end of life*. Washington: National Academy Press.

Foley, K.M. and Gelband, H. (2001) *Improving Palliative Care for Cancer. Summary and Recommendations from the National Cancer Policy Board, Institute of Medicine, and National Research Council*. Washington: National Academy Press.

Foundation for Hospices in sub-Saharan Africa (2002) *Challenging Times. FHSSA*: Liverpool, NY.

Goh, C.R. (2002) The Asia Pacific Hospice Palliative Care Network: a network for individuals and organisations. *Journal of Pain and Symptom Management*, 24(2): 128–33.

Grady, P.A. (2005) Introduction: Papers from the National Institutes of Health State-of-the-Science Conference on Improving End-of-Life Care. *Journal of Palliative Medicine*, 8(1): S1–S3.

ten Have, H. and Clark, D. (eds) (2002) *The ethics of palliative care. European perspectives*. Buckingham: Open University Press.

Harding, R., Stewart, K., Marconi, K., O'Neill, J.F. and Higginson, I.J. (2003) Current HIV/AIDS end-of-life care in sub-Saharan Africa: a survey of models, services, challenges and priorities. *BMC Public Health*, 3: 33.

Harding, R. and Higginson, I.J. (2005) Palliative care in sub-Saharan Africa, *The Lancet*, 365(9475): 1971–7.

Humphreys, C. (2001). 'Waiting for the last summons': the establishment of the first hospices in England 1878–1914. *Mortality*, 6(2): 146–66.

Hunt, R., Fazekas, B.S., Luke, C.G., Priest, K.R. and Roder, D.M. (2002) The coverage of cancer patients by designated palliative services: a population-based study, South Australia, 1999. *Palliative Medicine*, 16(5): 403–9.

James, N. and Field, D. (1992) The routinisation of hospice. *Social Science and Medicine*, 34(12): 1363–75.

Kubler Ross, E. (1969) *On Death and Dying*. London: Tavistock.

Luczak, J. and Kluziak, M. (2001) The formation of ECEPT (Eastern and Central Europe Palliative Task Force): a Polish initiative. *Palliative Medicine*, 15: 259–60.

Maruyama, T.C. (1999) *Hospice Care and Culture*. Aldershot: Ashgate.

McDermott, E., Selman, L., Wright, M.C. and Clark, D. (in press) Hospice and Palliative Care Development in India: A Multi-method Review of Services and Experiences. *Journal of Pain and Symptom Management*.

Mount, B. (1997) The Royal Victoria Hospital Palliative Care Service: a Canadian experience. In: C. Saunders and R. Kastenbaum (eds) *Hospice Care on the International Scene*. New York: Springer.

Morris, K. (2003) Cancer? In Africa? *The Lancet Oncology*, 4(1): 5.

Poznan Declaration (1998) *European Journal of Palliative Care*, 6(2): 61–5.

Radbruch, L., Foley, K., de Lima, L., Praill, D. and Fürst, C.J. (2007) The Budapest Commitments: setting the goals. A joint initiative by the European Association for Palliative Care, the International Association for Hospice and Palliative Care and Help the Hospices. *Palliative Medicine*, 21(4): 269–71.

Richardson, H., Praill, D. and Jackson, A. (2002) The UK Forum for Hospice and Palliative Care Overseas. *European Journal of Palliative Care*, 9(2): 72–3.

Sepulveda, C., Habiyambere, V., Amandua, J., Borok, M., Kikule, E., Mudanga, B., Ngoma, T. and Solomon, B. (2003) Quality care at the end of life in Africa. *British Medical Journal*, 327: 209–13.

Saunders, C. (1960a) *Care of the Dying*. London: *Nursing Times* Reprint.

Saunders, C. (1961) 'And from sudden death . . .' *Frontier*, 1–3.

Saunders, C. (1964) Care of patients suffering from terminal illness at St Joseph's Hospice, Hackney, London. *Nursing Mirror*, 14 February: vii–x.

Saunders, C. (2000) Global developments and the Hospice Information Service. Editorial. *Palliative Medicine*, 14: 1–2.

Shabeer, C. and Kumar, S. (2005) Palliative care in the developing world: a social experiment in India. *European Journal of Palliative Care*, 13(2): 76–9.

Stjernswärd, J., Bruera, E., Joranson, D., Allende, S., Montejo, G., Quesada Tristan,

L., Castillo, G., Schoeller, T., Rico Pazos, M.A., Wenk, R., Pruvost, M., de Lima, L., Mendez, E., Nunez Olarte, J., Olalla, J.F. and Vanegas, G. (1995). Opioid availability in Latin America: The Declaration of Florianopolis. *Journal of Pain and Symptom Management*, 10(3): 233–6.

Stjernswärd, J. and Clark, D. (2003) Palliative care – a global perspective. In: G. Hanks, D. Doyle, C. Calman and N. Cherny (eds) *Oxford Textbook of Palliative Medicine* (3rd edn). Oxford: Oxford University Press.

Swerdlow, M. and Stjernswärd, J. (1982) Cancer pain relief – an urgent public health problem. *World Health Forum*, 3: 329.

Wang, X.S., Yu, S., Gu, W. and Xu, G. (2002) China: status of pain and palliative care. *Journal of Pain and Symptom Management*, 24(2): 177–9.

Winslow, M. and Clark, D. (2005) *St Joseph's Hospice Hackney. A century of caring in the East End of London*. Lancaster: Observatory Publications.

Woodruff, R., Doyle, D., de Lima, L., Bruera, E. and Farr, W.C. (2001) The International Association for Hospice and Palliative Care (IAHPC): history, description and future direction. *Journal of Palliative Medicine*, 4(1): 5–7.

Worcester, A. (1935) *The Care of the Aged, the Dying and the Dead*. Springfield, IL: Charles C. Thomas.

Wright, M. and Clark, D. (2006) *Hospice and Palliative Care Development in Africa. A review of developments and challenges*. Oxford: Oxford University Press.

# 3

# Involving or using?

## User involvement in palliative care

*Tony Stevens*

---

**Key points**

- User involvement can be seen as a way to increase collective knowledge, by means of the distillation of the experience of individuals.
- Care should be taken not to exert any coercion to gain the involvement of users.
- Tokenistic attempts at involvement need to be avoided.
- Evaluations of the processes and outcomes of involvement are important.
- The increasing complexity of service delivery and research are major challenges to the involvement of palliative care users.
- Information and communication technologies have the potential to increase the scope and nature of involvement.
- Costs and benefits of user involvement should be carefully considered – user involvement is resource intensive, benefits may be hard to quantify and time is itself precious to users.

---

## What is user involvement?

User involvement has come to be regarded in many countries as a desirable aim, despite uncertainties as to what it is, how it can be measured and the outcomes that might be expected. It can be defined as a process to broaden collective knowledge, by the inclusion of individual experience as part of the underpinning evidence base. It can also be seen as a form of empowerment, whereby subjective truth becomes recognized as a constituent part of objective reality.

There are three principal areas in health care generally in which patients and members of the public can be involved. The first is involvement in the processes by which health care services are delivered. The second is through involvement in the design, development and management of research activities. The third area is involvement in the development and formulation of strategic decisions or policy. Some users may be involved in all these areas – others may decide to focus upon one particular aspect. In many Western industrialized countries there are opportunities for involvement in health care in its broadest sense and other opportunities focusing on particular diseases. Increasingly, national and international collaborations involving users are being established. However, there are fewer opportunities for the involvement of palliative care users and even less for those who have non-malignant disease.

Different levels of involvement have been identified according to how much power or control users have. One of the earliest, and still one of the most influential expositions of involvement was developed by Arnstein (1969). She put forward a typology of involvement based on the idea of a 'ladder of citizen participation', based on three categories of citizen power that included eight levels of participation: *non-participation* (manipulation and therapy), *tokenism* (informing, consulting and placation) and *citizen power* (partnership, delegated power and citizen control). Arnstein reasoned that for participation to be 'effective', then simply 'involving' people was insufficient. There must also be a sense of partnership where those involved are given real opportunities to exercise their influence. There have been a number of variants on Arnstein's model. For example, INVOLVE, a UK national advisory group that aims to promote active public involvement in research, has suggested a classification based upon three types of participation (INVOLVE 2003). At the lowest level of participation is *consultation*, whereby users are asked for their viewpoints with no assurances that these will be used. *Collaboration* is when professionals and users work together in partnership. *Control* is when users are able to direct and control the patterns of interaction. However, in all these typologies, power remains the key issue, in terms of how it is shared between professionals and users, or how much is devolved to users.

The involvement of users is a relatively recent phenomenon, with a history of barely 30 years. In a statement that many would tend to take for granted today, in 1978, the World Health Organization (World Health Organization 1978) stated that 'patients have a right and responsibility to be involved in their own care' (page 1). From the 1980s, the number of user-led movements and organizations focusing on welfare and social care grew at an unprecedented rate. Many of those early movements were based upon securing 'rights' of individuals, together with an acknowledgement of social justice and community responsibility (Bastian 1998). The constituents were principally disabled people, people with learning difficulties and mental health service users. Organizations also quickly grew among users of maternity services, and survivors and people living with HIV/AIDS. In the field of cancer, in North America, highly vocal and influential activists, like Deborah Collyar, formed groups dedicated particularly to raising issues of those affected by breast cancer, especially in regard to research (Collyar 2005). The pattern of the development of these groups was quickly replicated in Europe. However, patients who were near to the end of their lives and those caring for them, particularly those who were suffering from non-malignant disease, found it more challenging to organize on a similar scale, and to thus exert comparable influence.

During the 1990s there were many policy initiatives, particularly in the UK, reflecting the growth of interest in consumer choice, the need for higher quality information and patients' rights (Stevens and Wilde 2005). In 2004, the Department of Health published 'Patient and public involvement – a brief overview' (Department of Health 2004). This stated that 'The involvement of patients and the public in health decision making is now a central theme of national and local policy in the NHS. Involvement illumin-ates the patient experience and helps to shape a health service that is truly responsive to individual and community needs' (page 4). In addition, around this time, research funders began to recommend the involvement of users in funding applications or that users be included on their awards committees (Clinical Trials Awards and Advisory Committee 2006). It seemed that some users were beginning to be offered real opportunities to influence the processes of research and patterns of service delivery.

This chapter will seek to assess the nature and extent of these opportu-nities for palliative care users. It will address the identity of the palliative care 'user' population, define the purposes of involvement, examine the evidence of any benefits of involvement, identify some of the challenges and highlight examples of good practice.

## Who are the 'users'?

There has been much debate as to the terminology and language employed in defining those who are involved. The term 'lay people' is becoming less common, though still in use (Earl-Slater 2004), as some have argued that it is a typology based upon a lack of knowledge (Hogg and Williamson 2001). 'Patient experts' does not include people who are not patients. 'Users' or 'service users' can be criticized on the grounds that they exclude groups such as carers and relatives. Similarly, 'consumers' is also used less frequently (Telford *et al.* 2002). Other descriptors that have been used include citizens, clients, partners and stakeholders. 'Patients and the public' is the term currently employed by the UK Clinical Research Network and Macmillan Cancer Support, although many acknowledge there may be significant dif-ferences between the views of the public and the views of patients (Litva *et al.* 2002). Some authors have argued that 'users' should not include people who have at any point been health care professionals, professionally engaged as policy makers or researchers, or involved in the design or delivery of services, on the grounds that their perspectives and priorities may be skewed by their experiences (Earl-Slater 2004). It is clear that there is no single term that is acceptable to all, and a report by INVOLVE (2003) suggested 'we are all potential users' (page ii).

# What are the purposes of involvement?

There is evidence that users of palliative care do want to have involvement in research activity and the way that services are organized (Gott *et al.* 2002; Beresford 2005; Cotterell *et al.* 2005). There is also evidence that older people, for example, have concerns about death and dying and welcome the opportunity to express their views and put forward recommendations to improve care at the end of life (Seymour *et al.* 2002). However, the views that users may hold as to the purpose of their involvement may be very different to those held by professionals. For example, users may view their participation as part of a process to help improve services or treatments. This 'democratic approach' towards involvement is predicated on the belief that if individuals have more input, then services will improve and people will have greater control over their lives in general. Professionals, on the other hand, may see the input of users as part of a way to improve the efficiency of the system – the 'consumerist' approach (Beresford 2005). The 'involvement' of users in this way, without any real sharing of power, can be employed as a strategy to legitimize potentially unpopular decisions, such as restricting access to treatments, rather than to foster genuine consumer involvement. In such instances, a patient-centred approach is transformed into one in which there is pressure for user compliance within the existing bureaucratic structures, resulting in an 'illusion of influence' (Clayton 1988).

Other reasons favouring the involvement of users have been identified. There is an ethical dimension that is based upon the rights of the individual, community responsibilities and social justice, and the development of the democratic ideal of citizenship. In this context, it is regarded as ethically proper for consumers to be involved in how budgets are allocated, the way that services are delivered and the process by which research priorities are identified (see Boote *et al.* 2002).

It has also been argued that involving users can enhance the quality and effectiveness of decision-making or the research process. This is referred to as the 'patient expert' approach (Sitzia *et al.* 2006). The theoretical reasoning for this is based on conceptualizations of models of health. The World Health Organization (WHO) has identified two distinct paradigms, whereby disease is defined as 'physiologic and clinical abnormality' while illness is defined as the 'subjective experience of the individual' (Ong 1996). It is argued that the users can act as a bridge between these two perspectives and help develop a holistic interpretation of health (Entwistle *et al.* 1998). Mutual benefit is thought to follow – patients and the public become more informed about the process of disease, and health care professionals understand more about the experience of illness. The quality of both process and outcome is believed to improve.

# What is the evidence to support user involvement?

Intuitively one might expect that input from users into policy initiatives, new patterns of service delivery, or research protocols, would have some added value. Users will have been able to input their views that have been grounded in their own experience of the disease, its treatment and the nature of the delivery of services. Indeed, many organizations have issued broad statements advocating the benefits of user involvement. The WHO has stated that policy and decision makers should 'involve older people – as the users of services – in making decisions about the type and mix of services they want available to them towards the end of life and into bereavement' (World Health Organization 2004: 36). The Consumer Liaison Group of the UK National Cancer Research Institute and National Cancer Research Network has reported that the consumer involvement approach 'brings increased value to cancer research and for patient benefit' (National Cancer Research Institute 2006: 1). The United Kingdom Clinical Research Network, which will ultimately oversee all clinical research, has also stated 'active public involvement is needed if it is to encourage research which directly benefits and reflects the needs and views of patients and the public' (United Kingdom Clinical Research Network 2006: 2).

There is, however, a paucity of evaluative studies that have sought to identify whether the involvement of users has any significant effects. There are even fewer studies that have specifically examined the input of palliative care users. Beresford notes 'we have little systematic knowledge about what the gains and achievements of participation may actually be' (Beresford 2005: 6). This is partly due to lack of consensus about outcome measures, and partly due to the fact that user involvement has become accepted as intrinsically beneficial and/or politically desirable. In such instances, it needs to be documented that involvement has occurred in some form, rather than to demonstrate that it has had any effect.

The evaluations that have been conducted have occurred chiefly within cancer, but some important generic issues have been identified. Many of the service development evaluations reported that the involvement of users had limited impact, professionals were often reluctant to fully engage with users and there was inadequate resourcing. Evaluations of user involvement in cancer research have tended to be more positive, although little empirical evidence has been presented, and there remain no agreed outcome methodologies or measures for assessing the influence of users.

Within the field of service delivery, Tritter and Daykin (2003) conducted a review of user involvement within one of the 34 cancer networks in England. The authors noted that users had been involved in the accreditation of palliative care services, developed a questionnaire in conjunction with a local hospice and other palliative care teams designed to explore carers' perceptions of palliative care services, and had been involved in teaching palliative care to medical students. The user input into the medical education programme was rated very highly by the palliative care professionals involved.

Members of the Palliative Care Multi-Disciplinary Team were themselves interviewed. Some said they felt that the user involvement agenda was 'politically motivated', and that it was very difficult to recruit palliative care users because they are 'mainly elderly, mainly frail, mainly pretty poorly'. There was uncertainty as to the value of involving users, while those who had been recruited were felt to be unrepresentative because they were 'self-selected'. Users who had received training were treated with some degree of caution as they may have become 'professionalized' (Tritter and Daykin 2003: 23). Gold *et al.* (2005) reported on the outcomes of patient participation in the planning of three regional supportive care networks in Ontario, Canada. These attempts to involve patients were considered to be 'failures'. The causes were a lack of clear policy direction to develop patient participation, under-resourcing and difficulties in defining the role and responsibilities of patient participants. Sitzia *et al.* (2006) published an evaluation of the UK Cancer Partnership Project, which set up collaborative service improvement groups in each of the 34 cancer networks in England. They concluded that substantial changes in NHS systems and culture were required in order for the potential envisioned to be realized. Carlsson *et al.* (2006) reviewed seven associations for cancer patients collaborating with health care professionals over a three-year period with the aim of improving cancer care in Sweden. Although patient members reported an increase in knowledge, they also reported decreased feelings about possibilities to influence health care.

Within the field of research, the results of a questionnaire study indicated that 23 out of 62 clinical trial coordinating centres (who were conducting trials in a range of diseases) were involving users in their work. The authors concluded, possibly somewhat prematurely, that 'involvement seems likely to improve the relevance to consumers of the questions addressed and the results obtained in controlled trials' (Hanley *et al.* 2001: 519). The role of the 'lay reviewer' in the peer review process has also been examined. One study examining the process at the National Cancer Institute of Canada found that scientific members thought involvement was time-consuming, irrelevant and unhelpful (Monahan and Stewart 2003). 'Lay members', however, felt they brought a 'different perspective' to the meetings. Lay members felt it was more desirable for 'advocates' (that is, those active within a particular organization) to be involved rather than cancer patients or 'survivors'. Scientific members held the opposite view.

In the USA, there have been concerted efforts to integrate 'patient advocates' (the preferred descriptor) into many research committees and federal agencies. Within the National Cancer Institute, patient advocates have had particular influence in shaping research activity, particularly through the Director's Consumer Liaison Group and the Consumer Advocates in Research and Related Activities. A study carried out on the use of 'consumer reviewers' in the breast cancer research programmes found that although many scientists had originally thought that consumer reviewers would have a political agenda and be less predisposed to funding basic science studies, they subsequently changed their views (Andejeski *et al.* 2002a). However, the authors also reported that consumer involvement affected the overall score in only about a quarter of applications (Andejeski *et al.* 2002b). Collyar (2005), in a summary of the diverse initiatives that cancer patient advocates have participated in within the USA, concluded that 'advocate interactions have led to renewed scientific energy to find better ways to diagnose, treat and, eventually, prevent cancers' (page 77).

Some of those involved in cancer research have written about their experience of involvement. Professor David Cunningham, Chair of the UK National Cancer Research Institute Upper Gastrointestinal Cancer Clinical Studies Group has noted that:

> The integration of consumer perspective with expert opinion aids study selection and design, and therefore potential patient recruitment, which is vital if the study is to be answered accurately. Clinical endpoints help to define the importance of a study but without appropriate quality of life assessments they become meaningless. The development of patient centred outcomes is paramount and only possible with consumer input and advice.
>
> (Stevens and Wilde 2005: 103)

Not all users have reported wholly positive feelings regarding their involvement. Dawn Wragg, a breast cancer patient involved in a regional research panel in a UK cancer network has stated that 'I feel my involvement has given me the opportunity to do something positive with my experiences, hopefully helping others and influencing change in a very small way'. However, she added that 'consumers can be overwhelmed by unrealistic expectations, with no allowances made for their fatigue, or the amount of time they can actually give' (Stevens and Wilde 2005: 105). Users have also said they are uneasy at taking part in discussions where their own health provider is present, for fear that any reported criticisms may adversely affect their own care (Gott *et al.* 2002).

## Constraints on user involvement

The involvement of palliative care users can be highly challenging, necessitating a range of approaches in regard to differing conceptualizations of disease and illness, the relationship between personal experience and scientific objectivity, and ultimately about how to facilitate effective communication between powerful elites and individual representatives who may be near the end of their life. The practical issues of user involvement have been well documented in the literature (Earl-Slater 2004: 43–53). However, there are some particular challenges that need to be emphasized.

### Representativeness

The two key issues in relation to representativeness are generalizability (to what extent the views of users that are involved reflect those of all users) and constituency (whether users are regarded as individuals or representatives of, and therefore accountable to, an interest or pressure group). These issues often are poorly addressed at an organizational level, which can create confusion for both users and the organizations that have invited their participation (Sitzia *et al.* 2006).

Recruiting palliative care users can be difficult. Attempting to ensure that users are 'representative', or able to provide a range of perspectives, is even more of a challenge. 'Users' are not a homogeneous group – the views, experiences and priorities of patients may be very different from those who are care-givers or those who act as advocates (for example, in terms of priorities, language and potential solutions). There may also be differences between people from different socio-economic backgrounds and those with different diseases. Perspectives may change over time, or in relation to the information people have access to. The perspective of a single 'user' can never be held to be representative of a group or population, in the same way as the views of one doctor cannot be held to be representative of all clinicians. Concerns have also been voiced that those consumers who do become involved are a minority and their views are thereby held to be either unrepresentative, overly and overtly negative, or motivated by personal or political objectives (see Gott *et al.* 2000). Professionals have on occasion argued that users may make biased and erroneous generalizations from their own highly variable experiences, in a process that is the antithesis to knowledge generation in the medical and scientific community (Canter 2001). Users may feel inhibited in contributing to any debate if they feel their own perspective is the valuable thing they can provide, but is regarded as devoid of merit from the professionals' point of view. Many users, however, would argue that their strength *is* their own perspective, and their role is not to comment on the science underpinning a research proposal, or examine intricate details regarding project management or accounting (Taylor 2002).

Most professionals tend to recruit representatives from existing user groups, but only a small minority of palliative care users will ever join such groups (Stevens *et al.* 2003). Furthermore, palliative care services are not accessed equally, further complicating the question of representation. Older patients, those from black and minority ethnic communities and the poor are less likely to use palliative care services (Koffman *et al.* 2007). The reasons are complex and include lack of awareness, gatekeeping by services and, within some communities, a preference to care for patients within the extended family network (Dent 2007). Organizations may be dissuaded from involving users from these communities by basic logistical challenges. For example, it has been estimated that there are 300 languages spoken in London, and the potential costs of providing interpreting and translating services for members of these communities may be considerable (Dent 2007). In addition, the majority of attention to date has been upon developing user involvement in palliative care among those patients who have malignant disease. This is, in part, a reflection of the current patterns of delivery of palliative care services. In the UK, for example, 95 per cent of access to hospice and specialist palliative care is by people with a diagnosis of cancer, while it is estimated that annually about 300,000 people with life-threatening non-malignant conditions would benefit from palliative care but do not, or cannot, access it (National Council for Palliative Care 2005).

### The 'professional' consumer

Within any one disease type and, particularly among those who are near the end of their life, the number of people who wish to become involved in service development or research activities is going to be small. Over a relatively short period, this may result in the development of 'career' users, typically those who are most easily accessible to professionals, and who may have a tendency to become involved at the expense of others (see Gott *et al.* 2002). This process, however, may be beneficial to users in general because as a group of quasi-professional users evolves and develops skills to collect, coordinate and interpret individual experiences, they may become able to establish a more powerful relationship with the professionals they are liaising with. Users themselves have presented powerful arguments that this is indeed the case, arguing as individual users become more 'expert', the value of their contributions is enhanced (Taylor 2002; Thornton *et al.* 2006). Nevertheless, there is a possibility that users' views may become skewed, as they gradually tend to adopt the views of professionals, and their perspectives begin to diverge from those of the patient population who they are considered to represent, or be representative of. This issue is related to that of representativeness, and offers a reminder that a range of user perspectives should, in general, be sought.

### The burden of illness

Involving people with life-limiting illnesses is inherently challenging, with a range of 'practical, emotional and conceptual barriers' (Bradburn and Maher 2005). Patients and carers have the additional burden of coping with their own daily needs, which may inhibit their opportunities to participate. The disease trajectory for some may be short and not all users will have the inclination, time or capacity to engage with professionals. It is highly unlikely that participants in palliative care initiatives will benefit personally and may die before they see any changes come about at all. Indeed, their preferences for involvement, and physical and mental capacities to be involved, may change as their disease progresses. Some users may find it difficult to come to terms with their own prognosis, and not want to meet others who are in a more advanced stage of disease. It should not thereby be assumed that those who are receiving palliative care either do or do not want to be involved, or are deemed automatically capable or not capable, of such involvement. Some patients will die from their disease and where several users are involved, provision needs to be made for the unsettling effect this may have on other members of the group. On the other hand, participants may find support in being able to share their experience with others.

Participants must not feel they are working alone and have access to support mechanisms from health care professionals.

It is inevitable that on some occasions users may feel unwell and be unable to attend meetings, which contributes to their lack of formal contact. The current pattern of involvement for users tends to be discontinuous (for example, they may be asked to attend quarterly meetings). Three months between meetings may be an unrealistic option for some people who are near the end of their life. Professionals, on the other hand, tend to be seeing colleagues regularly and discussing issues, perhaps on a daily basis. Unless clearly and frequently informed and updated, users will suffer from a major disadvantage in trying to engage in dialogue with professionals. The dominant pattern of involvement has been asking users to attend face-to-face meetings, with often long periods of travel involved. For many palliative care users, particularly the most sick and the most vulnerable, this may be impossible. However, developments in information and communication technology are making virtual interactions much more feasible and mean that a physical presence at meetings is not always required (Street 2003).

Another important consideration concerns the timing of involvement, particularly in regard to involvement in research. It has been argued that users should be involved in the developmental stages of research protocols because at this point, they can exert more influence, for example in the establishment of study endpoints (Goodare and Smith 1995). However, research protocols can often take a substantial time to develop, they may involve technical discussions that users can have relatively little input into and many studies do not actually progress to receive funding. In addition, at the protocol development stage, there are usually no grant funds available to cover the costs of involvement. Judgements therefore need to be made as to the most effective use of users' time and users themselves need to be part of any such discussion.

How users feel about the nature and extent of involvement has received scant attention in the literature. It is important to take into account the emancipatory feelings that users may gain from the experience of taking part, particularly where they are able to exercise control over their influence, for example in user-initiated or user-controlled research (Beresford 2002; Wright *et al.* 2006). Care must be exercised in ensuring the processes of involvement do not become exploitative, in the sense that users feel an obligation to participate, or that professionals make excessive demands on vulnerable people (Payne 2002; Beresford 2005).

### The increasing complexity of involvement

Despite the powerful pressures to foster user involvement, some authors have argued that involvement remains tokenistic, focused on relatively insignificant 'process' issues and that users still have little real power (Lowes and Hulatt 2005). Some studies of user involvement have also shown that users were confused about the nature of their participation and unfamiliar with the procedures associated with committee working (Sitzia *et al.* 2006).

Yvonne Andejeski, program director of the US National Cancer Institute's liaison activities, has said that 'over and over again, we heard there was confusion about roles' (McNeil 2001: 257). It has also been argued that users may not have the necessary scientific, medical, financial, managerial or organizational knowledge to fully engage with professionals (see Boote *et al.* 2002).

Such views may be partly related to shifts in the ways that users are being asked to participate. First, the tasks that users are being asked to undertake are becoming increasingly complex. Second, the decision-making environment is changing and a much wider range of competing considerations need to be reviewed. Third, the role of users is altering – users are less likely to be engaged in making the case for involvement, but rather they need to be developing the skills to 'dialogue effectively' (McNeil 2001).

Users themselves have said that they want a better understanding of the technical and organizational issues. A veteran advocate of the US Food and Drug Administration drug advisory committee, Sandra Zook-Fischler, has stated that 'a good grasp on the language and literature of science is important' (McNeil 2001: 259). Susan Weiner, vice chair of advocacy for the North American Brain Tumour Coalition, has gone further, and suggested that 'putting a non-scientist into a complex bureaucracy with no sense of role or task or expectations is a recipe for disaster' (McNeil 2001: 259). The response from professionals has been to offer training and orientation programmes with the aim of enabling users to operate more effectively. High quality, and sometimes lengthy, programmes for users have been initiated in many countries. Project LEAD, for example, is a four-day course for users in the USA, developed by the National Breast Cancer Coalition. The US National Cancer Institute oversees the Patient Advocate Research Team training program that helps prepare patient advocates for their work in the many Specialized Programs of Research Excellence (McNeil 2001). In the UK, and also in Australia, Cancer Voices have produced an integrated package of resources that addresses training needs, personal support and good practice guidance (Macmillan Cancer Support 2007). User representatives participating in the UK National Cancer Research Institute and National Cancer Research Network activities have access to an induction programme and ongoing training that includes an overview of the cancer research community, research methodologies, and advice on maximizing effective input at meetings. Consumers also have access to a scientific mentor and are encouraged to attend national and international conferences (Stevens and Wilde 2005).

However, these current models of training and support may not necessarily be appropriate for many palliative care users, for whom time is short, and for whom attendance at a four-day training course may simply not be feasible. The implication is that those users who do not, or cannot, develop these higher level skills that are being demanded by professionals, will tend to remain in a less powerful position, with their views and experiences less likely to be of influence. An additional challenge is that the total number of users involved in palliative care initiatives is relatively small, and likely to be geographically spread. There is therefore only limited scope to take advantage of any economies of scale that may result from, for example, the organization of regional training events or conferences. However, as noted above, the opportunities that may arise from the application of information and communication technologies (such as online training and video conferencing) are likely to be significant in the future, particularly so within palliative care (Street 2003). The most sick and the most vulnerable may find the existing processes of participation to be a significant challenge, but the liberating potential of information and communications technologies should not be under-estimated. It is also essential that consumers have access to the same data (although the format may require some modification), as health care professionals, in order that they can make effective contributions. Providing users with electronic access to documentation and results of research are important tasks.

## Examples of good practice

Despite the constraints and challenges, examples of how palliative care users have been successfully involved in palliative care research and service development, nationally and internationally are given below.

---

**Case Study 3.1**    Local involvement in palliative care service development

User feedback systems, primarily through the use of questionnaires to bereaved relatives, was established at St Christopher's Hospice in London in 1998. A user's forum for patients and carers, meeting every four months, has also been convened (Kraus *et al.* 2003). Issues that the group has considered include signposting in the hospice, information provision for carers, food and transport. The authors of this report concluded that 'the holistic model of palliative care is enhanced by this other dimension into service planning, development and audit/clinical governance'. However, they also noted that 'professionals remain clearly in a powerful position and are able to control and manipulate the outcome of the user involvement activity' (page 377). Although the forum meets relatively infrequently and there are inherent limitations in the range of topics that can be addressed, this is nevertheless a significant development.

---

**Case Study 3.2**    National involvement in palliative care service development

The UK National Council for Palliative Care (NCPC) has an overall principle that patient and public involvement should be 'embedded' throughout all its activities. The opportunities for involvement have recently been expanded with the formation of a Service User Reference Forum, intended to provide a pool of expert users that can be involved in all activities of the Council, and a User Involvement Advisory Group, which will work more strategically. There are also opportunities to join the Policy Groups, Ethics Committee and the Board of Trustees. The NCPC has stated that: 'Palliative care service user experiences will be included in the list of expertise to be sought within the membership of all NCPC's standing groups' (National Council for Palliative Care 2007: 1). These are new developments and, as yet, there is no evidence as to their effectiveness.

---

**Case Study 3.3**   International involvement in palliative care research

Users are involved in the preparation of systematic reviews of the literature through the Cochrane Consumer Network. Health care providers, researchers and users work collaboratively to produce the reviews in order to develop evidence to guide well-informed decisions about health care. One of the Cochrane Collaborative Systematic Review Groups is the Pain, Palliative Care and Supportive Care Group (PaPaS). Currently, there are 70 completed reviews in the PaPaS database, with many focused upon non-malignant disease. The Group is committed to involvement at every level and users are encouraged to become involved. The remit of PaPaS is to address palliative and supportive care issues in the broadest sense, arguing that 'palliative and supportive care is not just for cancer, but extends to all chronic diseases, and affects not only patients but carers and professionals. Often it will be not just what we do but how we do it, so we would love to hear from groups which have found that through better organisation they can deliver a better quality of care' (Cochrane Pain, Palliative Care and Supportive Care Group 2007: 1). The work of PaPaS is of particular importance, as it has a commitment to search for a wide range of evidence for its reviews, including results from randomized trials as well as other study designs. In addition, users can work from their own homes at their own pace, with excellent training and support available from the Cochrane Collaborative Group.

---

# Conclusion

The opportunities for users to be involved in palliative care, particularly within cancer, have increased in large measure, especially over the past five years. This is true particularly in the UK, as well as in North America, Europe and Australia. Opportunities for involvement by those with non-malignant disease remain less well developed. The evidence base for all types of involvement remains low.

The roles that people are being asked to perform, and the settings in which these activities are conducted, are becoming more complex. The practical difficulties and competing considerations that govern the development of research strategies and the configuration of service delivery issues may seem overwhelming to users. Professionals must take care to support, and not to ask too much from those who have volunteered to help. The central philosophy of palliative care is based upon listening, responding and acting quickly at a time when the extent of life is limited. The principles of user involvement in palliative care should also be based upon similar foundations. Users can bring a perspective unavailable from any other sources and it is essential that their views should be incorporated into decision-making. The processes of change can be slow and users may die before the results of their engagement change practice. It is essential therefore that a sense of mutual engagement between professionals and users should be nurtured. The challenges are great and the price, to all parties, of user involvement can be high. However, the costs of not involving users, and in losing those unique insights, are likely to be considerably greater.

# References

Andejeski, Y., Bisceglio, I.T., Dickersin, K., Johnson, J.E., Robinson, S.I., Smith, H.S., Visco, F.M. and Rich, I.M. (2002a) Quantitative impact of including consumers in the scientific review of breast cancer research proposals. *Journal of Women's Health and Gender-Based Medicine*, 11(2): 379–88.

Andejeski, Y., Breslau, E.S., Hart, E., Lythcott, N., Alexander, L., Rich, I., Bisceglio, I., Smith, H.S. and Visco, F.M. (2002b) Benefits and drawbacks of including consumer reviewers in the scientific merit of breast cancer research. *Journal of Women's Health and Gender-Based Medicine*, 11(2): 119–36.

Arnstein, S. (1969) A ladder of citizen participation. *Journal of the American Institute of Planners*, 35(4): 216–24.

Bastian, H. (1998) The evolution of consumer advocacy in health care. *International Journal of Health Technology in Health Care*, 14(1): 3–23.

Beresford, P. (2002) User involvement in research and evaluation: liberation or regulation? *Social Policy and Society*, 1(2): 95–105.

Beresford, P. (2005) Theory and practice of user involvement, in L. Lowes and I. Hulatt (eds) *Involving service users in health and social care research*. Abingdon: Routledge.

Boote, J., Telford, R. and Cooper, C. (2002) Consumer involvement: a research and review agenda. *Health Policy*, 61(2): 213–36.

Bradburn, J. and Maher, J. (2005) User and carer participation in research in palliative care. *Palliative Medicine*, 19(2): 91–2.

Canter, R. (2001) Patients and medical power. *British Medical Journal*, 323(7310): 414.

Carlsson, C., Nilbert, M. and Nilsson, K. (2006) Patients' involvement in improving cancer care; experiences in three years of collaboration between members of patients associations and health care professionals. *Patient Education and Counseling*, 61(1): 65–71.

Clayton, S. (1988) Patient participation: an underdeveloped concept. *Journal of the Royal Society of Health*, 108(2): 55–6.

Clinical Trials Awards and Advisory Committee (2006) *Final Terms of Reference.* London: Cancer Research UK.

Cochrane Pain, Palliative Care and Supportive Care Group (2007) *Palliative and supportive care.* www.jr2.ox.ac.uk/bandolier/booth/booths/pall (accessed June 2007).

Collyar, D. (2005) How have patient advocates in the United States benefited cancer research? *Nature Reviews Cancer*, 5(1): 73–8.

Cotterell, P., Clarke, P., Cowdrey, D., Kapp, J., Paine, M. and Wynn, R. (2005) *Influencing palliative care project.* Worthing: Worthing and Southlands Hospital Trust.

Dent, E. (2007) Tales of the city. *Health Service Journal*, 117(6053): 24–6.

Department of Health (2004) *Patient and public involvement – a brief overview.* London: The Stationery Office.

Earl-Slater, A. (2004) *Lay involvement in health and other research.* Oxford: Radcliffe Medical Press.

Entwistle, V.A., Renfrew, M.J., Yearley, S., Forester, J. and Lamont, T. (1998) Lay perspectives: advantages for health research. *British Medical Journal*, 316(7129): 463–6.

Gold, S., Abelson, J. and Charles, C. (2005) From rhetoric to reality: including patient voices in supportive care planning. *Health Expectations*, 8(3): 195–209.

Goodare, H. and Smith, R. (1995) The rights of patients in research. *British Medical Journal*, 310(6990): 1277–8.

Gott, M., Stevens, T., Small, N. and Ahmedzai, S.H. (2000) *User Involvement in Cancer Care: Exclusion and Empowerment.* Bristol: Policy Press.

Gott, M., Stevens, T. and Small, N. (2002) Involving users, improving services: the example of cancer. *British Journal of Clinical Governance*, 7(2): 81–5.

Hanley, B., Truesdale, A., King, A., Elbourne, D. and Chalmers, I. (2001) Involving consumers in designing, conducting and interpreting randomized controlled trials: questionnaire survey. *British Medical Journal*, 322(7285): 519–23.

Hogg, C. and Williamson, C. (2001) Whose interests do lay people represent? Towards an understanding of the role of lay people as members of committees. *Health Expectations*, 4(1): 2–9.

INVOLVE (2003) *Involving the public in NHS, public health, and social care research: Briefing notes for researchers.* Eastleigh: INVOLVE.

Koffman, J., Burke, G., Dias, A., Raval, B., Byrne, J. and Daniels, C. (2007) Demographic factors and awareness of palliative care and related services. *Palliative Medicine*, 21(2): 145–53.

Kraus, F., Levy, J. and Oliviere, D. (2003) Brief report on user involvement at St Christopher's Hospice. *Palliative Medicine*, 17(4): 375–7.

Litva, A., Coast, J., Donovan, J., Eyles, J., Shepherd, J., Tacchi, J., Abelson, J. and Morgan, K. (2002) 'The public is too subjective': public involvement at different levels of health care decision-making. *Social Science and Medicine*, 54(12): 1825–37.

Lowes, L. and Hulatt, I. (2005) *Involving service users in health and social care research.* Abingdon: Routledge.

McNeil, C. (2001) Cancer advocacy evolves as it gains seats on research panels. *Journal of the National Cancer Institute*, 93(4): 257–9.

Macmillan Cancer Support (2007) *Training.* www.macmillan.org.uk/Get_Involved/cancerVoices/Resources/Training.aspx (accessed June 2007).

Monahan, A. and Stewart, D.E. (2003) The role of lay panellists on grant review panels. *Chronic diseases in Canada*, 24(2/3). www.phac-aspc.gc.ca/publicat/cdic-mcc/24-2/d_e.html (accessed June 2007).

National Cancer Research Institute (2006) *Consumer Liaison Clinical Studies Group 2005–6 Annual Report*. London: National Cancer Research Institute.

National Council for Palliative Care (2005) *Palliative care manifesto*. London: National Council for Palliative Care.

National Council for Palliative Care (2007) *User involvement in National Council*. www.ncpc.org.uk/policy_unit/user_involvement (accessed June 2007).

Ong, B.N. (1996) The lay perspective in health technology assessment. *International Journal of Technology Assessment in Health Care*, 12(3): 511–17.

Payne, S. (2002) Are we using the users? (editorial) *International Journal of Palliative Nursing*, 8(5): 212.

Seymour, J., Bellamy, G., Gott, M., Clark, D. and Ahmedzai, S.H. (2002) Using focus groups to explore older people's attitudes to end of life care. *Ageing and Society*, 22(4): 415–26.

Sitzia, J., Cotterell, P. and Richardson, A. (2006) Interprofessional collaboration with service users in the development of cancer services: the Cancer Partnership Project. *Journal of Interprofessional Care*, 20(1): 60–74.

Stevens, T., Wilde, D., Hunt, J. and Ahmedzai, S. (2003) Overcoming the challenges to consumer involvement in cancer research. *Health Expectations*, 6(1): 81–8.

Stevens, T. and Wilde, D. (2005) Consumer involvement in cancer research in the United Kingdom. In: L. Lowes and I. Hulatt (eds) *Involving service users in health and social cares research*. London: Routledge, pp. 97–111.

Street, Jr R.L. (2003) Mediated consumer-provider communication in cancer care: the empowering potential of new technologies. *Patient Education and Counselling*, 50(1): 99–104.

Taylor, K. (2002) Researching the experiences of kidney cancer patients. *European Journal of Cancer Care*, 11(3): 200–4.

Telford, R., Beverley, C.A., Cooper, C. and Boote, J.D. (2002) Consumer involvement in health research: fact or fiction? *British Journal of Clinical Governance*, 7(2): 92–103.

Thornton, H., Baum, M. and Clarke, M. (2006) Involvement of the consumer voice. *Health Expectations*, 9(1): 92–3.

Tritter, J. and Daykin, N. (2003) *Developing and evaluating best practice in user involvement in cancer services*. Bristol: Avon, Somerset and Wiltshire Cancer Services.

United Kingdom Clinical Research Network (2006) *Getting involved in clinical research*. London: United Kingdom Clinical Research Network.

World Health Organization (1978) *Declaration of Alma Ata: Report of the International Conference on Primary Health Care*. Geneva: World Health Organization.

World Health Organization (2004) *Better palliative care for older people*. Copenhagen: World Health Organization.

Wright, D., Corner, J., Hopkinson, J. and Foster, C. (2006) Listening to the views of people affected by cancer about cancer research: an example of participatory research in setting the cancer research agenda, *Health Expectations*, 9(1): 3–12.

# 4

# Referral patterns and access to specialist palliative care

*Julia Addington-Hall*

---

**Key points**

- Specialist palliative care availability varies between and across countries depending on the health care system, health care funding and both political and public support for these services.
- Access to the available services is determined by eligibility criteria, both explicit and implicit, which are themselves determined by beliefs about the purpose and benefits of palliative care.
- Palliative care in most, but not all, settings is focused on the care of terminally ill cancer patients. Patients dying from HIV/AIDS or from motor neurone disease often also access this care.
- In the UK, there has been a shift in the rhetoric of palliative care away from a focus on cancer and towards access being determined by need, not diagnosis.
- There is increasing evidence that people who die from other chronic and progressive conditions have physical, psychological, social and spiritual problems in the last weeks or months of life. It is not yet known whether specialist palliative care can address these problems successfully.
- Until there is evidence that specialist palliative care has benefits beyond cancer patients, then patients cannot be said conclusively to have specialist palliative care needs. Making access depend on need rather than diagnosis will not, therefore, necessarily change the characteristics of those receiving care.
- Barriers to extending specialist palliative care beyond cancer include a lack of funding, difficulties identifying suitable candidates because of prognostic uncertainty, a lack of skills in conditions other than cancer among specialist palliative care health professionals, and a lack of evidence that patients with other conditions would find referral to these services acceptable.
- Older people with cancer access specialist palliative care services less often than younger people with similar problems. This age differential may be justified: there is some limited evidence that older people need less

help to face death and that they may have fewer symptom control problems. Older people need to have their palliative care needs assessed
individually and not predetermined from their age or diagnosis.
- Cancer in older people often co-exists with other chronic and progressive
conditions. The lack of familiarity of many specialist palliative care services
with these conditions may explain in part the under-representation of older
cancer patients in these services.
- Differences between countries in the characteristics of patients receiving
palliative care demonstrate that specialist palliative care services need not
be focused on cancer or primarily serve younger patients.
- There will continue to be local and national variations in access to specialist palliative care, and there also needs to be continued reflection and
debate about whether these variations are justified or are a consequence
of stereotypical views of levels of palliative care need among different
demographic and diagnostic groups.

This chapter presents evidence on the availability of specialist palliative care
services and on who accesses them, drawing primarily, but not exclusively,
on data from the UK. The appropriateness or otherwise of these services
focusing primarily on cancer patients is discussed, as is the question of
whether older people are disadvantaged in terms of access to these services.
Variations in access to specialist palliative care by social class and ethnic
group are not considered here as they are discussed elsewhere in this book.

# Availability of specialist palliative care

Access to health services is determined both by availability and eligibility.
The availability of specialist palliative care services in the UK has increased
considerably over the past 20 years. In 1990, there were 124 inpatient units,
277 community palliative care teams and more than 40 hospital palliative
care teams (St Christopher's Information Service 1990). By 2005, this had
risen to 220, 358 and 361, respectively.[1] New forms of specialist palliative
care service have also developed, for example hospice day care, of which
there were 263 in 2005, and hospice at home services providing 24-hour
nursing care for limited periods, of which there were 104.

Much of the development of these services has taken place outside of
the National Health Service (NHS), although the NHS is playing an increasing role in the provision of these services, particularly of community and
hospital palliative care services. However, although there are 64 inpatient
units funded and managed by the NHS, most hospices are independent and
receive on average 32 per cent of their funding from the NHS, the rest
coming from local fund-raising and charitable contributions. These services
have been initiated by local enthusiasts in response to local perceived need,
rather than resulting from local or national health care planning. This has
given them the freedom to expand and to develop new initiatives without

having to compete with all other forms of health care for limited NHS funding. The reliance on non-NHS funding sources can threaten the financial viability of services, however, particularly in a time of reduced charitable giving and economic recession. Independent hospices in the UK are therefore campaigning for a larger contribution to their running costs from the NHS. Their success in achieving this, together with the state of the national economy, will impact on the availability of palliative care services, particularly inpatient care, across the UK.

Two national charities have played a significant role in increasing specialist palliative care in the UK: Macmillan Cancer Relief, which has provided initial funding and continued educational support for many palliative care nursing, medical and social work posts, has contributed to the costs of buildings and funded innovative services; and Marie Curie Cancer Care, which funds ten specialist palliative care inpatient units as well as providing night-sitting services. Lunt and Hillier observed in 1981 that the development of services by local groups in response to local need had led to considerable regional variations in services, with most being in the relatively affluent south. Macmillan Cancer Relief played an important role in funding services in less affluent areas and in reducing inequalities in service provision (Lunt 1985).

Despite this, and the increasing role played in the 1990s by local health authorities in assessing need for palliative care and developing local strategies (Clark *et al.* 1995), inequalities in the availability of specialist palliative care persist. In 1999, the Department of Health commissioned two surveys to provide a picture of the current level of provision for palliative care and health authority views about the need for such services (National Council of Hospice and Specialist Palliative Care Services 2000). The results identified widely differing volumes of service between regions, and even greater discrepancies at health authority level. The conclusion was that the differing levels of provision were unlikely to reflect differing levels of need. The government has used the New Opportunities Fund, money generated by the National Lottery, to fund new initiatives in palliative care aimed at reducing inequalities in provision. Given the major role played by local charities in both funding and running specialist palliative care services in the UK, unequal access to this care across the UK is likely to continue. Therefore, access to palliative care is not only determined by the characteristics of the individual and the 'match' between these and eligibility criteria for palliative care (discussed below), but also by local availability of these services.

This highlights how access to specialist palliative care cannot be fully explained by the criteria for eligibility developed by services themselves. Instead, the organization and funding of health care systems and the relationship of palliative care to these play a major role. Theoretically, access to this care in the UK might have been expected to be better if it had developed within the NHS via centralized planning, although the current debate about the 'postcode lottery' of health care in the UK and the development of national bodies such as the National Institute for Clinical Excellence aimed explicitly at reducing inequalities suggest that this would not have eliminated all local variations in care provision.

The influence of funding mechanisms on the availability of palliative care is illustrated by the example of the USA, where the Medicare hospice benefit was approved by the Health Care Financial Administration in 1983. This was designed specifically to increase access to hospice programmes and has enabled hospice programmes to grow on the basis of a predictable income flow. About 60 per cent of hospice patients are covered by the benefit (Field and Cassel 1997). Patients certified as having a life expectancy of six months or less and who waiver the right to standard Medicare benefits for curative treatments are eligible for the benefit, which provides a *per diem* payment. This covers short, inpatient stays (provided these do not exceed 20 per cent of the total hospice care days for the hospice) and a variety of medical and non-medical services at home. The benefit has influenced not only the speed of growth of hospice programmes but also their character-istics: services are expected to use volunteers and to limit inpatient care, while patients have to have a predictable prognosis and usually to have informal carers to share in the care. The characteristics of patients receiving hospice care in the USA differ in a number of ways from those of hospice patients in the UK: they are much more likely to have a diagnosis other than cancer, to be closer to death, to be at home rather than be an inpatient and to be in a nursing home. The benefit's availability has encouraged an entre-preneurial approach to the provision of hospices, with expansion into new markets (such as nursing homes and non-cancer patients) and the develop-ment of for-profit hospice chains. Initial enthusiasm for this benefit has changed in some quarters to opposition to the ways it constrains and shapes hospice provision.

As these examples illustrate, the availability of specialist palliative care services is largely determined by the health care system of the country in question and the level of health care funding. A third element is the political will to support these services. Palliative care has to compete with many other deserving recipients of the 'health pound', and its success or otherwise in gaining political support is an important determinant of the funding it receives and therefore of service availability. In many countries, including the UK and the USA, innovative services have been initiated by local sup-porters, but achieving acceptance within the health care system and political support are important if existing services are to be sustained and new ser-vices are to be developed. Italy and Canada are both examples of successful sustained attempts to gain political support and the impact of doing so on service provision, although, as with the Medicare benefit in the USA, the initial champions and initiators of palliative care do not always like the consequences of gaining political support and becoming more 'mainstream' within national health care provision (Toscani 2002).

The availability of specialist palliative care thus varies between and across countries depending on the health care system, health care funding and both political and public support for these services. Access to the avail-able services is determined by eligibility criteria, both explicit and implicit, which are themselves determined by beliefs about the purpose and benefits of palliative care. These are considered in the remainder of this chapter.

### Access to specialist palliative care

Most people who receive care from hospice and specialist palliative care services have a diagnosis of cancer: in 2004–2005, 95 per cent of patients receiving inpatient care or home care from a hospice had cancer, as did 89 per cent of patients receiving support from hospital palliative care teams (National Council for Palliative Care 2006). In the UK at least, specialist palliative care is largely synonymous with cancer care, in particular terminal cancer care.

This is not surprising given that a strong desire to improve care for dying cancer patients provided much of the motivation for founding St Christopher's Hospice, usually regarded as the first modern hospice, and accounts for the rapid uptake of the ideas developed by its founder, Dame Cicely Saunders. The number of people who died from cancer increased rapidly in the twentieth century as better public health and the development of effective treatments such as antibiotics led to a decline in the number of deaths from infectious diseases. The same period saw the development of modern, scientific medicine with its emphasis on cure rather than care, and the concomitant growth in hospital provision and utilization. Glaser and Strauss, in their seminal work in the 1960s (Glaser and Strauss 1965, 1968), observed how dying cancer patients were often ignored, particularly by medical staff and kept in the dark about their prognosis and isolated in hospitals. Dame Cicely's own observation of the neglect and poor symptom control experienced by these patients in hospitals while a medical almoner or social worker had earlier led her to undertake medical training to find ways to improve their care. The picture of poor communication with health professionals, of inadequate support and of distressing, uncontrolled symptoms was reinforced by the results of surveys of patients nursed at home (Marie Curie Memorial Foundation 1952), cared for in terminal care homes (Hughes 1960) and dying in hospital (Hinton 1963). Dying from cancer in the 1950s and 1960s could often be an appalling experience for patients and their families (as, of course, it can still be today in the absence of effective palliative care). The groundswell of public and professional support which made possible the opening of St Christopher's Hospice in 1967, and which fuelled the rapid spread of the hospice movement, is evidence of widespread dissatisfaction with the care these patients received.

The growth of hospice and specialist palliative care has led to improvements in the care that can be offered to terminally ill cancer patients and their families. Cancer pain can now be controlled in the majority of patients, and effective therapies are available – or are being developed – for other distressing symptoms (Doyle *et al.* 1998). Dame Cicely's concept of 'total pain' embraces psychological, social and spiritual as well as physical distress (Clark 1999), and expertise has also been developed in addressing these aspects of the patient's experience. Dame Cicely Saunders has argued that much less progress would have been made if hospices from the beginning had been open to all dying patients, regardless of diagnosis (personal communication). The initial focus of hospice services on terminal cancer care can therefore be explained by the overwhelming needs of these patients, and by a desire to focus on one group to make rapid progress in, for example, symptom control. Rapid progress in the understanding and treatment of pain at this time was also important.

From its inception, however, the relevance has been recognized of the principles and practice of hospice care to patients dying from other diseases. For example, Dame Cicely Saunders and Dr Mary Baines from St Christopher's Hospice wrote in 1983 that 'many of the symptoms to be treated and much of the general management will be relevant to other situations . . . Terminal care should not only be a part of oncology but of geriatric medicine, neurology, general practice and throughout medicine' (Saunders and Baines 1983: 2). The hope – and expectation – was that other medical specialties would take on the task of developing services specific to and appropriate for 'their' terminally ill patients. There is little evidence that this has happened in terms of service provision, although occasional publications have recognized the needs of dying patients (Graham and Livesley 1983; Wilkes 1984).

Some patients with conditions other than cancer have been cared for by hospice and specialist palliative care services. For example, St Christopher's Hospice initially provided care for some long-term chronically ill patients such as those with multiple sclerosis or motor neurone disease, mirroring the practice of St Joseph's Hospice where Dame Cicely had previously worked. It continues to care for motor neurone patients, as do other services.

### Challenges to the focus on cancer: AIDS/HIV

The focus of specialist palliative care services on terminal cancer care has been challenged, particularly in the past decade. The inception of the AIDS/HIV epidemic in the 1980s meant that there were growing numbers of predominately young terminally ill patients who, like cancer patients, experienced distressing physical, psychological, social and spiritual problems, compounded by the fear and stigma associated with an AIDS diagnosis. There was considerable debate as to whether these patients' needs could best be met within existing hospice and specialist palliative care services, or whether new AIDS/HIV-specific services needed to be developed. Initially, specific services were developed, in part because of the availability of ring-fenced funds for AIDS/HIV services. The characteristics of people with AIDS in the UK have, however, changed, with a growth in the proportion of sufferers who are women and who come from sub-Saharan Africa. These clients may not feel comfortable in services developed primarily for gay men and, because of the stigma attached to AIDS, may prefer to access generic services. This demographic shift, together with removal of ring-fenced funding and the decline in AIDS-related mortality due to use of the triple therapies, has led to increased use of generic hospice services and a decline in the availability of AIDS-specific services.

### NHS reforms

Changes to the organization of the NHS in the early 1990s also resulted in challenges to the focus of specialist palliative care services on cancer. District health authorities (forerunners of Primary Care Trusts) no longer managed patients directly, but instead were made responsible for assessing the need of their resident population for health care, and then purchasing (later commissioning) care from local health service providers to meet these needs. This led to interest in needs assessment, accompanied in palliative care by increasing recognition that cancer patients are not alone in needing palliative care. An expert report to the Department of Health in 1992 from the Standing Medical Advisory Committee and the Standing Nursing and Midwifery Advisory Committees on the Principles and Provision of Palliative Care (1992) recommended that 'all patients needing them should have access to palliative care services. Although often referred to as equating with terminal cancer care, it is important to recognise that similar services are appropriate and should be developed for patients dying from other diseases' (page 28). Here the emphasis is on separate services being developed for patients with conditions other than cancer, which is consistent with the approach adopted by the hospice movement since its inception. However, in 1996 an NHS Executive letter to health authorities stated that purchasers are asked to ensure that provision of care with a palliative approach is included in all contracts of service for those with cancer and other life-threatening diseases . . . although this letter is focused on services for cancer patients, it applies equally for patients with other life-threatening conditions, including AIDS, neurological conditions, and cardiac and respiratory failure.

This uses a model of palliative care that distinguishes between the palliative care approach, the responsibility of all health care providers, and specialist palliative care (NHS Executive 1996). It does not explicitly require either that separate services should be provided for patients with conditions other than cancer or that they should have increased access to existing specialist services, but it does redefine the boundaries of palliative care to include these patients. This is reflected in the epidemiologically based needs assessment for palliative care (Higginson 1997) that provided estimates of the number of people per one million population with cancer, progressive non-malignant disease and HIV/AIDS who may need palliative care. In 2000, the National Service Framework (NSF) for Cardiac Disease (Department of Health 2000a) reflected this boundary shift and, indeed, took it further by stating that patients with severe heart failure should have access to specialist palliative care services. Subsequent NSFs have also included a requirement that palliative care be made available to patients with conditions other than cancer. The NSF for Long-Term Conditions, for example, includes as one of its 11 quality requirements the requirement that people in the later stages of long-term neurological conditions receive 'a

comprehensive range of palliative care services when they need them ...'
(Department of Health 2005). The NSF for Renal Services similarly lists a
quality requirement for end-of-life care which requires those near the end of
life to have 'a jointly agreed palliative care plan' and proposes that the
expertise of palliative care terms is drawn on in developing these plans.
Political changes in the NHS, first producing the purchaser/provider split
and fuelling the development of needs assessments, and then commissioning
national service frameworks, have been influential in extending palliative
care beyond cancer. The extent of this change is evident in the most recent
policy documents from the Department of Health in the UK to refer to end-
of-life care which either emphasize the importance of improving end of care
for all regardless of diagnosis,[2] or make no mention of diagnosis at all
(Department of Health 2006).

## Palliative care needs beyond cancer

Stating that palliative care should be provided on the basis of need is not in
itself, however, sufficient to produce an increase in the numbers of patients
with conditions other than cancer accessing specialist palliative care services.
These patients may not have physical, psychological, social or spiritual needs
at the end of life, and thus may not require these services. Some evidence that
this is not the case comes from the increasing body of research into palliative
care needs beyond cancer. For example, the Regional Study of Care for the
Dying, a large population-based interview study of bereaved relatives of a
representative sample of deaths in England in 1990 (Addington-Hall and
McCarthy 1995; McCarthy *et al.* 1997a), found that people who died from
heart disease were reported to have experienced a wide range of symptoms,
which were frequently distressing and often lasted more than six months,
and which were associated with a decreased quality of life. Half were thought
to have known they were dying: most worked it out for themselves, a situation
similar to cancer in the 1960s (McCarthy *et al.* 1996, 1997b). Other papers
from the study highlighted the experiences of people who died from respiratory disease, stroke or dementia (Addington-Hall *et al.* 1995; McCarthy *et
al.* 1997a; Edmonds *et al.* 2001). At the same time, evidence was emerging
from a large US study, the SUPPORT study, of the poor quality of life,
uncontrolled symptoms and inadequate communication of people dying
from conditions such as severe heart failure, chronic obstructive pulmonary
disease (COPD) and cirrhosis of the liver (Lynn *et al.* 1997b).

Other studies have been reported more recently expanding on and refining these findings in heart failure (for example, Rogers *et al.* 2000; Boyd *et al.*
2004; Willems *et al.* 2004, 2006; Barnes *et al.* 2006; Gott *et al.* 2006); COPD
(for example, Gore *et al.* 2000; Weisbord *et al.* 2003; Elkington *et al.* 2005;
Knauft *et al.* 2005); chronic renal failure (for example, Murtagh *et al.* 2007);
and progressive neurological conditions (for example, Kristjanson *et al.*
2006; Clarke *et al.* 2005; Edmonds *et al.* 2007). Solano *et al.* (2006)

conducted a systematic review of the limited symptom prevalence data in AIDS, COPD, heart disease and renal disease and compared it to cancer. They found that pain, breathlessness and fatigue were found in more than half of patients in all five diseases, suggesting a common pathway towards death in all of these diseases and strengthening the case for the extension of palliative care beyond cancer. However, despite the growth in research many questions remain unanswered. Nevertheless, there is growing evidence that many people who die from causes other than cancer need in their last weeks and months of life better symptom control, more psychological and spiritual support, more open communication with health professionals, and more support for their families.

Establishing that some patients with conditions other than cancer have similar problems at the end of life as cancer patients is not in itself, however, sufficient to establish a *need* for specialist palliative care provision beyond cancer. According to the definition of need adopted in the influential publications on epidemiologically based needs assessment (Stevens and Raftery 1997), it is necessary to establish that someone will benefit from a health care intervention before describing them as needing that service. Evidence that non-cancer patients benefit from specialist palliative care services is sparse (Bosanquet and Salisbury 1999) and even sparser beyond HIV/AIDS and neurological conditions. Specialist palliative care services need to add to this evidence base by evaluating the impact of their care beyond cancer, and demonstration projects incorporating evaluation are needed of new innovative palliative care services for these patients. It is not self-evident that they will want or benefit from services developed primarily for cancer patients, and it is important to establish the costs and benefits of specialist palliative care outside cancer if harm to patients is to be avoided and resources are to be used efficiently.

There are a number of examples of good practice in this area, where novel services for patients with diagnosis other than cancer have been developed and subjected to evaluation. For example, the St James Place Foundation funded a programme of small grants to independent hospices in the UK to enable them to develop innovative, small services beyond cancer which have been independently evaluated (Frankland *et al.* 2007). Results from other pilot projects have been reported, for example, from a novel palliative care programme for renal patients (Weisbord *et al.* 2003), as have findings from randomized controlled trials of new service configurations for patients with diagnoses other than cancer (Aiken *et al.* 2006). On a smaller scale, individual services at the forefront of developing services beyond cancer have audited their services and reported their experiences (Daley *et al.* 2006; Johnson and Houghton 2006). The evidence for the benefits (or otherwise) of palliative care beyond cancer and, importantly, of the sorts of provision which work for which patient groups is, therefore, beginning to develop. It is, however, still inadequate and the case for palliative care benefits beyond cancer has not yet been proven.

## Use of palliative care services beyond cancer

The lack of evidence that specialist palliative care services benefit patients with conditions other than cancer may explain in part why, in the UK, the proportion of patients using these services who do not have cancer is rising slowly, if at all. This differs from the USA, where the proportion of hospice patients in 2005 who had a diagnosis other than cancer was 54 per cent, with 12 per cent having heart-related diagnoses, 10 per cent dementia, 9 per cent debility and 7 per cent lung disease.[3] Differences between the two countries illustrate the impact that funding systems have on access to palliative care, and it has been hypothesized that the number of patients with conditions other than cancer served by specialist palliative care services in the UK would rise more swiftly if additional funding were available. The Medicare hospice benefit has served this role in the USA, as discussed above, while ring-fenced funding for HIV/AIDS was important in encouraging the development of palliative care for these patients in the 1990s. Existing specialist palliative care services in the UK depend heavily on charitable fund-raising, much of it explicitly directed to the care of terminally ill cancer patients. Within the NHS, the National Cancer Plan, the development of supportive and palliative care guidance by the National Institute of Clinical Excellence (NICE 2004) and increased funding for cancer research and service provision (Department of Health 2000b) have again focused attention on cancer. Even if specialist palliative care services are shown to have benefits beyond cancer, demonstrating need will not be sufficient to increase access – the question of who will fund care for these patients will also need to be addressed.

Funding is not the only barrier to existing specialist palliative care services caring for patients with conditions other than cancer (Field and Addington-Hall 1999). An important difference between cancer and other conditions is the difficulty in judging prognosis and thus in identifying suitable candidates for palliative care. For example, the SUPPORT study used multivariate computer models based on clinical and biochemical indices to predict prognosis. On the day before death, lung cancer patients were estimated to have less than a 5 per cent chance of surviving for two months, while chronic heart failure patients had a more than 40 per cent chance (Lynn *et al.* 1997a). This causes several problems. For example, palliative care services are geared towards patients whose illness trajectory is characterized by a short period of evident decline, as in cancer. Patients with the illness trajectory of long-term limitations with intermittent serious episodes more commonly described in organ failure (Murray *et al.* 2005) do not necessarily fit well with the way palliative care services are organized. This may cause concern among these services about providing care for patients who may survive for months or years, limiting the care they can offer other patients. In addition, because of their different illness trajectory organ failure patients may never be viewed by their clinicians as 'dying' or having a limited prognosis, and they may consequently (and perhaps correctly) continue to receive intensive medical care until they die. The prognostic uncertainty associated with an organ failure trajectory is a barrier to many patients receiving palliative care until very close to death (as in the American hospice experience) or at all. Innovative models of care are needed such as, for example, providing palliative care alongside usual care (Aiken *et al.* 2006) or offering one-off consultations, short-term interventions with the possibility of re-referral if new problems develop, or 'full' palliative care depending on the complexity of the patient's problems (George and Sykes 1997).

Many nurses and doctors in palliative care have primarily trained and worked in cancer patient care and may rightly be concerned about whether they have the skills to care for other patient groups. As has happened with AIDS/HIV patient care, they will need to work in partnership with colleagues in, for example, cardiology or health care for older people. The importance of educating palliative professionals in conditions other than cancer has been demonstrated in the UK St James Place project (Frankland *et al.* 2007). Encouraging and facilitating health professionals from backgrounds other than cancer to train and work in palliative care will also be important.

A final barrier to extending specialist palliative care beyond cancer is the image of these services and their acceptability to, for example, patients with heart failure or chronic respiratory diseases. Cancer patients can be reluctant to accept referrals to hospices or other services because of their association with dying. Changes in terminology from 'hospice' to 'palliative care', in eligibility criteria to include patients earlier in the disease trajectory, and in patterns of service delivery (including joint clinics with oncologists in hospitals) have all helped to attract earlier referrals for terminally ill cancer patients, and to overcome the anxieties cancer patients and their families may have about accessing this care. Cancer, however, still has a close association with death and dying in the public imagination. Heart failure, like other chronic diseases, does not. The shock of being referred to a palliative care service may be even greater in these patients and needs very careful explanation. The acceptability of these services beyond cancer is largely unknown, and may represent a major challenge to increasing access for them. Again, innovative patterns of service provision with, for example, hospital and community palliative care teams working closely with the growing numbers of heart failure nurses (Blue *et al.* 2001) will be needed.

In summary, specialist palliative care provision in the UK is primarily used by cancer patients, with some AIDS/HIV and motor neurone disease patients also receiving care. The higher proportion of patients with other diagnoses in American hospice programmes shows that the focus on cancer is not inevitable. There is growing evidence of palliative care needs among patients with chronic progressive diseases such as chronic heart failure and COPD, although there is little evidence that specialist palliative care services benefit these patients. There are barriers to increasing access for chronic disease patients, including funding, the difficulty of identifying appropriate candidates because of prognostic uncertainty, the putative lack of appropriate skills among palliative care professionals, and unanswered questions about the acceptability of these services beyond cancer. Innovation and trial-and-error, accompanied by both summative and formative evaluations, will be needed to adapt palliative care to the needs of patients with conditions other than cancer and to the settings where they currently receive care.

Improving access for beyond cancer will not just – or, perhaps, even primarily – mean opening the doors of existing services to these patients, but will require adaptations to these services as well as the development of new services. It may mean a radical rethink about the nature of specialist palliative care and who should access it, with one suggestion being that it should be seen as a service for those with complex end-of-life symptoms or problems, regardless of diagnosis (Skilbeck and Payne 2005). However it is redesigned in the future, it will require a close partnership between palliative care and other specialities, particularly health care for older people (including nursing homes) given the ageing population and the higher incidence of chronic, progressive conditions in older people (Lye and Donnellan 2000). Indeed, discussing access for patients with conditions other than cancer to palliative care services without considering access issues for older people, including older cancer patients, is to oversimplify the issues. The access of older people to specialist palliative care services is therefore considered in the next section.

## Older people's access to palliative care

Causes of death vary significantly with age. While overall rates of heart disease remain fairly stable across age groups (unlike chronic heart failure rates, which increase with age: Lye and Donnellan 2000), the proportion of deaths from stroke increase from 5 per cent in those aged under 65 to 13 per cent in those aged 85 or over. Dementia accounts for less than 1 per cent of deaths in the youngest age group, compared with nearly 10 per cent in the oldest age group. The proportion of cancer deaths decreases significantly with age, from 37 per cent in those who die before age 65 to 12 per cent in those who survived to at least 85. This has led to the suggestion that age is the crucial factor in determining how people with cancer differ from other patients (Seale 1991a). While this is true when the proportion of deaths from each cause is considered, the total number of deaths increases with age. This means that the number of people aged 75 or older who die from cancer does not differ much from the number who die from it before the age of 75: 63,049 versus 70,397 in England and Wales in 1999. Patients with cancer differ from others at the end of life in a number of ways, including the pattern and severity of symptoms and their dependency levels (Addington-Hall and Karlsen 1999). This is true of patients under 65 as well as of older patients, and it is therefore not helpful to see age as the main difference between cancer patients and those who die from other causes. It risks obscuring the needs of younger patients in the latter group and of older people with cancer. Nevertheless, in terms of numbers, the limited access to specialist palliative care services beyond cancer has a greater impact on older people who die than it does on younger people. This is compounded by evidence that older cancer patients access specialist palliative care services less frequently than younger patients, at least in the UK.

Older people who are terminally ill with cancer are less likely to access hospice inpatient care than younger patients. In the Regional Study of Care for the Dying, patients under the age of 85 years at death were almost three times (2.82) more likely to have been admitted to a hospice than those over this age (Addington-Hall *et al.* 1998). Differences in site of cancer, dependency levels and reported symptoms were controlled for statistically and do not explain this finding. In health districts with a lower than average number of hospice beds, patients under the age of 65 were significantly more likely to access hospice care than those over this age. A recent systematic review of studies examining use of or referral to specialist palliative care services in adult cancer patients confirmed the finding of a statistically significant lower use of specialist palliative care among those aged 65 and above compared to younger patients (Burt and Raine 2006). Recent research has suggested that the age of the informal carer, as well as the age of the patient, may be important to explaining access to hospices (Grande *et al.* 2006).

Why might older cancer patients be less likely than younger ones to access inpatient hospice care? Hospices – or those making referrals – may be focusing a scarce resource on patients they believe to be most at need. Nursing homes may be an acceptable alternative for older people unable to remain at home, but be considered less suitable for younger patients who are therefore admitted to a hospice instead. This apparent use of inpatient hospices to provide care for younger patients who can no longer cope at home is out of step with the increasing emphasis of many UK hospices on short-term admissions to alleviate difficult physical or psychological symptoms. This cannot fully explain the evidence of age-related differences in access to specialist palliative care services, as the same pattern is found in community palliative care services as for inpatient hospices.

Why might being older affect access to these services? Again, older individuals may be seen – or see themselves – as being less in need of the expert support provided by specialist palliative care services. Early research suggested that they experience less symptom distress than younger patients (Degner and Sloan 1995) but more recent evidence does not support this (Teunissen *et al.* 2006; Holtan *et al.* 2007). Older people may be at increased risk of experiencing uncontrolled pain, with health professionals failing to detect or treat their pain, perhaps because of beliefs that it is less of a problem in this population. A seminal study of pain management in a large population of older patients with cancer concluded that daily pain is prevalent and often goes untreated (Bernabei *et al.* 1998). More information is needed on how the prevalence, perception and control of symptoms varies with age. The limited available evidence suggests that the relative under-utilization of specialist palliative care services in older people cannot be wholly explained by these factors, although health professional beliefs about symptom experience at different ages may play an important role.

Specialist palliative care includes psychological and spiritual support as well as the control of physical symptoms. Do older people need this type of support less than younger patients? Older patients with cancer are thought to be less troubled by a cancer diagnosis than younger people (Harrison and Maguire 1995) and are believed to be more accepting of death (Feifel and Branscomb 1973). Lower rates of death anxiety have indeed been reported for older people in some studies (for example, Russac *et al.* 2007); however, the evidence for this being a general characteristic of older age remains equivocal (Fortner and Neimeyer 1999). Some, perhaps many, older people do find it less difficult to face death than their younger counterparts. However, this is not true of all older people and some may benefit from the expertise of specialist palliative care teams in helping them to come to terms with their own mortality and to make some sense of their lives. Their families may also benefit from the care and continuing support these teams provide: although younger families with children have particularly acute social and psychological need, the devastation experienced by many older spouses and their adult children and the physical consequences of caregiving in older people with their own health problems should not be overlooked.

People who are admitted to a hospice in the last year of life are more likely than other cancer patients to have cancer alone recorded as cause of death on their death certificate (Seale 1991b). Older patients with cancer are likely to have co-morbidities, such as musculoskeletal, respiratory and circulatory conditions, and this may contribute to their under-utilization of specialist palliative care services. As discussed above, these services focus on patients for whom the consequences of cancer are the main problem, and who are often relatively unfamiliar with the management of other conditions. The higher incidence of dementia may also reduce hospice usage in the UK (but to a lesser extent in the USA; Hanrahan *et al.* 2001), as these services are reluctant or unable to care for patients with severe cognitive impairment (Addington-Hall 2000).

There is little evidence with which to address the question of whether the focus on cancer patients who have limited or no co-morbidities is appropriate or whether it discriminates against older people. A patient's age conveys little or no information about the needs of that individual, however much information it conveys about the needs of the total population of people of that age. Patients need to be assessed as individuals and to have their eligibility for specialist palliative care determined on the basis of this assessment, not on the basis of their chronological age.

This discussion presupposes that the age differential in access to specialist palliative care is a consequence solely of the admission policies and practices of these services. These are important, but the attitudes of those making referrals and of the patients themselves are also important in determining access to specialist palliative care. Older people aged over 75 do not seem to differ from those aged under 75 in their attitudes to palliative care services (Catt *et al.* 2005). Hinton (1994) reported that age differentials were evident in referrals to a palliative care community service, but not in referrals from that service to an inpatient hospice. Health professionals caring for these patients may not make referrals to specialist palliative care if they perceive the referral as being unlikely to be accepted, if they underestimate the patient's physical, psychological or spiritual needs, or if they (perhaps rightly) consider themselves to have superior skills in the management of the patient. They may also be caring for patients in a setting with limited access to palliative care services. More research is needed to explore further the attitudes of referrers to palliative care for older people, and to explore the attitudes of older people themselves. Many older people spend at least some time in a nursing home and current efforts in the UK and elsewhere to improve palliative care in these settings are therefore important (Maddocks and Parker 2001; Froggatt 2004).

# Conclusion

Access to specialist palliative care services is determined primarily by availability. This varies between and across countries depending on the health care system, health care funding and both political and public support for these services. Access to the available services is determined by eligibility criteria, both explicit and implicit, which are themselves determined by beliefs about the purpose and benefits of palliative care.

Older people are more likely than younger people to die from causes other than cancer and to have a number of co-morbidities alongside cancer. They are therefore disproportionately affected by the focus of specialist palliative care on cancer. Even those who die from cancer are less likely to access specialist palliative care than younger patients with similar dependency and symptoms. There is limited research evidence to justify either the focus on cancer or the age-related differentials in access to these services.

The evidence on palliative care needs beyond cancer supports the argument that many of these patients have unmet palliative care needs, but there is very limited evidence that they would benefit from specialist palliative care interventions. Establishing benefit is an essential stage in establishing need for specialist palliative care beyond cancer, and more innovative research and audit studies are needed to build the evidence base. Evidence is also lacking on older people's attitudes to specialist palliative care, their needs at the end of life and the reasons why older cancer patients are referred to these services less often than younger patients. Again, further research is needed. Access to specialist palliative care for beyond cancer patients and for older people are closely related issues and should not be considered in isolation.

The literature on access to these services illustrates the importance of assessing each individual's need for palliative care rather than making judgements based implicitly or explicitly on the basis of their age or diagnosis. This, however, presumes that 'palliative care needs' are easily defined and identified. The debate elsewhere in this book on definitions of palliative care shows that they are not. There will continue to be local and national variations in access to specialist palliative care, and there also needs to be continued reflection and debate about whether these variations are justified or are a consequence of stereotypical views of levels of palliative care need among different demographic and diagnostic groups.

# Notes

1   See Hospice Information Service (2007) Summary of UK hospice and palliative care units 2005 (www.hospiceinformation.info/factsandfigures/ukhospices.asp, accessed 24 October 2007).
2   See Department of Health (2006) 'Better end of life care for patients – Government announces strategy to improve end of life care'.
3   See National Hospice and Palliative Care Organization (www.nhpco.org/files/public/2005-facts-and-figures.pdf).

# References

Addington-Hall, J.M. (2000) *Positive Partnerships: Palliative Care for Adults with Severe Mental Health Problems. Occasional Paper No. 17*. London: National Council for Hospices and Specialist Palliative Care Services/Scottish Partnership Agency for Palliative and Cancer Care.

Addington-Hall, J.M. and Karlsen, S. (1999) Age is not the crucial factor in determining how the palliative care needs of people who die from cancer differ from those of people who die from other causes. *Journal of Palliative Care*, 15: 13–19.

Addington-Hall, J.M. and McCarthy, M. (1995) The Regional Study of Care for the Dying: methods and sample characteristics. *Palliative Medicine*, 9: 27–35.

Addington-Hall, J.M., Lay, M., Altmann, D. and McCarthy, M. (1995) Symptom control, communication with health professionals, and hospital care of stroke patients in the last year of life as reported by surviving family, friends and officials. *Stroke*, 26: 2242–8.

Addington-Hall, J.M., Altmann, D. and McCarthy, M. (1998) Who gets hospice inpatient care? *Social Science and Medicine*, 46: 1011–16.

Aiken, L.S., Butner, J., Lockhart, C.A., Volk-Craft, B.E., Hamilton, G. and Williams, F.G. (2006) Outcome evaluation of a randomized trial of the PhoenixCare intervention: program of case management and coordinated care for the seriously chronically ill. *Journal of Palliative Medicine*, 9: 111–26.

Barnes, S., Gott, M., Payne, S., Parker, C., Seamark, D., Gariballa. S. and Small, N. (2006) Prevalence of symptoms in a community-based sample of heart failure patients. *Journal of Pain and Symptom Management*, 32: 208–16.

Bernabei, R., Gambassi, G., Lapane, K., Landi, F., Gatsonis, C., Dunlop, R., Lipsitz, L., Steel, K. and Mor, V. (1998) Management of pain in elderly patients with cancer. SAGE Study Group: Systematic Assessment of Geriatric Drug Use via Epidemiology. *Journal of the American Medical Association*, 279: 1877–82.

Blue, L., Lang, E., McMurray, J.J., Davie, A.P., McDonagh, T.A., Murdoch, D.R., Petrie, M.C., Connolly, E., Norrie, J., Round, C.E., Ford, I. and Morrison, C.E.

(2001) Randomised controlled trial of specialist nurse intervention in heart failure. *British Medical Journal*, 323: 715–18.

Bosanquet, N. and Salisbury, C. (1999) *Providing a Palliative Care Service: Towards an Evidence Base.* Oxford: Oxford University Press.

Boyd, K.J., Murray, S.A., Kendall, M., Worth, A., Frederick Benton, T. and Clausen, H. (2004) Living with advanced heart failure: a prospective, community based study of patients and their carers. *European Journal of Heart Failure*, 6: 585–91.

Burt, J. and Raine, R. (2006) The effect of age on referral to and use of specialist palliative care services in adult cancer patients: a systematic review. *Age and Ageing*, 35: 469–76.

Catt, S., Blanchard, M., Addington-Hall, J., Zis, M., Blizard, R. and King, M. (2005) Older adults' attitudes to death, palliative treatment and hospice care. *Palliative Medicine*, 19: 402–10.

Clark, D. (1999) 'Total pain', disciplinary power and the body in the work of Cicely Saunders, 1958–1967. *Social Science and Medicine*, 49: 727–36.

Clark, D., Neale, B. and Heather, P. (1995) Contracting for palliative care. *Social Science and Medicine*, 40: 1193–202.

Clarke, D.M., McLeod, J.E., Smith, G.C., Trauer, T. and Kissane, D.W. (2005) A comparison of psychosocial and physical functioning in patients with motor neurone disease and metastatic cancer. *Journal of Palliative Care*, 21: 173–9.

Daley, A., Matthews, C. and Williams, A. (2006) Heart failure and palliative care services working in partnership: report of a new model of care. *Palliative Medicine*, 20: 593–601.

Degner, L.F. and Sloan, J.A. (1995) Symptom distress in newly diagnosed ambulatory cancer patients and as a predictor of survival in lung cancer. *Journal of Pain and Symptom Management*, 10: 423–31.

Department of Health (2000a) *National Service Framework for Coronary Heart Disease*. London: Department of Health.

Department of Health (2000b) *The NHS Cancer Plan: A Plan for Investment, A Plan of Reform*. London: Department of Health.

Department of Health (2005) *National Service Framework for Long-term Conditions*. London: Department of Health.

Department of Health (2006) *Our health, our care, our say: a new direction for community services*. London: Department of Health.

Doyle, D., Hanks, W.C. and MacDonald, N. (1998) *Oxford Textbook of Palliative Medicine*, 2nd edn. Oxford: Oxford University Press.

Edmonds, P., Karlsen, S. and Addington-Hall, J.M. (2001) Quality of care in the last year of life: a comparison of lung cancer and COPD patients. *Palliative Medicine*, 15: 287–95.

Edmonds, P., Vivat, B., Burman, R., Silber, E. and Higginson, I.J. (2007) 'Fighting for everything': service experiences of people severely affected by multiple sclerosis. *Multiple Sclerosis*, 13: 660–7.

Elkington, H., White, P., Addington-Hall, J., Higgs, R. and Edmonds, P. (2005) The health care needs of chronic obstructive pulmonary disease patients in the last year of life. *Palliative Medicine*, 19: 485–91.

Feifel, H. and Branscomb, A.B. (1973) Who's afraid of death? *Journal of Abnormal Psychology*, 81(3): 282–8.

Field, D. and Addington-Hall, J. (1999) Extending specialist palliative care to all? *Social Science and Medicine*, 48: 1271–80.

Field, M.J. and Cassel, C.K. (1997) *Approaching Death: Improving Care at the End of Life*. The Committee on Care at the End of Life, Division of Health Care Services, Institute of Medicine. Washington, DC: National Academy Press.

Fortner, B.V. and Neimeyer, R.A. (1999) Death anxiety in older adults; a quantitative review. *Death Studies*, 23: 387–411.

Frankland, J., Rogers, A. and Addington-Hall, J.M. (2007) Developing a non-cancer service – A resource for hospices. www.helpthehospices.org.uk/servicedev/downloads/hth_non_cancer_guide.pdf (accessed June 2007).

Froggatt, K.A. (2004) *Palliative Care in Care Homes for Older People*. London: The National Council for Palliative Care.

George, R. and Sykes, J. (1997) Beyond cancer? In: D. Clark, J. Hockley and S. Ahmedzai (eds) *New Themes in Palliative Care*. Buckingham: Open University Press.

Glaser, B.G. and Strauss, A.L. (1965) *Awareness of Dying*. Chicago, IL: Aldine.

Glaser, B.G. and Strauss, A.L. (1968) *Time for Dying*. Chicago, IL: Aldine.

Gore, J.M., Brophy, C.J. and Greenstone, M.A. (2000) How well do we care for patients with end stage chronic obstructive pulmonary disease (COPD)? A comparison of palliative care and quality of life in COPD and lung cancer. *Thorax*, 55: 1000–6.

Gott, M., Barnes, S., Parker, C., Payne, S., Seamark, D., Gariballa, S. and Small, N. (2006) Predictors of the quality of life of older people with heart failure recruited from primary care. *Age and Aging*, 35: 172–7.

Graham, H. and Livesley, B. (1983) Dying as a diagnosis: difficulties of communication and management in elderly patients. *The Lancet*, 2: 670–2.

Grande, G.E., Farquhar, M.C., Barclay, S.G. and Todd, C.J. (2006) The influence of patient and carer age in access to palliative care services. *Age and Ageing*, 35: 267–73.

Hanrahan, P., Luchins, D.J. and Murphy, K. (2001) Palliative care for patients with dementia. In: J.M. Addington-Hall and I.J. Higginson (eds) *Palliative Care for Non-Cancer Patients*. Oxford: Oxford University Press.

Harrison, J. and Maguire, P. (1995) Influence of age on psychological adjustment to cancer. *Psycho-Oncology*, 4: 33–8.

Higginson, I.J. (ed.) (1997) *Health Care Needs Assessment: Palliative and Terminal Care. Health Care Needs Assessment*, 2nd series. Oxford: Radcliffe Medical Press.

Hinton, J. (1963) The physical and mental distress of the dying. *Quarterly Journal of Medicine*, 32: 1–21.

Hinton, J. (1994) Which patients with terminal cancer are admitted from home care? *Palliative Medicine*, 8: 197–210.

Holtan, A., Aass, N., Nordoy, T., Haugen, D.F., Kaasa, S., Mohr, W. and Kongsgaard, U.E. (2007) Prevalence of pain in hospitalized cancer patients in Norway: a national survey. *Palliative Medicine*, 21: 7–13.

Hughes, H.L.G. (1960) *Peace at the last*. London: Gulbenkian Foundation.

Johnson, M.J. and Houghton, T. (2006) Palliative care for patients with heart failure: description of a service. *Palliative Medicine*, 20: 211–14.

Kristjanson, L.J., Aoun, S.M. and Oldham, L. (2006) Palliative care and support for people with neurodegenerative conditions and their carers. *International Journal of Palliative Nursing*, 12: 368–77.

Knauft, E., Nielsen, E.L., Engelberg, R.A., Patrick, D.L. and Curtis, J.R. (2005) Barriers and facilitators to end-of-life care communication for patients with COPD. *Chest*, 127: 2188–96.

Lunt, B. (1985) Terminal cancer care services: recent changes in regional inequalities in Great Britain. *Social Science and Medicine*, 20: 753–9.

Lunt, B. and Hillier, R. (1981) Terminal care: present services and future priorities. *British Medical Journal*, 283: 595–8.

Lye, M. and Donnellan, C. (2000) Heart disease in the elderly. *Heart*, 84: 560–6.

Lynn, J., Harrell, F. Jr., Cohn, F., Wagner, D. and Connors, A.F. Jr. (1997a) Prognoses of seriously ill hospitalised patients on the days before death: implications for patient care and public policy. *New Horizons*, 5: 56–61.

Lynn, J., Teno, J.M., Phillips, R.S., Wu, A.W., Desbiens, N., Harrold, J., Claessens, M.T., Wenger, N., Kreling, B. and Connors, A.F. Jr (1997b) Perceptions by family members of the dying experience of older and seriously ill patients. *Annals of Internal Medicine*, 126: 97–106.

Maddocks, I. and Parker, D. (2001) Palliative care in nursing homes. In: J.M. Addington-Hall and I.J. Higginson (eds) *Palliative Care for Non-Cancer Patients*. Oxford: Oxford University Press.

Marie Curie Memorial Foundation (1952) *Report on a National Survey Concerning Patients Nursed at Home*. London: Marie Curie Memorial Foundation.

McCarthy, M., Lay, M. and Addington-Hall, J.M. (1996) Dying from heart disease. *Journal of the Royal College of Physicians of London*, 30: 325–8.

McCarthy, M., Addington-Hall, J.M. and Altmann, D. (1997a) The experience of dying with dementia: a retrospective survey. *International Journal of Geriatric Psychiatry*, 12: 404–9.

McCarthy, M., Addington-Hall, J.M. and Lay, M. (1997b) Communication and choice in dying from heart disease. *Journal of the Royal Society of Medicine*, 90: 128–31.

Murray, S.A., Kendall, M., Boyd. K. and Sheikh, A. (2005) Illness trajectories and palliative care. *British Medical Journal*, 330: 1007–11.

Murtagh, F.E.M., Addington-Hall, J.M. and Higginson, I.J. (2007) The prevalence of symptoms in end-stage renal disease: a systematic review. *Advances in Chronic Kidney Disease*, 14: 82–99.

National Council for Palliative Care (2006) *National Survey of Patient Activity Data for Specialist Palliative Care Services*. London: NCPC.

National Council of Hospice and Specialist Palliative Care Services (2000) *The Palliative Care Survey 1999*. London: NCHSPCS.

National Institute for Clinical Excellence (NICE) (2004) *Guidance on cancer services: improving supportive and palliative care for adults with cancer – the manual*. London: NICE.

NHS Executive (1996) *A Policy Framework for Commissioning Cancer Services: Palliative Care Services*. EL(96)85. London: NHS Executive.

Rogers, A.E., Addington-Hall, J.M., Abery, A.J., McCoy, A.S.M., Bulpitt, C., Coats, A.J.S. and Gibbs, J.S.R. (2000) Knowledge and communication difficulties for patients with chronic heart failure; a qualitative study. *British Medical Journal*, 321: 605–7.

Russac, R.J., Gatliffe, C., Reece, M. and Spottswood, D. (2007) Death anxiety across the adult years: an examination of age and gender effects. *Death Studies*, 31: 549–61.

Seale, C. (1991a) Death from cancer and death from other causes: the relevance of the hospice approach. *Palliative Medicine*, 5: 12–19.

Seale, C. (1991b) A comparison of hospice and conventional care. *Social Science and Medicine*, 32: 147–52.

Skilbeck, J.K. and Payne, S. (2005) End of life care: a discursive analysis of specialist palliative care nursing. *Journal of Advanced Nursing*, 51(4): 325–34.

Solano, J.P., Gomes, B. and Higginson, I.J. (2006) A comparison of symptom prevalence in far advanced cancer, AIDS, heart disease, chronic obstructive pulmonary disease and renal disease. *Journal of Pain and Symptom Management*, 31: 58–69.

St Christopher's Hospice Information Service (1990) *Directory of Hospice and Specialist Palliative Care Services in the UK and the Republic of Ireland*. London: St Christopher's Hospice Information Service.

Standing Medical Advisory Committee and the Standing Nursing and Midwifery Advisory Committees (1992) *The Principles and Provision of Palliative Care*. London: SMAC/SNMAC.

Stevens, A. and Raftery, J. (1997) Introduction. In: I.J. Higginson (ed.) *Health Care Needs Assessment: Palliative and Terminal Care*. 2nd series. Oxford: Radcliffe Medical Press.

Teunissen, S.C., de Haes, H.C., Voest, E.E. and de Graeff, A. (2006) Does age matter in palliative care? *Critical Reviews in Oncology-Hematology*, 60: 152–8.

Toscani, F. (2002) Palliative care in Italy: accident or miracle? *Palliative Medicine*, 16: 177–8.

Weisbord, S.D., Carmody, S.S., Bruns, F.J., Rotondi, A.J., Cohen, L.M., Zeidel, M.L. and Arnold, R.M. (2003) Symptom burden, quality of life, advance care planning and the potential value of palliative care in severely ill haemodialysis patients. *Nephrology Dialysis Transplantation*, 18: 1345–52.

Wilkes, E. (1984) Dying now. *Lancet*, 1: 950–2.

Willems, D.L., Hak, A., Visser, F. and van der Wal, G. (2004) Thoughts of patients with advanced heart failure on dying. *Palliative Medicine*, 18: 564–72.

Willems, D.L., Hak, A., Visser, F.C., Cornel, J. and van der Wal, G. (2006) Patient work in end-stage heart failure: a prospective longitudinal multiple case study. *Palliative Medicine*, 20: 25–33.

# 5

# Dying
## Places and preferences

*Carol Thomas*

---

**Key points**

- The relationship between the quality of the dying experience and place of death.
- Research literature on place of death patterns.
- Research literature on patient preferences for place of death.
- Qualitative evidence on why patients hold the place of death preferences that they do.
- Reasons why terminally ill patients and their carers might prefer to die in a hospice rather than home setting.

---

## Introduction

As specialist palliative care has developed, the quality of the dying experience has remained at the top of this care sector's expanding agenda. It is a priority that is shared by professionals delivering specialist end-of-life care across the world, despite the marked international variations in the pattern of development and current configuration of palliative care services (Seale 2000; Clark 2007; International Observatory on End of Life Care 2007). The *location* of deaths – home, hospital, inpatient hospice, residential care institutions, other setting – is now an interwoven theme. *Where* people die matters. It is widely understood in both professional and lay circles across the globe that the quality of the dying experience frequently depends upon where dying and death occurs. Although patterns of 'place of death' differ between and within regions and nation states – reflecting oft-cited global East/West and first-world/third-world divides – contrasting dying settings are associated with remarkably common cultural markers of 'good' versus 'bad' deaths (Seale 2000): dying with loved ones in attendance versus dying alone; dying in pain versus dying in comfort; dying in emotional anguish versus dying in a calm and reconciled state of mind; dying in the impersonal technical jungle of hospital wards versus dying in more 'natural' settings.

In late capitalist societies, specialist palliative care services have developed with a particular focus on the support of patients with advanced cancer and their family carers (Clark 2007). Since the end of the twentieth century, the location of cancer deaths has constituted a practice, policy and research concern in many countries. The trend towards increasing proportions of cancer deaths in general hospital settings alarmed those who valued what they perceived to be the 'good death' and 'better death' possibilities offered by inpatient hospices or by professionally trained teams who were able to support cancer deaths in community settings. University and clinically based research continues to expand and to inform health policy makers on the location of formal end-stage care for dying patients and their informal carers. In the United Kingdom (UK), the past decade has witnessed the advocacy and implementation of a strong official policy drive toward supporting 'home' death options, fuelled by research evidence that over 50 per cent of cancer patients would prefer to die at home (Higginson and Sen-Gupta 2000). The next few years will reveal if the policy initiatives currently underway have been able to bring about the intended goal of boosting the proportion of supported cancer deaths that occur in home settings.

This chapter explores the location of deaths in two sections, focusing on cancer deaths. The first examines research literature from across the globe on what is commonly referred to as *actual* place of death. The second turns to the smaller body of literature on *preferences* for place of death held by cancer patients and their informal carers; this section has a UK focus, and features some of the findings generated in a research project that I directed on place of death.

## Actual place of cancer deaths

Compared to establishing the presence of disease or illness, the body's death has the merit of a yes/no certainty. In most societies, this allows deaths to be recorded, catalogued and counted. In countries where cancer deaths are carefully registered, together with key socio-demographic characteristics of the deceased, it becomes possible to track place of death and to undertake statistical analyses of national and regional data sets. Sophisticated statistical methods with large data sets using multiple regression analyses or multi-level modelling techniques can begin to tease out the 'factors' that are associated with, or 'predict', the location of cancer deaths. A sizeable body of published research of this socio-epidemiological character now exists.

### Trends

Turning first to simple trend and cross-sectional cancer data, the long-term trend in late capitalist societies has been away from deaths in home settings towards institutionally located deaths. For example, the proportion of cancer deaths in hospitals in England between 1967 and 1987 increased from 45 per cent to 50 per cent, and from 5 per cent to 18 per cent in hospices and other institutions (Cartwright 1991). The increase in hospice deaths is testimony to the rapid expansion and diversification of hospice services in the UK in the years following the opening of the landmark St Christopher's Hospice in 1967. However, regional variations are marked. In south east England, the years between 1985 and 1994 saw a trend away from hospital deaths (from 67 to 44 per cent), to home (from 17 to 30 per cent) and hospice deaths (from 8 to 20 per cent) (Davies *et al.* 2006: 593). This trend reversed partially after 1995, and by 2002 hospital deaths had risen to 47 per cent, with home deaths down to 23 per cent; hospice deaths had remained stable, while nursing home deaths had risen (from 3 to 8 per cent) (ibid.). In north west England in the early 1990s (1990–1994), the proportion of cancer deaths occurring at home ranged from 33 per cent in South Lancashire to 22 per cent in the coastal Morecambe Bay district in North Lancashire (Hospice Information Service data, in Higginson 1999).

By 2000, the proportion of cancer deaths in hospital in the UK stood at 55.5 per cent, with 23 per cent at home, 16.5 per cent in hospice and 5 per cent in other settings – principally nursing and residential homes (Ellershaw and Ward 2003). In 2004, the World Health Organization (WHO) reported that the majority of cancer deaths also occurred in hospital in the United States (US), Germany, Switzerland and France (cited in Gomes and Higginson 2006). Other less prosperous capitalist societies with Anglophile health care systems and ageing populations have been moving closer to this profile in the last two decades, though cancer deaths at home still predominate in many. In Italy, for example, a paper published in 2006 (Beccaro *et al.*) reported that a nationally representative follow-back survey of 2,000 cancer deaths found that hospital deaths had reached 34.6 per cent (hospice 0.7 per cent, nursing home 6.5 per cent) – with home deaths accounting for more than half (57.9 per cent). Regional variations in such countries are often stark, and usually associated with the degree of urban and industrial development: the proportion of cancer deaths in home settings in Italy between 1987 and 1995 achieved a high of 40 per cent in the province of Liguria compared with 73 per cent in Toscana (Costantini *et al.* 2000).

Overall, the wealthiest countries have witnessed the speediest institutionalization of cancer deaths in the last quarter of the twentieth century, though some are now trying to reverse this trend in favour of maximizing supported deaths in home settings. When deaths from *all causes* are examined, the proportion of deaths occurring in hospital generally mirrors and exceeds the pattern for cancer deaths.

### Factors associated with actual place of death

Many factors are associated with the trends and patterns in actual place of death outlined above. Key among these, on a global scale, are the prevalence of types of cancer and other life-threatening diseases, disease survival rates, the degree of development of hospital and specialist palliative care services – especially inpatient hospice and hospice-at-home services, and the commitment of health policy makers and professional groups to supporting deaths in home settings. These combine in complex ways with demographic factors such as: the age profile of populations; the gender and ethnic mix of populations (differential social status and age profiles); urban/rural residential profiles; socio-economic factors that determine income levels and income diversity/inequality; household and family structures; cultural values and attitudes to death and dying; cultural values and attitudes towards elderly people, especially women, living alone and unsupported by members of the next generation(s) (Seale 2000). Understanding the way that these and other factors interact, and separating out those that play a dominant determining role, presents researchers with a considerable challenge.

*Within* nations, studies of factors associated with the place of cancer deaths fall into two main categories. The first consists of epidemiological interrogations of the interaction of factors in routinely collected death registration data – at national, regional and local scales (Clifford *et al.* 1991; Hunt *et al.* 1993; Sims *et al.* 1997; Grande *et al.* 1998; Higginson *et al.* 1998, 1999; Duffy *et al.* 2002; Bruera *et al.* 2003; Gatrell *et al.* 2003). The second category comprises prospective and retrospective cohort studies of terminally ill cancer patients involving, in varying combinations, the analysis of individual-level data gathered from patients, their informal carers, their formal health care providers, and case records (Dunlop *et al.* 1989; Townsend *et al.* 1990; Hinton 1994a, 1994b; Brazil *et al.* 2002).

Both types of study have brought to light a wide range of place of death predictors. Epidemiological studies by Sims *et al.* (1997), Higginson *et al.* (1999) and Grundy *et al.* (2004) established the existence of marked socio-economic variations in place of death, with patients in socio-economically disadvantaged circumstances being more likely to die in hospital than in a hospice or at home. Other factors identified in this type of study are tumour type, gender, age and distance from services. Tumour type is a key determinant – it has an important bearing on the speed of disease development, the timing of palliative care referrals, and options for treatment and management at different disease stages (Gomes and Higginson 2006). In the UK, deaths from lymphatic, breast and haematological cancers are much more likely to occur in hospital than are deaths from other cancers (Higginson *et al.* 1998; Gatrell *et al.* 2003); deaths at home are most often associated with gastrointestinal, genitourinary and respiratory cancers (Hunt *et al.* 1993; Grande *et al.* 1998). Men are more likely than women to die at home, and older adults are less likely than their younger counterparts to die at home or in a hospice (Hunt *et al.* 1993; Grande *et al.* 1998; Higginson *et al.* 1998; Gatrell *et al.* 2003). At an individual level, Gatrell *et al.* (2003) measured proximity to hospices and hospitals in north west England and found this to be a significant influence on place of death: proximity to a hospice increases the probability that a cancer patient will die there, and the same is true of hospitals (see also Herd 1990).

Studies utilizing prospective and retrospective cohort designs have confirmed these findings and drawn attention to the importance of other factors in predicting the place of death of cancer patients in late capitalist societies. The relevance of the presence and characteristics of informal carers, and their ability 'to cope' with patients' symptoms and emotional states, has come to the fore in this research, something that cannot be identified in most routine mortality data sets.

In a prospective study of 160 patients referred to a hospice support team in the UK, Dunlop *et al.* (1989) identified the carer's inability to cope at home, usually in the face of deterioration in the patient's condition, to be a key factor leading to a hospital admission followed by a death in that setting. Hinton's prospective study confirmed this (1994a, 1994b) and pointed to other factors, often interrelated, precipitating admission to either hospice or hospital care: the need for specialist symptom control; further serious deterioration, typically involving severe pain; a request for admission by a patient, relative or GP; and the patient's emotional distress or confusion.

Prospective and retrospective studies in the US have produced similar results (see Brown and Colton 2001; Evans *et al.* 2006). In a retrospective cohort study in the USA, Brazil *et al.* (2002) found the odds of dying at home were lower when patients had care-givers whose own health was reported as being only fair to poor, and among patients who used hospital palliative care beds in the course of their illness. This finding was echoed in a UK study using a 1 per cent sample of the population of England and Wales: the odds of a home death among those dying of cancer in the 1990s were highest for those who lived with a spouse who had no limiting long-term illness (Grundy *et al.* 2004).

Some of the factors reported above are related to the nature of service infrastructures in a patient's area of residence, especially the availability of specialist inpatient and community based palliative care services. In their comprehensive review of the literature, Grande *et al.* (1998) concluded that 'Patients with certain characteristics may therefore be more likely to die at home by virtue of being more likely to access services which improve their chances of dying at home' (1998: 573). Higginson and Priest (1996) reported that home deaths in the UK were more likely when community palliative care nurses and Marie Curie nurses (offering care during the night) are involved in care arrangements. The involvement of a committed GP, confident in the support of dying patients, increases the chances of a home death (Thorpe 1993; Brazil *et al.* 2002). Symptom severity and the availability of specialist equipment for use in home settings is also found to be predictive of place of death; however, the use of social and health services for social care is associated with a decreased likelihood of home death in the UK (Karlsen and Addington-Hall 1998). The availability of specialist palliative care beds in hospitals in an area of residence predicted place of death, with higher bed levels associated with an increased proportion of hospital deaths (Pritchard *et al.* 1998). Such findings resonate with those reported above concerning distance to services.

Turning to another type of factor, prospective and retrospective studies in a range of countries have found that the strength and visibility (to professionals) of a patient's desire to die at home is associated with the actual location of death: the stronger the preference for a home death, the greater the chances of achieving it (Karlsen and Addington-Hall 1998; Cantwell *et al.* 2000; Brazil *et al.* 2002; Gyllenhammar *et al.* 2003). An 'open awareness' of dying, where patients and carers both acknowledge impending death and can discuss place of death options, increases the chance of dying at home or in a hospice (Seale *et al.* 1997). Other factors that have been found to influence the location of cancer deaths include the length of survival time from diagnosis (Hunt and McCaul 1996; Dunlop *et al.* 1989), marital status and rural residency (Moinpur and Polissar 1989).

In a recent systematic literature review of factors influencing cancer deaths at home, involving 58 studies in 13 countries, Gomes and Higginson (2006) synthesized the evidence and found that there was high-strength evidence for the effect of 17 factors on place of death – all of which are mentioned above. Six of these were strongly associated with home deaths: patients' low functional status; patients' preferences for place of death; the level of use and intensity of home care services; patient co-residence with relatives; and the presence of extended family support.

My own study on place of cancer deaths in north west England in 2000–2002 was unusual in that it made additional use of qualitative interview data to add to knowledge on *actual* place of death patterns (Thomas 2005). This aspect of the three-part study involved interviews with a set of palliative care professionals (n=15). The interviews generated findings that not only confirmed and considerably enriched understanding of factors that are known to predict actual place of death, but also brought new factors into view. New factors could be grouped under the following headings: 'service infrastructure', 'patient and carer attitudes' and 'cultures of professional practice'. It is useful to complete this section by including the summary table that was generated (Thomas 2005), with 'new' factors shown in italics (see Table 5.1). These new factors are now in need of confirmation through larger-scale studies, but provide useful pointers for further research on actual place of death.

## Preferences for place of death

The quantity of literature on actual place of death far exceeds that on patient or carer *preferences* for the location of final care and death. As well as reflecting the greater methodological and ethical challenges involved in identifying such preferences, this also reflects the fact that patient preferences and choices did not feature prominently in professional debates about

**Table 5.1** Key factors associated with the place of death of cancer patients, and how these predict a home death

Factors identified in the place of death research literature and confirmed in interviews are shown in normal text. New factors, or new dimensions of known factors arising from the interview data, are shown in *italics*.

| Group headings for key factors associated with place of death (not in order of importance) | Predicts a death at home |
| --- | --- |
| **Service infrastructure factors:**<br>– Health and social service provision (specialist palliative care beds in hospital and hospice; specialist and non-specialist palliative care staff in primary care and social services). | – A relatively small number of specialist palliative care beds (hospice, hospital) in a locality.<br>– A relatively high number of specialist palliative care professionals in community settings (e.g. nurses, doctors, social workers).<br>– Supportive input from non-specialist professionals in community contexts, especially GPs. |
| – *Service funding, budgets and priority setting.*<br>– *Micro-politics in play in the locality.* | – High levels of financial investment in care in home settings.<br>– *Cross-agency/sector, organizational and interprofessional agreement to invest in and support home deaths.* |
| – National cancer and palliative care policies.<br>– *Existence of multidisciplinary palliative care teams.* | – Policy directives in favour of increasing the proportion of home deaths.<br>– *All of the required skill-types are available to support patients and carers in home settings.* |
| **Informal carer characteristics** | – A carer is present, either co-resident or in close proximity.<br>– Absence of serious morbidity in carer; carer is female.<br>– High level of ability and motivation in the carer to deliver care at home, for as long as necessary.<br>– *High level of support for the main carer, from family, friends and professionals.* |
| **Symptom severity and management and case complexity** | – Symptoms are under control because equipment and drugs are available for use in home settings.<br>– There is recourse to rapid assistance at home if symptoms suddenly deteriorate and crises arise, e.g. severe pain.<br>– *Cancers do not present too much complexity in their medical and nursing management.* |

**Table 5.1** *Continued*

Factors identified in the place of death research literature and confirmed in interviews are shown in normal text. New factors, or new dimensions of known factors arising from the interview data, are shown in *italics*.

| Group headings for key factors associated with place of death *(not in order of importance)* | Predicts a death at home |
|---|---|
| **Patient and carer attitudes:**<br>– Strength of place of death preference.<br>– Changes in place of death preference.<br>– Patient and carer attitude to dying.<br>– *Strength of patient desire not to be a burden upon the carer.*<br>– *Degree of trust invested in individual professionals.* | – A strongly expressed preference to die at home.<br>– A consistent preference to die at home.<br>– An open awareness and acceptance of dying.<br>– *Patient and carer acceptance that caring is not too burdensome.*<br>– *Patients and carers invest a great deal of trust in individual professionals attending in home settings.* |
| **Cultures of practice**<br>– *Quality of interprofessional relationships.*<br>– *The ethics and habits of professional practice.*<br>– *Changing nature of practice within hospices (medical specialization and increased patient throughput).* | – *Team working, especially across organizational and specialist/non-specialist boundaries, is of high quality.*<br>– *Professionals' ideas of best practice and of a 'good death', and their routines of professional behaviour, are facilitative of home deaths.* |
| **Patient demographic and socio-economic characteristics** | – Younger, male, married. Higher socio-economic status, *but home deaths can be supported if extended family networks exist among those of lower socio-economic status.* |
| **Tumour type** | – Gastrointestinal, genitourinary, respiratory cancers. |
| **Distance to services** | – Inpatient care (hospital, hospice) is at some geographical distance, e.g. rural residential location. |

Source: Thomas 2005.

the quality of dying until the last quarter of the twentieth century. The change occurred at a time when the wider cultural context in late capitalist societies encouraged individuals to 'know their rights' and to expect services to respond to their needs as 'users'. In the UK in the 1990s, the National Health Service (NHS) was instructed by politicians and leading policy makers to 'listen' and 'respond' to patient voices. Picking up this theme, the NHS Cancer Plan (Department of Health 2000), while focusing on cancer treatment services, acknowledged that most patients with advanced cancer would prefer to die at home but that only about a quarter were able to do so.

In their systematic review of the published literature on patient preferences for place of final care and death at the start of this century, Higginson and Sen-Gupta (2000) found strong evidence that over 50 per cent of cancer patients would prefer to die at home, with the figure rising to over 70 per cent in some studies; inpatient hospices were the second most preferred site. Hospitals were not favoured, though Hinton (1994b) had noted that the acceptability of a death in hospital rose as time progressed for those with terminal cancer, particularly as problems with self-care increased and relatives' fatigue worsened.

Even less is known about the factors *that shape* the place of death preferences held by terminally ill patients and their informal carers. *Why* do patients and carers hold the preferences that they do? Some of the studies featured in Higginson and Sen-Gupta's review (2000) referred, in rather speculative terms, to an association between the type of preference held and factors such as: the difficulty of symptom management (especially pain); changing disease status; the gender of the patient or carer; whether a religious faith is in evidence; patients' and carers' previous personal experience of death and dying. Nevertheless, we do know from some of the actual place of death research literature, reviewed above, that the *strength* of a place of death preference has been found to play an important role in determining where patients do end their days: a *strong* patient preference for a death at home – known both to the family members and health professionals involved – can raise the probability of its achievement.

### Qualitative data on preferences for place of death

In my own social scientific research on the location of cancer deaths in recent years, referred to above, my research team was interested in taking up the challenge posed in Higginson and Sen-Gupta's (2000: 299) conclusion: that 'No consistent conceptualisation of the factors that determine preferences for place of terminal care of patients with cancer emerged from the studies reviewed and this should be the focus for future work'.

With my co-researchers, I developed and presented a conceptual framework based on the analysis of conversational style interviews with a relatively small number of terminally ill cancer patients (n=41) and their co-resident informal carers (n=18) in one health district (Thomas *et al.* 2004). The cancer patients involved were estimated by clinicians to have up to three months of life remaining. The conceptual framework comprised four categories of factors, containing 13 factors in all: i) the informal carer resource, ii) the management of the body, iii) patients' experience of services, iv) patients' existential perspectives (see Table 5.2). Of course, as a conceptual framework generated in a small qualitative study, testing is required by larger-scale research using both qualitative and quantitative research designs to identify its wider robustness and utility. In my view, such research would confirm the robustness of this framework or 'model', though there are, no doubt, other factors to add.

Before reviewing the factors in brief, it is important to note that we found preferences most commonly take the form of a *leaning* (sometimes strong) in a particular direction; preferences rarely constitute categorical certainties. Moreover, preferences could be 'positive' choices or could express resigned acceptance that there were no other options 'given the circumstances'.

## Category 1: the informal care resource

The presence or absence of informal carers in the end-of-life care scenario is not only key to determining where patients actually die, but also shapes patients' preferences for place of death. The patients in our study assessed the care resource available to them – both its quality and quantity – and only contemplated a home death if they thought the person or persons close to them could manage or cope. Difficult questions had to be faced about the practical and emotional support offered by spouses, other family members

**Table 5.2**   Factors shaping cancer patient and carer place of death preferences

**Factors shaping preferences:**

*Category 1: The informal care resource*
  1. Patient's social network and living arrangements
  2. Patient's assessment of the carer's capacity to care
  3. Patient concern for the welfare of the family/carer
  4. Carer's attitude and willingness to care

*Category 2: Management of the body*
  5. Symptom management
  6. Patient's fear of loss of dignity

*Category 3: Experience of services*
  7. Perceptions of the reliability of services and the degree of 'safety' offered
  8. Patient's attitude to the hospice
  9. Patient's experience of hospitals
  10. Patient's knowledge and experience of community services
  11. Patient's attitude to nursing homes

*Category 4: Experiential perspectives*
  12. Patient's attitude to death and dying, including religious faith
  13. Previous experience of facing death and dying

Source: Thomas *et al.* 2004

and friends. Carers, too, found themselves assessing their own capacity to cope with a patient's worsening illness and impending death. If the informal care resource was found to be wanting in some way, then, in our study, minds turned towards the hospice as a potential place of care and death. The hospice also became an attractive option for patients who were particularly eager to spare their loved ones 'the burden' of caring for them 'at the end'. It is helpful to appreciate that this latter stance was a means by which patients could sustain their own identities and roles as family stalwarts and former carers in the face of death.

### Category 2: the management of the body

We found that place of death preferences were greatly influenced by a range of 'body matters' – factors bound up with symptom management and the maintenance of personal dignity and identity in the face of an increasingly unruly and unreliable body. Patients expressed much uncertainty about what the progression of their illness would bring, and this could lead to indecision about place of death. Worries about the management of incontinence and other culturally stigmatized symptoms – bound up with ideas of unacceptable mess and disgust – led some patients to consider placing their bodies in the hands of professionals in a hospice when 'the time came'. Professionals, it was said, could cope with such things, so minimizing embarrassment. A hospice death was certainly a preference for those patients who thought it 'not right' that a son, daughter or sibling should be required to engage in intimate care tasks such as toileting, body washing, or clearing up faeces and vomit.

### Category 3: experience of services

If a service had been found to be 'good' during patients' illness journey (or in a past illness), then the setting involved – a hospice, the community, a hospital – might be considered an acceptable place of death option; if aspects of a service were experienced as 'bad' or indifferent, then it was ruled out. In patients' interview accounts, the qualities that constituted 'good services' and 'good professionals' included: being reliable, trustworthy, safe and secure, 'caring', 'understanding', available, accessible, and responsive to calls for help. Services that provided individualized care and demonstrated an appreciation of the needs of carers were also highly valued. Services and their staff were deemed to be 'poor' if these qualities were perceived to be absent.

Evaluated by these criteria, the users of hospice services in our study formed very favourable opinions, and this often translated into a hospice place of death preference. Most community based nursing services and some GP services were thought to be of high quality, giving some patients and carers the confidence to make and stick with a home death preference. In contrast, while some features of hospital services were reported to be excellent, many aspects of hospital care were viewed as problematic and distressing. Very few looked favourably upon nursing and residential care homes.

*Category 4: existential perspectives*

Place of death preferences in our study were also bound up with patients' and carers' attitudes to death and dying, their previous exposure to the deaths of others, and to their own earlier encounters with serious illness. Having or not having a religious faith was also of relevance. Such concerns could lead to a strong place of death preference, or, alternatively, to the view that where one dies is of little or no consequence. A stoical stance towards life's closure sometimes meant that such matters were thought to be of no great concern.

Of course, these categories and factors usually work in combination in real-life contexts. They interact, producing a rich and potentially shifting mix of reasons for particular preferences. Overall, preferences have a socially contingent character – they are informed by personal biographies, assessments of present social circumstances, as well as by speculations about the effects that the disease will have upon the body and mind as life's closure approaches. Preferences for place of death among cancer patients in our small sample were overwhelmingly in favour of *either* a home or hospice death (sometimes an equal preference); no-one wished to die in hospital[1] (see Thomas *et al.* 2004). Only four patients altered (as opposed to completely changing) their preference over time: two who had favoured a home death became more oriented toward a hospice death, one leaned from 'hospice if I'm bad' towards home, and one expanded his preference from hospice to 'hospice or local hospital'. When preferences were matched against actual place of death, a clear picture emerged. Patients who wished to die at home were not always able to do so; in contrast, patients who preferred to die in a hospice were all able to do so. If a patient had an equal preference for a home or hospice death, all deaths, with one exception, occurred in a hospice rather than at home. A fifth of patients ended their lives in one of the three hospitals in the study area.

# Conclusion

This chapter has explored place of death from two angles, focusing on cancer deaths: *actual* place of death, and lay *preferences* for place of death. The overriding message is that in the shadow of international trends towards the institutionalization of dying, people with terminal diseases such as advanced cancers are often unable to die in preferred settings. In an attempt to increase the proportion of supported deaths that can occur 'at home', policy makers and practitioners in some countries with anglophile health care systems and ageing populations are currently committed to promoting the philosophy and delivery of specialist palliative care services in the community.

However, my own research, reported briefly above, strikes a note of caution about the current policy push in the UK towards raising the proportion of home deaths. It warns that patients and carers may have sound reasons for desiring end of life options *other than home*, particularly the opportunity to die in a hospice. The reasons given for wanting to die in a hospice make perfect sense in many circumstances, whether formulated positively or in the spirit of resigned acceptance. These include: the limitations imposed by the quantity and quality of the informal care resource; individuals' living circumstances; the drive to protect loved ones and relieve them of the burden of care; the desire to sustain personal dignity once bodily control is lost; and the attraction of what is perceived to be very 'safe' professional care in the face of pain and other distressing symptoms. In a larger study, such reasons would no doubt manifest themselves in some patients expressing a preference to die in other institutional settings, especially in hospitals with specialist palliative care beds and services on site. One thing is certain: dying of cancer at home places demands on patients and informal carers that usually take them very far outside realms of 'normality' in their daily routines and emotional scales. The difficulties faced are often immense.

Given this, there ought, perhaps, to be a greater critical examination of the 'home is best' assumption. At the very least, service providers and planners everywhere should attempt to identify what the place of death preferences of their patients and carers are, *and to understand why these choices are made* – a prerequisite to meaningfully responding to them.

## Note

1   It should be noted that there were no specialist palliative care beds in the hospital sector in the study area at the time of the study.

## References

Beccaro, M., Costantini, M., Rossi, P.G., Miccinesi, G., Grimaldi, M. and Bruzzi, P. (2006) Actual and preferred place of death of cancer patients. Results from an Italian survey of the dying of cancer (ISDOC). *Journal of Epidemiology and Community Health*, 60: 412–16.

Brazil, K., Bedard, M. and Willison, K. (2002) Factors associated with home death for individuals who receive home support services: a retrospective cohort study. *BMC Palliative Care*. http://www.biomedcentral.com/1472-684X/1/2 (accessed July 2007).

Brown, M. and Colton, T. (2001) Dying epistemologies: an analysis of home death and its critique. *Environment and Planning*, 33: 799–821.

Bruera, E., Sweeny, C., Russell, N., Willey, J. and Palmer, J. (2003) Place of Death of Houston Area Residents with Cancer over a Two-Year Period. *Journal of Pain and Symptom Management*, 26(1): 637–43.

Cantwell, P., Turco, S., Benneis, C., Hanson, J., Neumann, C.M. and Bruera, E.

(2000) Predictors of home death in palliative care patients. *Journal of Palliative Care*, 16(1): 23–8.

Cartwright, A. (1991) Changes in life and care in the year before death 1969–1987. *Journal of Public Health Medicine*, 13(2): 81–7.

Clark, D. (2007) From margins to centre: a review of the history of palliative care in cancer. *Lancet Oncology*, 8: 430–8.

Clifford, C.A., Jolley, D.J. and Giles, G.G. (1991) Where people die in Victoria. *Medical Journal of Australia*, 155(7): 446–51.

Costantini, M., Balzi, D., Garroncc, E., Orlandini, C., Parodi, S., Vercelli, M. and Bruzzi, P. (2000) Geographical variations of place of death among Italian Communities suggest an Inappropriate hospital use in the terminal phase of cancer disease. *Public Health*, 114(1): 15–20.

Davies, E., Linklater, K.M., Jack, R.H., Clark, L. and Moller, H. (2006) How is place of death from cancer changing and what affects it? Analysis of cancer registration and service data. *British Journal of Cancer*, 95: 593–600.

Department of Health (2000) *The NHS Cancer Plan: A plan for investment. A plan for reform.* London: Department of Health.

Duffy, J.A., Irvine, E.A. and Shaw, D.R. (2002) Cancer deaths in Dundee – a Comparative Study. *Progress in Palliative Care*, 10(6): 280–2.

Dunlop, R.J., Davies, R.J. and Hockley, J.M. (1989) Preferred versus actual place of death: a hospice palliative care team experience. *Palliative Medicine*, 3: 197–210.

Ellershaw, J. and Ward, C. (2003) Care of the dying patient: the last hours or days of life. *British Medical Journal*, 326: 30–4.

Evans, W.G., Cutson, T.M., Steinhauser, K.E. and Tulsky, J.A. (2006) Is There No Place Like Home? Caregivers Recall Reasons for and Experience upon Transfer from Home Hospice to Inpatient Facilities. *Journal of Palliative Medicine*, 9(1): 100–10.

Gatrell, A.C., Harman, J.C., Francis, B., Thomas, C., Morris, S.M. and McIllmurray, M.B. (2003) Place of death: analysis of cancer deaths in part of north-west England. *Journal of Public Health Medicine*, 25(1): 53–8.

Gomes, B. and Higginson, I.J. (2006) Factors influencing death at home in terminally ill patients with cancer: systematic review. *British Medical Journal*, 332: 515–21.

Grande, G.E., Addington-Hall, J.M. and Todd, C.J. (1998) Place of death and access to home care services: are certain patient groups at a disadvantage? *Social Science and Medicine*, 47: 565–79.

Grundy, E., Mayer, D., Young, H. and Sloggett, A. (2004) Living arrangements and place of death of older people with cancer in England and Wales: a record linkage study. *British Journal of Cancer*, 91: 907–12.

Gyllenhammar, E., Thoren-Todoulos, E., Strang, P., Strom, G., Eriksson, E., and Kinch, M. (2003) Predictive factors for home deaths among cancer patients in Swedish palliative home care. *Supportive Care in Cancer*, http://www.springerlink.com/content/upmluthdrk35h3dx (accessed July 2007).

Herd, E.B. (1990) Terminal care in a semi-rural area. *British Journal of General Practice*, 40: 248–51.

Higginson, I.J. (1999) Which cancer patients die at home? District Data for North West Region, *Fact Sheet No. 31, Hospice Information Service*. London.

Higginson, I.J., Astin, P. and Dolan, S. (1998) Where do cancer patients die? Ten-year trends in the place of death of cancer patients in England, *Palliative Medicine*, 12: 353–63.

Higginson, I.J., Jarman, B., Astin, P. and Dolan, S. (1999) Do social factors affect where patients die: an analysis of 10 years of cancer deaths in England, *Journal of Public Health Medicine*, 21: 22–8.

Higginson, I. and Priest, P. (1996) Predictors of family anxiety in the weeks before bereavement. *Social Science and Medicine*, 43(11): 1621–5.

Higginson, I.J. and Sen-Gupta, G.J.A. (2000) Place of care in advanced cancer: a qualitative systematic literature review of patient preferences, *Journal of Palliative Medicine*, 3: 287–300.

Hinton, J. (1994a) Can home care maintain an acceptable quality of life for patients with terminal cancer and their relatives? *Palliative Medicine*, 8: 183–96.

Hinton, J. (1994b) Which patients with terminal cancer are admitted from home care? *Palliative Medicine*, 8: 197–210.

Hunt, R., Bonnett, A. and Roder, D. (1993) Trends in the terminal care of cancer patients: South Australia, 1981–1990. *Australian and New Zealand Journal of Medicine*, 23(3): 245–51.

Hunt, R. and McCaul, K. (1996) A population based study of the coverage of cancer patients by hospice services. *Palliative Medicine*, 10: 5–12.

International Observatory on End of Life Care (2007) www.eolc-observatory.net (accessed February 2008).

Karlsen, S. and Addington-Hall, J. (1998) How do cancer patients who die at home differ from those who die elsewhere? *Palliative Medicine*, 12: 279–86.

Moinpour, C. and Polissar, L. (1989) Factors affecting place of death of hospice and non-hospice cancer patients. *American Journal of Public Health*, 79: 1549–51.

Pritchard, R., Fisher, E., Tento, J., Sharp, S., Reding, D. and Knaus, W. (1998) Influence of patient preferences and local health system characteristics on the place of death. *Journal of the American Geriatric Society*, 46: 1242–50.

Seale, C. (2000) Changing patterns of death and dying. *Social Science and Medicine*, 51: 917–30.

Seale, C., Addington-Hall, J. and McCarthy, M. (1997) Awareness of Dying: Prevalence, Causes and Consequences. *Social Science and Medicine*, 45(3): 477–84.

Sims, A., Radford, J., Doran, K. and Page, H. (1997) Social class variation in place of cancer death. *Palliative Medicine*, 11: 369–73.

Thomas, C. (2005) The Place of Death of Cancer Patients: Can Qualitative Data Add to Known Factors? *Social Science and Medicine*, 60(11): 2597–607.

Thomas, C., Morris, S.M. and Clark, D. (2004) Place of death: preferences among cancer patients and their carers. *Social Science and Medicine*, 58(12): 2431–44.

Thorpe, G. (1993) Enabling more dying people to remain at home. *British Medical Journal*, 307: 915–18.

Townsend, J., Frank, A., Fermont, D., Dyer, S., Karran, O., Walgrove, A. and Piper, M. (1990) Terminal cancer care and patients' preferences for place of death: prospective study. *British Medical Journal*, 301(6749): 415–17.

# 6

# An uncertain journey

## Coping with transitions, survival and recurrence

*Margaret O'Connor*

---

**Key points**

- There are different models of illness in relation to experiences of chronic illness, prognostication, transition, survival and recurrence.
- Patients encounter a number of transitions as a dynamic experience of changes in illness.
- Survival and living with chronic illness has implications for the person adapting to changes in their life.
- In cancer, recurrence triggers the prospect of facing an early death and seeking meaning.

---

## Introduction

Traditional understandings of illnesses like cancer being a 'death sentence' are continually challenged as contemporary health care confronts new frontiers of treatment and cure. However, even though death rates of once predictable terminal illnesses are falling, many people are living with the aftermath of the illness itself and/or the treatment regimens. Chronic illness and associated morbidities, together with ageing populations in many industrialized countries, have the potential to change the community's demands on health care systems.

If we acknowledge that the illness experience includes a longer period of *living with* illness and its effects, a longitudinal understanding of illness that incorporates the whole illness 'journey' is appropriate. This requires consideration of various illness models as well as the personal implications of the end point – survival or recurrence.

This chapter examines a range of models and understandings of illness that contribute to how we both understand and manage chronic illness remission and recurrence. It is the transition response that is important rather than a focus on the outcome – further illness or survival.

# Chronic illness

Contemporary health care has seen exponential shifts in both the treatment and survival rates of illnesses like cancer that were once regarded as terminal, meaning more people are now living longer with the after-effects of their illness. This raises a related issue about the implications of care and care-giving for communities, as dependencies increase (Payne and Ellis-Hill 2001). Even cancer registries have not yet adjusted to monitoring the longer-term cancer survival rates, of 15 years or more (Brenner and Hakulinen 2002).

The presence of chronic illness in the community is increasing, if only because of advances in health technology and because people are living longer. Field and Cassell (1997) note that in countries like the United States of America, most people die of chronic illness. They suggest that 'many people are fearful that a combination of old age and modern medicine will inflict on them a dying that is more protracted and in some ways more difficult than it would have been a few decades ago' (p. 14). In the United Kingdom, people are also living longer especially because of improved cancer survival rates (CancerStats 2005).

In Australia, deaths from cardio-vascular disease have reduced by about 10 per cent; breast cancer death rates have fallen by nearly 20 per cent and cervical cancer death rates have fallen by about 40 per cent (Cresswell 2007). The consequence of falling death rates is greater numbers of people living with these illnesses for longer, with varying degrees of morbidity. Described as the 'tsunami of chronic illness' (Cresswell 2007: 29), this has meant that significant strategic planning is required. In public discourse about chronic illness, there appears to be a connection between encouraging population management of chronic illness rates and the adoption of national screening, awareness and health prevention strategies (Cresswell 2007). In other parts of the world, early detection and treatment programmes are regarded as strategies more likely to achieve successful outcomes. Bury (1997) suggests that falling death rates, together with more public health attention to particular illness risk factors, have led to an emphasis on health promotion strategies and surveillance or 'control' activities. The key tasks of these activities are:

> . . . to identify the disease or the risk of the disease at the earliest possible stage; to get patients to their doctors as soon as the disease, or the possibility of disease, was identified; and to ensure their early treatment by experts using a recognised means of treatment – generally surgery, radiotherapy, chemotherapy, or some combination thereof.
>
> (Cantor 2007)

Chronic illness may manifest in many forms – sudden or insidious onset, with episodic symptoms or remission, various trajectories and, perhaps, with the presence of co-morbidities. Chronic illness remains part of the person's life experience; there is no return to 'normal' life. Due to the uncertainty of the illness trajectory, the interface with palliative care services may be problematic, if referral is based on prognosis. People who have illnesses with the characteristics of chronicity may benefit from palliative care but may not be perceived as appropriate, because of a lengthy or uncertain prognosis. The individual experience of *living* with chronic illness is one that encompasses all aspects of the person's life, as well as the lives of those who support them and care for them (Kleinmann 1988). Chronic illness becomes a part of the person's current identity as well as part of projecting their life's journey looking into the future. Levealahti *et al.* (2007) describe this as the person's 'biographical map' as they look to a 'different destination' in terms of health outcomes (p. 471). The illness trajectory may vary in prediction and control and is both 'the pattern of illness and the work involved in managing the illness and treatment' (Germino 1998).

# Illness as a total experience

An aspect of meaning in chronic illness is for health professionals to seek understanding of the illness from *inside* an individual's experience, which necessarily requires taking a longitudinal view of issues like when the illness began, how the person understands their illness, how it affects them, what adaptations they have made – in other words, listening to their narrative. The individual meanings given to living with a chronic illness are shaped particularly by relationships to other people and the expectations shared in those relationships (Kleinman 1988). While each person's story will be highly individual, Bury (1997) highlights the importance for a lay person of 'labelling' their illness, at various stages along the illness trajectory; that is, the attribution of the disease identity and its social, biological and cultural consequences. Labelling forms an important part of the individual's illness narrative (Young 2004). Frank (1995) suggests that the activity of telling the illness story removes its passivity by providing an opportunity for healing, creating empathetic bonds between the teller and the listener, and thus widening the 'circle of shared experience' (p. xii). The gathering of these stories of individual experience, as opposed to seeking one common and dominant cultural experience, may assist others in understanding the illness journey. But individual stories many also add to the disparate postmodern view of illness and death, usually by emphasizing the highly personal nature of their individual experiences (Seale 1998). Kellehear and Howarth (2001) also describe uncertainty as part of illness – an 'unscheduled journey' in terms of near-death experiences and related illness experiences of other people (p. 71). The tension of holding the individual and the collective experience is one that Kellehear (2007) suggests is like 'gazing into a reflecting pool' – that beneath the individual images of self, lies the common influences of history and culture, which both shape our identity.

Illness narratives in the popular literature provide insight into the ways that people view the experience of illness (Kellehear and Ritchie 2003). For some, illness may be one continuous journey (Bayley 1998); for others, it may be viewed as a series of un/related acute episodes (Birnie 1998). These stories illustrate highly individual examples of coping (de Beauvoir 1964; Shields 1994); creating meaning from difficulty (Orchard 2003); the importance of resilience (Deveson 2003); emergent understandings of oneself (Deveson 2003; Orchard 2003) and the consequent changes in life roles (Jennings 2002). Responses to living with chronic illness, evidenced in narratives, encompass aspects like physical, behavioural, cognitive and emotional responses, which reflect the complexity of its impact on not just the physical person, but their mind and spirit as well.

A total view of illness needs to encompass understandings of the chronic characteristics of illness; balancing the simultaneous treatments aimed at cure and symptom management; the day-to-day management of unstable symptoms; redefining the individual's view of themselves; exerting control; and the ongoing social and psychological adjustments that may be required (Corbin and Strauss 1988; Germino 1998). Many types of illness including cancer, once treated with the goal of seeking cure (and death was regarded as almost inevitable but nevertheless, a failure when it occurred), now undergo treatments aimed at enabling people to live longer, to increase their quality of life and to experience periods of remission. Thus people are *living* with their illnesses, with the associated issues of treatment and lifestyle limitations, not necessarily *dying* from them. A more active community perception of chronic illness, rather than being a reminder of illness and death, can challenge general cultural and social dimensions of death (McNamara 2001).

This understanding of the individual's broad experience, offers the health professional a different world view than one that concentrates on the current clinical manifestation of disease; a view that is particularly pertinent in the practice of palliative care. In clinical encounters, it may be expedient to filter all information that is extraneous to the presenting clinical issue. However, this approach risks a limited view of the person's individual response to their illness and the immediacy of its impact on their lives.

A longitudinal view of illness affords a different understanding of the impact of illness on a person's life. This may be particularly pertinent if the person is older and/or has an uncertain diagnosis or prognosis. Instead of considering the different aspects that make up the total person – physical, social, spiritual, emotional, cultural – this view takes account of the person's whole experience of life, situating illness as part of that experience, which will necessarily involve all aspects of the person. In viewing illness this way, transition then becomes a phase along that trajectory – be it from health to illness, illness to further illness leading to death, or illness to remission or cure (O'Connor 2004).

# Prognostication

Models that recognize different illness trajectories and patterns of functional decline in relation to different illnesses have been postulated over many years. Glaser and Strauss (1965) first described three different illness trajectories – abrupt, surprise deaths; expected deaths (both short term and long term; and entry-reentry deaths, where the person slowly declines over time and intermittently accesses care as required. It is suggested that diagnosing 'incurable, progressive disease that is expected to prove fatal is among the most difficult and sobering judgements that physicians make' as well as 'an exercise in uncertainty' (Field and Cassell 1997: 30). Having said that, however, predicting the course of an illness and prognostication is sometimes utilized as the basis for funding; thus with implications for policies about end-of-life care (Field and Cassell 1997). Prognostication may involve anticipating the length of life as well as the impact of illness on quality of life. Nevertheless there is an acknowledgement that any measures of prognosis are 'inherently imperfect' (Thibault 1997).

Goldstein (2006) challenges the community stereotype of the dying trajectory – the illness decline, taking to one's bed and dying on time – but suggests that this is where the model of hospice care arose. Lunney *et al.* (2003) studied functional decline before death, the results suggesting a sharper decline in function for those with cancer than for those people with other chronic illnesses, with age and medical condition affecting some differences. They also added another category of illness – that of those with diseases like heart disease who decline functionally, but retain a reasonably high level of performance, continuing many activities of life while coping with the prospect of death at any time.

Measuring their results against the United States Government Medicare funding for hospice care, Lunney *et al.* (2003) argue that funding models based on a predicted trajectory and prognosis are inappropriate. Suggesting that their work is based on 'clinical intuition' (p. 2390), they challenge the 'one-size-fits-all' models of end-of-life and palliative care, particularly when diseases like cancer, which are to some extent predictable, represent a comparatively small number of the cause of overall deaths.

# The 'sick role'

Parsons' (1951) seminal writing began a discussion of the mainly acute illness experience through connecting the disciplines of medicine and sociology. Drawing on psychoanalytic theory, he proposed that 'the sick role' was in deviance to societal norms because the sick person is unable to fulfill their obligations to society, by way of work and other responsibilities (Lupton 1997). In this understanding of illness, being healthy is the ideal or 'good'; ill health is thus 'bad' or negative and connotes individual loss of control of one's life (Lupton 1997). Within this framework one can understand the development of illness discourses utilizing combative language like 'fighting the battle' and 'the war on cancer'.

In Parsons' view (1951), the sick person is not necessarily in possession of the wherewithal to get well, being reliant on the medical role to provide such expertise and knowledge. In psychoanalytic terms, this is understood as an unequal, dependent relationship, not unlike that of the parent–child relationship. It is the doctor who facilitates the person's new identity into the sick role and who controls when they move out of the role in pronouncing recovery (Lupton 1997). Because Parsons' work was with acute illness, the illness experience was time limited and passing; once over, the person returns to their life's routine. Parsons further developed his concept of illness as an option for the individual to withdraw from their responsibilities in a socially acceptable way, provided it is not for too long; the goal always being the patient's duty to get completely well or at the very best to 'manage' their chronic illness (Parsons 1975: 259).

Moving away from the negative connotations of Parson's sick role as deviance, Kleinman (1988, 1992) and Fife (1995) emphasize the all-encompassing meanings of illness – the individual understandings of the implications of illness, changes in their sense of identity, their social world and interpersonal relationships. Kleinman (1988) has described this shift in perceptions of illness thus:

> Unlike cultural meanings of illness that carry significance *to* the sick person, this intimate type of meaning transfers vital significance from the person's life to the illness experience (p. 31).

More recent critiques of Parson's work centre around the passive interpretations of the sick role, where the doctor knows best, to the detriment of the ill person's inherent knowledge and ability to take control of their own situation (Lupton 1997; Rier 2000). Rier (2000) attributes shifts in the doctor–patient relationship to influences like feminism, consumerism, self-help and patient groups and ideologies of empowerment (p. 74). More ready access to information sources like the Internet presents the semblance of increased personal control.

# Biographic disruption

Of particular note arising from the developing literature about a more active response to the experience of chronic illness, is the notion of 'biographical disruption'. Bury (1991) suggests that this occurs as a consequence of the uncertainty, rather than the predicted trajectory, of chronic illness. Coming to terms with chronic illness involves understanding of both the meaning and the context of the illness. For the individual, biographical disruption encompasses changes to the body, and changes in the social and cultural constructions of their life (Bury 1991).

Bury (1997) describes the consequences and the significance as two concerns of chronic illness. Consequences involve adaptation to the way that the illness disrupts the everyday activities of family life and work. A concern about the significance of illness means coming to terms both with the impact of illness on individual identity, as well as communal understandings (real and symbolic) of the particular illness. For example, a community misperception that cancer is contagious may prevent a person's return to work.

Even though the naming of a condition with a particular diagnosis may alleviate anxiety about what is unknown, adaptation becomes continuous as an illness progresses. And meanings also change over the trajectory of illness; the individual may test out altered meanings within their surroundings; and the perception of others about the individual's illness may change over time, from being chronic to terminal.

Uncertainty about the course of an illness may involve 'watchful waiting', or watchfulness, an approach to care that involves 'unobtrusive supervision' (*Mosby's Dictionary* 2002) and observation of an illness before further testing or treatment options are considered. Much of the literature using this term is related to the treatment of prostate cancer (Steinbeck *et al.* 2002) where it may be a strategy employed when there is no harm in waiting, where treatment directions are unclear or where there are significant risks in treatment, which outweigh the potential benefits. However, Payne (2007) suggests that for an individual, balancing the incongruence of medical surveillance in conjunction with no treatment may cause anxiety. Indeed, the uncertainty of the disease status, coupled with the need for regular checkups, may cause more anxiety than undergoing active treatment (Jones and Payne 2000).

# Transition

> passage . . . change from one place or state to another
> (*The Australian Oxford Dictionary* 2004)

By its very definition transition is a dynamic experience; that is, it involves movement and change within the person. Transitions are part of life's journey, and a familiar term in developmental theory (Erikson 1968), to be expected along life's course.

Transition is common to many experiences in life, in response to either natural and expected phases or unexpected occurrences (Bridges 1996); illness may be one such occurrence. Transition in illness may either be in relation to surviving and coping with the chronicity of illness or facing the implications of recurrence. It is a major transition when a person has been chronically ill for some time and then the illness becomes terminal and, in particular, the tangible reminder of the limitations of treatment options.

Bridges (1996) suggests that rather than identifying periods of specific change in life (for example, the mid-life crisis), adulthood is at once a continuous process which 'unfolds its promise in a rhythm of expansion and contraction, change and stability' (p. 42). Transition is a highly individual experience, involving different experiences of illness, particularly 'the unpredictable timing of death' (Lunney *et al.* 2003); over which the person has little control (O'Connor 2004). All transitions involve letting go, which may be a most difficult and ambiguous task because one may be surprised to 'discover that some part of us is still holding on to what we used to be' (Bridges 1996: 12).

This creates disorientation, the loss of meaning in life and a consequent fear of the emptiness created. This is described as 'disidentification' (Bridges 1996: 96); that is, not being able to identify *oneself* anymore; this may be most readily seen externally, through changes in social roles, particularly work or when illness necessitates an inability to perform certain roles. A period of 'inbetween-ness' is characterized by an inability to draw on familiar patterns of behaviour and psychological supports, because they either do not work, or are not appropriate any more. The onset of illness can be an unfamiliar experience for the individual, creating uncertainty in the previously familiar patterns of life, changes in one's view of their physical self, and social disruption.

Part of the confusion of transition is not that of facing new beginnings; rather, it is the loss of what has gone before, even if it is of little use in the movement forward and a task of transition becomes unlearning, not necessarily to learn anew. One way to assist an individual in the illness transition, to understand their response to letting go, is to recall other experiences of transition in their life that are not necessarily illness related. Other strategies utilized in transition may involve the individual seeking information about what is happening, and creating substitute activities for what they are no longer able to undertake. Even developmental experiences of letting go, shared by all as we grow from one stage of life to another, can provide the individual with insight into their own pattern of response to letting go – from fully grappling with the challenge of change, to a response arising from anxiety and fear.

'Endings' in the experience of transition, may occur throughout the illness trajectory – but particularly at diagnosis, when one begins to grapple with its meaning, marking the beginning of a distinctive journey. Ending a treatment cycle may also be a trigger, when one is declared to be in remission; or when disease recurs, because each of these events demands a re-thinking of what was before in order to move into the future.

The person may experience discomfort, characterized by them needing to shift their priorities in response to reflection on what has occurred for them. Described as 'endings' by Bridges (1996), this can be a chaotic experience, a time when one's familiar life patterns and personal supports do not appear to work any more and choices appear to narrow (Germino 1998). In the illness experience, this time can be felt when one receives a new diagnosis, when the person is grappling with the implications of recurrence or remission, or when someone is recovering from illness but is not fully recovered. A tangible example of discomfort may be when the person experiences the irreversibility of changes that have occurred, like not being able to shower independently. This time may also involve re-evaluating one's personal goals in relation to the medical goals (Bury 1991).

Re-evaluation may mean a threat to the person's identity; many patients may 'report feeling fragile; their ongoing sense of identity, of who they are, has been drastically affected by the disruption to their lives' (Germino 1998: 581). Coping with a new identity is evidenced in a variety of ways, from directly confronting the circumstances, accepting the permanency of the changed circumstances, or conditionally acknowledging that maybe their condition will improve. But Germino (1998) suggests that a failure to acknowledge change prevents the person from moving through this time of transition.

New beginnings only occur when the endings have been completed and may appear to be a time of starting life again, perhaps in fulfilment of long-held dreams, or of changing direction in work or lifestyle. Some people may use the illness experience as the impetus for creating long-yearned-for changes in their lives. Beginnings may offer an individual time to attain some perspective about their illness, to 're-establish their credibility in the face of the assault on self-hood . . .' (Bury 1991: 456). This may involve taking risks, returning from the isolation of the illness experience, to grapple with what life now offers.

> Endings and beginnings, with emptiness and germination in between. That is the shape of the transition periods in our lives, . . . the same process is going on continuously in our lives.
>
> (Bridges 1996: 150)

New beginnings during illness may commence when a person has negotiated a treatment regime, when active treatment is ceased and when a period of remission is begun. For some people, beginnings may involve the realization that life will be shortened if treatment has not succeeded; thus the challenge is to use the remaining time as they wish. One may also begin to consider oneself a cancer survivor if treatment has been successful, and commence to negotiate life with a changed outlook or values.

# Survival

Due to increasing recognition of public health policy in screening and early detection, together with more effective treatment, increasing numbers of people in industrialized countries with once terminal illnesses like cancer consider themselves to be survivors. Seeking a definition of a survivor is difficult, since there is subjectivity to this status, as well as a changing understanding, depending on different phases of illness and treatment. Frank (1995) describes the 'remission society' in reference to those people who, though not considered cured of their illness, were nevertheless well. Payne (2007: 430) suggests that survivors 'have to simultaneously inhabit the world of the "healthy" population and the world of the "patient" ' in the follow-up medical surveillance they undergo. Mullen (1985) used the term 'seasons of survival' to connote that survival is cyclical and that it is not uniquely attached to a cured state. He described three states of survival – acute, extended and permanent.

There appears to be a dearth of research in relation to survivorship; reports appear mainly in the psychosocial literature, suggestive of a lack of recognition of issues of survival in mainstream medicine (Schou and Hewison 1999). The difficulties of finding oneself as a survivor are compounded at a communal level, since Little *et al.* (2001) also suggest that the shared discourse on survival is underdeveloped (p. 139).

Theoretical work on the relationship between stress and illness may also provide a basis for understanding individual responses to being a survivor. In particular, Taylor's model (1983) of cognitive adaptation is pertinent. This involves the individual's search for meaning in attempting to understand what has happened to them; gaining control in order to manage what has happened or keep it from recurring; and the process of self-enhancement whereby coping strategies involve restoring the individual's self-esteem (Feuerstein *et al.* 1987).

The work of Little *et al.* (2001) has contrasted the inspirational literature about individual resilience, with that of the difficulty of being a survivor. Individual survivor difficulties arise because the person is unable to completely move to new beginnings. This is why when listening to their narrative, survivors describe their illness experience as integral to their identity, especially in relation to being vulnerable to the possibility of recurrence and the subsequent impact on all aspects of their social life.

Little (2001) suggests that in developing a discourse of survivorship, there are several important factors:

- 'the way we construct our identities and the multiple selves we express in our relationships;
- some of the categories of the survival experience, including vulnerability, disempowerment, the need to preserve "face", the need for approval and the pressure survivors feel to pay something back for their survival;
- the nature of extreme experience and the effect it has on identity' (p. 18).

Personal identity, understood simply as 'the core of our being in the world' (Little *et al.* 2001: 19), is essential in understanding the way that surviving occurs. Continuity of memory is a distinctive part of identity, which among other things serves to construct the individual's narrative of illness (Little *et al.* 2002). One aspect of memory that is important in understanding survival is described by Little as 'future memory' (p. 171), which involves the individual imagining looking back at stages of life that are yet to occur – a young man with a poor prognosis imagining himself as a grandfather, for example, and placing a value on what he anticipates that experience to mean. This loss is significant because it arises from the meaning that is applied to the expectations of a predictable life span. The discontinuities in narratives reflect discontinuity in identity, especially if these anticipated life experiences are important aspects of the individual's identity.

Coming to terms with one's identity as a survivor may take considerable time, with many unable to complete this journey. In the process of becoming a survivor, the individual may experience anger, restlessness, alienation and dislocation and Little *et al.* (2002) suggest that this is because continuity of identity has been interrupted, impaired or alienated. If the community narrowly interprets survival to mean cure, there is an underlying expectation that survival means that the person's life will return to 'normal' – relationships will be resumed, work will re-commence and the patterns of life will be restored. 'The sense of continuity is of central importance in the experience of survivorship, whatever adaptive direction is taken' (Little *et al.* 2002: 176).

Some work has addressed the difficulties of cancer survivors in their return to normal life, in particular their working life (Tehan 2006). Spelten *et al.* (2002) studied the experiences of the return to work of cancer survivors, finding a lack of systematic research had been undertaken. They suggest that return to work rates varied considerably, with influencing factors like a supportive work environment that facilitates ease of return. Visible cancers (e.g. head and neck) disadvantage the person's return to their workplace, but age was not found to be a factor. Most employers were accommodating, particularly if the illness involved disability. It has also been postulated that:

> Perhaps maintaining their employment after diagnosis is entangled with access to comprehensive health insurance and treatment, as well as psychological reasons such as empowerment and the ability to maintain a sense of control.
>
> (Bradley and Bednarek 2002: 197)

It is a challenge for the survivor to make a new beginning, all the more so because of a lack of communal discourse about survival. Some survivors may be regarded as fortunate, 'lucky' to be alive, when others have died; others may remain in dependency relationships adopted during the illness. The beginning phase of transition however, challenges the person beyond old roles and expectations, to develop a new identity, new values, altered relationships and social roles (Little *et al.* 2001). These adaptations may be difficult, simply because of the ever-presence of the illness experience as integral to identity; and the sense that at some level, many people never move beyond the neutral (liminal) stage, remaining caught in a partial adaptation.

The most important assistance one can be to a survivor, is in the development of a discourse of survival – helping people to articulate their own narrative. Individual narratives will contribute to the development of a communally understood framework for articulating the experience, thus legitimizing the survivor state (Little *et al.* 2001).

# Recurrence

If the period of transition turns into the person needing to face an early death, Davies *et al.* (1995) suggest that change is integral – in one's social life, relationships, family life and work; as well as in roles and responsibilities. There is considerable literature that suggests that while the prospect of an untimely death is distressing for people to consider, what causes more distress is the process of dying – the prospect of dependency, a slow decline and social disengagement (Lawton 2000; Pollard and Swift 2003). A major task at this stage of life is searching for meaning – to put the experience 'in context and endure the turmoil' . . . 'connecting with their inner and spiritual selves, connecting with others or with nature' (Davies *et al.* 1995: 43).

Day-to-day living becomes the important concern and the goal of each day may change as the impact of disease progression is felt. Literature describes this phase as one where discussion about the transition to palliative care may be appropriate (Pollard and Swift 2003). There may, however, be confusion in the person's mind about what this transition means, because of disagreements between health professionals over the goal of care, the false dichotomizing of palliative care and treatment for cure, and ambiguous language (Pollard and Swift 2003; Seymour 2004; O'Connor 2005). Continuous conversations with different members of the health care team at this stage of the person's disease may assist in clarifying care goals and who might be the most appropriate person to offer such care.

Ideally, the transition from active treatment to palliative care should occur over a period of time, involving the person and other decision-makers in every step. Nurses may find themselves acting as 'coaches' in facilitating the person and their family members in this journey and in assisting them to express uncertainties, to gain as much information as they need and to adjust to their changing circumstances (Aranda and Kelso 1997). Clinicians need to undertake their own reflective exploration of how they understand this coaching role in their encounters with those in their care and not be afraid to take the conversational opportunities that present themselves in providing understanding and guidance as the person negotiates their transition.

With recurrence, there will necessarily be an experience of a 'cascade of losses' (Payne 2007) as part of what is happening to the person and their family. The consistent and ongoing relationship of the nurse may be pivotal in assisting the ill person and their family members to understand what is happening, to validate mixed emotions and to facilitate communication as they address issues relevant to their future.

The ill person and their family members will have varying needs for information about how the illness will progress, especially the various support roles that may be expected of them. They especially require reassurance of ongoing support in all settings of care – at home, in the acute hospital or the hospice – and of the range of choices that are available to them. Accurate and timely information is an essential part of care at this stage of life and the nurse needs to keep information sources up to date.

It is not uncommon for the ill person to seek information and assistance about what may occur at the end of life, which may involve statements requesting assistance to die. The reasons for these requests are highly personal and need to be understood from the perspective of the individual. It has been noted that requests may also fluctuate over time (Hudson *et al.* 2006). Nurses need to purposely develop a sensitive ear in picking up requests for assistance in dying and ensure they are skilled in responding appropriately.

In addition to providing reassurance about symptom management and other aspects of the process of dying, if requested, the nurse may facilitate discussion about planning for the funeral, and seek assistance with financial matters and making a will.

# Conclusion

This chapter has highlighted the complex issues in seeking understandings of illness, particularly in relation to chronic illness, remission and recurrence. With changes in medical treatment and improved survival rates, the line between cure and remission may sometimes not be as clear as it once was. Viewing shifts in illness as part of the overall illness experience creates an encompassing framework that promotes continuity of experience rather than highlighting separate stages. For the individual, however, it is their own experience of illness and transition, as they *cope with* and *live with* the effects of illness; as its centrality ebbs and flows within the total pattern of their life, rather than necessarily being focused on the outcome.

# References

Aranda, S. and Kelso, J. (1997) The nurse as coach in care of the dying. *Contemporary Nurse*, 6: 117–22.

Bayley, J. (1998) *Iris*. London: Abacus.

Birnie, L. (1998) *A good day to die*. Melbourne: Text Publishing Company.

Bradley, C.J. and Bednarek, H.L. (2002) Employment patterns of long-term cancer survivors, *Psycho-Oncology*, 11: 188–98.

Brenner, H. and Hakulinen, T. (2002) Very long-term survival rates of patients with cancer, *American Journal of Clinical Oncology*, 20(21): 4405–8.

Bridges, W. (1996) *Transitions: making sense of life's changes*. London: Redwood Books.

Bury, M. (1991) The sociology of chronic illness: a review of research and prospects. *Sociology of Health & Illness*, 13(4): 451–68.

Bury, M. (1997) *Health and illness in a changing society*. London: Routledge.

CancerStats (2005) *UK Incidence London*. Cancer Research UK.

Cantor, D. (2007) Introduction: cancer control and prevention in the twentieth century. *Bulletin of the History of Medicine*, 81(1): 1.

Corbin, J. and Strauss, A. (1988) *Unending work and care: managing chronic illness at home*. San Francisco, CA: Jossey-Bass.

Cresswell, A. (2007) Preventing heart disease offers the biggest saving. *The Australian*, Canberra, 29.

Davies, B., Reimer, J.C., Brown, P. and Martens, N. (1995) *Fading away: the experience of transition in families with terminal illness*. New York: Baywood.

de Beauvoir, S. (1964) *A very easy death*. London: Penguin.

Deveson, A. (2003) *Resilience*. Crows Nest: Allen & Unwin.

Erikson, E. (1968) *Identity, youth and crisis*. New York: W. W. Norton.

Feuerstein, M., Labbe, E.E. and Kuczmierczyk, A.R. (1987) *Health psychology: a psychobiological perspective*. New York: Pelium Press.

Field, M.J. and Cassell, C.K.E. (1997) *Approaching death: improving care at the end of life*. Washington: National Academy Press.

Fife, B.L. (1995) The measurement of meaning in illness. *Social Science and Medicine*, 40(8): 1021–8.

Frank, A. (1995) *The wounded storyteller: body illness and ethics*. London: University of Chicago Press.

Germino, B.B. (1998) When a chronic illness becomes terminal. *American Nephrology Nursing Journal*, 25(6): 579–82.

Glaser, B. and Strauss, A. (1965) *Awareness of dying*. Chicago: Aldine.

Hudson, P., Kristjanson, L., Ashby, M., Kelly, B., Schofield, P., Hudson, R., Aranda, S., O'Connor, M. and Street, A. (2006) A systematic review of the desire for hastened death in patients with advanced disease and the evidence base of clinical guidelines. *Palliative Medicine*, 20: 703–10.

Jennings, K. (2002) *Moral hazard*. Sydney: Pan McMillan.

Jones, G.Y. and Payne, S. (2000) Searching for safety signals: the experience of medical surveillance amongst men with testicular teratomas. *Psycho-Oncology*, 9(5): 385–94.

Kellehear, A. (2007) *A social history of dying*. Port Melbourne: Cambridge University Press.

Kellehear, A. and Howarth, G. (2001) Shared near-death and related illness experiences: steps on an unscheduled journey. *Journal of Near Death Studies*, 20(2): 71–85.

Kellehear, A. and Ritchie, D. (2003) *Seven dying Australians*. Bendigo Innovative Resources.

Kleinman, A. (1988) *The illness narratives: suffering, healing and the human condition*. New York: Basic Books.

Kleinman, A. (1992) Local worlds of suffering: an interpersonal focus for ethnographies of illness experience. *Qualitative Health Research*, 2(2): 127–34.

Lawton, J. (2000) *The dying process: patients' experiences of palliative care*. London: Routledge.

Levealahti, H., Tishelman, C. and Ohlen, J. (2007) Framing the onset of lung cancer biographically: Narratives of continuity and disruption. *Psycho-Oncology*, 16: 466–73.

Little, M., Paul, K, Jordens, C. and Sayers, E.J. (2001) *Surviving survival: life after cancer*. Sydney: Choice Books.

Little, M., Paul, K, Jordens, C. and Sayers, E.J. (2002) Survivorship and discourses of identity, *Psycho-Oncology*, 11: 170–8.

Lunney, J., Lynn, J., Foley, D., Lipson, S. and Guralnik, J. (2003) Patterns of functional decline at the end of life. *Journal of the American Medical Association*, 289(14): 2387–91.

Lupton, D. (1997) Psychoanalytic sociology and the medical encounter: Parsons and beyond. *Sociology of Health and Illness*, 19(5): 561–79.

McNamara, B. (2001) *Fragile lives: death, dying and care*. Crows Nest: Allen & Unwin.

*Mosby's Medical, Nursing & Allied Health Dictionary* (2002) St Louis, Mosby Inc.

Mullen, F. (1985) Seasons of survival: reflections of a physician with cancer. *New England Journal of Medicine*, 313: 270–3.

O'Connor, M. (2004) Transitions in status from wellness to illness, illness to wellness – coping with recurrence and remission. In: J. Seymour, S. Payne and C. Ingleton (eds) *Palliative Care Nursing* (1st edn). Maidenhead: Open University Press, pp. 126–41.

O'Connor, M. (2005) Mission statements: an example of exclusive language in palliative care? *International Journal of Palliative Care Nursing*, 11(4): 190–6.

Orchard, S. (2003) *Something More Wonderful*. Sydney: Hodder.

Parsons, T. (1951) *The Social System*. New York: The Free Press.

Parsons, T. (1975) The sick role and the role of the physician reconsidered. *Millbank Memorial Fund Quarterly*, 53: 257–78.

Payne, S. (2007) Living with advanced cancer. In: M. Feuerstein (ed.) *Handbook of Cancer Survivorship*. Springer: New York, 24: 429–46.

Payne, S. and Ellis-Hill, C. (2001) *Chronic and terminal illness: new perspectives on caring and carers*. Oxford: Oxford University Press.

Pollard, A. and Swift, K. (2003) Communication skills in palliative care. In: M. O'Connor and S. Aranda (eds) *Palliative Care Nursing: A Guide to Practice*. Melbourne: Ausmed.

Rier, D.A. (2000) The missing voice of the critically ill: a medical sociologist's first-person account, *Sociology of Health & Illness*, 22(1): 68–93.

Schou, K.C. and Hewison, J. (1999) *Experiencing cancer*. Buckingham: Open University Press.

Seale, C. (1998) *Constructing death: the sociology of dying and bereavement*. Cambridge: Cambridge University Press.

Seymour, J. (2004) What's in a name? In: J. Seymour, S. Payne and C. Ingleton (eds) *Palliative Care Nursing* (1st edn). Maidenhead: Open University Press, pp. 55–75.

Shields, C. (1994) *The stone diaries*. New York: Penguin.

Spelten, E.R., Sprangers, M.A.G. and Verbeek, J.H.A. (2002) Factors reported to influence the return to work of cancer survivors: a literature review, *Psycho-Oncology*, 11(2): 124–31.

Steinbeck, G., Helgesen, F., Adolfsson, J., Dickman, P., Johansson, J.E., Norlen, B.J. and Holmberg, L. (2002) Quality of life after radical prostatectomy or watchful waiting. *The New England Journal of Medicine*, 347(11): 790–6.

Taylor, S.E. (1983) Adjustment to threatening events: A theory of cognitive adaptation. *American Psychologist*, 38: 1161–73.

Tehan, M. (2006) *Developing a best practice support model for life-threatening illness in the workplace: a literature report*. Melbourne: Palliative Care Victoria.

*The Australian Oxford Dictionary* (2004) South Melbourne: Oxford University Press.

Thibault, G.E. (1997) Prognosis and clinical predictive models for critically ill patients. In: M.J. Field and C.K. Cassel (eds), *Approaching death: improving care at the end of life*. Washington: National Academy Press, pp. 358–62.

Young, J.T. (2004) Illness behaviour: a selective review and synthesis. *Sociology of Health & Illness*, 26(1): 1–31.

# 7

# Communication
## Patient and family

*Sue Duke and Christopher Bailey*

---

**Key points**

- Communication is fundamental to both health and effective health care.
- There are particular challenges to effective communication in palliative care that are raised by the threat of death inherent in life-threatening illness.
- Most definitions of communication emphasize information giving and emotional support: both are important to communication being perceived as effective.
- Communication is complex and influenced by a range of contextual factors.
- Skills training has been shown to be beneficial, though application in practice may be problematic.
- Support for practitioners (clinical supervision) is an essential part of effective palliative care.

---

## Introduction

Effective communication is fundamental to health. It provides a means by which people relate to each other and through which social relationships are built. Such relationships provide a sense of belonging and security and contribute to how people define themselves and how they describe their identity. In addition, relationships provide social support networks that can be drawn on at times of difficulty. Such networks have been shown to be one of the most important resources available to people to mitigate the impact of illness or bereavement (Osterweis *et al.* 1984). When these relations are jeopardized by illness or bereavement, social isolation and loneliness, fear, anxiety and depression can result.

Apart from positively influencing patient satisfaction, communication is central to the effectiveness of treatment, care and outcome (Davis and Fallowfield 1991) and to people's psychological health (Fallowfield and Jenkins 1999). In research examining palliative care nursing, effective communication has been shown to influence a person's sense of well-being (Richardson 2002), enable needs to be identified and met (Aranda and Street 1999; Bortoff *et al.* 2000; Morgan 2001; Mok and Chiu 2004), put people at ease so that their fears can be addressed (McLoughlin 2002; Houtepen and Hendrikx 2003) and to mitigate isolation and helplessness (Dunne and Sullivan 2000; Dunniece and Slevin 2002).

Poor health care communication, on the other hand, is associated with erosion of trust and misunderstanding of illness (Thorne *et al.* 2005). It invalidates personal experience, negatively influences an individual's ability to manage their illness in the context of their everyday lives (Thorne *et al.* 2004), and contributes to a feeling that 'nobody understands' (Okon 2006). It also decreases the likelihood that patients will disclose their concerns and so reduces the likelihood of clinicians recognizing psychological consequences of illness (such as anxiety and depression) (Thorne *et al.* 2005). Ineffective communication also has consequences for health care professionals, which include increased stress, lack of job satisfaction and burnout (Wilkinson *et al.* 2002). Indeed, as Thorne *et al.* (2005) conclude in their detailed review of the communication literature in cancer care, the costs of poor communication are 'potentially enormous' and include 'economic, social, psychological, emotional, and collateral costs to the patient, the patient's support network, the clinicians, the . . . care system and to . . . society' (pp. 880–1).

The threat of death that accompanies life-threatening illness raises particular challenges to effective communication in palliative care. Okon (2006) points to the difficulty of understanding and putting into words the experience of dying and the suffering that can result both from the experience (and from not being able to communicate this experience) and from health care professionals being reluctant to listen to this experience. In addition, dying threatens (since death severs) the social bonds that provide comfort, security and support and makes self-identity harder to hold together (Seale 1998), particularly when this is associated with a physically disintegrating body (Seale 1998; Kearney 2000; Lawton 2000). It signals 'the end of everything that we have known and lived' and consequently brings intensity to what is perceived as precious and meaningful (Cobb 2001: 49). Effective communication in palliative care needs to attend to the meaning of the threat of death to an individual and the people important to them and the associated losses, potential regrets and anxieties that may be raised as a consequence (Kearney 2000; Cobb 2001; Okon 2006). However, talking about death and dying with patients is difficult and complex. Not only is it difficult because it is hard to imagine what the experience is like (Okon 2006) but it needs sensitivity and careful timing (McGrath 2004).

# Defining communication

There are many definitions of communication in health care and nursing (see McCabe and Timmins 2006 for an overview and critical debate). One definition that has been influential in nursing communication research is provided by Wilkinson who sees effective communication as a two-way process in which patients are informed about the nature of their disease and treatment and are encouraged to express their anxieties and emotions (Wilkinson 1991, 1992; Kruijver *et al.* 2000).

While this definition is disease and treatment focused, which may or may not be relevant to people with palliative care needs depending on their illness progression, it emphasizes two common goals of communication – providing information and giving emotional support. These goals require different but complementary communication behaviours. Kruijver *et al.* (2001) describe those related to informing patients about their disease and treatment as 'instrumental behaviours' and those related to providing emotional support (for example, showing respect and providing comfort and trust) as 'affective behaviours'.

The process of providing information and support is emphasized within the definition provided by Davis and Fallowfield (1991), according to which communication means 'enabling individuals to describe their problems, and listening sufficiently well that the helper can grasp the meaning and offer appropriate advice' (p. 24). Davis and Fallowfield draw on the distinction between surface and deep learning, the former being associated with advice that is constituted by informational facts and the latter focused on enabling understanding by taking account of personal meaning and significance. They stress the importance of the latter: 'nothing can occur except in the context of the individual's understanding, values, desires, expertise and environment' (p. 26) and point to the importance of working in partnership with people.

Most definitions of communication include three concepts: sender, message and receiver. In its simplest form communication is conceived as a linear process in which a sender transmits a message to a receiver (Figure 7.1). Although the one-directional nature of communication depicted in this model is characteristic of certain kinds of communication, such as information-giving or email correspondence, it is inadequate to explain the complexities of health care communication. There are a number of issues that influence the sender, the message and the receiver and how these inter-relate to ensure patient-focused and effective communication. These need to be taken into account in any theory of health care communication.

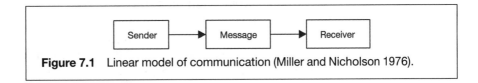

**Figure 7.1**   Linear model of communication (Miller and Nicholson 1976).

# Issues influencing communication

### *'Noise'*

DeVito (2002) describes four sources of 'noise' in communication:

- Physical noise in the environment such as patient call bells, bleeps, tele-phone calls, monitor and infusion pump alarms. As well as having the potential to distract or interrupt communication, there is some evidence that these stimuli are associated with clinical errors, and health care professional and patient/family member stress (Donchin and Seagull 2002). Furthermore, bleeps and pagers contribute to what Coiera and Tombs (1998) describe as an 'interruptive workplace' and can hinder communication between colleagues because the importance of the mes-sage has to be inferred from (insufficient) information conveyed by these forms of contact.

- Physiological noise, such as hearing loss for example, as well as fatigue and physiological illness, both of which make concentration and reten-tion of information difficult.

- Psychological noise, such as sender/receiver beliefs and values. Infor-mation about disease progression and symptom management is likely to be influenced by a person's perceptions of illness and their beliefs about nurses' willingness to discuss health, illness and dying. For exam-ple, people with chronic heart failure interviewed in a study by Rogers *et al.* (2000) attributed their symptoms to age rather than to their illness and as a consequence believed nothing could be done about their symptoms.

- Semantic noise, or how words are understood in different ways in differ-ing contexts. Fallowfield *et al.* (2002a) provide an example of this in relation to a doctor–patient interaction discussing the decision not to continue with chemotherapy because things were 'progressing'. When the patient was asked immediately after the consultation what the doctor had said, he said that it had been good news. The word progressing had been seen as positive, meaning that his cancer was improving.

### *Communication medium*

In addition to 'noise', communication is also influenced by the medium used to send the message:

- Written information – information given verbally and reinforced with written information is more likely to be remembered than information given only verbally, although this is dependent on issues such as the readability and comprehensibility of the written information (Ley 1988).

- Internet – health information provided on the internet tends to be used to assess or to add detail to the information provided by health care professionals, rather than being used as a sole source of information

(Herxheimer and Ziebland 2004). Although the internet predominately presents information in a linear way, when information is expressed in lay terms and through personal experience narratives, it becomes a means of providing emotionally supportive communication by enabling people to see their experience in relation to others' (Herxheimer and Ziebland 2004).

- Telephone – Street and Blackford (2001) found that personal visits were more effective than telephone contact for nurses trying to establish successful community palliative care networks, as communication by phone can easily be thwarted (for example, by receptionists 'protecting' their GP). Breaking bad news by phone should be avoided because personal contact provides much greater scope for providing support or assessment (Von Gunten *et al.* 2000). In some circumstances, however, telephone communication has been used as part of successful palliative care interventions. In their comparison of nurse-led follow-up and medical follow-up for patients with advanced cancer, for example, Moore *et al.* (2002, 2006) included telephone monitoring for patients receiving nurse-led follow-up to identify progression, symptoms requiring further intervention, or serious complications. Satisfaction scores for patients in the nurse-led group were significantly higher than those for the group receiving medical follow-up.

### Clinical context

Communication is also influenced by the setting in which it takes place. Clinical environments can often be geographically distant and difficult to reach (Rogers *et al.* 2000) and have financial implications, such as travel and parking costs that can be prohibitive to patients and families wishing to talk face-to-face with clinicians. In addition, poor signage, lack of assistive communication technology and bad customer care make them physically and emotionally daunting places to navigate (Freeney *et al.* 1999).

This lack of attention to facilitating access can be complicated by organizational processes that are designed for professional rather than patient and family/carer benefit (Allen 2001) and that are often focused on treatment and outcome rather than on care (Allen 2001; Foster and Hawkins 2005). Such processes foster a nursing focus on physical care and 'getting the work done' (McCabe 2004; Clarke and Ross 2006). This focus prevents patients and family members/carers with palliative care needs from communicating and participating in decision-making (Dunne and Sullivan 2000; Clover *et al.* 2004; Willard and Luker 2006).

Central to addressing these contextual influences on communication is the emotional climate valued and nurtured within clinical settings. Smith (1992) found that if ward sisters demonstrated emotional concern for staff and modelled psychosocial support through their relationships with them, the ward nurses were more likely to work with patients in a way that explored their emotional concerns. On the other hand, if a ward sister demonstrated an instrumental approach ('getting the work done'), nurses were more likely to avoid working with patients' emotional experience.

Studies of nurses in palliative care highlight the experience of 'being pulled in all directions' (Thompson *et al.* 2006) and the tension between operational expectations and the desire to meet people's emotional and palliative care needs (Seymour *et al.* 2002; Willard and Luker 2006). The extent to which this tension can be balanced is influenced by the distribution of nursing care – how far it has to stretch. When it is stretched too far in the direction of operational priorities rather than the emotional support needs of patients and family members, then communication becomes superficial and ineffective, not least because nurses' emotional resources are outstripped by the physical energy needed to get through the day (Clarke and Ross 2006).

### Patient-centredness of health care professionals

Communication is not only influenced by the emotional climate of care but also by the nature of the relationship between patients and professionals. More will be said about this in relation to nursing a little later but, in summary, where communication is patient-focused and occurs within a relationship conceived as a partnership, then communication is likely to be effective and appropriate to an individual's need for information and emotional support (see De Valck *et al.* 2001 for a discussion of this in relation to the World Health Organization Model of Breaking Bad News). When this is the case, knowledge is likely to be managed by both the patient and the professional. If, however, the relationship is conceived as either led by the doctor (paternalistic, the knowledge is owned by the doctor who decides what to tell the patient) or led by the patient (as in consumerist models of care, according to which the patient is told everything and expected to manage this knowledge), then communication is likely to focus on facts and information to the exclusion of emotional support (Ford *et al.* 1996; De Valck *et al.* 2001; Clover *et al.* 2004).

Communication with patients is also influenced by the relationship between professionals. Where a good working relationship exists, communication between team members and with patients and their family/carers is likely to be appropriate and effective (Allen 2001). On the other hand, if working relationships are characterized by discouragement of inter-professional discussion, then the quality of communication with patients and their family/carers will be negatively influenced (Allen 2001; Coombs 2004).

### Communication behaviour

Communication is facilitated by both verbal and non-verbal (or para-linguistic) communication. Speech rate and volume, facial expression, eye contact, posture, gesture and touch are important in establishing rapport and showing empathy and support (Kruijver *et al.* 2000). Personal and professional qualities such as kindness, warmth, compassion and genuineness are also important (Mok and Chiu 2004; Johnston and Smith 2006) as is being perceived as being confident and having expertise (Randall and Wearn 2005).

These behaviours need to be shaped to meet the needs of a particular patient or family member. In palliative care nursing this has been described as a balance between being authentic (true to self, personally and professionally) and being a chameleon, the type of nurse that a patient wants for a particular moment of care (Aranda and Street 1999), and as a balance between the values of palliative care and being adaptable to a person's way of life (Brännström *et al.* 2005). This combination of behaviours and qualities may help patients feel more able to disclose those concerns raised by being confronted with a life-threatening illness.

Communication behaviour is also influenced by health care professionals' perception of their ability (self-efficacy), the outcome that they anticipate, and the support they perceive or consider to be available to them. Parle *et al.* (1997) consider these influences to be inter-related and together they influence health care professionals' discussion of patient concerns (Figure 7.2). The success of communication behaviour is 'multi-determined' in the sense that levels of knowledge and skill, self-efficacy, outcome expectancies, and practical and psychological support all have a part to play (Parle *et al.* 1997).

## Theories of communication

The influences on communication, discussed above, have been variously accounted for within general communication theories by circular or feedback

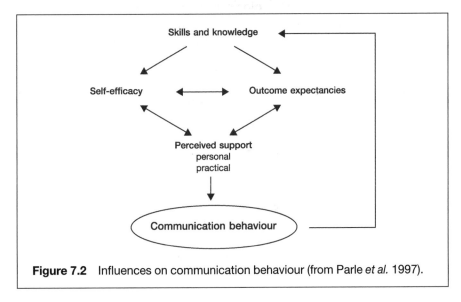

**Figure 7.2**   Influences on communication behaviour (from Parle *et al.* 1997).

models of communication, as summarized in Figure 7.3 (see Guirdham 1995 or McCabe and Timmins 2006 for an overview) or, alternatively, within psychological theories of communication (see Rungapadiachy 1999 for an overview) or organizational change theories (for example, Egan's (1985) systems model of communication and change).

In nursing, these influences have been theoretically situated within discussion of nurse–patient relationships. Communication is portrayed as central to nurse–patient/carer relationships and, in turn, relationships are conceived as the means by which care, comfort and self-management or independence are fostered (Morse *et al.* 1992; Haggerty and Patusky 2003; Edwards *et al.* 2006). This link has been supported in palliative care nursing research in studies from nurses' perspectives (Aranda and Street 1999; Luker *et al.* 2000; Dunniece and Slevin 2002; Mok and Chiu 2004), patient and carers' perspectives (Dunne and Sullivan 2000; McLoughlin 2002; Mok *et al.* 2002; Richardson 2002; Mok and Chiu 2004), and in studies that have considered both nurse and patient perspectives (Bottorff *et al.* 2000; Morgan 2001; Johnston and Smith 2006).

Nursing theories of communication have tended to focus on classifying varying kinds of nurse–patient relationships. For example, Haggerty and Patusky (2003) propose a theoretical model based on the degree of relatedness and comfort provided by nurse–patient communication. They describe four states of relatedness:

- Connection – the active involvement between nurse and patient which promotes comfort and a sense of well-being.
- Disconnection – the lack of active involvement between nurse and patient with concomitant anxiety, distress or lack of well-being.
- Parallelism – partial involvement between nurse and patient which, if wished by the patient, can have positive results by promoting solitude and psychological and physical renewal.
- Enmeshment – intense involvement between nurse and patient, characterized by anxiety, distress and functional difficulties.

While such categorizations are helpful in making the connection between communication and a person's well-being they have the disadvantage of polarizing different kinds of relationships – 'connected' and 'disconnected',

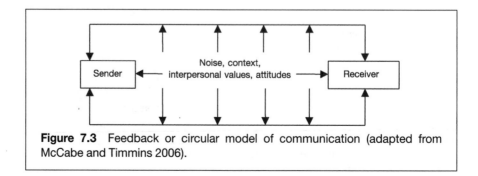

**Figure 7.3** Feedback or circular model of communication (adapted from McCabe and Timmins 2006).

for example, or 'enmeshed' and 'parallel'. As a consequence one kind of relationship can easily be perceived as being better than another (connected is good, disconnected is bad) without consideration of either patient preference (a patient may not want to develop a relationship with a particular practitioner, for example) or the contextual influences required to support effective communication. A further consequence of this theoretical categorization is that responsibility for the quality of the relationship and an individual's care appears to lay only with the nurse, rather than the nature of the relationship being seen as a consequence of interpersonal and contextual processes.

Furthermore, nursing communication theories do not account for the communication undertaken by nurses acting as intermediaries or in a liaison capacity to influence the context of communication in order to ensure good palliative and end-of-life care. As noted by Coombs (2004) this work is fundamental to clinical decision-making. However, since much of it takes place away from the bedside its contribution is less likely to be recognized by nurses, other health care professionals or patients (Corner *et al.* 2003; Coombs 2004) and yet this is often emotionally and morally difficult work (Seymour *et al.* 2002; Varcoe *et al.* 2004; Brännström *et al.* 2005). This 'invisible' communication practice has been shown in palliative care nursing to positively influence:

- coordination and continuity of care (Street and Blackford 2001; Skilbeck and Seymour 2002; Corner *et al.* 2003);
- change in direction of care – referral and support of patients and family in the transition to palliative care (Shotton 2000; Ronaldson and Devery 2001; Thompson *et al.* 2006);
- education and development of other professionals' understanding of palliative care (Jack 2002; Mytton and Adams 2003).

# The process of communication

### Common sequence of communication processes

One other shortcoming of theories of communication is that they do not always describe the process of communication as it happens on the ground between people when they communicate, or explore what fosters and hinders this process. To summarize, in nursing care communication can be seen as consisting of five interconnected sequences (synthesized from Egan 1985; Baile *et al.* 2000; Kendrick and Robinson 2002; Hudson *et al.* 2006):

- greetings and introductions
- listening to and understanding the other person's story
- exploring how this story might change and what this possibility feels like
- agreeing a plan to manage the things that might cause the story to change

- summarizing, providing follow-up and contact details, saying goodbye.

This process is inherent in assessment, the process of eliciting patient and family members/carers concerns, breaking bad news, and managing difficult conversations, such as desire to die statements (see Table 7.1).

A range of skills are required to facilitate the process of communication described above (summarized in Table 7.1), such as the ability to ask open questions, to seek clarification and to provide emotional comfort. Hudson *et al.* (2006) provide good examples of these skills in relation to palliative care practice but they are best learnt through skills-based education. Using these skills appropriately depends on being able to understand the patient or family members'/carers' perspective and on having empathy with another person's concerns, viewpoints and experiences.

### Perspective taking

Empathy is the process of imaginatively, sensitively and emotionally sensing another person's world. It involves being able to separate aspects of ourselves from aspects of others ('decentring') and the ability to accurately perceive other people's feelings. Lobchuk (2006) and others make an important distinction between *empathy* ('feeling into') and *sympathy* ('feeling with'). Whereas empathy involves sensing *another person's* perspective, sympathy is more a matter of imagining how *you* would feel if you were in another person's situation. It is argued on this basis that it is empathy that supports the exchange of thoughts, feelings and information that characterizes good communication, rather than sympathy.

Lobchuk (2006) speaks of sympathy as possibly leading to over-involvement with or attachment to others, and points out that this may have unwanted consequences in terms of distorted perceptions of other people's experiences; she also identifies a 'dysfunctional' form of empathy, or 'empathetic distress', which may arise when care-givers experience other people's suffering and are motivated as a result to alleviate their own distress through attending to others.

Research by Lobchuk and Vorauer (2003) with family care-givers has sought to test whether taking the patient's perspective is more effective than taking one's own perspective in terms of estimating cancer symptom experiences. The researchers compared care-givers' estimates of patients' lack of energy and worrying when using 'imagine-self' perspective-taking (i.e. imagining oneself with the patient's diagnosis) with estimates when using 'imagine-patient' perspective-taking (i.e. imagining how the patient feels and thinks, or putting oneself 'in the patient's shoes'). 'Imagine-patient' instructions were found to consistently increase the accuracy of estimates of patients' self-reported lack of energy and worrying relative to estimates following 'imagine-self' instructions, leading the researchers to conclude that engaging in some level of patient perspective-taking allows care-givers to achieve more accurate estimates of symptom experiences.

Lobchuk (2006) views perspective-taking as a key part of effective care-giving but raises questions about how well it is understood and suggests that a better understanding is required to support the development of care-giving skills and the monitoring and assessment of patients' experiences. Patient-orientated perspective-taking is seen as part of the sensitivity needed for 'seeing the patient's world from the patients' cognitive or emotive viewpoint' and providing effective assessment and symptom management (Lobchuk *et al.* 2006). 'Imagine-self' perspective-taking, on the other hand, tends to produce overestimates of patient symptom experiences and greater discrepancy between care-giver assessments and patient's self-reports, and therefore may increase the possibility of 'suboptimal' symptom management (Lobchuk *et al.* 2006).

These discussions of perspective-taking have important implications for palliative care nursing practice. First, they offer a way to enhance the symptom management care provided by family members by encouraging family members to use 'imagine-patient' perspectives rather than 'imagine-self' perspectives. Second, they offer a way of enhancing nurse–patient communication. The skill to imagine what an experience is like for a particular patient or a family member is a crucial part of ensuring that communication and the care subsequently offered is congruent with the person's experience, that it is patient-centred. This skill is fundamental to breaking bad news and to managing difficult conversations in palliative care.

## Breaking bad or significant news

Bad news is defined as 'any information which adversely and seriously affects an individual's view of his or her future' (Buckman 1992). This definition emphasizes the unknowable impact that news might have on an individual and this is central to the difficulty of communicating significant information to patients and families.

However, bad news has a salience in people's stories of their illness and this makes it possible to understand the potential impact of such information. Bad news features in particular places in illness stories, contributing to the structure of these stories. People often commence their illness story by relating the events experienced in relation to being told that they have an illness (diagnosis) and the development of this story is organized in relation to the points at which progress is medically assessed (for example, response to treatment, prognosis). Whether someone can make sense of these parts of their story is very much dependent on the quality of communication that occurs at the time the news is discussed and on whether opportunities are available to rehearse the news subsequently.

Very often palliative care nursing involves listening to people's accounts of what they have been told in the course of their illness. Listening carefully to people's stories provides ways in which nurses can support patients and family members. Providing an opportunity for a person to tell their story enables that person to tell the story out loud and to hear the story for

**Table 7.1** Common processes of communication and related skills

| General pattern of communication process | Communication process (Egan 1998) | Breaking bad news – SPIKES protocol (Baile et al. 2000) | Managing difficult conversations – e.g. responding to desire to die statements: general recommended principles (Hudson et al. 2006) | Skills needed to achieve processes involved |
|---|---|---|---|---|
| Greetings and introductions | | Set up the interview | Be alert to your own responses | Environmental awareness Awareness of social support needs Safety awareness Self-awareness |
| The story so far | Current scenario – a) listening to a person's story | Assess the patient's perception | Be open to hearing concerns | Active listening Reflecting Paraphrasing |
| | b) exploring the story from different angles (clarifying, exploring contradictions) | | Assess the potential contributing factors | Checking understanding Asking open questions Summarizing Gently challenging and exploring |
| | c) focusing and moving forward | Obtain the patient's invitation | | Facilitating focusing and prioritizing (giving a warning in breaking bad news, or making a list of things that need addressing and which is most pressing in assessment) |

| | | | | |
|---|---|---|---|---|
| How this might change or be thought about differently | Preferred scenario:<br>a) imagining how something might be different<br>b) reality testing and goal setting<br>c) moving forward | Give knowledge and information to the patient<br><br>Address the patient's emotions | Respond to specific issues | Giving information in language that can be understood<br>Pacing information<br>Knowing when to be quiet<br>Recognizing a person's emotional reaction<br>Validating a person's feelings<br>Responding to a person's emotional reaction<br>Helping a person to imagine what the new information means<br>Answering questions |
| Plan for next steps | Action strategies:<br>a) exploring possibilities<br>b) deciding what to do and how it can be done<br>c) deciding what things need to be done and in what order | Plan a strategy and summarize | Conclude the discussion (summarize, offering follow-up and support) | Summarizing<br>Action planning |
| Conclude – endings | | Document, liaise with others | Document, liaise with others | Skills in managing confidentiality appropriately<br>Skills in liaison |

themselves, something that helps make the story believable (Mok and Chiu 2004). It also provides an opportunity for refining how to tell the story – what words to use and what information it is important to tell. In this way, listening to patient and family members'/carers' stories is a way of helping them, to use Thorne *et al.*'s (2004) phrase, 'craft a life' that is inclusive of their illness, to rewrite their biography. In addition, it provides an opportunity for nurses to understand what else is needed for the person to make sense of the story – helping them to fill in the gaps by providing missing information and helping to reframe the information that was provided.

There is much discussion about how best to communicate news that could be considered significant or bad. Clearly, the emphasis here is on what Berry (2007) refers to as 'human understanding', rather than technical information. Lloyd and Bor (1996) suggest that breaking bad news should start with what patients already know and understand and then move on to finding out what they want to know (Berry 2007). A number of models have been developed to assist health care professionals. The SPIKES protocol provides a process for breaking bad news (Baile *et al.* 2000) (Box 7.1), the ABCDE model consists of techniques to guide the environmental and communication conditions for delivering bad news (Rabow and McPhee 1999) (Box 7.2), and there are others that have drawn on key principles (for example, Randall and Wearn 2005) (see below).

The SPIKES protocol (Baile *et al.* 2000) was, according to the authors, developed in response to advances in the treatment and care of people with cancer that, while offering more hope, have also increased the need for skills in discussing recurrence, spread, failure of treatment, serious side effects,

---

**Box 7.1**   Summary of SPIKES protocol for delivering bad news (Baile *et al.* 2000)

**Step 1: S – Setting up** the interview
**Step 2: P** – Assessing the patient's **Perception**
**Step 3: I** – Obtaining the patient's **Invitation**
**Step 4: K** – Giving **Knowledge** and information to the patient
**Step 5: E** – Addressing the patient's **Emotions** with empathic responses
**Step 6: S – Strategy** and **Summary**

---

**Box 7.2**   Summary of ABCDE model of breaking bad news (Rabow and McPhee 1999)

**A**dvance preparation
**B**uild a therapeutic environment relationship
**C**ommunicate well
**D**eal with patient and family reactions
**E**ncourage and validate emotions (reflect back emotions)

results of genetic tests, hospice care and resuscitation. Randall and Wearn (2005) focus on 'receiving bad news' rather than 'breaking bad news', which, they suggest, is doctor- rather than patient-centred, as it is doctors or other health care professionals who break the news and patients who receive it. Following a series of interviews with patients with haematological cancers, they highlighted a number of important points based on the patient's perspective, including:

- the bad news consultation is the beginning of a journey not an isolated event and sets the scene for the future
- the consultation should not be rushed and the patient should be allowed to express their feelings and ask questions
- feelings about 'touch' are mixed: there is no 'recipe' that can be applied to all individuals
- the term 'disease' was unpopular and patients wanted explanations in familiar language
- being given adequate factual information reduced fear of their condition
- discussing treatment options was seen as positive, but the question of who should take the lead in decision-making was less easily resolved
- information leaflets were valued, as were continuity and the development of a relationship
- patients were strongly in favour of a companion being present
- the setting should be private and preferably familiar.

Much of what has been said in the earlier part of the chapter about the process of communication and the issues that influence it is also of value in managing the communication of bad news. Some useful interactive resources on communication skills, including breaking bad news, can be accessed via the EDINA website based at the University of Edinburgh in the UK (www.edina.ac.uk).

# Managing difficult conversations

Difficult questions in palliative care have been described as conversations that are associated with feelings of discomfort and inadequacy on the nurse's part (McGrath *et al.* 1999). They are typically related to discussing death and dying with patients and their family members/carers. Communication skills training and experience can provide confidence in dealing with these kinds of conversations. However, most difficult conversations in palliative care are characterized by existential concerns (Houtepen and Hendrikx 2003). As a consequence, although the process of communication is similar to that described above and in Table 7.1, they have particular characteristics that skills training cannot mitigate. The nature of the dynamics within such conversations evokes strong feelings associated with being a witness to the suffering experienced by another person and with being unable to change the circumstances that are at the centre of this suffering. As they are associated with the experience of suffering, the issues that are raised in these conversations are often expressed with a sense of immediacy and urgency about them: they are expressed 'from the heart'. These kinds of concerns need communication skills that are about being sensitive to the meaning of what is being raised and being able to discern how and why it is of importance to that person's experience. There is no ready set of responses that will provide a nurse with these skills, although there is guidance in the literature about the types of replies that might be helpful (for example, see Hudson *et al.* 2006 for possible ways in which to respond to statements about desire to die). Rather more importantly this work is about communicating a willingness to stay with someone while they are suffering. In addition, it requires an ability to 'hold' someone's distress, to experience the feelings associated with the distress experienced by someone else and to be willing to work with these feelings (Jones 1999).

# Communication skills training

Good communication between health care professionals and patients is recognized as essential for quality care and, as discussed above, there is much that is known about what characterizes good communication. However, clinicians still lack adequate skills, patients continue to be unhappy with the amount of information they are given and the way in which it is given to them (Fallowfield *et al.* 2002b), and there is a lack of attention to emotional consequences of this information (Ford *et al.* 1996).

One explanation for this has been the lack of communication skills training provided for health care professionals and the fear of the consequences of talking to patients about their predicament (Maguire *et al.* 1996a, 1996b; Booth *et al.* 1999). Furthermore, research has shown that the more effective health care professionals become in eliciting patient concerns, the more worried they are about undertaking this work (Booth *et al.* 1996; Maguire *et al.* 1996a, 1996b). For example, the number of blocking behaviours (responses that inhibit further discussion) employed by hospice nurses increased in patient interactions following communication skills training (Booth *et al.* 1996). This indicates the complexity of enhancing communication through skills training and emphasizes the importance of considering all of the issues that influence communication when assessing the effectiveness of this training and in instigating practice development.

While good communication between health professionals and patients is a core clinical skill and essential for the delivery of high quality care (Department of Health 2000), communication skills do not improve reliably with time or experience alone (Cantwell & Ramirez, 1997; Fallowfield *et al.* 2002b; Fellowes *et al.* 2004). Consequently, there has been an increased effort in recent years in the UK to improve training in this area and to evaluate the effects of training programmes (Department of Health 2000; Fellowes *et al.* 2004; Gysels *et al.* 2004, 2005).

Booth and Maguire (1989) produced a detailed framework for evaluating assessment interviews with patients that has been used widely in subsequent research into the effects of communication skills training (see, for example, Razavi *et al.* 1993; Razavi *et al.* 2002; Liénart *et al.* 2006). Using this framework, interviews with patients can be assessed in terms of interviewer techniques, content, level of psychological disclosure (i.e. the extent to which feelings are disclosed) and 'blocking' tactics (i.e. when the interviewer moves the discussion away from issues raised by the patient or sidesteps distressing material). The process of facilitating disclosure of key concerns is seen as being undermined by leading questions, questions with a physical focus, clarification of physical issues, and premature advice, but as being supported by open directive questions, questions with a psychological focus, clarification of psychological aspects, educated guesses and empathic statements (Booth *et al.* 1999).

Fellowes *et al.* (2004) conducted a systematic review of communication skills training for health care professionals working with cancer patients, families or carers to assess the effectiveness of communication skills training in changing health professionals' behaviour. They identified three randomized controlled trials (Razavi *et al.* 1993; Fallowfield *et al.* 2002b; Razavi *et al.* 2002) and concluded that there is evidence that communication skills training can have a beneficial effect on the behaviour of trained health care professionals. The study by Fallowfield *et al.* (2002b) was highlighted in particular as showing that oncologists' skills improved following communication skills training. In this study, 160 oncologists were allocated to one of four groups: written feedback followed by three-day course, course only, written feedback only, and a control. The three-day course was residential and learner-centred, with participants working in groups of three to five led by an experienced facilitator with a team of patient simulators who provided constructive feedback. Filmed clinic consultations were reviewed at the beginning of the course to help participants to identify the communication problems most important to them. This was followed by role-play with simulated patients, video review and group discussion to work on ways of resolving problems (Fallowfield *et al.* 1998, 2002b). Feedback packs included analysis of participants' communication skills, satisfaction scores and comments from patients, and a measure of how closely participants' rating of patients' distress and understanding of information accorded with patients' own reports.

Results from the study suggest that those who attended the course were more patient-centred after it than they were before, and used more focused questions, expressions of empathy, and appropriate responses to patients' cues, compared with those who did not attend. These changes were felt to offer a number of benefits to patient care:

- fewer leading questions and more appropriate use of open or focused open questions improves dialogue with the patient and may provide better information about symptoms and side effects

- more expressions of empathy encourage a better relationship with the patient who may feel more valued and able to disclose important information
- summarizing complex information may assist patients' understanding of treatment advice and support informed decision-making (Fallowfield *et al.* 2002b).

In a recent review of the effectiveness of methods used in communication training courses Gysels *et al.* (2004, 2005) considered 16 papers covering 13 different interventions. They pointed out that all studies demonstrated some significant improvements, although in one (Heaven and Maguire 1996) levels of blocking behaviour increased following the intervention.

Overall, they suggest that health professionals can learn to communicate more effectively with patients who have cancer, although there are some important qualifications. While studies that focus on enhancing attitudes or objective skills have positive results, the evidence that improved skills are applied in practice is less clear. It is possible, however, that interventions that take attitudes and beliefs into account produce better results, and that an integrated approach that includes areas such as death and dying and raising self-awareness can significantly improve the confidence of nurses in key areas of their practice (Gysels *et al.* 2004).

## Conclusion

Communication is fundamental to health because it enables people to develop relationships that are important for a sense of belonging and a sense of identity. Effective communication is essential because it underpins effective treatment and care and contributes to psychological well-being and patient satisfaction. Poor communication, on the other hand, can undermine trust, spread misunderstanding and negatively influence job satisfaction among health care professionals. In palliative care, the work of communicating effectively is complicated by the knowledge that death may be close, and requires sensitivity, timing and compassion. Communication in these circumstances should convey the message that patients are safe and treasured as individuals (MacDonald 2004), and both patients and their families need to feel that death and dying will be a dignified, comfortable and caring process (Berry 2007).

Communication in health care involves both giving information and providing emotional support, and each of these requires different skills. Providing emotional support by showing respect or establishing trust requires, in particular, that we take account of personal significance – the things that mean something or matter to someone – and that we work with people in caring partnerships. Communication in health care is more complex than a simple linear relationship between sender, message and receiver would suggest, and we should take the many influences on communication into account (including the various forms of 'noise' and the clinical context) when considering theoretical models.

Communication involving significant or bad news can be particularly demanding for health care professionals. A number of models have been suggested that may help us to manage this process, and understanding the human need to tell and re-tell our stories of receiving difficult news and to be listened to as this story unfolds and gradually takes account of life-changing events is important. Communications skills training has been found to be beneficial in a number of research studies, although it is less clear that the benefits are transferred from research to practice settings. There are some aspects of palliative care, including the witnessing of suffering, that require a particular kind of expertise that has to do with a willingness to stay with and 'hold' the distress of others.

The nature of communication in palliative care nursing makes it important that professional support is available to practitioners. Jones (1999), quoting Lerner (1978), describes caring for the dying as a 'heavy and blessed experience'. He emphasizes the importance in psychological and emotional nursing of listening carefully to patients' stories and allowing them to talk about their suffering, and argues that supervision, guidance and support are essential to successful involvement in such difficult work. This is a point that is also apparent in some evaluations of communication skills training, which suggest that the courses with the clearest benefits also have a strong element of guided review and reflection (see Fallowfield *et al.* 2002b, for example). In palliative care nursing, which frequently takes place in close proximity to illness, grief and sometimes bereavement, an appropriate form of supervision, in which nurses are able to process and refine the thoughts, feelings and impressions from clinical practice (Jones 1999), is probably essential to effective practice.

# References

Allen, D. (2001) *The Changing Shape of Nursing Practice*. London: Routledge.

Aranda, S. and Street, A.F. (1999) Being authentic and being a chameleon: nurse–patient interaction revisited. *Nursing Inquiry*, 6: 75–82.

Baile, W.F., Buckman, R., Lenzi, R., Glober, G., Beale, E.A. and Kudelka, A.P. (2000) SPIKES – A six step protocol for delivering bad news: Application to the patient with cancer. *The Oncologist*, 5: 302–11.

Berry, D. (2007) *Health Communication: Theory and Practice*. Maidenhead: Open University Press.

Booth, K. and Maguire, P. (1989) *Workshop Evaluation Manual*. Report to Cancer Research Campaign.

Booth, K., Maguire, P.M., Butterworth, T. and Hillier, V.F. (1996) Perceived professional support and the use of blocking behaviours by hospice nurses. *Journal of Advanced Nursing*, 24: 522–7.

Booth, K., Maguire, P. and Hillier, V.F. (1999) Measurement of communication skills in cancer care: myth or reality? *Journal of Advanced Nursing*, 30(5): 1073–9.

Bottorff, J., Steele, R., Davies, B., Porterfield, P., Garossino, C. and Shaw, M. (2000) Facilitating day-to-day decision making in palliative care. *Cancer Nursing*, 23(2): 141–50.

Brännström, M., Brulin, C., Norberg, A., Boman, K. and Strandberg, G. (2005) Being a palliative care nurse for persons with severe congestive cardiac failure in advanced homecare. *European Journal of Cardiovascular Nursing*, 4: 314–23.

Buckman, R. (1992) *Breaking Bad News: A Guide for Health Care Professionals*. Baltimore: Johns Hopkins University Press.

Cantwell, B.M. and Ramirez, A.J. (1997) Doctor–patient communication: a study of junior house officers. *Medical Education*, 31(1): 17–21.

Clarke, A. and Ross, H. (2006) Influences on nurses' communications with older people at the end of life: perceptions and experiences of nurses working in palliative care and general medicine. *International Journal of Older People Nursing*, 1: 34–43.

Clover, A., Browne, J., McErlain, P. and Vandenberg, B. (2004) Patient approaches to clinical conversations in the palliative care setting. *Journal of Advanced Nursing*, 48(4): 333–41.

Cobb, M. (2001) *The Dying Soul*. Buckingham: Open University Press.

Coiera, E. and Tombs, V. (1998) Communication behaviours in a hospital setting: an observational study. *British Medical Journal*, 316: 673–6.

Coombs, M. (2004) *Power and Conflict between Nurses and Doctors*. London: Routledge.

Corner, J., Halliday, D., Haviland, J., Douglas, H-R., Bath, P., Clark, D., Normand, C., Beech, N., Hughes, P., Marples, R., Seymour, J., Skilbeck, J. and Webb, T. (2003) Exploring nursing outcomes for patients with advanced cancer following intervention by Macmillan specialist palliative care nurses. *Journal of Advanced Nursing*, 41(6): 561–74.

Davis, H. and Fallowfield, L. (1991) *Counselling and Communication in Health Care*. Chichester: Wiley.

Department of Health (2000) *The NHS Cancer Plan*. Department of Health, London. http://www.dh.gov.uk/en/Publicationsandstatistics/Publications/PublicationsPolicyAndGuidance/DH_4009609 (accessed 10 July 2007).

De Valck, C., Bensing, J. and Bruynooghe, R. (2001) Medical students' attitudes towards breaking bad news: an empirical test of the World Health Organisation Model. *Psycho-Oncology*, 10: 398–409.

DeVito, J.A. (2002) *Human Communication – The Basic Course* (9th edn). Massachusetts: Allyn and Bacon.

Donchin, Y. and Seagull, F.J. (2002) The hostile environment of the intensive care unit. *Current Opinion in Critical Care*, 8(4): 316–20.

Dunne, K. and Sullivan, K. (2000) Family experiences of palliative care in the acute hospital setting. *International Journal of Palliative Nursing*, 6(4): 170–8.

Dunniece, U. and Slevin, E. (2002) Giving voice to the less articulated knowledge of palliative nursing: an interpretive study. *International Journal of Palliative Care*, 8(1): 13–20.

Egan, G. (1985) *Change Agent Skills in Helping and Human Service Settings*. Monterey, CA: Brookes/Cole.

Edwards, N., Peterson, W.E. and Davies, B.L. (2006) Evaluation of a multiple component intervention to support the implementation of a 'Therapeutic Relationship' best practice guideline on nurses' communication skills. *Patient Education and Counselling*, 63: 3–11.

Fallowfield, L., Lipkin, M. and Hall, A. (1998) Teaching senior oncologists communication skills: results from phase I of a comprehensive longitudinal program in the United Kingdom. *Journal of Clinical Oncology*, 16: 1961–8.

Fallowfield, L. and Jenkins, V. (1999) Effective communication skills are the key to good cancer care. *European Journal of Cancer*, 35(11): 1592–7.

Fallowfield, L.J., Jenkins, V.A. and Beveridge, H.A. (2002a) Truth may hurt but deceit hurts more: communication in palliative care. *Palliative Medicine*, 16: 297–303.

Fallowfield, L., Jenkins, V., Farewell, V., Saul, J., Duffy, A. and Eves, R. (2002b) Efficacy of a Cancer Research UK communication skills training model for oncologists: a randomised controlled trial. *Lancet*, 359: 650–6.

Fellowes, D., Wilkinson, S. and Moore, P. (2004) Communication skills training for health care professionals working with cancer patients, their families and/or carers. *Cochrane Database of Systematic Reviews*, Issue 2. Art. No.: CD003751. DOI: 10.1002/14651858.CD003751.pub2.

Ford, S., Fallowfield, L. and Lewis, S. (1996) Doctor–patient interactions in oncology. *Social Science and Medicine*, 42(11): 1511–19.

Foster, T. and Hawkins, J. (2005) The therapeutic relationship: dead or merely impeded by technology? *British Journal of Nursing*, 14(13): 698–702.

Freeney, M., Cook, R., Hale, B. and Duckworth, S. (1999) *Working in Partnership to Implement Section 21 of the Disability Discrimination Act 1995 Across the NHS*. London: Department of Health.

Guirdham, M. (1995) *Interpersonal Skills at Work* (2nd edn). Oxford: Prentice Hall.

Gysels, M., Richardson, A. and Higginson, I.J. (2004) Communication training for health professionals who care for patients with cancer: a systematic review of effectiveness. *Supportive Care in Cancer*, 12: 692–700.

Gysels, M., Richardson, A. and Higginson, I.J. (2005) Communication training for health professionals who care for patients with cancer: a systematic review of training methods. *Supportive Care in Cancer*, 13: 356–66.

Haggerty, B.M. and Patusky, K.L. (2003) Reconceptualising the nurse–patient relationship. *Journal of Nursing Scholarship*, 35(2): 145–50.

Heaven, C. and Maguire, P. (1996) Training hospice nurses to elicit patients' concerns. *Journal of Advanced Nursing*, 23(2): 280–6.

Herxheimer, A. and Ziebland, S. (2004) The DIPEx project: collecting personal experiences of illness and health care. In: B. Hurwitz, T. Greenhalgh and V. Skultans (eds), *Narrative Research in Health and Illness*. Oxford: BMJ Books, Blackwell, pp. 115–31.

Houtepen, R. and Hendrikx, D. (2003) Nurses and the virtues of dealing with existential questions in terminal palliative care. *Nursing Ethics*, 19(4): 377–87.

Hudson, P., Kelly, B., Street, A., O'Connor, M., Kristjanson, L.J., Ashby, M. and Aranda, S. (2006) Responding to desire to die statements from patients with advanced disease: recommendations for health professionals. *Palliative Medicine*, 20: 703–10.

Jack, B. (2002) Do hospital-based palliative care clinical nurse specialists de-skill general staff? *International Journal of Palliative Nursing*, 8(7): 336–40.

Johnston, B. and Smith, L. (2006) Nurses' and patients' perceptions of expert palliative nursing care. *Journal of Advanced Nursing*, 54(6): 700–9.

Jones, A. (1999) 'A heavy and blessed experience': a psychoanalytical study of community Macmillan nurses and their roles in serious illness and palliative care. *Journal of Advanced Nursing*, 30(6): 1297–303.

Kearney, M. (2000) *A Place of Healing. Working with Suffering in Living and Dying*. Oxford: Oxford University Press.

Kendrick, K.D. and Robinson, S. (2002) ' "Tender Loving Care" as a relational ethic in nursing practice'. *Nursing Ethics*, 9(3): 291–300.

Kruijver, I.P.M., Kerkstra, A., Francke, A.L., Bensing, J.M. and van de Wiel, H.B.M. (2000) Evaluation of communication training programs in nursing care: a review of the literature. *Patient Education and Counseling*, 39: 129–45.

Kruijver, I.P.M., Kerkstra, A., Bensing, J.M. and van de Wiel, H.B.M. (2001) Communication skills of nurses during interactions with simulated cancer patients. *Journal of Advanced Nursing*, 34(6): 772–9.

Lawton, J. (2000) *The Dying Process*. London: Routledge.

Lerner, G. (1978) A death of one's own. In: S. Bertman (ed.) *Facing Death: Images, Insights and Interventions*. New York: Hemisphere.

Ley, P. (1988) *Communicating with Patients*. London: Croom Helm.

Liénart, A., Merkaert, I., Libert, Y., Delvaux, N., Marchal, S., Boniver, J., Etienne, A-M., Klastersky, J., Reynaert, C., Scalliet, P., Slachmuylder, J-L. and Razavi, D. (2006) Factors that influence cancer patients' anxiety following a medical consultation: impact of a communication skills training programme for physicians. *Annals of Oncology*, 17(9): 1450–8.

Lloyd, M. and Bor, R. (1996) *Communication Skills for Medicine*. Edinburgh: Churchill Livingstone.

Lobchuk, M.M. (2006) Concept analysis of perspective-taking: meeting informal caregiver needs for communication competence and accurate perception. *Journal of Advanced Nursing*, 54(3): 330–41.

Lobchuk, M.M. and Vorauer, J.D. (2003) Family caregiver perspective-taking and accuracy in estimating cancer patients symptom experiences. *Social Science and Medicine*, 57: 2379–84.

Lobchuk, M.M., Degner, L.F., Chateau, D. and Hewitt, D. (2006) Promoting enhanced patient and family caregiver congruence on lung cancer symptom experiences. *Oncology Nursing Forum*, 33(2): 273–82.

Luker, K.A., Austin, L., Caress, A. and Hallett, C.E. (2000) The importance of 'knowing the patient': community nurses' constructions of quality in providing palliative care. *Journal of Advanced Nursing*, 31(4): 775–82.

MacDonald, E. (2004) *Difficult Conversations in Medicine*. Oxford: Oxford University Press.

McCabe, C. (2004) Nurse–patient communication: an exploration of patients' experiences. *Journal of Clinical Nursing*, 13(1): 41–9.

McCabe, C. and Timmins, F. (2006) *Communication Skills for Nursing Practice*. Basingstoke: Palgrave.

McGrath, P. (2004) Affirming the connection: comparative findings on communication issues from hospice patients and haematology survivors. *Death Studies*, 28: 829–48.

McGrath, P., Yates, P., Clinton, M. and Hart, G. (1999) 'What should I say?': Qualitative findings on dilemmas in palliative care nursing. *The Hospice Journal*, 14(2): 17–33.

McLoughlin, P.A. (2002) Community specialist palliative care: experiences of patients and carers. *International Journal of Palliative Nursing*, 8(7): 344–53.

Maguire, P., Faulkner, A., Booth, K., Elliot, C. and Hillier, V. (1996a) Helping cancer patients disclose their concerns. *European Journal of Cancer*, 32A(1): 78–81.

Maguire, P., Booth, K., Elliot, C. and Jones, B. (1996b) Helping health professionals involved in cancer acquire key interviewing skills. *European Journal of Cancer*, 32A(9): 1486–9.

Miller, G.R. and Nicholson, H.E. (1976) *Communication Inquiry: A Perspective on Process*. Reading: Addison-Wesley.

Mok, E. and Chiu, P.C. (2004) Nurse–patient relationships in palliative care. *Journal of Advanced Nursing*, 48(5): 475–83.

Mok, E., Chan, F., Chan, V. and Yeung, E. (2002) Perception of empowerment by family caregivers of patients with a terminal illness in Hong Kong. *International Journal of Palliative Nursing*, 8(3): 137–45.

Moore, S., Corner, J., Haviland, J., Wells, M., Salmon, E., Normand, C., Brada, M., O'Brien, M. and Smith, I. (2002) Nurse led follow-up in management of patients with lung cancer: randomised trial. *British Medical Journal*, 325(7373): 1145–7.

Moore, S., Wells, M., Plant, H., Fuller, F., Wright, M. and Corner, J. (2006) Nurse specialist led follow-up in lung cancer: The experience of developing and delivering a new model of care. *European Journal of Oncology Nursing*, 10: 364–77.

Morgan A.K. (2001) Protective coping: the grounded theory of educative interactions in palliative care nursing. *International Journal of Palliative Nursing*, 7(2): 91–9.

Morse, J.M., Bottorff, J., Anderson, G., O'Brien, B. and Solberg, S. (1992) Beyond empathy: expanding expressions of caring. *Journal of Advanced Nursing*, 17: 809–21.

Mytton, E.J. and Adams, A. (2003) Do clinical nurse specialists in palliative care de-skill or empower general ward nurses? *International Journal of Palliative Nursing*, 9(2): 64–72.

Okon, T.R. (2006) 'Nobody understands': On a cardinal phenomenon of palliative care. *Journal of Medicine and Philosophy*, 31: 13–46.

Osterweis, M., Soloman, F. and Green, M. (1984) *Bereavement Reactions, Consequences and Care*. Washington: National Academy Press.

Parle, M., Maguire, P. and Heaven, C. (1997) The development of a training model to improve health professionals' skills, self-efficacy and outcome expectations when communicating with cancer patients. *Social Science and Medicine*, 44(2): 231–40.

Rabow, M.W. and McPhee, S.J. (1999) Beyond breaking bad news: how to help patients who suffer. *Western Journal of Medicine*, 171: 260–3.

Randall, T. and Wearn, A.M. (2005) Receiving bad news: patients with haematological cancer reflect on their experience. *Palliative Medicine*, 19: 594–601.

Razavi, D., Delvaux, N., Marchal, S., Bredart, A., Farvacques, C. and Paesmans, M. (1993) The effects of a 24-h psychological training program on attitudes, communication skills and occupational stress in oncology: a randomised study. *European Journal of Cancer*, 29A(13): 1858–63.

Razavi, D., Delvaux, N., Marchal, S., Durieux, J-F., Farvacques, C., Dubus, L. and Hogenraad, R. (2002) Does training increase the use of more emotionally laden words by nurses when talking with cancer patients? A randomised study. *British Journal of Cancer*, 87: 1–7.

Richardson, J. (2002) Health promotion in palliative care: the patients' perception of therapeutic interaction with the palliative nurse in the primary care setting, *Journal of Advanced Nursing*, 40(4): 432–40.

Rogers, A.E., Addington-Hall, J.M., Abery, A.J., McCoy, A.S.M., Bulpitt, C., Coats, A.J.S. and Gibbs, J.S.R. (2000) Knowledge and communication difficulties for patients with chronic heart failure: qualitative study. *British Medical Journal*, 321: 605–7.

Ronaldson, S. and Devery, K. (2001) The experience of transition to palliative care services: perspectives of patients and nurses. *International Journal of Palliative Nursing*, 7(4): 171–7.

Rungapadiachy, D.M. (1999) *Interpersonal Communication and Psychology*. London: Butterworth-Heinemann.

Seale, C. (1998) *Constructing Death. The Sociology of Dying and Bereavement*. Cambridge: Cambridge University Press.

Seymour, J., Clark, D., Hughes, P., Bath, P., Beech, N., Corner, J., Douglas, H-R., Halliday, D., Haviland, J., Marples, R., Normand, C., Skilbeck, J. and Webb, T. (2002) Clinical nurse specialists in palliative care. Part 3. Issues for the Macmillan nurse role. *Palliative Medicine*, 16: 386–94.

Shotten, L. (2000) Can nurses contribute to better end-of-life care? *Nursing Ethics*, 7(2): 134–40.

Skilbeck, J. and Seymour, J. (2002) Meeting complex needs: an analysis of Macmillan nurses' work with patients. *International Journal of Palliative Nursing*, 8(12): 574–82.

Smith, P. (1992) *The Emotional Labour of Nursing*. London: Macmillan Educational Ltd.

Street, A. and Blackford, J. (2001) Communication issues for the inter-disciplinary community palliative care team. *Journal of Clinical Nursing*, 7(6): 273–8.

Thompson, G., McClement, S. and Daeninck, P. (2006) Nurses' perceptions of quality end of life care on an acute medical ward. *Journal of Advanced Nursing*, 53(2): 169–77.

Thorne, S., Con, A., McGuinness, L., McPherson, G. and Harris, S.R. (2004) Health care communication issues in multiple sclerosis: An interpretive description. *Qualitative Health Research*, 14(1): 5–22.

Thorne, S.E., Bultz, B.D. and Baile, W.F. (2005) Is there a cost to poor communication in cancer care? A critical review of the literature. *Psycho-Oncology*, 14: 875–84.

Varcoe, C., Doane, G., Pauly, B., Rodney, P., Storch, J., Mahoney, K., McPherson, G., Brown, H. and Starzomski, R. (2004) Ethical practice in nursing: working the in-between. *Journal of Advanced Nursing*, 45(3): 316–25.

Von Gunten, C.F., Ferris, F.D. and Emanuel, L.L. (2000) Ensuring competency in end-of-life care: communication and relational skills. *Journal of the American Medical Association*, 284(23): 3051–7.

Wilkinson, S. (1991) Factors which influence how nurses communicate with cancer patients. *Journal of Advanced Nursing*, 16: 677–88.

Wilkinson, S. (1992) Good communication in cancer nursing. *Nursing Standard*, 7(9): 35–9.

Wilkinson, S.M., Gambles, M. and Roberts, A. (2002) The essence of cancer care: the impact of training on nurses' ability to communicate effectively. *Journal of Advanced Nursing*, 40(6): 731–8.

Willard, C. and Luker, K. (2006) Challenges to end of life care in the acute hospital setting. *Palliative Medicine*, 20: 611–15.

# 8

# Clinical assessment and measurement

*Michael I. Bennett and S. José Closs*

**Key points**

- Accurate assessment and measurement contribute to improved patient care.
- Remember that capturing complex subjective experience as simple numbers on a scale is not always meaningful.
- Measure what is important and do not assume that something is important because it can be measured.
- When using a measurement tool, ask whether it is valid and reliable for the task.
- Frequency and duration of measurement needs to adapt to the patient's changing condition.

## Principles of clinical assessment

Careful, individualized clinical assessment of health is a necessity to provide the best available planned palliative care. Clinical assessment is undertaken in varied ways depending on the specific health needs of the individual, their stage on the illness trajectory and their social or institutional context. The health outcomes of choice need to be monitored using instruments which have been developed with scientific rigour to reflect the goals of palliative care. The selection of instruments should be based on evidence of their appropriateness and validity, and the reliability of the instrument for use with the patient group to be assessed and the practical issues related to its use by specific individuals.

It is, perhaps, worth tempering this recommendation to use assessment instruments with some thoughts about their appropriate use in palliative care settings. Central to the WHO definition of palliative care is the aim of improving quality of life:

> Palliative care is an approach that improves the quality of life of patients and their families facing the problems associated with life-threatening illness through the prevention and relief of suffering by means of early identification and impeccable assessment of pain and other problems, physical, psychosocial and spiritual.
>
> (WHO 2007)

This encapsulates the huge range of possible factors which may need to be considered in providing care, but while factors such as pain, nausea and physical function may be measured fairly straightforwardly, quality of life is a broad, complex and highly individual concept which is not simply an item on a list, but a value judgement resulting from a total assessment of all aspects of daily life. It cannot be simply measured in any meaningful way.

Randall and Downie (2006: 20) point out that there is often a 'sad delusion' that assessment tools in themselves are an effective intervention. In parallel with the evidence-based medicine movement of the past decade or more, there has been an increasing tendency to require 'objective' assessments of almost any aspect of health or related factors which can be measured. The early, more holistic traditions of palliative care have been overtaken by an emphasis on generalizability and adherence to rules, guidelines and protocols which tend to ignore individual patients' very different experiences, needs and desires. Clinical judgement is necessary in the selection of what should usefully be measured, and what it is not necessary to measure. While many patients might benefit from various kinds of psychosocial or spiritual support, there are others who may have no interest in them whatsoever. The majority have the potential to benefit from symptom management (e.g. pain, depression, nausea), and it may be here that clinical assessments are of greatest importance.

### Measure what is important

> 'When you can measure what you are speaking about and express it in numbers, you know something about it.' Lord Kelvin

> 'Not all things that can be counted count, and not all things that count can be counted.' Albert Einstein

These different views of measurement are useful reminders of both the benefits and limitations of clinical measurement. In the quest to provide data on health care activity, it is easy to be drawn into measuring some aspect that is, in fact, not valuable. This then is the most important concept of clinical measurement – measure something important and do not assume that something is important because it can be measured.

There are many factors which are of importance to those receiving palliative care and, as we have mentioned, there is a bewildering array of different assessment instruments available to measure these. Some of these are appropriate for use in research studies, some for audit and others have a greater clinical utility. Numerous assessment instruments have been devised to measure aspects of pain, nausea, fatigue, mood, cognitive status and other factors. Some are well validated and widely used while others are newer and may be less thoroughly tested, or only tested with specific types of patients with specific conditions in specific settings. The selection of any of these instruments for clinical use requires consideration of these factors. Although many factors are relevant to palliative care, in this chapter we are going to focus mainly on the major issues of pain, nausea and functioning.

# Practical issues in measurement

### *Subjective or objective measurement?*

Much health care activity is directed towards measuring an aspect of patient experience. This is very much the case in palliative care where assessment and measurement of symptoms and quality of life (QOL) are core. This already presents a fundamental problem in that both symptoms and QOL are, by definition, subjective experiences and cannot be objectively measured, in contrast for example to the height or weight of the patient.

Subjective experiences such as symptoms are complex phenomena. As such, a number of psychological and social influences impact on the interpretation and expression of physical sensations by the patient. This results in one person's experience being difficult to compare to that of another, and even harder to conceptualize either of their experiences as a number. This also applies when measuring clinicians' 'objective' views of these same patients' experiences. Yet, comparing experiences using numbers is largely what clinical measurement seeks to achieve in the context of palliative care.

### *When should assessments be made?*

Clinical assessments may be undertaken at the time of diagnosis, during treatments, after treatments (long-term survival or terminal phase) and during active dying. While the benefits of structured assessments are clear in terms of providing professionals with information to inform health care, there is also the possibility of imposing a burden on patients when lengthy or numerous assessment instruments are used to elicit diagnostic information. For example, the assessment of nausea may not be needed at the point of initial diagnosis, while it would be important for cancer patients during certain treatments. Clinical measurement at initial consultations may be more comprehensive when the patient may have more physical and psychological concerns, is not fatigued, and can concentrate. When their health fails, fatigue increases and concentration inevitably declines, this results in the need for shorter measures administered less frequently. At some point, subjective measurement is no longer possible and measurement either ceases or proxies are used such as relatives or staff. A balance should therefore be struck between detailed assessment requiring the completion of lengthy instruments and the burden this may impose on patients.

### Who should undertake assessments?

Since palliative care is a multidisciplinary enterprise, different professionals are likely to be making different assessments at different points in the illness trajectory. Palliative medicine and other specialist physicians are likely to undertake the more detailed physical assessments, while nurses and other allied health professionals may be involved in the assessment of pain and other symptoms which may require regular and frequent monitoring. In hospitals, hospices and the community, nurses have a major role; while in care homes, it may be care assistants who undertake these activities. There are likely to be educational needs for many of those involved.

## Developing or selecting a measuring tool

### Key criteria

When selecting a patient-focused assessment instrument, the following seven questions should be considered:

1   Does the instrument adequately cover the health outcomes of interest?
2   Is there evidence of validation of the instrument with the patient group and within the setting in which it is to be used?
3   Is there evidence of the validity of the instrument with the intended population (does it measure what it claims to measure)?
4   Is there evidence of the reliability of the instrument with the intended population (are results reproducible and internally consistent)?
5   Is the instrument able to detect changes over the time-frames relevant to palliative care (is it sensitive enough)?
6   Is the instrument easy to complete, score and analyse?
7   If the patient is required to complete it, does it present an unacceptable burden in terms of what is required of them?

Assessment instruments should obviously not be used in clinical practice simply because they are easily available, or a particular consultant prefers them or they have 'always' been used in a specific setting. The seven questions above provide a guide for selecting the most appropriate for specific situations.

### Validity

Validity refers to the degree to which the instrument being used captures the experience or concept that it is intended to measure. In other words, does a certain pain scale accurately reflect a patient's pain experience or is it measuring anxiety or some other experience?

There are various aspects of validity to consider but the following six validity criteria are most commonly described (Streiner and Norman 2003):

- *Face validity* – whether the measure appears relevant, reasonable and is acceptable to those using the test.
- *Content validity* – the measure should reflect what is under study and sample all relevant or important domains in a balanced way (e.g. does a measure for psychological distress ask about mood, behaviour, thoughts, etc.?).
- *Construct validity* – the extent to which the measure is based on theoretical considerations that have been tested and include the types and degrees of associations between variables (e.g. has a measure of fatigue been constructed from items that have been shown independently to have statistically significant associations with fatigue?).
- *Criterion validity* – the extent to which the measure correlates with another criterion considered as the gold standard (e.g. do the scores on a breathlessness scale correlate closely with time to walk a certain distance, or levels of blood oxygen?).
- *Convergent validity* – the extent to which the measure agrees or correlates with other measures designed to measure the same concept or experience (e.g. does a new scale to measure mood agree with an established measure such as the Hospital Anxiety and Depression scale?).
- *Discriminant validity* – the extent to which the scale can distinguish between groups (e.g. does a prognostic index accurately identify patients that are likely to die within the next month compared to those that will survive longer?).

It is tempting to conclude that a measure is either valid or invalid but in reality, a continuum exists in which a particular measure is more or less valid in a particular population, in a particular context, at a particular time, etc. For example, many symptom measurement tools have been developed for use in resource-rich settings, establishing the validity of these tools in resource-poor settings is essential (Pappas *et al.* 2006).

### Reliability

Although a measure may be more or less valid, this is not enough to make it useful in clinical practice. Reliability refers to the quality control aspects of the measure – that is, its consistency or repeatability.

Reliability, like validity, can be assessed in various ways. The most frequently used methods are:

- *Internal consistency* – the extent to which all items in the measure are measuring the same concept ('items' refers to questions, statements or other components on a measurement tool to which a patient responds). For example, are all the questions on a pain scale assessing the intensity or sensation of pain, or are some simply measuring the impact of pain on daily living such as mood or reduced mobility? Statistically, this is represented by Cronbach's alpha – a high alpha score for a measure (between 0.7 and 0.9) indicates good internal consistency.

- *Test-retest reliability* – the extent to which the measure produces the same results from the same sample if repeated after a specific interval (and assuming that the underlying experience has not changed).

- *Inter-rater reliability* – the extent to which the measure will produce the same results from the same sample if used by two different observers.

Aspects of repeatability, such as test-retest or inter-rater, are often assessed statistically using Cohen's kappa. A high kappa score indicates good agreement and Streiner and Norman (2003) recommend that reliable scales have values for kappa > 0.5.

A much cited illustration of the relationship between reliability and validity is that of an archery target. Here, the bulls-eye is the concept or experience that the measure is targeting. The closer that the measurements (or shots) are to the centre, the more valid the measure. In this scenario, the closer the measurements are to each other (and perhaps from different 'archers' or at different time intervals), the more reliable the measure. Some would argue that if a measure is not reliable, it cannot be said to be valid either.

### Mode of collection

Measurement tools that capture subjective information are usually formatted as questionnaires and these can vary from simple linear scales (see

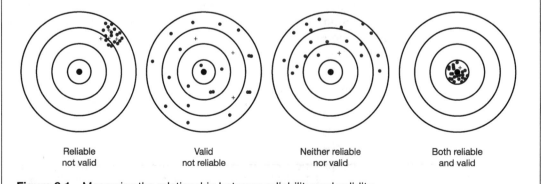

| Reliable not valid | Valid not reliable | Neither reliable nor valid | Both reliable and valid |

**Figure 8.1**   Measuring the relationship between reliability and validity

examples related to pain or nausea in the following section) to longer multi-item lists with different response categories for example, yes or no; mild, moderate or severe, etc. Commonly, these questionnaires are presented to patients on paper and either completed through an interview process or patients themselves are asked to complete them unaided (usually described as 'self-report' measures).

Increasingly, pen and paper measures are being replaced by alternatives. In clinical contexts where face-to-face contact exists these include touch-screen computers and hand-held devices (personal digital assistant or PDA). These have been used in palliative care settings within research studies and in clinical practice and have proved to be acceptable to patients and are usually easier to manage. An advantage is that the electronic screen shows one question at a time and patients are not subject to a whole page of questions which can overwhelm and lead to missed items. More complex measurement programmes are able to evaluate responses to initial screening questions and then present subsequent questions that are more specific to that particular patient (computer adaptive testing) (Cella *et al.* 2007).

Methods to capture clinical measures when the patient is remote from the clinical base include internet based tools and phone calls. The latter can range from a clinician or researcher phoning the patient and interviewing the patient, to automatic systems in which the patient inputs responses to a computer voice using the phone key pad.

### Level of measurement

Another important concept of clinical measurement relates to the type or level of measurement. Understanding the level of measurement of a particular tool will determine how the results of the measurement are analysed or used.

A hierarchy exists of four generally recognized levels of measurement:

- *Nominal* – this refers to 'names' of different categories such as recoding the district where a palliative care patient lives, or whether they suffer with nociceptive pain or neuropathic pain. This information can be coded 1, 2, etc. to represent different districts or pain type but these numbers cannot be ordered. That is, a higher number does not represent a better or worse place to live or a worse type of pain.

- *Ordinal* – this refers to categories that can be ordered or ranked. For example, whether a patient has mild, moderate or severe intensity pain (coded 1, 2, 3, etc.). Although 'moderate' pain represents more pain than 'mild' pain, it is impossible to conclude that it is twice as much pain. Similarly, the difference in pain intensity between mild and moderate categories may not be the same as between moderate and severe.

- *Interval* – this refers to attributes in which the difference between numbers does have meaning, for example temperature measured in Celsius. At this level of measurement, it is possible to compute a mean or average where it is impossible to do this for ordinal measures (in the latter case, calculating a median value might be more appropriate).

- *Ratio* – in ratio measurement there is always an absolute zero that is meaningful, e.g. a 100 mm visual analogue scale where zero equals no pain and 100 equals worst possible pain. This means that it is possible to state a ratio; for example, that a patient whose pain score was 60 mm but is now 30 mm has experienced 50 per cent pain relief.

# Measuring pain

Pain is the most common and probably the most feared symptom requiring management in palliative care. At all stages of illness, regular and systematic assessments which involve believing the pain reports of the patient and family are essential. A comprehensive assessment of pain should include:

- A detailed history including an assessment of pain location, intensity and characteristics.
- A physical examination which may be supplemented by a neurological examination, especially if neuropathic pain is suspected.
- A psychosocial and cultural assessment may also be undertaken, since the experience, expression and management of pain vary according to factors such as social support and religious beliefs.

At diagnosis an extremely thorough and comprehensive initial assessment is required, and is undertaken by the physician. All professionals involved in care should be party to this information, and should undertake repeated assessments at appropriate times, particularly of pain location, intensity and characteristics. Some pain may be due to the patient's condition, often changing as the illness proceeds, and some pain may be due to the treatments given. Assessment processes need to be tailored to fit with these events.

### Initial pain assessment

An initial pain assessment could begin with a general enquiry, such as 'Could you tell me about any pain you have had in the last week?'. This gives clear 'permission' to talk about pain, while being sufficiently open-ended that individuals can start with the aspects of pain (or related issues) which are of greatest importance to them. These issues can then be pursued on an individual basis.

Pain location may be assessed simply by asking the patient to indicate the source/s of pain, either verbally or by pointing. A body map may be used to record the location and extent of pain.

Intensity is the most common aspect of pain to be measured routinely. If someone has more than one source of pain, it may be useful to assess all of them. There are many scales available, but the simplest and most successful with a wide range of patient groups are the numerical and verbal rating scales (NRS Figure 8.2 and VRS Figure 8.3).

The NRS is the more sensitive of the two to changes in intensity, with a 10-point horizontal scale ranging from 0 (no pain) to 10 (worst possible pain). This is recommended for situations where getting pain under control is the priority, and pharmacological and other interventions can be introduced and their effectiveness assessed at regular intervals until acceptable control is achieved. A simpler five-point verbal rating scale (none, mild, moderate, severe, excruciating) can also be used and is particularly useful when pain levels have been stabilized to a great extent.

Visual analogue scales are commonly used in acute settings, and are even more sensitive to changes in intensity than an NRS. Unfortunately, they are conceptually difficult to use for some older people and those with cognitive impairments (Closs *et al.* 2004; Herr *et al.* 2004), and difficult to mark accurately if the patient has poor eyesight or difficulty holding a pen due to arthritic joints, etc. Monitoring of pain intensity is important at all stages of illness.

### Multidimensional pain assessment

The characteristics of pain can be extremely varied and sometimes bizarre in nature. The only well-validated instrument available to describe pain qualities is the McGill pain questionnaire (MPQ, Melzack 1975). Some of the words selected from this may suggest the presence of neuropathic pain, which may require specialist treatment. Words such as shooting, burning and electric are often used to describe it. There are several screening tools available which aim to identify neuropathic pain, five of which have recently been reviewed (Bennett *et al.* 2007). All use similar language to discriminate the neuropathic element of pain and demonstrate good validity and reliability for this approach. Unfortunately it is not yet clear which is the most appropriate for different groups and settings.

'Which number best describes your pain?'

No pain | 0 | 1 | 2 | 3 | 4 | 5 | 6 | 7 | 8 | 9 | 10 | Worst possible pain

**Figure 8.2**   Numerical rating scale

'How severe is your pain today?'

❑ None

❑ Mild

❑ Moderate

❑ Severe

❑ Excruciating

**Figure 8.3**   Verbal rating scale (5 points)

The most widely used multidimensional pain assessment instrument is the Brief Pain Inventory (BPI, Cleeland and Ryan 1994). This measures not only location and intensity, but also factors which improve or worsen pain and the effectiveness of medications. It also provides a useful overview of the impact of the pain on factors such as general activity, mood, relationships, enjoyment of life and sleep. It has been well validated for use with patients with cancer, and is also widely used in other long-term painful conditions. The original version requires self-completion of a fairly detailed six-page questionnaire, which makes it unsuitable for those in frail health or with poor concentration. Fortunately, a more user-friendly two-page version is also available. Both versions are available via the internet at no cost at: http://www.mdanderson.org/departments/prg/dindex.cfm?pn=0ee78204-6646-11d5-812400508b603a14.

### *Observational pain assessment*

Observational approaches to the identification of pain may be used when difficulties in self-report assessments of pain arise. This is usually when the patient is unable to communicate successfully, either verbally, through scale completion or other method (depending on the individual). While self-report is accepted to be the most accurate, there are some 15 or more observational scales available which could be used to assist in the identification of pain. All tend to use a selection of behaviours which are indicators of the potential presence of pain. Seven main types of observation occur within most of these pain assessment tools:

- physiological observations, e.g. breathing pattern, sweating
- facial expressions, e.g. wincing, grimacing, frowning, rapid blinking
- body movements, e.g. guarding, altered gait, pacing, rocking, hand-wringing, repetitive movements
- verbalizations/vocalizations, e.g. moaning, groaning, asking for help, screaming, aggressive or offensive speech
- changes in interpersonal interactions, e.g. aggression, withdrawal, resisting care
- changes in activity patterns or routines, e.g. wandering, altered sleep pattern, altered rest patterns
- mental status changes, e.g. crying, tears, increased confusion, irritability.

Most of the available observational scales are relatively new, having been developed during the past five years or so. There is as yet no single instrument that has been shown to have psychometric properties sufficient for it to be recommended for general clinical use. Examples of these range from the PAINAD Scale (Warden *et al.* 2003), which is a brief, simple five-item observational tool, to the longer, more comprehensive Pain Assessment Check List for Seniors with Severe Dementia (PACSLAC) (Fuchs-Lacelle and Hadjistavropoulos 2004), which includes a total of 60 items covering subtle as well as common pain behaviours. Detailed critiques of currently available scales can be found in Herr *et al.* (2006) and Hadjistavropoulos *et al.* (2007).

There may be difficulty in interpreting the meaning of these behaviours, which may indicate not only the presence of pain, but also other problems, such as anxiety, itching, an uncomfortably full bladder, etc. It may be possible to interpret at an individual level with the help of carers who are familiar with a particular patient's behaviour; for example, for one person pacing and hand-wringing may indicate pain, while in another it may indicate constipation.

In summary, pain assessment requires a tailored approach, depending on individual patients, the complexity of their pain/s and their point on the illness trajectory. A general question to introduce the topic of pain is a good starting point, and may be followed by more specific information about location, intensity and quality. Observation of pain behaviours may be the only method of identifying the presence of pain in those who are unable to communicate successfully.

# Measuring nausea and vomiting

Palliative care patients frequently experience nausea, retching and vomiting (Curtis *et al.* 1991; Fainsinger *et al.* 1991; Vainio and Auvinen 1996) and these are often taken to represent different intensities of a common underlying mechanism. In reality, these features should be regarded as a symptom cluster (often referred to as emesis) as nausea may exist without vomiting and vice versa. This means that measurement of each component is necessary for valid and reliable assessment. Vomiting is an observable and measurable phenomenon in terms of frequency, consistency and volume but nausea is subjective and hence reliant on self-report by patients. Nausea has dimensions of frequency, intensity and duration as well as quantitative and qualitative aspects (Rhodes and McDaniel 2001).

### *Specific tools*

In common with measures of pain, measures of emesis often consist of specific uni-dimensional scales of intensity. Categorical verbal (marked none, mild, moderate or severe nausea) and numerical rating or visual analogue scales (anchored 0 = no nausea to 10 = worst possible nausea) are the simplest tools to use. These have similar advantages and limitations to those used to measure pain discussed earlier.

In contrast to the measurement of pain however, very few multidimensional scales exist for the assessment of emesis. One example is the revised Rhodes index of nausea, vomiting and retching (INV-R) (Rhodes and McDaniel 1999) which provides information on the frequency, the amount, the duration and the distress caused by each of the three symptoms. The revised form is relatively simple and easy to use and comprises eight five-point Likert type scales with check boxes. It has been used in trials of anti-emetics in chemotherapy induced nausea and vomiting with only short-term follow-up (72 hours). Validation in a palliative care population would be needed before recommending it for routine use.

### Global symptom assessment tools

Assessment of emesis is also a component of several global symptom assessment tools. These tools may provide more limited information on prevalence only and can take longer to complete, which may make it difficult for frail patients or those with cognitive impairment. Examples of tools validated or developed for use in palliative care populations include the Edmonton Symptom Assessment Scale (ESAS), revised Rotterdam Symptom Checklist (RSCL), the Palliative Care Assessment tool and the EORTC QLC-30 (Ahmedzai 1995; Ellershaw 1995; Rees *et al.* 1998; Hardy *et al.* 1999).

The ESAS is brief and easy to use, is established in clinical practice and consists of nine 10cm visual analogue scales relating to specific symptoms, including nausea. Vomiting can be inserted as an additional symptom. It is designed for longitudinal assessment over time and can be completed by the patient alone, the patient with help or by a care-giver alone. In a study of oncology patients (Chang *et al.* 2000) that compared several global symptom assessment tools, all could be completed in five minutes but more explanation was required for the ESAS than for the other two. Difficulty in understanding the ESAS was more pronounced in elderly and severely ill patients, and Rees *et al.* (1998) did not find ESAS a practical tool in patients with poor performance status.

The PACA is concise and easy to use (Ellershaw 1995). It is completed by a health care professional who asks specific questions of the patient and has been validated in the hospital setting. There are anecdotal reports of the use of PACA in other care settings but formal validation of use in these areas has not been undertaken.

## Measuring mobility

The ability to move independently is often seen as a significant component of quality of life. In the context of life-threatening disease, assessment and maintenance of mobility is a key area for health professionals to focus upon. Mobility is usually measured on performance across a range of tasks and maintaining mobility is important because it prevents de-conditioning and delays dependency on others (and hence influences place of care such as home or institution). Measurement of performance is more easily undertaken by an observer in contrast to the measurement of symptoms such as pain and nausea where subjective ratings are more valid.

### Karnofsky Performance Status Scale (KPS)

The original Karnofsky Performance Status Scale was developed to measure the impact of cancer and its treatment on function in some of the first patients with cancer to receive chemotherapy in the USA (Karnofsky *et al.* 1948). The KPS has since been widely used in cancer and palliative care and is now considered one of the 'gold standard' methods of quantifying functional status in cancer patients.

In its original form the KPS consists of 11 categories with scores divided into deciles ranging from 100 (asymptomatic, normal function) to 0 (death). Each category combines information on the patient's ability to function, ability to work, the severity of symptoms and the need for care. It provides a global assessment of mobility but does not record information regarding specific mobility impairments or ability to carry out particular activities of daily living. The KPS can be used to measure mobility through interview, observation, examination or a combination of all methods and it is quick and easy to complete. The KPS has been shown to provide a more accurate measure of prognosis than clinical estimation in terminally ill patients (Evans and McCarthy 1985) and is still commonly used to stratify and select patients in chemotherapeutic trials (Boeck *et al.* 2007). The ability of the KPS to monitor change is less certain and Kaasa *et al.* (1997) stated that in their experience KPS scores for patients with terminal cancer tended to cluster at the low end of the scale (at 30 or below), therefore limiting the sensitivity to change.

### Eastern Cooperative Oncology Group Performance Status Scale (ECOG-PS)

The Eastern Cooperative Oncology Group Performance Status Scale was also developed for cancer patients (Oken *et al.* 1982) and consists of six categories which measure a patient's ability to function and ability to self-care, with a focus on activity. Total scores range from 0 (fully active) to 5 (dead). The ECOG-PS is self-explanatory and very easy to complete, requiring no formal training and has been shown to have good validity and reliability in cancer patients (Roila *et al.* 1991; Buccheri *et al.* 1996). It is now widely used in cancer and palliative care to compare functional outcome following cancer treatment, to select patients for clinical trials, and to predict survival. Comparisons of the ECOG-PS with the KPS have described them as comparable but the ECOG-PS was shown to have lower inter-rater variability and greater predictive validity (Buccheri *et al.* 1996).

### Barthel Index (BI)

The Barthel Index was first published in 1965 (Mahoney and Barthel 1965) and was originally developed and used to monitor functional independence in self-care and mobility activities for patients with paralytic conditions undergoing inpatient rehabilitation. Use of the index has now been extended to many contexts including cancer and palliative care. Moderate to severe functional disability in stroke and elderly patients as measured by the BI has been shown to be predictive of hospital mortality, prolonged stay in hospital, discharge destination, early emergency hospital readmission, use of home health care services, future social functioning and mortality within six months of discharge (Alarcon *et al.* 1999; Chu and Pei 1999; Thomassen *et al.* 1999; Bohannon *et al.* 2002; Bohannon and Lee 2004). The rate of change of the BI has been shown to be an important indicator of survival in hospice patients (Bennett and Ryall 2000).

Although several versions of the BI exist, the most commonly used version consists of ten items scored on a three-point scale: dependent, partially dependent and independent. Items generally assess mobility and aspects of self-care. It is quick to complete and scoring is relatively straightforward although it does require some calculation by adding the individual ADL sub-scores. The BI has been widely tested for reliability and validity (Granger and Greer 1976; Collin *et al.* 1988; Shah *et al.* 1989) and several studies have confirmed high inter-rater agreement, good internal consistency and test-retest reliability. Collin *et al.* (1988) showed good agreement in the measurement of ADL between self-report, clinical observation, nurse examination, and physiotherapist examination. Telephone scoring with the help of relatives has also been shown to be reliable (Shinar *et al.* 1987).

# Conclusion

Clinical assessment and measurement is an important aspect of modern health care and is increasingly applied to palliative care activity at the level of symptom management or satisfaction with services. Despite these apparent pressures, it is still essential to discriminate between measuring something important, and only valuing something because it can be measured.

Measurement tools need to be valid and reliable for their purpose and these concepts may be true in one context but not necessarily hold in another context. For example, between oncology patients newly diagnosed versus frail patients in the last days of life. Evolving issues in measurement, such as computer adaptive testing, and improvements in data capture, such as automated telephone calling and touch-screen computers, are likely to be features of palliative care practice in the future. Although clinical measurement is an established component of patient assessment in palliative care, it is but one part of this process alongside aspects of communication, wisdom and compassion.

# References

Ahmedzai, S. (1995) Feasibility of self-rating questionnaires for quality of life evaluation in palliative care. *Palliative Medicine*, 9: 64–5.

Alarcon, T., Barcena, A., Gonzalex-Montalvo, J.I., Penalosa, C. and Salgado, A. (1999) Factors predictive of outcome on admission to an acute geriatric ward. *Age and Ageing*, 28: 429–32.

Bennett, M. and Ryall, N. (2000) Using the modified Barthel Index to estimate survival in cancer patients in hospice: observational study. *British Medical Journal*, 321: 1381–2.

Bennett, M.I., Attal, N., Backonja, M.M., Baron, R., Bouhassira, D., Freynhaen, R., Scholz, J., Tölle, T., Wittchen, H. and Jensen, T. (2007) Using screening tools to identify neuropathic pain. *Pain*, 127(3): 199–203.

Boeck, S., Hinke, A., Wilkowski, R. and Heinemann, V. (2007) Importance of performance status for treatment outcome in advanced pancreatic cancer. *World Journal of Gastroenterology*, 13: 224–7.

Bohannon, R.W. and Lee, N. (2004) Association of physical functioning with same-hospital readmission after stroke. *American Journal of Physical Medicine and Rehabilitation*, 83(6): 434–8.

Bohannon, R.W., Lee, N. and Maljanian, R.R.N. (2002) Post admission function best predicts acute hospital outcomes after stroke. *American Journal of Physical Medicine and Rehabilitation*, 81(10): 726–30.

Buccheri, G., Ferrigno, D. and Tamburini, M. (1996) Karnofsky and ECOG performance status scoring in lung cancer: a prospective, longitudinal study of 536 patients from a single institution. *European Journal of Cancer*, 32(7): 1135–41.

Cella, D., Gershon, R., Lai, R.S. and Choi, S. (2007) The future of outcomes measurement: item banking, tailored short-forms, and computerized adaptive assessment. *Qual Life Res*, 16 Suppl 1: 133–41.

Chang, V.T., Hwang, S. and Feuerman, M. (2000) Validation of the Edmonton Symptom Assessment Scale. *Cancer*, 88(9): 2164–71.

Chu, L.W. and Pei, C.K.W. (1999) Risk Factors for Early Emergency Hospital Readmission in Elderly Medical Patients. *Gerontology*, 45(4): 220–6.

Cleeland, C.S. and Ryan, K.M. (1994) Pain assessment: global use of the Brief Pain Inventory. *Annals of the Academy of Medicine of Singapore*, 23: 129–38.

Closs, S.J., Barr, B., Briggs, M., Cash, K. and Seers, K. (2004) A comparison of five pain assessment scales for nursing home residents with varying degrees of cognitive impairment. *Journal of Pain and Symptom Management*, 27: 196–205.

Collin, C., Wade, D.T., Davies, S. and Horne, V. (1988) The Barthel Index: a reliability study. *International Journal of Disability Studies*, 10(2): 61–3.

Curtis, E., Krech, R. and Walsh, D. (1991) Common Symptoms in Patients with Advanced Cancer. *Journal of Palliative Care*, 7: 25–9.

Ellershaw, J.E. (1995) Assessing the effectiveness of a hospital palliative care team. *Palliative Medicine*, 9: 145–52.

Evans, C. and McCarthy, M. (1985) Prognostic uncertainty in terminal care: can the Karnofsky index help? *Lancet*, 1(8439): 1204–6.

Fainsinger, R., Miller, M.J., Bruera, E., Hanson, J. and Maceachern, T. (1991) Symptom Control During the Last Week of Life on a Palliative Care Unit. *Journal of Palliative Care*, 7: 5–11.

Fuchs-Lacelle, S. and Hadjistavropoulos, T. (2004) Development and preliminary validation of the pain assessment checklist for seniors with limited ability to communicate (PACSLAC). *Pain Management Nursing*, 5(1): 37–49.

Granger, C.V. and Greer, D.S. (1976) Functional status measurement and medical rehabilitation outcomes. *Archives of Physical Medicine and Rehabilitation*, 57(3): 103–9.

Hadjistavropoulos, T., Herr, K., Turk, D.C., Fine, P.G., Dworkin, R.H., Helme, R. *et al.* (2007) An interdisciplinary expert consensus statement on assessment of pain in older persons. *Clinical Pain Journal*, 23 Suppl 1: S1–43.

Hardy, J.R., Edmonds, P., Turner, R., Rees, E. and A'Hern, R. (1999) The use of the Rotterdam Symptom Checklist in Palliative Care. *Journal of Pain and Symptom Management*, 18(2): 79–84.

Herr, K.A., Spratt, K., Mobily, P.R. and Richardson, G. (2004) Pain intensity assessment in older adults: use of experimental pain to compare psychometric properties and usability of selected pain scales with younger adults. *Clinical Journal of Pain*, 20(4): 207–19.

Herr, K., Bjoro, K. and Decker, S. (2006) Tools for assessment of pain on nonverbal older adults with dementia: a state-of-the-science review. *Journal of Pain and Symptom Management,* 31(2): 170–92.

Kaasa, T., Loomis, J., Gillis, K., Bruera, E. and Hanson, J. (1997) The Edmonton Functional Assessment Tool: preliminary development and evaluation for use in palliative care. *Journal of Pain and Symptom Management*, 13(1): 10–19.

Karnofsky, D.A., Abelmann, W.H., Craver, L.F. and Burchenal, J.H. (1948) The use of the nitrogen mustards in the palliative treatment of carcinoma. *Cancer*, 1: 634–56.

Mahoney, F.I. and Barthel, D. (1965) Functional evaluation: the Barthel Index. *Maryland State Medical Journal*, 14: 56–61.

Melzack, R. (1975) The McGill Pain Questionnaire: major properties and scoring methods. *Pain*, 1: 277–99.

Oken, M.M., Creech, R.H., Tormey, D.C., Horton, J., Davis, T.E., McFadden, E.T. and Carbone, P.P. (1982) Toxicity And Response Criteria Of The Eastern Cooperative Oncology Group. *American Journal of Clinical Oncology*, 5(6): 649–55.

Pappas, G., Wolf, R.C., Morineau, G. and Harding, R. (2006) Validity of measures of pain and symptoms in HIV/AIDS infected households in resource-poor settings: results from the Dominican Republic and Cambodia. *BMC Palliative Care*, 5: 3.

Randall, F. and Downie, R.S. (2006) *The Philosophy of Palliative Care, Critique and Reconstruction*. Oxford: Oxford University Press.

Rees, E., Hardy, J., Ling, J., Broadley, K. and A'Hern, R. (1998) The use of the Edmonton Symptom Assessment scale within a palliative care unit in the UK. *Palliative Medicine*, 12(2): 75–82.

Rhodes, V.A. and McDaniel, R.W. (1999) The Index of Nausea, Vomiting and Retching: A New Format of the Index of Nausea and Vomiting. *Oncology Nursing Forum*, 26(5): 889–94.

Rhodes, V. and McDaniel, R. (2001) Nausea, Vomiting and Retching: Complex problems in Palliative Care. *CA: Cancer Journal for Clinicians*, 51: 232–48.

Roila, F., Lupatteli, M. and Sassi, M. (1991) Intra- and interobserver variability in cancer patient's performance status according to Karnofsky and ECOG scales. *Annals of Oncology*, 2(6): 437–9.

Shah, S., Vanclay, F. and Cooper, B. (1989) Improving the sensitivity of the Barthel Index for stroke rehabilitation. *Journal of Clinical Epidemiology*, 42(8): 703–9.

Shinar, D., Gross, C.R., Bronstein, K.S., Licata-Gehr, E.E., Eden, D.T., Cabrera, A.R., Fishman, I.G., Roth, A.A., Barwick, J.A. and Kunitz, S.C. (1987) Reliability of the activities of daily living scale and its use in telephone interview; a modified Barthel Index. *Archives of Physical Medicine and Rehabilitation*, 68(10): 723–8.

Streiner, D.L. and Norman, G.R. (2003) *Health Measurement Scales: a practical guide to their development and use*. Oxford: Oxford University Press.

Thomassen, B., Bautz-Holter, E. and Laake, K. (1999) Predictors of outcome of rehabilitation of elderly stroke patients in a geriatric ward. *Clinical Rehabilitation*, 13: 123–8.

Vainio, A. and Auvinen, A. (1996) Prevalence of Symptoms Among Patients with Advanced Cancer: An International Collaborative Study. *Journal of Pain and Symptom Management*, 12(1): 3–10.

Warden, V., Hurley, A.C. and Voicer, L. (2003) Development and psychometric evaluation of the pain assessment in advanced dementia (PAINAD) scale. *Journal of American Medical Directors Association*, 4(1): 9–15.

WHO Definition of Palliative Care – http://www.who.int/cancer/palliative/definition/en/ (accessed 24 July 2007).

# 9

# Adapting complementary therapies for palliative care

*Ann Carter and Peter Mackereth*

---

**Key points**

- Clarification of terminology in providing clear information about interventions and their role to patients, carers and health professionals.
- Popularity of complementary therapies (CTs) and the potential for greater integration.
- Examination of the nurse's role in assessing, developing and supporting the provision of complementary therapies.
- The importance of appropriate training, therapeutic skills, ability to adapt interventions, and continuing education and clinical supervision for therapists.
- The need to evaluate the evidence of safety, efficacy and outcomes for complementary interventions within palliative care services.
- Consideration of the value and appropriateness of providing access to complementary therapies for carers and staff.
- Recommendations for future research and practice development.

---

# Introduction

In this chapter the focus is on complementary therapies (CTs), which are presented as adjunctive therapies aimed at symptom management and enhancement of quality of life. This understanding of purpose has been clarified by Corner and Harewood (2004) who have categorized under two separate headings the use of CTs by patients living with cancer. The first category includes those therapies adopted by patients to treat the underlying disease, usually referred to as 'alternative' treatments. The second category, the focus of the chapter, includes 'complementary' therapies which support ongoing medical care by way of easing symptoms and improving well-being.

In the United Kingdom there has been a rapid increase in the use of such complementary therapies in palliative and supportive care in the past decade (Kohn 2002; Tavares 2003). In a study across 14 countries in Europe, there was evidence of complementary therapies use among people (n=956) living with cancer, which ranged from 14.8 per cent to 73.1 per cent (mean 35.9 per cent) (Molassiotis *et al.* 2005). In two separate studies from the United States of America, 63 per cent of cancer clinical trial patients surveyed had used at least one CT (Sparber *et al.* 2000), while in another survey of patients attending an outpatient cancer clinic, 83 per cent of respondents had used CTs (Richardson *et al.* 2000). A Canadian study identified a similar prevalence of the use of CTs (67 per cent) in breast cancer patients (Boon *et al.* 2000)

While the popularity of complementary therapies has grown, an increase in provision could be compromised by funding issues, given growing health care costs. As a 'Cinderella' service, it is often largely dependent on charitable funding, together with the contribution of part-time volunteer therapists, and a small but growing number of professional skilled practitioners and coordinators (Carter and Mackereth 2006). The evidence base for complementary therapies is complicated by limited research funding and expertise. Despite these challenges, the research effort is increasing as the public, therapists and health professionals recognize the needs to critically appraise the value of these interventions (Field 2000; Mackereth and Stringer 2005).

## Defining key terms

The terms 'alternative' and 'complementary' are frequently used incorrectly as being interchangeable. The British House of Lords Select Committee Report has investigated and classified Complementary and Alternative Medicine (CAM) (HoL 2000 – see Box 9.1) and concluded that the purpose

---

**Box 9.1**   House of Lords Report on CAM divided therapies into three groups

1   Professionally organized alternative therapies, e.g. acupuncture, chiropractic, osteopathy, homeopathy and herbalism
2   Complementary therapies, e.g. aromatherapy, reflexology and massage
3   Alternative disciplines:

   (a)   traditional systems of health care, such as Ayurvedic medicine, Chinese herbal medicine and Eastern medicine.
   (b)   other alternative disciplines, e.g. crystal healing, iridology and kinesiology.

(House of Lords 2000)

of providing complementary therapies is to support, improve and maintain well-being, and where possible help with symptoms and quality of life. Key questions raised by this report relevant to this chapter are: 'Is the therapy safe in practice?' and 'Does it provide the benefits claimed?' and 'Is the therapy cost-effective compared to other tried and tested interventions?'

The term 'alternative', however, suggests choice to a patient. It has also usually been associated with the rejection of conventional medical treatments in favour of interventions that may not be deemed efficacious in the wider medical community. Concern has been raised by researchers that the internet is often used 'unwisely' as a source of information about 'alternative cures' for cancer (Schmidt and Ernst 2004). Apart from raising false hopes, safety and cost are key concerns for health professionals faced with patients and carers desperate to try anything in pursuit of a cure. If interventions fail to 'work' then individuals can rightly feel they have wasted precious time, money, effort and emotional investment.

Traditionally, therapies have evolved through trial and error. For example, remedies with a herbal origin have formed the basis of many medical treatments today, e.g. foxglove (digitalis), periwinkle (vinicristine) and aspirin from willow bark. Herbal remedies are popular with some patients living with cancer (Molassiotis and Cubbin 2004). However, evidence of effectiveness of many remedies is unclear and concerns have been raised as to their safety and interactions with conventional medication, including chemotherapy and narcotics (Ernst 2001). St John's Wort is an example of a herbal remedy that is thought to be useful for mild, but not for major, depression but is known to interact with other medication (HDTSG 2002, see chapter by Lloyd Williams and Hughes). The ancient practice of acupuncture is receiving wider research interest and growing application in health care settings, for example in helping to alleviate chronic pain (Ezzo *et al.* 2000).

The most common therapies provided by nurses are 'complementary' as opposed to 'alternative'. However, there is a grey area where some nurses use techniques as a therapeutic tool, such as acupressure to help relieve nausea and essential oils, for example lavender, to help with sleep (Tavares 2003). Here, the difference is that interventions are intended as adjuncts, rather than replacements for medication. However, complementary therapies, such as massage, are not necessarily so specific in their goals. First, the primary intention of touch therapies and relaxation techniques may be to improve well-being, reduce anxiety and manage distress in the short term. Some secondary benefits could be experienced by the patient; these can include reduction in pain perception, improved sleep, and amelioration of some side effects of treatment. The comforting effects of complementary therapies are beginning to be appreciated by the multidisciplinary team as both therapeutic and improving the patient experience of health care. There is also a growing body of evidence to suggest that touch therapies may have longer-term benefits through improving immune function associated with reduction in anxiety (Field 2000). The mind–body association linked to health changes and stress is based on the concept of psychoneuroimmunology (see Further reading).

# Complementary therapies and the nurse

It could be argued that nurses who carry out complementary therapy interventions wish to be seen as a new breed of health practitioner, much in the way that professional physiotherapy emerged from nursing. Some advocates of nurses using complementary therapies argue that there is an historical precedence for these techniques and approaches; for example, in the therapeutic use of touch (Wright and Sayre-Adams 2000) and the philosophy of 'holism' in nursing care (Dossey 1995). Conversely, Tovey and Adams (2003) have argued that an 'affinity between nursing and CAM is virtually non-existent' (p. 1469) and that some sections of the nursing world are uncomfortable with an affiliation to complementary therapy practices.

Traditional approaches to ill health, such as spa treatments, convalescent homes, invalid diets, recuperative health resorts, use of poultices and steam inhalations have lost popularity as medicine has become more technical. It could be argued that in pursuing the science of medicine, the ethos of the healing arts have been diminished. The resurgence of interest in complementary therapies among nurses provides opportunities to reassess the contribution these interventions have to make to health 'care'. This growing interest in CAM by nurses may be a reflection of the professional's desire and interest for a greater therapeutic role (Wright and Sayre-Adams 2000; Rankin-Box 2001).

The expansion of the nurse's role to include complementary therapies is not fully embraced by all in the profession. Ersser (2000) believes that any expansion of the therapeutic role of the nurse needs to be debated on how such core developments can be effectively integrated and balanced. It has been argued that nurses should not be wasting their time on training in complementary therapies; rather they should focus on spending time with patients and providing effective listening and touch which is supportive and comforting (Rayner 1999). This is an important point. When providing massage, for example, the treatment has to be planned, contracted and consented for intervention, which is different from 'hand-holding'. Massage can comfort an individual, and at the same time its goal is to promote deep relaxation through rhythmic strokes and gentle manipulation of soft tissue. Unfortunately, touch is commonly associated with a medical task, such as taking a pulse, rather than providing comfort. Touch deprivation, an issue for those marginalized by age, disability and infection is further compromised by fears that physical contact may be misinterpreted. These concerns need to be considered and put in perspective when working with those who are in need of supportive and palliative care.

It has been suggested that nurses are ideally placed to provide information about therapies through their clinical contact with patients and carers. Molassiotis and Cubbin (2004) recommend that a great deal more needs to be done to educate health professionals, including nurses, about complementary therapies. A key issue is being able to talk from experience, as well as from an understanding of theories and philosophies. It is argued here that nurses may also need to observe and receive therapies to begin to understand the contribution that they can make to health care.

# Therapeutic role, training and support for complementary therapists

According to Ong and Banks (2003) a number of surveys have identified that the public are attracted to complementary therapies because of the quality of the practitioner's interpersonal skills, touch, and the time given to consultations and treatment. Conventional health care professionals are often frustrated by the demands of workload that limit time spent with patients. Many health professionals, including nurses, are attracted to complementary therapies as a means of improving job satisfaction, being able to spend quality time with patients and expand their range of therapeutic skills to humanize health care. There are key professional issues to consider when providing complementary therapies to patients.

## *Professional and safe working*

Health professionals have an ethical duty to provide benefit to patients, which is enshrined in the legal concept of duty of care. Therapists, whether nurses or not, need to ensure that any interventions are provided on the basis of doing benefit not harm. Most complementary therapies used in supportive and palliative care involve physical touch. It is essential that therapists ascertain that consent is established prior to and during treatment. The civil action of battery (or trespass to the person), which upholds respect for the patient's bodily autonomy, is of importance here. A battery is said to occur when touch is given to a patient, for example in the course of the treatment, without first having obtained consent (Stone 2002). Complementary therapists can be asked to intervene in situations where consent is not clear and where care and sensitivity are needed in understanding verbal and non-verbal cues (see Case study 9.1).

---

**Case Study 9.1**

A referral for massage was received for a patient with brain metastases. At times, he was restless, agitated and disorientated. After careful consideration, the therapist offered to teach Rosie, his partner, how to give a simple ten-minute foot massage. Three teaching sessions were provided. This support and guidance included how to identify non-verbal cues which may suggest the need to stop or to take a break from the massage.

Rosie reported that the twice daily massages were well received. On a couple of occasions she had picked up the need to wrap his feet in a towel and leave him to rest and sleep, which he did.

In situations when ongoing consent is difficult to assess, it may be appropriate to decline to treat or, if appropriate, a therapist could teach and support a family member, partner or close friend in giving gentle massage (Mackereth *et al.* 2005a, 2005b). It is important for the complementary therapist to inform the referrer about how he or she has responded to the referral. A team approach, which includes the family, is essential to support a patient's autonomy and safety.

### The importance of the coordinator role

There is a need to foster a culture where facilitating innovation and leadership in complementary therapies are valued. However, the status of the service first needs to be established by asking, are these treatments recognized as a core activity or are they merely 'cherries on the cake'? To move forward with an integrated provision requires a number of essential stages. First, a steering group or committee needs to be created to gather information, assess need, identify resources (including funds), as well as gathering information about good practice from other centres offering similar services (Tavares 2003). Second, it has been suggested that the appointment of a suitably qualified and experienced coordinator is pivotal in securing and developing an accountable service (Carter and Mackereth 2006). Third, a team of skilled and dedicated therapists is required to provide a range of therapeutic interventions, ideally accessible to all patients using services. Where a complementary therapy team has become established, provision of treatments can be expanded to include carers and staff (Kohn 1999).

If a nurse is appointed to the coordinator role, this can present challenges as well as benefits to both the organization and the individual. For example, exposure to health care practice in clinical settings can provide knowledge and skills to inform safe delivery of treatments. Conversely, nurses may have problems when colleagues expect them to perform nursing duties or get overly involved in emergency situations.

### The need for audit and evaluation of services

Increasingly, any service development is required to demonstrate its effectiveness, as well as safe practice. The British House of Lords Science and Technology Report (2000) recommended that the complementary (and alternative) professions should work towards ensuring that the therapeutic claims for their treatments should be supported by quality evidence of benefit and safety. Audit and evaluation should be an integral part of any CT service, with defined aims and objectives implicit from the beginning. Methodology needs to be effective for the intervention and also needs to be credible to satisfy scrutiny and to provide credible evidence for the continuation and development of the service. There may be a need to involve research and development expertise, either within the institution or externally, so that professional time is utilized to maximum benefit. There is also a need for therapists to keep up to date with research and development in their field to ensure evidence-based practice and safety in delivery of the therapies.

## Research evidence for touch therapies

The evidence for benefit has, in the past, been largely anecdotal. Increasingly, research studies suggest that these therapies can help to improve physical symptoms and immunological parameter, for example lymphocyte activity and count. The evidence-based culture, a professional emphasis on research work, and historical interest in touch as means of support and communication have contributed to the emerging research base for touch therapies in clinical practice.

Recent qualitative work on reflexology suggests that these interventions can be a transformative experience with effects on the emotional and spiritual well-being. In the UK, Gambles *et al.* (2002) used a semi-structured questionnaire with a convenience sample (n=34) of patients attending for between four and six reflexology treatments at a hospice. Patients reported relief from anxiety, improved well-being, increased ability to cope with the diagnosis and prognosis, as well as feeling supported and comforted by the therapists.

Grealish *et al.* (2000) used a quasi-experimental design to evaluate the outcomes of foot massage provided by nurse reflexologists. Inpatients with cancer (n=87) were randomized to receive two massages and one resting period, but in three different orders or arms of the trial. Visual analogue scales (VAS) were used to measure pain, nausea and relaxation. Significant differences were found in scores, demonstrating improved relaxation and reduced nausea and pain for the massage intervention.

Stephenson and Weinrich (2000) used a cross-over trial with patients (n=23) living with lung or breast cancer to evaluate reflexology. Patients were randomized to receive a) 30 minutes of reflexology followed by a 30-minute control time after a two-day break or b) 30 minutes of control time, a two-day break and then 30 minutes of reflexology. There was a significant decrease in anxiety reported following the reflexology treatment, but effects on pain were less apparent.

Smith (2002), investigating the outcomes of reflexology for women with breast cancer (n=150) receiving radiotherapy, reported significant differences for both reflexology and foot massage (given by the same therapist) compared to standard care in some sub-scales of the mood scale and fatigue checklist. Additionally, for reflexology a trend for a possible effect on lymphocyte activity, worthy of further investigation, was identified.

Morris *et al.* (2000), in a postal survey enquiring about use of complementary therapies, received a total of 617 replies from the original 1,935 questionnaires sent to a random selection of cancer patients attending their centre. Fifty-three per cent of these patients reported using massage. Given the context for this survey, the response rate is not unusual.

In the USA, Post-White *et al.* (2003) showed that massage reduced ratings in several measures, including anxiety and perception of pain, in patients living with cancer (n=230). Cassileth and Vickers (2004) have also reported effects of massage in a larger study of over 1,000 cancer patients attending the Sloan-Kettering Cancer Centre over three years. Reductions in symptoms of anxiety, depression, pain and nausea were reported.

In the University of Miami, Florida, United States of America (USA), Hernandez-Reif *et al.* (2004) completed a study on the effects of massage in women (n=34) with early stage (I and II) breast cancer. Their results identified that massage was linked to significant reductions in anxiety and depression scores ($p < 0.05$) and enhancement of immune function through increase in numbers of Natural Killer (NK) cells in the massage group ($p < 0.05$). An analysis of co-variance performed on NK-cells numbers from the first to the last day of the five-week study period disclosed a significant group effect ($p < 0.05$), which reflected a significant positive change ($p < 0.05$) in NK-cell numbers for the massage arm and a negative change for the control arm. These papers are examples of a growing body of evidence that touch therapies can have psychological and immunological benefits.

## Relaxation and creative imagery techniques

Techniques which help patients to access a state of relaxation can be very useful and there are both physical and 'imagery' interventions that nurses may wish to offer to patients. A useful neuromuscular approach is the Adapted Progressive Muscle, which involves tightening and releasing muscle groups combined with breathing techniques developed by Edmund Jacobson (Freeman 2001). There are many techniques which are based on creative imagery. In working with people with cancer and other debilitating diseases, creative imagery can provide a useful resource, not only as distraction, but also as a means of deepening relaxation and helping with reducing anxiety and other symptoms (Vickers and Zollman 1999). Both approaches can be taught as self-help techniques to help patients manage, for example, distressing medical procedures, such as dressing a wound and draining ascites. Hypnotherapy, which utilizes a 'trance' state may also be of value in managing existential anxiety and other treatment related concerns in a palliative setting. This needs to be provided by a skilled therapist with the appropriate training (Rankin-Box 2001).

It does need to be acknowledged that many nurses and other health practitioners are already skilful in facilitating relaxation in their work with patients. For example, this could happen when a nurse comforts and soothes a distressed patient; helping by establishing rapport, listening calmly, and only talking in a paced manner attuned to the individual. It is recommended that training is essential to maximize the therapeutic benefits of these interventions, and also to identify when they would not be appropriate.

# 'Healing' modalities

'Healing' is a term which is often used generically to describe specific 'healing' practices (Rankin-Box and Williamson 2006). The most frequently used therapies in this category which are used in palliative care settings include therapeutic touch, reiki and spiritual healing (Kohn 1999; Tavares 2003). These therapies are based on the concept that energy flows through the body, which is surrounded by an energy field, sometimes referred to as the 'aura'. The aim of the therapies is to detect and modulate imbalances in the 'energy' flow in the physical body or the aura by using the hands. Fundamental to the practice of 'healing therapies' is a therapist's conscious intention to 'heal'; the healing may happen on physical, emotional, mental or spiritual levels. The term 'healing' can be confusing as for some patients 'healing' is synonymous with 'curing' (see Further reading).

# Caring for carers

Cancer diagnosis, treatments and the uncertainty of the process of the illness is extremely stressful, not only for patients, but for families, friends and work colleagues (Faulkner and Maguire 1994; Mackereth and Campbell 2002). Often carers place their own lives on hold as they cope with a roller coaster of emotions – the hopes of a cure, the possibility of losing someone close to them, dealing with the constant readjustment of hopes and fears, and maybe having to stop work all together, which leads to financial problems. Other stressors experienced by carers, wanting to do their best to help, include physical problems due to lifting, having to stay alert, and sitting by the bedside for long hours. These can lead to lack of sleep, exhaustion and mental health problems such as anxiety, depression and feeling isolated from the usual situations of everyday life (Carers UK 2001).

Carers may feel that they have limited time to receive massage, often because they are reluctant to spend time away from their loved ones (see Case study 9.2). Sometimes, they may not want to 'take treatments away from other patients', so they may refuse the offer of having some complementary therapy for themselves. A service project providing massage to carers has been the subject of a published evaluation in the USA (Macdonald 1998). Thirteen care-givers were given an average of six massages, after which 85 per cent reported emotional and physical stress level reduction, 77 per cent reported physical pain reduction and 54 per cent reported better patterns of sleep. In the UK, a massage service for family members of patients receiving palliative care has been well evaluated by subjects participating in focus groups (Penson 1998).

---

**Case Study 9.2**

Marion had been caring for her son, Mark, aged 46, who had been admitted to the hospice with metastatic disease. Marion kept a vigil at the bedside as Mark was at times very anxious and restless. She was offered a chair massage at the bedside. At the beginning of the treatment, Mark watched what was happening and then dozed off. Following the 30-minute treatment, Marion reported an immediate improvement in neck and shoulder tension. She talked openly about how hard it had been for her seeing the rapid deterioration in Mark's health, and how relieved she was to see Mark sleeping. The nurse reported the next day that Marion had a night of undisturbed sleep as she slept near to Mark on a fold-up bed.

---

## Involving carers in complementary therapies

Carers can feel hopeless and helpless as they observe health professionals delivering treatment, care and comfort to their loved ones. Partners, close friends and family members may wish to be involved in treatments. They can work alongside a therapist, and/or give a simple treatment following guidance from a skilled therapist (see Case study 9.3). Importantly, this requires therapists to be comfortable in a teaching and support role, taking into account the carer's individual needs as a learner in a sometimes difficult and stressful situation.

---

**Case Study 9.3**

Jill, a therapist working in a hospice, noticed that Martin's daughter, Sandra, observed her closely while she massaged his feet. Jill asked her if she wanted to learn massage. Sandra said she had always wanted to learn but she had not got around to it. With Martin's permission Jill taught Sandra a simple ten-minute massage routine using a guidance sheet with drawings and written instructions. First, they massaged one foot each, enabling Martin to give feedback to Sandra about the depth and speed of the massage strokes.

During their second practice session, Martin closed his eyes and relaxed. After the session he said, 'I didn't know who was massaging which foot!' Sandra beamed.

## Complementary therapies: providing services for staff and volunteers

Nurses, doctors and other health professionals working in supportive and palliative care settings can experience high stress levels. A major concern for all formal carers is the exposure to repeated loss, the distress of patients and their carers, and feelings of not being able to do enough to help. These challenges can result in emotional and physical exhaustion, problems with sickness and the retention of staff and volunteers. Burnout is a recognized result of being overwhelmed by the demands of being a professional carer (Barrett and Yates 2002).

Aside from managerial support, clinical supervision and counselling, CTs can provide physical and emotional support (Field *et al.* 1997; Katz *et al.* 1999). Having a separate service for staff, possibly subsidized by the organization, can help to combat stress, provide time out from busy shifts and acknowledge the need to support staff in a practical way.

Researchers have reported that 15-minute sessions of chair massage can reduce stress and enhance electroencephalogram patterns of alertness in health care professionals. Field *et al.* (1997) identified that a group of 26 nurses receiving a chair massage twice a week for five weeks had more reduced anxiety levels, lowered cortisol readings, improved alertness and higher scores in computational tasks after treatment than the control group of 24 subjects. Importantly for health care workers, Field *et al.* (1997) conducted a study in which hospital workers were given a ten-minute chair massage. Decreases in anxiety, depression and fatigue were reported at the end of the massage as well as increases in vigour. An example of how complementary therapy can support nurses is given below.

---

**Case Study 9.4**

Sandra, aged 47, had been working in a hospice for ten years. Following the loss of her father six months previously, she had been on sick leave with depression and low back pain. She was provided with vouchers by her organization to attend a subsidized complementary therapy service.

After receiving six weekly sessions of massage lasting approximately one hour each, Sandra reported that this had helped her to return to work and to express her grief to family and friends. She reported that the massage had provided relief from her back pain. Sandra had also taken up yoga and had renewed her interest in gardening.

# Managerial and political issues

The provision of complementary therapies in the British NHS is largely restricted to hospice settings, and as such provides an opportunity to examine how these interventions can contribute to care in the UK (Wilkinson 2002; Roberts *et al.* 2005). If services are to expand, for example as part of community palliative care or within an acute hospital, then service providers need to consider clinical governance in developing employment contracts for complementary therapists. Stanton (2004) states that supervisory and managerial processes are needed to 'identify (and differentiate between) safe, suboptimal and unsafe performance' (p. 1) in clinical practice. A recent report on clinical governance and CAM to the Department of Health identified that there was an 'emerging landscape of opportunities' for complementary therapists to be included in the NHS mainstream (Wilkinson *et al.* 2004: 1). The report, based on the University of Westminster study *Clinical Governance for Complementary and Alternative Medicine in Primary Care* (Wilkinson *et al.* 2004), mapped complementary health care in primary care. Evidence was gathered from 73 per cent (221) of Primary Care Trusts in England. The study revealed that complementary treatments are being provided by lay therapists (54 per cent) as well as health professionals with further training. Wilkinson *et al.* (2004) recommend that lay therapists employed on NHS contracts will require good systems of registration, revalidation and local accountability (clinical governance). The report also makes recommendations on the clinical governance issues and supervision needs of therapists, with a 'toolkit' to support best practice.

Currently, complementary therapies exist on the boundaries of health care, viewed by some individuals as no more than a treat or a placebo (Rayner 1999). Ernst (2001), commenting on patient choice and its limitation, distinguished wants from needs by saying: '. . . needs can only extend to treatments whose value has been firmly established; wants can be satisfied outside the NHS' (p. 41). According to Field, Director of the Touch Research Institute, it is the patients who are driving forward the integration of complementary therapies, and the medical community (including nurses) 'need to have an educated discussion' with patients about the benefits of these interventions (Mackereth 2001).

# Conclusion

Complementary therapies are increasingly being accepted as beneficial interventions in supportive and palliative care. This chapter has covered some of the main aspects of integrating complementary therapies into patient care. The use of the terms 'alternative' and 'complementary' has been clarified along with the need for health professionals and therapists to be accurate in the information they give to their patients and carers. The nurse's role in assessing, developing and supporting the provision of complementary therapies has been explored. Other areas on which the chapter has focused include ethical practice, clinical leadership and management of services, professional boundaries, and the importance of appropriate training and supervision. There is a need to evaluate the outcomes for complementary interventions within palliative care services. Recommendations for future research and practice development have been made below. These recommendations are based on existing literature and the author's experience (see Further reading).

---

**Recommendations**

- It is essential that health care workers and therapists are aware of the philosophical difference between 'complementary' and 'alternative' therapies and feel confident to discuss the implications of these terms with colleagues, patients, family and friends.
- Therapists need to take account of health concerns. For example, if lymphoedema is present it is essential to seek advise and, where possible, assessment from a specialist prior to treatment.
- Treatments require adaptation to ensure safety, comfort and effectiveness. For example, offering short and gentle sessions for patients with fatigue.
- It is important to involve and empower clients, this could include patients (and their carers) being taught simple techniques with supervision.
- There needs to be clinical leadership in complementary therapies to enable the development and effective running of a complementary therapy service.
- Therapists and health care professionals must be aware of multidisciplinary team working and professional roles and boundaries.
- Further research is essential in evaluating interventions and services, this must be done without burdening patients in palliative care settings.

---

# Further reading

Field, T. (2000) *Touch Therapy*. London: Harcourt Press.

Mackereth, P. and Carter, A. (eds) (2006) *Massage & Bodywork – adapting therapies for cancer care*. London: Elsevier Science.

Rankin-Box, D. (ed.) (2001) *The nurse's handbook of complementary therapies*. Edinburgh: Ballière Tindall.

# References

Barrett, L. and Yates, P. (2002) Oncology haematology nurses: a study of job satisfaction, burnout and intention to leave the speciality, *Australian Health Review*, 25(3): 109–21.

Boon, H., Stewart, M., Kennard, M.A., Gray, R., Sawka, C., Brown, J.B., McWilliam, C., Gavin, A., Baron, R.A., Aaron, A. and Haines-Kamka, T. (2000) Use of complementary/alternative medicine by breast cancer survivors in Ontario: prevalence and perceptions. *Journal of Clinical Oncology*, 18(13): 2515–21.

Carers UK (2001) *Taking a Break*. Information Leaflet for Carers, Ruth Pitter House.

Carter, A. and Mackereth, P. (2006) Clinical leadership: developing the role of complementary therapy coordinators. *Complementary Therapies in Clinical Practice*, 12(2): 80–2.

Cassileth, B.R. and Vickers, A.J. (2004) Massage Therapy for Symptom Control: Outcome Study at a Major Cancer Centre. *Journal of Pain and Symptom Management*, 28(3): 244–9.

Corner, J. and Harewood, J. (2004) Exploring the use of complementary and alternative medicine by people with cancer. *Journal of Research in Nursing*, 9(2): 101–9.

Dossey, B.D. (1995) Visions of healing. In: B.D. Dossey, L. Keegan, C.E. Guzzetta and L.E. Kolkmeier (eds) *Holistic Nursing: a handbook for practice* (2nd edn). Gaithersburg, MD: Aspen Publications.

Ernst, E. (ed.) (2001) *The desktop guide to complementary medicine*. London: Mosby.

Ersser, S. (2000) Editorial. *Journal of Clinical Nursing*, 9: 655–7.

Ezzo, J., Berman, B., Hadhazy, V.A., Jadad, A.R., Lao, L. and Singh, B.B. (2000) Is acupuncture effective for the treatment of chronic pain? – a systematic review. *Journal of Pain*, 86(3): 217–25.

Faulkner, A. and Maguire, P. (1994) *Talking to cancer patients and their relatives*. Oxford: Oxford University Press.

Field, T. (2000) *Touch Therapy*. London: Harcourt Press.

Field, T., Quintino, O., Henteleff, T., Wells-Keife, L. and Delvecchio-Feinberg, G. (1997) Job stress reduction therapies. *Alternative Therapies*, 3(4): 54–6.

Freeman, L.W. (2001) Research on mind-body effects. In: L.W. Freeman and G.F. Lawlis (eds) *Complementary and Alternative Medicine: a research based approach*. London: Mosby.

Gambles, M., Crooke, M. and Wilkinson, S. (2002) Evaluation of a hospice based reflexology service: a qualitative audit of patient perceptions. *European Journal of Oncology Nursing*, 6(1): 37–44.

Grealish, L., Lomasney, A. and Whiteman, B. (2000) Foot massage: a nursing intervention to modify the distressing symptoms of pain and nausea in patients hospitalised with cancer. *Cancer Nursing*, 23(3): 237–43.

Hernandez-Reif, M., Ironson, G., Field, T., Hurley, J., Katz, G., Diego, M., Weiss, S., Fletcher, M.A., Schanberg, S., Kuhn, C. and Burman, I. (2004) Breast Cancer Patients have Improved Immune and Neuroendocrine Functions Following Massage Therapy. *Journal of Psychosomatic Research*, 57(1): 45–52.

House of Lords Select Committee on Science and Technology (2000) *6th Report on Complementary and Alternative Medicine*. HL. 118. London: HMSO.

Hypericum Depression Trial Study Group (HDTSG) (2002) Effect of Hypericum perforatum (St. John's Wort) in major depressive disorder: a randomized, controlled trial. *The Journal of the American Medical Association*, 287(14): 1807–14.

Katz, J., Wowk, A., Culp, D. and Wakeling, D. (1999) Pain and tension are reduced amongst hospital nurses after on-site massage treatments: a pilot study. *Journal of Perianesthesia Nursing*, 14(3): 128–33.

Kohn, M. (1999) *Complementary therapies in cancer care: abridged report of a study produced for Macmillan Cancer Relief*. London: Macmillan Cancer Relief.

Kohn, M. (2002) *Directory of Complementary Therapy Services in UK Cancer Care*. London: Macmillan Cancer Relief.

MacDonald, G. (1998) Massage as a respite intervention for primary caregivers. *American Journal of Hospice and Palliative Medicine*, 15(1): 43–7.

Mackereth, P. (2001) Touch Research Institutes: an interview with Dr Tiffany Field. *Complementary Therapies in Nursing and Midwifery*, 7: 84–9.

Mackereth, P. and Campbell, G. (2002) Chair massage: attention and touch in 15 minutes. *Palliative and Cancer Matters*, 25: 2 and 6.

Mackereth, P. and Stringer, J. (2005) CAM and cancer care: champions for integration. *Complementary Therapies in Clinical Practice*, 11(1): 45–7.

Mackereth, P., Sylt, P., Weinberg, A. and Campbell, G. (2005a) Chair Massage for Carers, *European Journal of Oncology Nursing*, 9(2): 167–79.

Mackereth, P., Cawthorn, A., White, K. and Lynch, B. (2005b) Improving stressful working lives: complementary therapies, counselling and clinical supervision for staff. *European Journal of Oncology Nursing*, 9(2): 147–54.

Molassiotis, A. and Cubbin, D. (2004) 'Thinking outside the box': complementary and alternative therapies use in paediatric oncology patients. *European Journal of Oncology Nursing*, 8(1): 50–60.

Molassiotis, A., Fernadez-Ortega, P., Pud, D., Ozden, G., Scott, J.A., Panteli, V., Margulies, A., Browall, M., Magri, M., Selvekerova, S., Madsen, E., Milovics, L., Bruyns, I., Gudmundsdottir, G., Hummerston, S., Ahmad, A.M.-A., Platin, N., Kearney, N. and Patiraki, E. (2005) Use of complementary and alternative medicine in cancer patients: a European survey. *Annals of Oncology*, 16(4): 655–63.

Morris, K.T., Johnson, N., Homer, L. and Walts, D. (2000) A comparison of complementary therapy use between breast cancer patients and patients with other primary tumour sites. *The American Journal of Surgery*, 179(5): 407–11.

Ong, C. and Banks, B. (2003) *Complementary and alternative medicine: the consumer perspective*. Occasional Paper 2. London: The Prince of Wales's Foundation for Integrated Health.

Penson, J. (1998) Complementary therapies: making a difference in palliative care. *Complementary Therapies in Nursing and Midwifery*, 4(3): 77–81.

Post-White, J., Kinney, M.E., Savik, M.S., Berntsen Gau, J., Wilcox, C. and Lerner, I. (2003) Therapeutic Massage and Healing Touch Improve Symptoms in Cancer. *Integrative Cancer Therapies*, 2(4): 332–44.

Rankin-Box, D. (2001) Hypnosis. In: D. Rankin-Box (ed.) *The nurse's handbook of complementary therapies*. Edinburgh: Ballière Tindall.

Rankin-Box, D. and Williamson, E.M. (2006) *Complementary medicine: a guide for pharmacists*. London: Churchill Livingstone.

Rayner, C. (1999) Stuff and nonsense. *Nursing Standard*, 13(39): 22–33.

Richardson, M.A., Sanders, T., Palmer, J.L., Greisinger, A. and Singletary, S.E. (2000) Complementary/alternative medicine use in a comprehensive cancer center and the implications for oncology. *Journal of Clinical Oncology*, 18(13): 2505–14.

Roberts, D., McNulty, A. and Caress, A. (2005) Current issues in the delivery of complementary therapies in cancer care, policy, perceptions and expectations: an overview. *European Journal of Oncology Nursing*, 9(2): 115–23.

Schmidt, K. and Ernst, E. (2004) Assessing websites on complementary and alternative medicine for cancer. *Annals of Oncology*, 15: 733–42.

Smith, G. (2002) A randomised controlled clinical trial of reflexology in breast cancer patients, to reduce fatigue resulting from radiotherapy to the breast and chest wall. Unpublished PhD thesis, University of Liverpool.

Sparber, A., Bauer, L., Curt, G., Eisenberg, D., Levin, T., Parks, S., Steinberg, S.M. and Wootton, J. (2000) Use of complementary medicine by adult patients participating in cancer clinical trials. *Oncology Nurse Forum*, 27(4): 623–30.

Stanton, P. (2004) Executive Summary. *The strategic leadership of clinical governance in PCTs*. NHS Modernisation Agency. Clinical Governance Support Team, National Primary Care Trust Development Programme.

Stephenson, N.L.N. and Weinrich, S.P. (2000) The effects of foot reflexology on anxiety and pain in patients with breast and lung cancer. *Oncology Nursing Forum*, 27(1): 67–72.

Stone, J. (2002) *An ethical framework for complementary and alternative therapies*. London: Routledge.

Tavares, M. (2003) *The National Guidelines for the Use of Complementary Therapies in Supportive and Palliative Care*. The Foundation for Integrated Health.

Tovey, P. and Adams, J. (2003) Nostalgic and nostophobic referencing and the authentication of nurses' use of complementary therapies. *Social Science and Medicine*, 56: 1469–80.

Vickers, A. and Zollman, C. (1999) ABC of complementary therapies – Hypnosis and relaxation therapies. *British Medical Journal*, 319: 1346–9.

Wilkinson, J., Peters, D. and Donaldson, J. (2004) *Clinical governance for complementary and alternative medicine (CAM) in primary care*. University of Westminster.

Wilkinson, S. (2002) Complementary therapies – patient demand. *International Journal of Palliative Nursing*, 8(10): 468.

Wright, S.G. and Sayre-Adams, J. (2000) *Sacred space – right relationship and spirituality in health care*. Edinburgh: Harcourt Brace.

# PART TWO

**Transitions into the terminal phase**

# 10

## Overview

*Jane Seymour and Christine Ingleton*

One of the only certainties in life is that we will all die, and yet death is both a 'fact of life and a profound mystery' (Field and Cassell 1997: 1); we cannot report back once we have gone through the process of dying; we cannot evaluate the care that we were given or suggest ways in which it might have been done better. Although dying is regarded as one of the most critical stages of life, the quality of the experience of dying very largely depends upon others. At a societal level, value is placed on a humane approach to dying: there is a desire to care for people well when they die, in ways that protect their dignity and give comfort to them and their companions when they most need it. However, the way in which these aims are achieved has been radically transformed over the past century. Until the fairly recent past, death was something that took place at home within the family. There may not have been much that could be done to relieve physical suffering, but people knew how to manage death and how to behave around a dying person, who was embraced as part of the family unit and ministered to by relatives, friends and loved ones. A religious leader may have been called, and perhaps a doctor, but they would not be central figures in this scene (Ariès 1981). Moreover, death was a frequent visitor across the generations, not something that tends to happen primarily to older people as in modern society. Nowadays, in spite of efforts to the contrary, death at home in many resource-rich countries is less common than institutional death. Even when death does occur at home, it tends to be overseen by technical and clinical 'experts'. Modern dying has some particular features that can make caring for dying people difficult:

- Clinical technologies and the potential of new treatments to offset death have made a diagnosis of dying difficult and the process of dying much longer than it used to be. Not recognizing imminent death means that some people die in pain and distress which could otherwise be relieved.

- Clinical training in the twentieth and twenty-first centuries has tended to encourage the view that death is a failure and has, to some extent, prioritized bodily or physical care rather than spiritual, social or family care, which may be just as or even more important to the dying person.

- The management of modern dying is fraught with ethical difficulties: poor understanding of ethics and law at the end of life can make good care at the end of life difficult to achieve.

Hospice and palliative care has, it might be argued, become synonymous with 'good death'. As Clark and Seymour (1999) note, this concept stands now not only as a 'symbolic critique' (McNamara 1997: 3) of medicalized, institutionalized death, but also as a central point of reference for popular expectations of dying and of standards of care at the time of death. These are, however, expectations that remain unfulfilled for the vast majority of the dying population across the world. Of the 54 million deaths that occur annually, 46 million take place in the low- and middle-income countries of the world (Stjernswärd and Clark 2005), meaning that there are fundamental inequalities in state-provided health and social care that the dying receive and in the resources that their family carers are able to mobilize in delivering care to them. In spite of these inequalities, it is now recognized that, ideally, we should all be able to expect a death that involves privacy, dignity, good quality care in comfortable surroundings, adequate pain relief and appropriate support (General Medical Council 2006). The following principles can be identified as characterizing 'good' care of people approaching death and their companions:[1]

- Care for those approaching death is an integral and important part of health care. Care for the dying should involve and respect patients and those close to them.

- Care at the end of life depends upon health care professionals having strong interpersonal skills and clinical knowledge, and is informed by ethical understanding and personal and professional values and experience.

- Good care for dying people is a team endeavour and depends as much on the organization of health care as it does on individuals.

- Nurses have special responsibilities in caring for dying people, since they most commonly have closest contact with the seriously and terminally ill.

In this chapter, we examine some of these important issues about death and dying, focusing in particular on: selected key concepts; processes leading to the definition of dying; ethical issues related to end-of-life care decision-making, focusing particularly on assisted dying and advance care planning; evidence about the experience of dying in different cultures and settings of care; and nursing care during dying. The chapter draws on research studies and 'critical cases' throughout.

# Key concepts

Since we published the first edition of this book, the term *'end-of-life care'* has gradually begun to supplant the more familiar terms of 'hospice' and 'palliative' care, featuring commonly in both research and policy reports internationally. The term originates from North America, where it has been used particularly in the context of the care of older people and relates to an '. . . approach that treats, comforts and supports older individuals who are living with, or dying from, progressive or chronic life-threatening conditions. Such care is sensitive to personal, cultural and spiritual values, beliefs and practices and encompasses support for families and friends up to and including the period of bereavement' (Ross *et al.* 2000). End-of-life care is an appropriate term to capture care given when a person is known to be in the last stages of their life but is not clearly 'dying'. In the UK during 2007, work to develop an 'end-of-life care strategy' followed recognition of the need to respond more appropriately to the changes in epidemiological trends which mean that, at the start of the twenty-first century, most deaths follow a period of chronic illness such as heart disease, cancer, stroke, chronic respiratory disease, neurological disease or dementia. Trajectories of dying associated with these diseases, and the needs associated with them, do not fit with the classic 'cancer journey' or model of care on which the hospice and palliative care movement was originally based.

The concept of *'trajectories'* of dying is useful to help us understand what might be the different experiences and needs of people as they approach the end of life. This concept was first discussed by two sociologists, working in the USA in the 1960s (Glaser and Strauss 1965). Depending on the cause of death and the type and availability of treatment, the trajectory of a dying process may be slow, sudden, or take the shape of a series of relapses and recoveries. One conceptual model depicting different trajectories of dying has become popular over the last few years (Lynn and Adamson 2003). Lynn and Adamson suggest that there are three 'ideal type' trajectories which can be described to help us understand the similarities and differences among those people who are likely to need palliative and end-of-life care: those who have a short period of decline before death, for example the typical case of a person dying from cancer; those who have long-term limitations with periods of relapse and remission before what is often a sudden death, for example as may be the case for people living with lung or heart disease; and 'prolonged dwindling' before death, as may be the case for older people living with extreme frailty or cognitive impairment.

Improved understanding of the trajectories of illness progression may help to plan end-of-life care for persons in need more effectively, providing a 'broad time frame and patterns of probable needs and interactions with health and social services that can, conceptually at least, be mapped out towards death' (Murray *et al.* 2005: 1007), and enabling patients and caregivers to prepare as far as possible for future challenges in their own unique circumstances. It has been argued that these 'ideal types' (conceptual tools to help us to think about reality but do not exactly mirror it) can help in thinking about the planning of services at a population level to meet a range of needs (Dy and Lynn 2007).

Another concept about which much has been written and which has been used to strengthen the claims of those taking quite different positions on the continuum between the 'right to die' and 'right to life' lobbies, is that of *'dignity'*. 'Dignity' is a concept applied very frequently to describe an idealized 'good death'. De Raeve (1996: 71), writing about the links between 'death with dignity' and 'good death', notes that we need to think carefully and reflectively about the term 'dignity' in order to move away from prevalent 'crude images' of the good death in which people are manoeuvred through predetermined 'stages'. She suggests that we consider 'dignity' in terms of its contribution as a quality or aspect of nursing care given to people who are seriously ill or dying, and whose sense of innate dignity or personal, spiritual and physical integrity may be under threat:

> . . . what sense can be made of the idea of death with dignity? Could it escape the good death straitjacket by being construed not as a manner of dying but as a way of treating the dying? Dying and seriously ill people perhaps deserve to be treated with dignity in such a way as to try to preserve the dignity that they have and help them regain the sense of dignity that feels lost.
>
> (de Raeve 1996: 71)

In a phenomenological study with patients and nurses in a hospital, Walsh and Kowanko (2002) show that nurses and patients agree on the key elements of dignity and the sorts of nursing care practices that support or detract from it. In both nurses' and patients' accounts in this study, the body, its treatment and its exposure were central themes, with maintenance of privacy being inextricably linked to perceptions of respect, consideration and personhood. Threats to dignity were perceived to emanate from a neglectful attitude to patients and their bodies; for example, where nurses forgot, or saw others forget, to extend ordinary everyday civilities to their patients (such as a greeting or polite request to enter a room) that are taken for granted outside of the health care system. Incursions of this type, which may seem relatively trivial, were seen to lead to more fundamental breaches of personhood, such as being left exposed to view, or not having one's permission asked before medical students witnessed embarrassing procedures, or having one's feelings disregarded.

Walsh and Kowanko (2002) note the powerful way in which structural and environmental influences make it hard for nurses to treat patients as people all of the time. They observe how the 'system', and how it militates against maintaining patients' and nurses' dignity, has been an enduring theme in commentaries about health and health care. Within these commentaries, objectification of the patient is seen as a strategy with which nurses engage to protect themselves from personal involvement in situations where they are relatively powerless to influence patients' treatment or inexorable progress through the bureaucracy of health care (see, for example, Menzies

1970). Maintaining patients' dignity is perhaps especially difficult in the context of the complex and paradoxical nature of demands facing contemporary health care professionals who have the responsibility for the treatment and care of dying people in an era of rapid change and scarce nursing resources.

The concept of perhaps most resonance for those facing the end of life or charged with providing care for those approaching the end of life is that of *'suffering'*. In his study of suffering, the physician Eric Cassell argues that suffering is experienced by persons, occurs when an impending destruction of the person is perceived and continues until the integrity of the person can be restored in some manner (Cassell 2004: 32). The experience of suffering is not dependent upon or directly linked to the severity of pain or the status of illness. Rather, it is dependent upon the meanings that illness and pain have for the person experiencing them. Kleinman (1988) in his seminal text 'The Illness Narratives: Suffering, Healing and the Human Condition' notes that: 'it is possible to talk to patients, even those who are most distressed, about the actual experience of illness, and that witnessing and helping to order that experience can be of therapeutic value' (Kleinman 1988: xii).

Making sense of suffering and helping the person who is suffering involves understanding what may be a unique and highly personal reaction to illness and distress. For some people, the experience of suffering is linked to a need to find meaning and to search for spiritual or religious explanations for questions that emerge from the experience of suffering: Why me? Why now? Why like this? Much has been written about the possibility of personal transformation through suffering and how this is related to predominant cultural mores. One well-known depiction is that posited by Arthur Frank who, drawing on his own experience of suffering from cancer and heart disease, describes particular types of narratives of suffering that tend to be associated with mortal illness in the modern world:

> Restitution narratives attempt to outdistance mortality by rendering illness transitory. Chaos stories are sucked into the undertow of illness and the disasters that attend it. Quest stories meet suffering head on; they accept illness and seek to use it.
>
> (Frank 1995: 115)

Frank suggests that for some people, suffering leads them to 'construct new maps and new perceptions of their relationships to the world' (1995: 3). To some extent, the notion of 'narrative' stances can be compared and contrasted with the notion of 'trajectory', with the first being useful perhaps in thinking about the heterogeneity of experience and the different personal responses to illness and the second being valuable for understanding the broad patterns of illness which may be associated with the personal experience of suffering.

Writing about the socially shaped nature of suffering, Wilkinson (2005) draws our attention to the importance of taking a historical, sociological and cultural studies perspective to what is a universal human experience.

Although not writing directly about end-of-life care, Wilkinson gives a number of examples (the phenomenon of 'Live Aid' in the 1980s, for example) which show that it is possible to create social movements that mobilize our common feelings of compassion and bonds of humanity to support the relief of suffering at a global level. Arguably, we have not yet managed to do this in relation to end-of-life care, although the public support of the early hospice movement suggests that there is an as yet untapped source of support for a new movement which better responds to the myriad dilemmas, problems and needs associated with death and dying in the late modern world. We turn now to review some of these.

# Defining dying

Field, writing in 1996, argued that 'modern' dying is characterized by what Glaser and Strauss called a 'status passage' (Glaser and Strauss 1965, cited in Field 1996), in which there are four major characteristics: first, dying is linked to a medical definition of terminal disease; second, dying is linked to a loss of activities and social roles, with little or no new activities; third, there is little prior socialization to the role; and fourth, there are few 'rites of passage' to signal the person's transition to the dying role. Here, we focus on the first of these, the medical definition of dying. Here, we look especially closely at the consequences that flow from the peculiarly modern problem of *defining* dying.

## Medical definitions of dying

With advances in medical technology becoming of widespread application in the developed world, diseases that are potentially life-threatening can be diagnosed at an early stage even to the point of identifying a genetic predisposition to developing such a disease in the future, where none may yet exist. Our awareness of our mortality is, as a result (at an intellectual level at least) highly developed. For example, many of us will be aware of familial dispositions to particular types of chronic disease that could contribute to our eventual demise, and many of us spend a great deal of energy in trying to minimize such risks through attention to diet, weight control, screening opportunities and other similar devices. Yet, ironically, receiving a medical diagnosis of *dying* as a result of chronic disease is perhaps less likely now than at any time hitherto. In the not too distant past, serious illness led to death quite quickly. Dying was encapsulated into a few weeks or days and there were fairly clear norms of social and clinical behaviour surrounding the person who was dying and their companions. Now, with the rise of what has been called the 'indistinct zone' of chronic illness and the concentration of death in older age (Lynn 2005), things have fundamentally changed: we tend to live for a long time with illnesses that are eventually fatal and die without ever having the label 'dying' attached to us.

Bauman (1992) identified two strategies which are employed by developed societies to ward off 'the problem' of death that results from the technical abilities that we now possess to diagnose disease. One strategy attempts to 'deconstruct' death into individual problems of health and disease that we conceive of as potentially soluble, given adequate knowledge, resources, effort and time. In this strategy, the problem of death becomes contained by the specific medical explanation of its cause; for example, cardiac arrhythmias at the late stages of heart disease may be dealt with as discrete problems rather than as indicators of any more general movement towards death. Thus we have a situation in which disease detection is highly developed, but the definition of dying is highly complex because of the extensive attempts made to defer, through a search for 'cure', any manifestations of dying (Lofland 1978; Bauman 1992). Even when it is recognized that death is a likely outcome of disease, widespread access to life-supporting interventions (such as artificial feeding or chemotherapy) may radically transform the life expectancy of some dying people from the few days or weeks usually associated with a terminal disease to the several months or years more often associated with a chronic disease (Jennett 1995). Questions about the withdrawal or withholding of life-supporting interventions (Hopkins 1997), and arguments about the best way in which to break the news to patients that dying may be inevitable, give rise to intense debate and ethical conjecture. Nicholas Christakis, a physician and sociologist, examined how doctors 'prognosticate' in cases of life-limiting and terminal illness (Christakis 1999). Christakis's thesis is that of the three main tasks of the physician – diagnosis, treatment and prognosis – the last was neglected during the twentieth century. This means that care and treatment options for people facing life-limiting illness are not always assessed, planned and evaluated appropriately. Christakis's observations are paralleled closely by those of Ellershaw and Ward (2003), who link quality of end-of-life care to the 'diagnosis of dying':

> In order to care for dying patients it is essential to 'diagnose dying'. However, diagnosing dying is often a complex process. In a hospital setting, where the culture is often focused on 'cure', continuation of invasive procedures, investigations, and treatments may be pursued at the expense of the comfort of the patient. There is sometimes a reluctance to make the diagnosis of dying if any hope of improvement exists and even more so if no definitive diagnosis has been made. When recovery is uncertain it is better to discuss this rather than giving false hope to the patient and family. This is generally perceived as a strength in the doctor–patient relationship and helps to build trust.
>
> (Ellershaw and Ward 2003: 30)

Ellershaw and Ward (2003) identify a range of barriers to the diagnosis of dying, including, among others: hope that the patient may get better; disagreements about the patient's condition; medico-legal issues; and fears of foreshortening life.

The consequences that result from the problems that doctors have with defining dying and with prognostication are illuminated well by the findings from a well-known North American study: the Study to Understand Prognoses and Preferences for Outcomes and Risks of Treatment (SUPPORT Principal Investigators 1995, see Box 10.1). This study, which began in 1989, had the stated aim of achieving a clearer understanding of the character of dying in American hospitals.

Christakis, in his commentary on the SUPPORT study, notes that:

> it is clear that discussion of prognosis occurred insufficiently frequently, since a majority of these seriously ill patients said they would have

---

**Box 10.1**  Highlight on research: the Study to Understand Prognoses and Preferences for Outcomes and Risks of Treatment

SUPPORT enrolled a total of 9,105 patients suffering from life-threatening illness in five hospitals in the USA over a four-year period. Each patient's illness was judged to be such that they had a 50 per cent chance of death within the next six months. In the first phase of the study, the care and treatment that 4,301 patients received was documented:

- 80 per cent of those who died during phase one had a 'do-not-resuscitate' order, but almost half of these orders were written within two days of death.
- 31 per cent of patients in phase one expressed a preference (to researchers) not to be resuscitated, but this was understood by slightly less than half of their lead clinicians.
- Of those patients who died in phase one, 38 per cent spent ten or more days in intensive care units.
- 50 per cent of all conscious patients who died in phase one were reported by their families as having moderate or severe pain.

The second phase of the study was the implementation and evaluation of an intervention aimed at resolving the problems highlighted in phase one. The remaining 4,804 patients were involved in this phase. An intervention was designed that was aimed at improving communications between the relevant parties. First, researchers provided doctors with brief written reports on their patients' probability of surviving up to six months, likelihood of being functionally impaired at two months and probability of surviving cardiopulmonary resuscitation. Second, doctors were provided with brief written reports regarding patients' views on life-sustaining treatment, presence of pain and desire for information. Third, specially trained nurse facilitators were given responsibility for initiating and maintaining communication between patients, their carers and their health care team. Patients were randomized to receive either the intervention or to continue with the usual medical care. Data pertaining to the key issues highlighted in phase one were then gathered from the two groups and the results compared. The results indicate that there were no significant differences between the two groups regarding the four key issues: the timing of do-not-resuscitate orders remained the same; patient–physician communication did not improve; reported pain levels remained static; and high levels of technology attended a significant proportion of deaths.

desired a discussion of the prognosis. Moreover, all had an objectively high risk of death within a few months, so *the prognosis was material to their care*, and there was ample opportunity for them to be provided with prognostic information, given that they were in hospital being seen daily by physicians . . . [as a result] patients generally had substantially unduly optimistic expectations about their prospects for recovery. These false prognostic impressions apparently influenced the choices that patients made, tilting patients in favour of active treatment of their illnesses rather than palliative care.

(Christakis 1999: 188–9, our emphasis)

One of the problems associated with achieving a medical definition of dying, and how and when it occurs, is that there is still a myth that dying is essentially a 'natural' phenomenon that exists independently of the activities and beliefs of those caring for the dying person. However, an examination of how matters of team interaction determine the status of ill persons as 'dying' reveals that dying is a fluid state heavily dependent not only on the technical and clinical work that informs prognostication, but also the social interaction between clinicians and their colleagues at the bedside of patients.

### Interactional issues in defining dying

Writing in 1996, Turner made the sharp observation that it is illusory to think that the problem of recognizing imminent death is merely a matter of the inaccuracy of our *technical* abilities to define or diagnose dying:

the problem, however, is not simply technical since there is an essential difference between medical death and social death. Dying is a social process, involving changes in behaviour and a process of assessment which do not necessarily correspond to the physical process of bodily death. Death, like birth, has to be socially organized and, in the modern hospital, is an outcome of team activities.

(Turner 1996: 198)

Turner is arguing here that clinical work transforms the body and invokes, or produces, dying as an identity through the activities of teamwork and team discussions. The PhD research of one of us (Seymour 2001), summarized in Box 10.2, applied this latter insight to interpret the interactional processes that precede the withdrawal or withholding of life-prolonging treatments from people dying in intensive care units. In this study, the largely unspoken negotiation that occurs between medicine and nursing during interaction was explored, with a focus on how the seemingly contradictory 'whole person work' of nursing and 'medical-technical' work of medicine are balanced during the care of dying patients.

In Seymour's study, the recognition that there are two potentially divergent trajectories of dying in intensive care ('technical' and 'bodily' dying) and two opposing foci of work ('whole body' and 'medical-technical')

> **Box 10.2**   A summary of Seymour's research (Seymour 2001)
>
> Seymour's ethnographic research examines the way in which problems of defining dying are resolved during medical work within the adult intensive care unit. She argues that issues of non-treatment in intensive care are emotive and, at times, contentious matters which hinge upon the resolution of 'problem[s] of social definition' (Glaser and Strauss 1965: 16). She then explores the way in which such resolution occurs and examines the navigation of 'uncertain death at an unknown time' (Glaser and Strauss 1965: 16) for people who were patients in the intensive care units of two city hospitals in the UK during the mid-1990s. At the outset, the study was envisaged as an attempt to slow down and dwell upon fast-moving action in intensive care to better understand the social processes that culminate in a definition of dying and precipitate an application of human agency (in the form of withholding or withdrawing life support) such that death can follow dying. Seymour presents an analysis of observational case study data and suggests that the definition of 'dying' in intensive care hinges upon four strategies. These are presented as a framework with which to interpret social interaction between physicians during end-of-life decision-making in intensive care. They are as follows: First, the establishment of a 'technical' definition of dying – informed by results of investigations and monitoring equipment – over and above 'bodily' dying informed by clinical experience. Second, the alignment of the trajectories of technical and bodily dying to ensure that the events of non-treatment have no perceived causative link to death. Third, the balancing of medical action with non-action, allowing a diffusion of responsibility for death to the patient's body. Last, the incorporation of the patient's companions and nursing staff into the decision-making process.

allows for an examination of the consequences for the care of (probably) dying patients and their families. The study shows clearly the deleterious outcomes for nurses as they struggle to achieve the 'good death' for patients in circumstances in which, because it is difficult to align technical and bodily dying, death is either precipitated or delayed. We see also the problems that result in trying to advance and protect the rights of families to participate in the decision-making process, when much of the interactional work that leads to critical decisions about the withdrawal and withholding of treatment takes place 'behind the scenes' and thus is insulated from all but the most determined of family members (Seymour 2001).

It might be easy to think that intensive care is somehow a 'special case', in which death is indeed profoundly problematic but has little relevance for other settings of care, and can therefore be set aside. More recently published work in the anthropological tradition seems to suggest that this is not the case and that similar problems frequently attend the definition of dying in less technological environments of care, and even at home. For example, Kaufman's (2003) study of a long-term care facility in North America for people in near persistent vegetative states alerts us very movingly to some of the ethical complexities that attend dying in our developed world. She speaks of the suffering endured by the sister of a man who exists, by virtue of severe brain injury as a result of a failed suicide attempt and the indecision of those caring for him about continuation or cessation of life-prolonging treatments, in the twilight world between living and dying. The sister feels that he should be allowed to die and is deeply distressed about the possibility that he is suffering even more profoundly than at the time of his unsuccessful suicide attempt. The team, having failed to resolve questions of decision-making through reference to ethical principles, decide to 'wait and see' for another few months. Kaufman argues that

> medicine ponders a cluster of questions, constructed through the frame of bioethics, whose very formulation minimizes or ignores location and context. For example, how can professionals promote 'quality of life' when the idea is itself debatable? What is in the patient's 'best interest'? Those questions, based on the primacy of patient autonomy, underlie every medical intervention and every interaction even though patients' identities are actually invoked through inter-subjective relations ... those questions and the rationalist, utilitarian moral philosophy from which they derive cannot, by themselves, reveal medicine's complicated ethical role in transforming and fabricating persons through its examinations and treatments. Nor do those questions speak to the realm of compassion and emotional connection felt toward very impaired persons. Those questions, as debated in the public sphere, ignore a powerful and essential dimension of human relations.
>
> (Kaufman 2003: 2259–60)

The questions that Kaufman raises here about 'bioethics', 'autonomy', 'quality of life', 'best interests' and the potential schism between the medical interpretations of an ill person's identity and those of others with an emotional attachment to the person, underpin much ethical and moral debate in palliative care and beyond. We turn now to look at a few selected issues in more detail.

## Ethical issues in clinical practice at the end of life

As the means have become available to support life and to defer death for prolonged periods, so the moral and ethical complexities surrounding clinical practice at the end of life have multiplied. In palliative care, ethics centre on 'decisions which will enable us to satisfy the criteria for a peaceful death, dignified and assisted by a helpful society' (Roy and MacDonald 1998: 97). Medical and clinical ethics are those values and obligations of a moral nature that govern the practice of medicine and are enshrined in professional codes and standards of practice. *Medical ethics* change over time, although medicine in the UK has been guided by the Jewish/Christian and Hippocratic traditions, in which doctors' obligations to the sick have been emphasized. *Clinical ethics* are of more relevance when thinking about the nature of interdisciplinary teamwork in palliative care, and the need to engage with ethical issues across disciplinary and professional boundaries in order to give good care to dying patients. The field of *bioethics*, in which the rights of the individual are emphasized, emerged following the Second World War. Bioethics is rooted in the reaction to the 'medical' experiments conducted in Germany by scientists during the war and exposed during the Nuremberg Trials. In its contemporary form, bioethics focuses on the consequences for people of new health technologies and other scientific developments (ten Have and Clark 2002; Dingwall 2003). An alternative ethical framework which has been gaining ground in latter years, particularly in the nursing and social science literature, is that of *'care ethics'* which focuses on how ethical problems and their solutions are always embedded in, and contingent upon, a network of relationships and contextual circumstances (Gastmans 2006). In the latter, interpretation of stories and of personal narratives in order to work out what is the best thing to do in the particular circumstances at hand, are as important as appealing to universal principles.

Below, we provide a brief review of two particular issues in palliative and end-of-life care that are the subjects of wide debate: advance care planning and assisted dying. This choice is necessarily highly selective and we refer readers to the texts referenced at the end of this chapter for further study of ethical issues in end-of-life care. However, to begin with we will discuss three critical cases to highlight for readers some of the wider issues involved in end-of-life care decision-making (see Box 10.3).

### Assisted dying

The cases of Diane Pretty and Miss 'B' in the UK highlight the clinical and public dilemmas that can surround caring for people at the end of their life. In particular, questions of how refractory symptoms can be managed, what should be done when a person no longer wants to live, or the person's life appears to be so tortured with suffering that death could be in that person's best interest. Is there a right to death, and does it ever outweigh the right to life? When a life has become unbearable, is it ever permissible to choose a path of clinical action or non-action that ends that life? Should a doctor ever help a patient die? How are we to understand the relationship between the moral principles of sanctity of life, autonomy, mercy and justice (Cobb 2003)? The differential resolutions of the cases of Miss B (who was taken off a ventilator at her own request and died shortly afterwards) and of Diane Pretty (whose husband was not allowed to assist her to commit suicide) provoked a storm of controversy, with some saying that there was little between the cases and that the judgments showed how disadvantaged certain groups of terminally ill people are by the laws surrounding the withdrawal and withholding of treatment. The distinction between the two cases hung on the difference perceived in English law between *acts of commission* (i.e. killing) and *acts of demission* (i.e. 'pulling the plug' or withdrawing treatment)

**Box 10.3** Ethical issues at the end of life: four critical cases

### Diane Pretty (UK)

Diane Pretty was a woman of 43 who had late-stage motor neurone disease and applied during 2002 to the European Court of Human Rights to allow her husband to help her to commit assisted suicide. The application, which was rejected, was surrounded by publicity. Mrs Pretty eventually died in a hospice. It was widely reported that, in the days before her death, she had suffered the very symptoms she had feared, although these had eventually been well controlled. The case was supported by the Voluntary Euthanasia Society and the civil rights group 'Liberty'.

(BBC News, Monday, 13 May 2002: http://news.bbc.co.uk/1/hi/health/1983941.stm)

### Miss B (UK)

A quadriplegic woman who fought and won a legal battle for the right to come off the ventilator which kept her alive, has got her wish and died peacefully in her sleep. Miss B, a former senior social worker, was moved three weeks ago to a London hospital where doctors had agreed to carry out her wishes, after those caring for her at another hospital for more than a year refused to take a step they regarded as killing her. Last-ditch attempts were made to persuade her to try rehabilitation, which would not have improved her physical condition but might have increased her quality of life through the use of mechanical aids. But 43-year-old Miss B, who was unmarried, was adamant that she did not want to live, as she was paralysed from the neck down and reliant on others for all her personal care. She died last Wednesday, but the death was announced yesterday. Miss B, who was paralysed after a blood vessel burst in her neck, made UK history last month as the first non-terminally ill patient to ask to be withdrawn from a ventilator. The Department of Health announced yesterday: 'Miss B has died peacefully in her sleep after being taken off the ventilator at her request.' Dame Elizabeth Butler-Sloss, President of the High Court's family division, ruled in the High Court in London last month that Miss B had the 'mental capacity to give consent or refuse consent to life-sustaining medical treatment'.

(Dyer 2002)

### Terry Schiavo (USA)

Terry Schiavo, a 41-year-old Florida woman, who was in a persistent vegetative state[1] for 15 years before her death on 31 March 2005, was at the centre of a political, legal and media tempest over the removal of a feeding tube. Hyperbole has run high on both sides of the controversy. Religious conservatives have decried the removal of her feeding tube as a 'mortal sin'; defenders of the 'right to die' have claimed that 'Congress will now go trampling into the most private, personal and painful decisions that families must ever make'. At the centre of the storm lay Terry Schiavo, her husband and her parents – all grievously struck by a tragedy 15 years ago. Unable to agree how to move forward, Schiavo's husband and parents sought remedy in the courts. . . . Recalling a statement that his wife had once made [Michael Schiavo] refused further life-prolonging treatments on her behalf. However, her parents, Bob and Mary Schindler, never accepted the diagnosis of persistent vegetative state and vigorously opposed their son-in-law's decision. Seven years of litigation generated 30 legal opinions, all supporting Michael Schiavo's decision on his wife's behalf.

(Weijer 2005)

1 Schiavo's arrest was caused by hypokalaemia induced by an eating disorder.

(Shaw 1995). Shaw also refers to *acts of omission*, which relate to situations where treatments judged to be able to confer no benefit to a person are withheld. A further distinction relates to the way in which the courts used the principles of autonomy and sanctity of life in making their judgments. In Miss B's case, autonomy was prioritized, whereas in Diane Pretty's case, sanctity of life, and the need to be seen to protect this for the good of society, triumphed (Huxtable and Campbell 2003).

Many cases which give rise to disputes over decision-making at the end of life involve families who are struggling to find the 'right' thing to do for a person close to them who lost capacity due to catastrophic illness. These personal and family dilemmas and their consequences for persons tend to be neglected in bioethical analyses of end-of-life care decision-making. The case of Terry Schiavo in the USA, who died in 2005 following the withdrawal of her artificial feeding after 15 years in a persistent vegetative state, is an exemplar of the passions and difficulties that such struggles produce. It involved a battle in the courts between her husband and her parents, in which their personal desires to do the best thing for a person they all loved were hijacked by powerful media and ideological lobbies and dissected in legal and ethical terms which arguably contributed little to finding a solution which may have kept the family intact. Commentating on this case from a care ethics perspective, Weijer notes that legal solutions should be a last resort and that end-of-life care in cases such as that of Terry Schiavo should rather be directed at helping the family reach consensus using arbitration, negotiation and facilitation. Weijer concludes that the case of Terry Schiavo was a double tragedy: 'a death in the family, and the death of a family' (2005: 1198).

As medical technology increasingly exists not only to relieve the suffering associated with dying, but to prolong life or to procure early death, the clarification of the distinction between 'killing' and 'letting die' which beset the Schiavo case is perhaps one of the most pressing concerns facing society today. In most of the developed world, it is now recognized that where death is inevitable, then life-prolonging treatments such as resuscitation, artificial ventilation, dialysis, artificial nutrition and hydration can be withdrawn or withheld, and the goal of medicine redirected to the palliation of symptoms and the provision of 'basic care' and comfort, which are mandatory (see, for example, British Medical Association 2007). One device which is increasingly promoted as a means of ensuring appropriate levels of intervention in accordance with the wishes of persons is that of the 'advance statement' drafted as a result of a process of 'advance care planning'.

### Advance care planning

Advance care planning (ACP), usually defined as a process of discussion between an individual, their family and care providers, has been widely promoted as one means of addressing the dilemmas associated with what are appropriate levels of intervention in life-limiting illness. The term first appeared as an umbrella term describing a range of interventions and associated outcomes in the literature in the early 1990s (Teno *et al.* 1994). ACP has been promoted as a means of setting on record the views, values and specific treatment choices of those living with serious, progressive conditions that are likely to cause incapacity or loss of the ability to communicate wishes to others in the future. The goals of advance care planning have been identified as: ensuring that clinical care is in keeping with patient preferences when the patient has become incapable of decision-making; improving the health care decision-making process by facilitating shared decision-making; improving patients' well-being by reducing the frequency of either under- or over-treatment (Teno *et al.* 1994).

Advance care planning commonly results in one or more outcomes, all of which are well described in the literature. In summary, these are:

- An instructional directive: often known as a 'living will', which sets on record positive or negative views about specific life-prolonging treatments such as CPR or ventilation, in defined circumstances. Those that set out an advance refusal now have legal force in most countries when assessed as valid and applicable. In the UK, these are called 'advance decisions'. Both generic and disease specific directives are described in the literature (e.g. Singer 1994).

- The nomination of a proxy: often known as an 'attorney', who then has the authority to represent the patient once they have lost capacity in relation to decisions surrounding their medical treatment. In the UK, the introduction of provisions for 'lasting powers of attorney' under the Mental Capacity Act of 2005 (Department of Constitutional Affairs 2005) is one example.

- The setting out of general values and views about care and treatment. In the UK, these are known as statements of 'wishes and preferences', and are promoted as a useful record to guide future care (Henry and Seymour 2007).

Various initiatives in law, policy and health care systems are actively and strongly promoting practice, together with strategic initiatives to support implementation of ACP, although the exact form of implementation and the terms used differs across states and countries (Dunbrack 2006).

The evidence to support the use of advance care planning and to understand the range of outcomes associated with their use, is sparse with most evidence coming from the few countries that have established patterns of use (USA and Canada primarily). This seems to point to the possibility that advance care planning, particularly when it goes beyond the narrow objective of drafting an instructional directive, may contribute to a sense of control among some patients, may engender better understanding between them, their families and care providers, and may in some cases increase a sense of well-being through promoting hope (Seymour 2007).

However, some difficulties have been associated with advance care planning and the statements that may result. One concern relates to the status and relevance of choices about treatment expressed by a person when well, to the later situation of their grave illness when they are no longer able to confirm such expressions. Other concerns relate to the potential use of the advance statement as a form of health care rationing and evidence of little professional or public understanding or inclination to use or discuss them (see, for example, the review by Seymour *et al.* 2004). Many people, because of their social structural location, may never have had any opportunity to 'choose' what happens to them: to then be presented with 'choices' in end-of-life care does not fit with their wider experience and may therefore be exceedingly difficult to engage with. In some countries, the idea of advance care planning may be counter-cultural, and seen as contradicting deeply held notions about family obligations, religious beliefs and medical duties to care for dying persons.

# Euthanasia[2]

As far as humans are concerned, the protection of innocent human life is regarded as the central principle to morality asserted in the United Nations' Universal Declaration of Human Rights (General Assembly of the United Nations 1948) and, in the UK, in the Human Rights Act of 1998 (Office of Public Sector Information 2007). If we accept that all persons have full and equal moral status, then we also have to accept our obligations to one another, specifically to do no harm. However we may regard euthanasia, it is an act that violates this fundamental human right to life, and for this reason alone it is a highly contested subject. Causing the death of someone is usually considered wrong, but not always – take, for example, self-defence or war. Killing is therefore sometimes permitted, but in health care it seems to contradict the very purpose of what we set out to do, to save lives and bring about healing. Some argue, however, that under certain conditions, ending the life of a terminally ill patient in extreme suffering is consistent with the ethic of beneficence in that it is a compassionate and merciful response that brings relief. In the UK, the broad definition of euthanasia adopted by the House of Lords says that euthanasia is 'a deliberate intervention undertaken with the express intention of ending a life to relieve intractable suffering' (House of Lords 1993–94: 10). When there is a request for euthanasia from the patient who is a mentally competent adult, who is fully informed and who has arrived at a reasoned decision without coercion, then the act of euthanasia in response to the patient may be termed 'voluntary'. The act is 'non-voluntary' when the patient does not have the capacity to express a reasoned preference to request, agree or refuse to be killed.

When considering euthanasia, we become aware of the conflicts that can exist between an individual's call to be released from suffering and society's efforts to protect and sustain life. Clinically, this tension becomes focused in the health professional's duty to provide beneficial care to those in need, to refrain from harming them, and to respect an individual's choices.

### Arguments for euthanasia: appealing to 'mercy', 'autonomy' and 'justice'

*Mercy*

Those who prioritize the moral value of 'mercy' in arguing for euthanasia assert that allowing euthanasia would produce more good than harm, since it would relieve uncontrolled suffering and reassure others that death is not painful. Proponents of this position argue that while modern medicine can, in most cases, relieve pain and suffering, it still cannot do so in all cases. For example, while most patients dying of cancer have little or no pain, some have pain that is erratic and very difficult to control. Those taking this position often also argue that there is no substantive distinction between 'killing' and 'letting die', and that the maintenance of this distinction disadvantages some groups of dying people because it leads to all sorts of difficulties about what should be withdrawn, when and how. The published critiques of the legal judgment on the Diane Pretty case (summarized by Huxtable and Campbell 2003) use these sorts of arguments. It is arguably the case that ethical confusion over these issues means that clinical behaviour can lurch from 'the abrupt cessation of treatment, minimalist palliative care and treatment directed at bringing about a rapid dying process, to excessive caution about being seen to be instrumental in causing death' (Ashby 1998: 74, cited in Seymour 2001). Most commonly, many of those who support the legalization of euthanasia on the grounds of 'mercy' suggest that it is a necessary solution to the problem of containing the unintended effects of 'medical heroism', in which dying may be prolonged in a profoundly undignified way. Le Fanu (1999, cited in Seymour 2001), in commenting on the 'transforming power' of the technological innovation of artificial ventilation and oxygenation that heralded the development of intensive therapy in the early 1950s, notes that 50 years later those same life-saving therapies have also become a means of prolonging the 'pain and misery of terminal illness' for many.

In Belgium and the Netherlands, euthanasia at the voluntary request of a competent adult is now legal under very tightly defined circumstances (Broeckaert and Janssens 2005). The position taken in the latter countries is that under certain conditions, ending the life of a terminally ill patient in extreme suffering is consistent with the ethic of beneficence in that it is a compassionate and merciful response that brings relief, and is consistent with the ethic of autonomy, which allows people who competently request euthanasia to have their wish respected.

*Autonomy*

Clearly then, the principle of mercy is tied conceptually to the principle of autonomy (Pabst-Battin 1994). To impose 'mercy' on someone who wishes to live regardless of their pain and suffering would clearly be a contradiction of the mercy principle. Autonomy – meaning informed consent to treatment and the respect of a person's competent wishes where these do not violate other moral obligations or cause harm to others – is also crucially important. The 'right to die' lobby in both the USA and the UK use this principle to underpin their argument that individual choice for euthanasia should be respected and the law changed to ensure that medical actions to help people to die are permissible. In the UK during 2004–2006, there were a number of attempts to change the law to permit assisted dying using arguments about autonomy.

### Justice

A final key principle that has been used to support euthanasia is that of justice. Here it is argued that some people have a 'meaningless existence' – those in deep, irreversible comas, for example, or suffering from late-stage Alzheimer's disease – and that in the interests of the fair distribution of scarce resources, laws against euthanasia should be relaxed to embrace these groups. One famous argument that has been used to back up this position has been put forward by an American ethicist, Daniel Callahan (1987), who argues that when people have had 'their fair innings' it should be recognized that health resources are better spent on younger people who are more likely to benefit and contribute to the overall wealth of a society. It is perhaps a short jump from this argument for rationing based on age to an extension of the same argument as a justification for euthanasia.

## Arguments against euthanasia: the 'slippery slope'

Those who argue against the legalization of euthanasia suggest that such legalization will mean that there will inevitably be abuses of the law, and that vulnerable people will be put at risk. These arguments are known collectively as 'slippery slope' arguments. Slippery slope arguments recognize that individual treatment decisions are always constrained to a greater or lesser extent by wider economic and social factors. Proponents of this position suggest that there is a possibility that wholesale discrimination on a societal level may be unleashed against those considered, possibly arbitrarily, as an economic or social burden. A particularly powerful argument against the legalization of voluntary euthanasia has come from those who point to the possibility of 'coerced' altruism becoming a significant element in requests for euthanasia. This theme was a major consideration in the rejection of euthanasia by the House of Lords Select Committee on Medical Ethics (1993–94) in the UK and in a subsequent review of the law following debate of a bill to support assisted dying presented to the UK government during 2005 (Finlay *et al.* 2005).

Many in the hospice and palliative care movement also reject euthanasia for precisely these reasons. They argue that there is a risk that euthanasia may become an easy alternative to the difficult challenge of addressing care delivery and planning for people as they approach the end of their lives. The general stance of the hospice and palliative care movement in the UK is summarized by Robert Twycross (1995). He responds to the arguments for euthanasia based on 'mercy' by saying that good palliative care for patients and families will mean that suffering can be relieved and the fears of dying and death greatly lessened. He frames the problem of euthanasia in terms of inadequate provision of palliative care services together with a lack of knowledge about how to respond appropriately to requests for euthanasia.

Twycross's position is similar to that of Roy and Rapin (1994), who compiled the First Position Paper on Euthanasia at the behest of the European Association for Palliative Care. In this, they argued unequivocally that 'we should firmly and without qualification, oppose the legalisation of euthanasia as both unnecessary and dangerous' (Roy and Rapin 1994: 58). Roy and Rapin used a definition of euthanasia which was very close to the UK definition put forward by the House of Lord's Select Committee on Medical Ethics, and to which we referred above.

A task force set up by the European Association for Palliative Care in 2002 set out a revised position paper on euthanasia (Materstvedt *et al.* 2003). This was in response to rapid social and clinical changes since 1994 when the first statement was issued; in particular, the legalization of euthanasia in Belgium and the Netherlands subject to strict constraints, its brief legalization in the Northern Territories of Australia, and the legalization of physician-assisted suicide in Oregon, USA. The statement perhaps overturns the traditional opposition between palliative care and euthanasia, since it suggests that the two can, in certain circumstances, co-exist. It adopts a much narrower definition of euthanasia: 'Euthanasia is killing on request and is defined as: a doctor intentionally killing a person by the administration of drugs at that person's voluntary and competent request' (Materstvedt *et al.* 2003: 98). Following this definition, the position paper sets out a number of key issues, and calls for dialogue between the opposed camps in this debate. This provoked a huge commentary from across the world (*Palliative Medicine* 2003: 17(2)), showing that the issue is set to continue to arouse debate and contention well into the twenty-first century.

## Experiences of dying

The individual experience of dying is shaped, at least in part, by a myriad of complex factors, all of which interrelate. Depending on the cause of death, and the type of treatment being given to a person, the trajectory of the dying process may be slow, sudden or take the form of a series of relapses and recoveries. As we have discussed above, in contemporary society, death has particular features which makes 'dying' difficult to anticipate, diagnose and plan for. The lack of recognition of dying associated with some chronic illnesses, for example heart failure, is arguably a major factor in the death experience for many. The place of death varies, and different places tend to give rise to different care practices and interpersonal relationships: these can fundamentally influence what sort of death experience a person has. For example, in spite of rhetoric to the contrary (and as we have discussed elsewhere in this book), to be in receipt of specialist palliative care in an inpatient hospice or at home remains largely dependent on having a diagnosis of cancer. Those dying of other diseases tend to die in hospitals or, when dying is associated with advanced old age, in care homes. The structure and organization of formal health care systems, and aspects of the dying person's social networks and living arrangements, are thus critically important. Beyond these lie wider belief systems, attitudes to death and the complex, shifting tapestry of meanings, values and representations of death in modern society. Age, gender, ethnicity, social class and culture, these have all been shown to affect the experience of dying, both in the sense of the access a person has to the material and social resources that can support them during dying and, existentially, in terms of the meaning and sense that a person makes of their dying (Field *et al.* 1997). Most notably, dying is part of the biography of an individual and will be seen by them in that context: the sorrows, regrets, joys and achievements of life, whether or not the dying person has lived through war, the way in which they have seen others close to them die, how they have experienced bereavement, their experience of family life. These are but a few of the many biographical factors that are likely to have a powerful influence on the experience of dying. By way of pointing out that death falls into recognizable categories or types, such as the 'gradual' death, the 'catastrophic' death or the 'premature' death, Clark and Seymour (1999) analyse how 'the social' interweaves with 'the individual' in powerfully shaping the experience of death and dying.

The most common contemporary experience of dying is that associated with chronic disease, especially in older age. This type of dying process may create dependencies on others, which can be experienced at one and the same time (by the dying person as well as their carers) as a welcome intimacy and a burdensome trouble. It may involve an increasing struggle to do those things on which everyday life depends, and the dying person's carers will be drawn, inexorably, into gradually assuming more and more caring responsibilities whether or not this is welcomed. For many, a sense of 'social death' may be experienced (Mulkay 1993) as a result of feeling that one is of diminishing importance to the lives and concerns of other people and no longer an active participant in the affairs of daily life. This is not something that just affects older people: it has been shown to be of relevance to children and young adults suffering from cancer and for whom the lack of sustained contact with friends is a significant contributor to their experience of suffering (Hodgson and Eden 2003). Lawton (2000), in a powerful ethnography of patients' experiences of dying in a hospice, argues that bodily unboundedness (incontinence and other problems encountered during the late stages of terminal illness) is a particularly powerful determinant of 'social death'. She claims, controversially, that hospices could be seen as places of 'sequestration', taking in patients who, because of their lack of bodily control, are no longer regarded as people. Lawton thus theorizes that 'self' is determined by the ability to control one's body, rather than the ability to maintain social relationships.

As Clark and Seymour (1999) have observed, death may be 'experienced as sheer hard work – as the illness advances and as the burdens of caring grow; but it may also be experienced as an opportunity – for personal development or fulfillment in relationships with others' (p. 12).

Sociologists draw our attention to the social-symbolic nature of human interaction (Leming and Dickenson 2002). This means that how death and dying are experienced is shaped by the way in which others react to a person once they know, or suspect, that individual is dying. To this extent, dying is a shared event. Leming and Dickenson (2002) identify a number of issues that are raised by the interactions that dying people have with their family, their friends and others. They list these from the perspective of how the dying person perceives others' behaviour:

- What people are willing to talk about with me and what they avoid.
- Whether they are willing to touch me, and how they touch me when they do.
- Where I am, or maybe where others have located me – hospital, nursing home, intensive care unit, isolation unit, or my room at home.
- Tangible and verbal gifts that others give to me.
- What people will let me do, or expect me to do, or will not let me do.
- The tone of voice that people use when they talk to me.
- The frequency and length of visits from others.
- Excuses that people make for not visiting.
- The reactions of others to my prognosis.

Taking a broader perspective beyond the close interaction emphasized by Leming and Dickenson, Kellehear (1990) has argued, on the basis of interviews with 100 people dying of cancer, that the social experience of dying is marked by five features. He argues that these are likely to be universal across cultures:

- Awareness: whether or not a person knows that they are dying.
- Social adjustments and preparations: the making of a will or preparing one's funeral, for example.
- Public preparations.
- Relinquishing of roles: one person may have many different roles, and their dying may leave many 'gaps'.
- Formal and informal farewells.

Kellehear argues that these are:

> Central recurrent concerns of organising dying despite variations to the content of that organisation ... individual styles of dying are bounded by the shape of that person's social and cultural existence.

Cultures provide behavioural possibilities. In other words they supply broad prescriptions for how to act. In turn, individuals provide unique variations.

(Kellehear 1990: 34)

In addition to Kellehear's classic study, there have been a number of fascinating studies that allow us to gain a perspective on the experience of dying, and which have been written drawing on accounts from dying persons (as opposed to being an account proffered by the analyst, or constructed through the 'proxy' accounts of the dying person's carers). We highlight one of these studies here (see Box 10.4). The objective of the study highlighted in Box 10.4 was to describe the experiences of illness and needs and use of services in two groups of patients with incurable cancer, one in a developed country (Scotland) and one in a developing country (Kenya) (Murray *et al.* 2003). In Scotland 20 patients with inoperable lung cancer and their carers were interviewed, while in Kenya 24 patients with various advanced cancers and their carers were interviewed. The study found that people dying in Scotland were primarily concerned with the emotional pain of facing death, whereas those in Kenya were much more concerned about physical pain and financial issues. The district in Kenya where the research took place was an area of abject poverty, and what few health care services there were could only be accessed on payment of a fee, with the cost of admission to hospital

---

**Box 10.4**   Summary of the issues raised by respondents in the study of Murray *et al.* (2003)

| *Scotland* | *Kenya* |
|---|---|
| • Main issue is the prospect of death | • Main issue is physical suffering, especially pain |
| • Pain is unusual | • Analgesia unaffordable |
| • Anger in the face of illness | • Acceptance rather than anger |
| • Just keep it to myself | • Acceptance of community support |
| • Spiritual needs evident | • Patients comforted by belief in God |
| • Diagnosis brought active treatment and then a period of watching and waiting . . . | • Diagnosis signalled waiting for death |
| • Patients concerned about how carer will cope in the future | • Patients concerned about being a physical and financial burden to their family |
| • Support from hospital and primary care teams | • Lack of medical support, treatment options, equipment and basic necessities |
| • Specialist palliative care available | • Specialist palliative care services not available in the community |
| • Cancer a national priority | • Cancer not a national priority |

the equivalent of seven months' wages for an unskilled worker. In contrast, in Scotland, people had access to primary and secondary care free at the point of delivery and a social security system. Running water and all other domestic facilities that we take for granted in the West were available in Scotland but lacking in Kenya. In their conclusion, Murray *et al.* note that:

> Though living in a resource rich country, Scottish patients described unmet psychosocial needs. Meeting physical needs did not alone ensure a good death. In developing countries, while physical needs often go unmet, the family and local religious community can and do meet many of the psychological, social and spiritual needs: 'higher order' needs can be met amid physical distress inverting Maslow's typology of need.
>
> (Murray *et al.* 2003: 367)

At the beginning of this section, we drew attention to the myriad of factors that shape the experience of death. Murray and co-workers' study demonstrates this powerfully through the comparison of patients' experiences in a developed and a developing country, where vividly contrasting social, economic, political, cultural and spiritual contexts led to very different concerns and priorities among two groups of people dying from the same disease.

Using a very different methodology, Heyland *et al.* (2006) surveyed what 596 seriously ill patients and 176 family members ranked as most important in care at the end of life. They devised a structured questionnaire which listed 28 items drawn from the existing literature, finding that the most important elements related to trust in their treating physician, avoidance of unwanted life support, effective communication, continuity of care and life completion. Having 'control' over treatments or where a patient died, were chosen infrequently. Heyland *et al.* note that '. . . quality in end of life care has more to do with enhancing relationships and improving communication between the attending physician and family [therefore] promoting autonomy with tools such as advance directives or living wills may not be the optimal approach' (page 7). Similar critiques of the assumed importance of autonomy come from studies of older people's understandings of end-of-life care technologies and their views about good care at the end of life (see, for example, Clarke *et al.* 2006; Vandrevala *et al.* 2006).

# The nurse's role in caring for dying people

Of all those involved with the care of dying persons, except for close companions and friends, nurses have the closest and most sustained contact with them. Indeed, it has been claimed that care of the dying is the 'quintessential' expression of nursing care (Bradshaw 1996). However, as we have seen elsewhere in this book, caring has not traditionally been afforded a high priority in developed health systems and this poses fundamental problems for nurses as they care for the dying. The early work of Quint (1967) was particularly influential in revealing how the lack of education given to nurses about how to care for dying patients in hospitals demonstrates the low status afforded to 'caring' work, and the negative impact of this on the physical and psychological care of those people.

In the UK, Field's (1989) study of nurses' experiences of caring for dying patients demonstrated that attitudes to disclosure of terminal prognoses had changed by the 1980s, with open awareness regarded as a necessary component of humane care. However, Field showed that nurses had relatively little autonomy in their work. This was especially the case on general surgical and medical wards, where medical staff exerted considerable power. This constrained nurses' ability either to communicate openly to dying patients or to respond to their needs in an individualized way. The enduring relevance of Field's work has been confirmed by similar findings in other contexts (Kiger 1994; Beck 1997).

At about the same time as Field's work was published, Degner and Beaton (1987) published their four-year study of life and death decisions in acute care settings in Canada. Like Field, they suggested that nurses' conceptualization of their work leads frequently to disagreements, which were often not verbalized, with medical staff over the continuation of treatment for patients. Drawing on a follow-up study, Degner went on to publish a paper with colleagues (Degner *et al.* 1991) in which they identified a list of seven critical nursing behaviours in care for the dying. This was based on interviews with nurse-educators and palliative care nurses. The behaviours identified were:

- *Responding to the death scene*: maintaining a sense of calm, involving the family.

- *Providing comfort*: reducing discomfort, especially pain.

- *Responding to anger*: showing respect and empathy even when anger is directed at the nurse.

- *Enhancing personal growth*: showing that the nurse has defined a personal role in caring for the dying.

- *Responding to colleagues*: providing emotional support and critical feedback to colleagues.

- *Enhancing quality of life*: helping patients to do those things which are important to them.

- *Responding to the family*: responding to the need for information; reducing the potential for future regret; including the family in care or relieving them of responsibility according to their needs.

While other studies have identified further dimensions of the nurses' role in palliative care, this list seems to capture very well the complex responsibilities of nurses at the critical time of a patient's death. What stands out is the way in which competing demands and high levels of emotional engagement must be managed for death to be well managed. This is 'work' that involves the nurse relating not only to patients, but also to the patient's family and close companions and to other professional colleagues. De Raeve (1996) argues that nursing the dying involves a degree of professional self-exposure that makes the nurse vulnerable to harm.

In a classic empirical study of nurses' responses to exposure to repeated death, Saunders and Valente (1994) examined the relationship between nurses' perceptions of 'good death' and the maintenance of nurses' 'professional integrity, personal wholeness and self esteem' (page 321). In their study, nurses delineated certain key conditions that characterize a 'good death': all relate to a protection of their patient's physical, psychological safety, to the appropriate location of death in time and space, and to a maintenance of 'family' and professional relationships. In a similar way to Field (1989) and Degner and Beaton (1987), Saunders and Valente identified that those situations where deaths were perceived by nurses as 'difficult' were marked by unresolved conflicts between health care staff over issues such as continuation of treatment or resuscitation. This issue of team relationships has been highlighted elsewhere as a problem among nurses in acute settings caring for the dying (Copp and Dunn 1993).

Whatever problems nurses face in caring for dying people, they need to be able to bring some sense of meaning to the experience. Maeve (1998) has suggested that nurses 'weave a fabric of moral meaning' into their work with dying people; in this, nurses use the dilemmas of their patients' lives to inform their own personal and professional lives, and thus come to terms with their own mortality and with the universal experience of suffering. Reflection on experiences of caring for dying patients and their families, then, clearly has the potential to become a reservoir of personal development. It also can be one valuable way in which nurses learn to provide high-quality and sensitive care. Wong (2001) reports on work with student nurses in Hong Kong, in which the latter attended problem-based learning sessions focused on group discussion of some fictional scenarios involving death and dying. The students documented their learning in reflective journals focusing on the care they gave to dying patients. Within these journals, there was compelling evidence that the nurses experienced anxiety about death and felt inadequate in dealing with dying patients. However, the dual processes of engaging in problem-based learning and of writing about their clinical experiences emerged as an effective strategy to enhance their awareness and sensitivity to dying patients and to facilitate their formulation of appropriate care plans for the dying.

## Overview of chapters in Part Two

It has been our intention to provide a broad overview of the issues with which the authors of the subsequent chapters in this part of the book are concerned. We turn now to introduce these.

In Chapter 11, Michael Wright examines how, through facing the inevitability of one's own mortality, spiritual activity occurs. Wright shows that as dying patients begin to address their religious and spiritual needs across many dimensions, health professionals have an opportunity to play a supportive and important role. Jessica Corner's chapter turns to examine the challenge of managing difficult symptoms from which dying patients may suffer. She takes a critical approach to symptom control and, rather than offering a 'tool kit', explores how symptom control has become a dominant construct in palliative care in which 'personal' knowledge is marginalized *vis-à-vis* 'scientific' knowledge. She shows that symptoms are a product of mind *and* body, and that their control takes place in a social and cultural context, which itself shapes the experience of the symptom and the way in which it is managed. She concludes by drawing attention to the importance of developing an understanding of *why* a symptom is perceived as difficult and of listening to patients' stories in developing, with them, a meaningful approach to control in which 'self-management' is enhanced.

Silvia Paz and Jane Seymour follow Corner by focusing on pain. They look at pain and its management drawing on theoretical and historical perspectives to show how pain management has evolved across the twentieth and early twenty-first centuries. They explore the distinction between chronic and acute pain states, and review the evidence about controlling cancer pain. They explore the role of the nurse in pain control, drawing attention to the importance of pain assessment and measurement. Throughout they emphasize the experience of pain as a multidimensional phenomenon that requires the very best standards of multidisciplinary teamwork for its management.

In Chapter 14, Mari Lloyd-Williams continues the theme of the interconnectedness of body and mind through an examination of how we may help and support patients who are facing feelings of depression and sadness at the end of their lives. She draws our attention to the impact that poor communication practices can have on patients and how important it is to recognize that not all suffering is physical. Lloyd-Williams' chapter is complemented by Chapter 15 in which Lee and Hoptof examine some of the other key psychiatric problems which are presented in palliative care. They explore problems of delirium, dementia and psychosis, as well as giving guidance on when to refer to psychiatric care and the structure of psychiatric services.

The next chapter focuses on family care-givers, in recognition that most of the care that dying people receive in the last year of life takes place within their own home, and that family care-giving is absolutely essential in helping patients remain at home if this is what they wish to do. Smith and Skilbeck explore the rewarding and challenging process of working with family care-givers, and examine how they perceive and shape their role. Picking up the theme of interrelatedness in the experience of end-of-life care, Jenny Hockey then discusses themes of identity and personhood in Chapter 17. She argues that identity can be seen as an active process, rather than a 'thing' and that it arises out of interaction between our view of 'self' and others' views. She points to the possibility that by drawing from non-Western models of self, there is scope for moving beyond ideas of 'social death' or 'stigma' that have often characterized the experience of life-limiting illness.

Koffman and Camps offer, in Chapter 18, an analysis of social exclusion in end-of-life care, noting that there is no second chance to improve the care of individuals who are dying, and argue that it remains the case that significant 'silent' sections of the community are inadequately served at the end of life. This is a timely reminder of the way in which ethical issues are integral to palliative care. Bert Broeckaert's chapter follows this by examining closely, from a largely ethical and philosophical perspective, but also drawing on historical and cultural issues, debates surrounding treatment decisions at the end of life. He offers a typology about the different kinds of treatment decisions that can be taken in advanced stages of life-threatening illness and shows how these relate to international legislation and research in this difficult area.

This part of the book concludes with a chapter from Jeanne Katz, who examines the organization and delivery of palliative care in different types of institution. Katz picks up many of the issues explored elsewhere and shows how these translate into particular care practices and experiences for the dying person. Katz compares and contrasts hospices, hospitals, prisons, community hospitals and care homes in terms of the services they can provide to the dying, the social relationships they engender, and the constraints on quality of care imposed by their particular cultures and wider missions. Her analysis and description of initiatives in the USA to introduce hospice concepts into prisons show how it is possible to radically transform the quality of the dying experience even in the most difficult of circumstances.

## Notes

1   These principles are broadly based on those identified by Field and Cassell (1997: 4–5) in their report published by the Institute of Medicine in the USA: 'Approaching death: Improving care at the end of life'.
2   We are grateful to Mark Cobb for allowing us to draw on his lecture notes on the historical, social and clinical aspects of euthanasia delivered to medical students at the University of Sheffield between 2002 and 2003.
3   See the Guidance from the Standards Committee of the General Medical Council (2006) *Withholding and Withdrawing Life-Prolonging Treatments: Good Practice in Decision-Making* (http://www.gmc.org.uk).

## References

Ariès, P. (1981) *The Hour of Our Death*. London: Allen Lane.
Ashby, M. (1998) Palliative care, death causation, public policy and the law. *Progress in Palliative Care*, 6: 69–77.

Bauman, Z. (1992) *Mortality, Immortality and Other Life Strategies*. Oxford: Polity Press.

Beck, C.T. (1997) Nursing students' experiences caring for dying patients. *Journal of Nursing Education*, 36: 408–15.

Bradshaw, A. (1996) The spiritual dimension of hospice: the secularisation of an ideal. *Social Science and Medicine*, 43(3): 409–20.

British Medical Association (2007) *Withholding and Withdrawing Life-Prolonging Medical Treatment*. London: BMA.

Broeckaert, B. and Janssens, M.J.P.A. (2005) Palliative care and euthanasia. Belgian and Dutch perspectives. In: P. Schotsmans and T. Meulenbergs (eds) *Euthanasia and palliative care in the low countries*. Leuven: Peeters, pp. 35–70.

Callahan, D. (1987) *Setting Limits: Medical Goals in an Ageing Society*. New York: Simon & Schuster.

Cassell, E. (2004) *The Nature of Suffering and the Goals of Medicine*. Oxford: Oxford University Press.

Christakis, N. (1999) *Death Foretold: Prophecy and Prognosis in Medical Care*. Chicago, IL: University of Chicago Press.

Clark, D. and Seymour, J. (1999) *Reflections on Palliative Care*. Buckingham: Open University Press.

Clarke, A., Seymour, J.E. and Welton, M. (2006) *Opening the door for older people to explore end of life issues*. London: Help the Aged.

Cobb, M. (2003) *Euthanasia: historical, social and clinical issues*. Lecture delivered to the School of Medicine, University of Sheffield, March.

Copp, G. and Dunn, V. (1993) Frequent and difficult problems perceived by nurses caring for the dying in community, hospice and acute care settings. *Palliative Medicine*, 7: 19–25.

de Raeve, L. (1996) Dignity and integrity at the end of life. *International Journal of Palliative Care Nursing*, 2(2): 71–6.

Degner, L.F. and Beaton, J.I. (1987) *Life and Death Decisions in Health Care*. New York: Hemisphere.

Degner, L.F., Gow, C.M. and Thompson, L.A. (1991) Critical nursing behaviours in care of the dying. *Cancer Nursing*, 14(5): 246–53.

Department of Constitutional Affairs (2005). *Mental Capacity Act*. London, HMSO.

Dingwall, R. (2003) Bioethics. In A. Pilnick (ed.) *Genetics and Society*. Buckingham: Open University Press.

Dunbrack, J. (2006) *Advance care planning: the Glossary project*. Health Canada. http://www.hc-sc.gc.ca/hcs-sss/alt_formats/hpb-dgps/pdf/pubs/2006-proj-glos/2006-proj-gloss_e.pdf (accessed 15 May 2007).

Dy, S. and Lynn, J. (2007) Getting services right for those sick enough to die, *British Medical Journal*, 334: 511–13.

Dyer, C. (2002) Miss B dies after winning fight to end care. *Guardian*, Tuesday 30 April.

Ellershaw, J. and Ward, C. (2003) Care of the dying patient: the last hours or days of life. *British Medical Journal*, 326: 30–4.

Field, D. (1989) *Nursing the Dying*. London: Tavistock/Routledge.

Field, D. (1996) Awareness and modern dying. *Mortality*, 1(3): 255–65.

Field, D., Hockey, J. and Small, N. (1997) *Death, Gender and Ethnicity*. London: Routledge.

Field, M.J. and Cassell, C.K. (1997) *Approaching Death. Improving Care at the End of Life*. Washington: National Academy Press.

Finlay, I.G., Wheatley, V.J. and Izdebski, C. (2005) The House of Lords Select Committee on the 'Assisted Dying for the Terminally Ill Bill': implications for specialist palliative care. *Palliative Medicine*, 19, 444–53.

Frank, A. (1995) *The Wounded Storyteller. Body, Illness and Ethics*. London and Chicago: University of Chicago Press.

Gastmans, C. (2006) The care perspective in health care ethics. In: A. Davis, V. Tschudin and L. de Raeve (eds) *Essentials of Teaching and Learning in Nursing Ethics, Perspectives and Methods*. Edinburgh: Elsevier.

General Assembly of the United Nations (1948) *Universal Declaration of Human Rights*. Available at: http://www.un.org/Overview/rights.html (accessed 22 November 2007).

General Medical Council (2006) *Withholding and Withdrawing Life-Prolonging Treatments: Good Practice in Decision-Making. Guidance from the Standards Committee of the General Medical Council*. London: GMC.

Glaser, B. and Strauss, A. (1965) *Awareness of Dying*. Chicago, IL: Aldine.

Henry, C. and Seymour, J.E. (2007) *Advance Care Planning: a guide for health and social care professionals*. NHS End of Life Care Programme.

Heyland, D.K., Dodek, P., Rocker, G., Groll, D., Ggafni, A., Pichora, D., Shortt, S., Tranmer, J., Lazar, N., Kutsogiannis, J. and Lam, M. (2006) What matters most in end of life care: perceptions of seriously ill patients and their family members. *CMAJ*, 174(5). DOI:10.1503/cmaj.050626 (accessed 15 November 2007).

Hodgson, A. and Eden, O.B. (2003) *'Everything has changed': experiences of young people with recurrent or metastatic cancer*. Paper presented to the Palliative Care Research Society Annual Scientific Meeting, Royal College of Physicians, Edinburgh, 25 June.

Hopkins, P.D. (1997) Why does removing machines count as 'passive' euthanasia? *Hastings Center Report*, 27: 29–37.

House of Lords (1993–94) *Report of the Select Committee on Medical Ethics* (HL Paper 21-I). London: HMSO.

Huxtable, R. and Campbell, A.V. (2003) The position statement and its commentators: consensus, compromise or confusion? *Palliative Medicine*, 17: 180–3.

Jennett, B. (1995) High technology therapies and older people. *Ageing and Society*, 15(2): 185–98.

Kaufman, S. (2003) Hidden places, uncommon persons. *Social Science and Medicine*, 56: 2249–61.

Kellehear, A. (1990) *Dying of Cancer: The Final Year of Life*. Reading, PA: Harwood Academic.

Kiger, A.M. (1994) Student nurses' involvement with death: the image and the experience. *Journal of Advanced Nursing*, 20: 679–86.

Kleinman, A. (1988) *The Illness Narratives. Suffering, Healing and the Human Condition*. New York: Basic Books.

Lawton, J. (2000) *The Dying Process: Patients' Experiences of Palliative Care*. London: Routledge.

Le Fanu, J. (1999) *The Rise and Fall of Modern Medicine*. London: Little, Brown & Company.

Leming, M.R. and Dickenson, G.E. (2002) *Understanding Death, Dying and Bereavement*. Fort Worth, TX: Harcourt College Publishers.

Lofland, L. (1978) *The Craft of Dying*. Beverley Hills, CA: Sage.

Lynn, J. (2005) Living long in fragile health: The new demographics shape end of life care. In: Improving end of life care: Why has it been so difficult? *Hastings Center Report*, Special Issue, 35(6): S14–S18.

Lynn, J. and Adamson, D.M. (2003) *Living Well to the End of Life: Adapting Health Care to Serious Chronic Illness in Old Age*. Arlington, VA: Rand Health.

Maeve, M.K. (1998) Weaving a fabric of moral meaning: how nurses live with suffering and death. *Journal of Advanced Nursing*, 27(2): 1136–42.

Materstvedt, L.J., Clark, D., Ellershaw, J., Forde, R., Boeck Gravgaard, A-M., Christof Müller-Busch, H., Porta i Sales, J. and Rapin, C-H. (2003) Euthanasia and physician assisted suicide: a view from an EAPC Ethics Task Force. *Palliative Medicine*, 17(2): 97–101 (discussion 102–79).

McNamara, B. (1997) A good enough death? Paper presented to the Third International Social Context of Death, Dying and Disposal. Conference, Cardiff, April.

Menzies, I. (1970) *The Functioning of Social Systems as a Defence Against Anxiety* (reprint of Tavistock Pamphlet No. 3). London: Tavistock Institute.

Mulkay, M. (1993) Social death in Britain. In D. Clark (ed.) *The Sociology of Death*. Oxford: Blackwell/The Sociological Review.

Murray, S.A., Grant, E., Grant, A. and Kendall, M. (2003) Dying from cancer in developed and developing countries: lessons from two qualitative interview studies of patients and their carers. *British Medical Journal*, 7385: 326–68.

Murray, S.A., Kendall, M., Boyd, K. and Sheikh, A. (2005) Illness trajectories and palliative care. *British Medical Journal*, 330: 1007–11.

Office of Public Sector Information (2007) *Human Rights Act, 1998*. Available at: http://www.opsi.gov.uk/ACTS/acts1998/19980042.htm (accessed 22 November 2007).

Pabst-Battin, M. (1994) *The Least Worst Death: Essays in Bioethics on the End of Life*. Oxford: Oxford University Press.

Quint, J.C. (1967) *The Nurse and the Dying Patient*. New York: Macmillan.

Ross, M., Fisher, R. and McClean, M.J. (2000) *A Guide to End-of-Life Care for Seniors*. Ottawa: Health Canada.

Roy, D.J. and MacDonald, N. (1998) Ethical issues in palliative care. In D. Doyle, G.W.C. Hanks and N. MacDonald (eds) *Oxford Textbook of Palliative Care*. Oxford: Oxford University Press.

Roy, D.J. and Rapin, C-H. (1994) The EAPC Board of Directors: regarding euthanasia. *European Journal of Palliative Care*, 1: 57–9.

Saunders, J.M. and Valente, S.M. (1994) Nurses' grief. *Cancer Nursing*, 17: 318–25.

Seymour, J.E. (2001) *Critical Moments: Death and Dying in Intensive Care*. Buckingham: Open University Press.

Seymour, J.E. (2007) Into the unknown: advance care planning at the end of life. *10th Congress of the European Association of Palliative Care*, Budapest, 7–9 June.

Seymour, J., Gott, M., Bellamy, G., Ahmedzai, S.H. and Clark, D. (2004) Planning for the end of life: the views of older people about advance care statements. *Social Science and Medicine*, 59(1): 57–68.

Shaw, A.B. (1995) Acts of commission, omission and demission or pulling the plug. *Journal of the Royal Society of Medicine*, 88: 18–19.

Singer, P.A. (1994) Disease specific advance directives. *Lancet*, 244(8922): 594–6.

Singer, P. (1994) *Rethinking Life and Death: The Collapse of Our Traditional Ethics*. Oxford: Oxford University Press.

Stjernswärd, J. and Clark, D. (2005) Palliative medicine. A Global perspective. In:

D. Doyle, G. Hanks, N. Cherny and K. Calman (eds) *Oxford Textbook of Palliative Medicine* (3rd edn). Oxford: Oxford University Press, pp. 1199–224.

SUPPORT Principal Investigators (1995) A controlled trial to improve care for seriously ill hospitalized patients: the study to understand prognoses and preferences for outcomes and risks of treatment (SUPPORT). *Journal of the American Medical Association*, 174: 1591–8.

ten Have, H. and Clark, D. (eds) (2002) *The Ethics of Palliative Care: European Perspectives*. Buckingham: Open University Press.

Teno, J.M., Nelson, H.L. and Lynn, J. (1994) Advance care planning: priorities for ethical and empirical research. *Hasting's Center Report* [special supplement]; 24: S32–36.

Turner, B.S. (1996) *The Body and Society*. London: Sage.

Twycross, R.G. (1995) Where there is hope, there is life: a view from the hospice. In J. Keown (ed.) *Euthanasia Examined: Ethical, Clinical and Legal Perspectives*. Cambridge: Cambridge University Press.

Vandrevala, T., Hampson, S.E., Daly, T., Arber, S. and Thomas, H. (2006) Dilemmas in decision making about resuscitation: a focus group study of older people. *Social Science and Medicine*, 62(7): 1579–94.

Walsh, K. and Kowanko, I. (2002) Nurses' and patients' perceptions of dignity. *International Journal of Nursing Practice*, 8: 143–51.

Weijer, C. (2005) A death in the family. Reflections on the Terry Schiavo case. *CMAJ*, 172(9): 1197–8.

Wilkinson, I. (2005) *Suffering. A sociological introduction*. Cambridge: Polity Press.

Wong, F.K.Y. (2001) Educating nurses to care for the dying in Hong Kong: a problem based learning approach. *Cancer Nursing*, 24(2): 112–21.

# 11

# Good for the soul?

The spiritual dimension of hospice and palliative care

*Michael Wright*

---

**Key points**

- Religion and spirituality have come to be regarded as separate entities.
- When the narrative of illness places mortality centre stage, an increase in spiritual activity may be detected among patients and relatives.
- Many patients who describe themselves as 'not-religious' believe in God and pray regularly.
- A key element of spiritual care provision is the expertise of staff and the creation of a spiritual ethos.
- A broadly based role that relates to the spiritual activities of becoming, transcending, finding meaning and connecting has come to attract a wide ownership within palliative care.
- The challenge for those charged with spiritual care delivery is how to blend a cohesive team of spiritually aware personnel that meets the patient with affirmation and understanding at the point of need.

---

Confronting mortality in the face of approaching death can be a deeply disturbing experience (Ainsworth-Smith and Speck 1999). Yet amidst the imminence of separation and the incremental disintegration of self, a well-spring of spiritual activity may frequently be found. Here, this activity is addressed from three standpoints. First, I explore the concept of spirituality, its nature and essence, and outline an inclusive model of the spiritual domain. Next, there is an examination of the ways in which life-limiting illness influences the perceptions and spiritual needs of patients and their relatives. Then, I consider how hospices and hospitals provide spiritual care in an institutional setting. Importantly, I will demonstrate that as dying patients address their spiritual and religious needs, health professionals have an opportunity to play a supportive and vital role.[1]

# The conceptual perspective

## *Background*

When Cicely Saunders founded St Christopher's Hospice (London) in 1967, she sought to recapture the spirit of the former Christian 'hospes', welcoming the sick and performing the works of mercy found in Matthew 25 verses 35 and 36 (Saunders 1986). But as hospice philosophy developed, questions came to be asked about its religious foundation: was the Christian perspective part of the essence of hospice; or might there be a group of spiritual issues, evident towards the end of life, which transcends their meaning in a particular religious tradition? In effect, these questions echo the late twentieth century debate about religion and what has come to be termed 'spirituality' – and the nature of the relationship between them.

Currently, fewer people in Europe seem inclined to become religious. A survey (Gallup 1999) of 50,000 people across 60 countries found that only 20 per cent of respondents in Western Europe and 14 per cent in Eastern Europe worship on a weekly basis. In the same year, the figure for the established church in Britain was estimated at 8 per cent (Brierley 1999). Yet in this changing scenario, data from the 2001 census indicate that about 70 per cent of the population describe themselves as Christian. This endorses previous research undertaken by Davie (1994) which led her to identify a contemporary population 'believing without belonging'.

Paradoxically, as religious observance has declined, interest in the spiritual has increased, producing a form of spirituality that is considered to be 'religion-free'. Dictionary definitions relate 'spirituality' to its root – 'spirit' – locating it within the non-physical aspects of humankind. Seen as a universal human attribute, spirituality has come to be regarded as somehow 'purer' than religion: further 'upstream', freer to access and more personally relevant. In essence, this represents a rejection of life lived in external roles and obligations and a movement towards a different life: a life lived by reference to one's own experiences and rendered authentic by connection with one's inner depths. Identified as a subjective 'turn', it has been described as 'the defining cultural development of modern Western culture' (Heelas and Woodhead 2005: 5).

This relational, ontologically based perception of spirituality has found a ready acceptance within health care (DoH 1992; Ronaldson 1997; Swinton 2001; Jewell 2003; McSherry 2006). Nevertheless, it remains a contested area. Markham (1998) points to the strong association between spirituality and Christianity and wonders whether the term is recognized equally by other religious traditions. For Pattison, it is the lack of conceptual clarity which causes him to liken spirituality to 'intellectual Polyfilla, changing shape and content conveniently to fill the space its users devise for it' (Pattison 2001: 37).

### Meaning of spirituality

In the light of these divergent views, I conducted a phenomenological enquiry designed to identify the meaning of spirituality among a sample of spiritual care stakeholders. Participants included representatives of major world faiths and those of no faith who nonetheless regarded themselves as spiritual. Based on the philosophy of Husserl (1962) and developed by Heidegger (1962) and Merleau-Ponty (1962), phenomenology seeks to describe the meaning of a phenomenon through the lived experience of human beings. Such approaches have been used both in health care research (Styles 1994; Hallorsdottir and Hamrin 1996) and in enquiries into the essence of religious experience (Otto 1902; Buber 1970). A summary of interviewee perceptions is shown in Table 11.1.

An analysis of these perceptions produced the following taxonomy:

- *Personhood*: values, beliefs, achievements.
- *Relationships*: with self, others, the universe, a 'life force' or God.

**Table 11.1** Spiritual care stakeholders' perceptions of spirituality

*Synthesis of statements: Spirituality*

1 All people are spiritual beings; spirituality recognizes each individual as a unique person
2 Spirituality is a life orientation shaped by culture and history, incorporating values and beliefs, practices, customs and ritual
3 Spirituality is about understanding suffering, preparing to die and letting go
4 Spirituality is like being on fire; all that's possible are flowing and quickening
5 Spirituality is being at one with the universe and in touch with nature and creation
6 Spirituality is concerned with something other than just the body; it is concerned with feelings, relationships, personal awareness and the mystery of our understanding of ourselves
7 Spirituality is concerned with the soul and its link with the spirit
8 Being spiritual is not the same as being religious
9 Spirituality can be expressed religiously or non-religiously
10 Spirituality is a submission to the commands of God
11 Spirituality is related to God's call and to the effects of that call
12 Christian spirituality orientates towards a life that is linked to the Holy Spirit and is patterned by Christ
13 Spirituality is expressed in worship, devotion and prayer
14 Spirituality is about questing and searching – that journey, that struggle – addressing the big questions of life, death, another life and the universe
15 Spirituality is an awakening to life and a focus upon the meaning, direction, purpose and achievements of individual lives
16 Spirituality is concerned with the intangibility of transcendence and the tuning in to something both beyond and within, something deeper, something wider
17 Spirituality is being aware of a life force – sometimes called God

- *Religion*: prayer, vocation, commitment and worship.
- *Search for meaning*: the 'big questions' of life and death, mortality.
- *Transcendence*: something beyond/something within.

It is striking that 'spirituality' was meaningful to all the participants, indicating an element of commonality. The conclusion may be drawn, therefore, that whatever the differences of faith (or lack of it) the term had assumed potency in the lived experience of this group of stakeholders (Wright 2002).

### Model of the spiritual domain

The above typology is emblematic of the range of perceptions summarized in the following model of the spiritual domain (Figure 11.1): a construction based on a synthesis of key elements of health care and related literature. This inclusive, overarching model recognizes that spirituality may be expressed *both* religiously *and* humanistically. It acknowledges the dynamic relationship between the dimensions of 'self', 'others' and the 'cosmos' and the questions of life and death that spring from these interactions. The spiritually related activities of 'becoming', 'connecting', 'finding meaning' and 'transcending' are highlighted, and their key elements itemized (Wright 2001b).

While there is no evidence of a universal belief in God or adherence to a religious faith, it is apparent that in some instances, religion and spirituality not only have a connection but have become inseparable (Hollins 2005). As a result, religious devotees are provided with an all-encompassing vehicle to encounter the mysteries of their life, their relationships and their death (Butler and Butler 1996). Mark Jacobson, the medical director of Selian

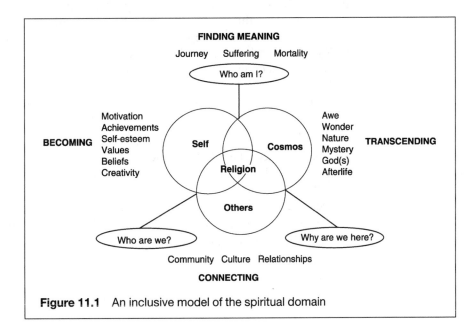

**Figure 11.1**    An inclusive model of the spiritual domain

Hospital in Arusha, tells how this connectedness is evident among his patients in Tanzania.

> For a very long time in Africa, people have sought to die at home and be buried on their home property. They belong to the traditional religions that see the spiritual world as being located in the place of your home; so ancestors and family that are buried together is a very important part of the many traditional religions.
>
> (Jacobson 2004)

In the multi-faith country of India, Firuza Patel, president of the Indian Association of Palliative Care, speaks of the importance of religion and how, at Chandigarh Hospice, all faiths are acknowledged and welcomed. 'The hospice is open to all religions and we have made a logo of a caring hand with a hospice hut on top of it; and then we have the four religious signs with it – the Hindu, the Sikh, the Muslim and the Christian' (Wright *et al.* 2004: 223).

During its global spread, the hospice-palliative care ideal has come to interface with a broad spectrum of faiths, prompting a profound religious debate. Central to this debate is the recognition of shared values. In her study of the Koruna Hospice Service (Australia), McGrath (1998) notes how the Buddhist metaphysic resonates with the ethos of hospice, apparent in the concept of universal compassion. In Budapest, Katalin Hegedus tells how a common purpose has been found between hospice philosophy and Jewish spirituality: to cherish each moment of a person's life (Clark and Wright 2003: 201). A harmonious relationship has also been sought in Saudi Arabia, with its strong Islamic culture and the submission of its people to the will of God (Gray *et al.* 1997); and in Hong Kong, with its diverse religious practices and differing approaches to death (Chung 1997). Christian spirituality is exemplified by hospices with a Christian foundation and expressed through organizations such as St Columba's Fellowship (UK), the Sisterhood of St Elizabeth (Russia) and the Sisters of Charity (global). In its many forms, the religious articulation of hospice continues to feature prominently, both in Britain and worldwide.

The spiritual activity of becoming centres on the unfolding life involving reflection, creativity and a sense of who one is (Ferrucci 1993). Within this activity are a number of discreet models, including:

- Developmental models – founded on the premise that as there are stages in physical growth, so there are stages in spiritual growth (Scott Peck 1987).
- Needs-based models – suggesting that human beings have a need for meaning, purpose and fulfilment in life (Renetzky 1979).
- Values-based models – associated with the 'ultimate' values of love, truth, forgiveness and reconciliation (Stoll 1989).
- Personhood models – relating to that which characterizes human beings: embodiment, cognition, the emotions and relationships (Wilson 1999).

Spirituality has become associated with connectedness, where meaning and fulfilment are found in loving relationships (Burkhardt 1994). In essence, the spiritual life is a community life (Erricker and Erricker 2001), a life with opportunities for belonging through the vehicles of language, ritual and art (Helman 1990). Within the activity of connecting, relationship and cultural models are particularly relevant. Relationship models are exemplified by the notion of 'being there', an activity that involves sharing the patient's space, hopes and fears (Speck 1995). Cultural models occur at both macro and micro levels. A macro example is Danièle Hervieu-Léger's (2000) notion of a chain of memory connecting past, present and future members of a community. This has relevance to the care of the dying, having parallels with the growing interest in patient-centred care shown during the past decade by countries of the former Soviet Union. Rights of passage associated with hospice admission procedures exemplify the micro level. These procedures contextualize a ritual entry into a unique space – described as sacred and transitional – as people cross boundaries between one status and another (Froggatt 1997).

In the West, finding meaning has come to be regarded as a central feature of spirituality, due partly to the influence of Frankl (1959), a holocaust survivor who formed the view that the purpose of human beings is not to avoid pain but to find meaning in life. Metaphors of journey acknowledge the impact of illness upon the individual, likening the search for meaning to a sacred quest to discover the mysteries of life (Hawkins 1999). On this journey, suffering and mortality occupy a special place. The journey into death is considered by some to be the ultimate vehicle for spiritual discovery (Singh 1999).

Transcending the self has been described as 'going beyond' – an action or state of being that exceeds the usual limits of human experience (Page 1995). It is associated with a sense of awe and wonder in the presence of mystery and the beauty of nature, prompting questions about the existence of a creator and life after death. Within health care, writers frequently favour the 'vertical' idea of transcendent space: a dualist worldview in the Cartesian tradition that regards the natural and supernatural as essentially different from one another (Harrison 1993). Gill (1998) argues for a re-thought, postmodern view of 'mediated transcendence' – a phenomenon whereby intangible reality can be encountered *in and through* the particulars of tangible reality. This fusion of the tangible and intangible suggests the possibility of fresh insights into patient transcendence and resonates with Kellehear's (2000) pragmatic view that transcendence may be achieved by searching for meanings in situations, in moral or biographical contexts and in religious beliefs.

John Hunt, a hospice nurse drawn to the Buddhist tradition, explains how a broad view of spirituality has become integrated into his clinical practice:

> It's about caring for the person – whether it's going back after a while to ask whether the pain is less, or sitting with somebody whilst they cry or

they laugh. It's about being able to engage in the big questions with people, things like: 'why is this happening to me?' – enabling them to talk about their fears and anxieties about the process of dying, and what will happen to them as well as to those who are left behind. For some people, it's about supporting them in trying to leave things, or say things, or do things, which they feel are important to leave or say or do before they die. It's trying to listen to people properly. Where possible, we try and let people tell us how they want things to be, and we try and make it be that way. I also think it's important that when a person can't communicate with us any more as themselves, that we continue to respect them as themselves up to the point at which they die.

(Wright 2001a)

A postmodern description of the spiritual domain might liken it to a diamond, its multiple facets revealed or concealed depending on the viewer's angle of observation. At best, inclusive models resonate with concepts of holism and the values of acceptance and non-judgemental compassion. Such models recognize that among patients drawn from pluralistic societies, there is no single spiritual source but multiple explorations, multiple interpretations and multiple expressions.

# Patient and family perspectives

### *Patient narratives*

The spiritual needs of patients relate in no small part to their encounter with their illness. Within a whole-life context, these needs are grounded in the successes, failures, hopes and dreams of individual biographies. A feature of the late twentieth century has been the willingness of patients and their relatives to reveal the experience of illness and what it has come to mean. Despite his faith, Michael Mayne – a former Dean of Westminster – was no stranger to uncertainty as cancer of the jaw led him to contemplate mortality and determine the ultimate meaning of his life.

We each have our own story to tell, like and unlike everyone else's story. We each need to discern it and marvel how, in retrospect, it begins to make sense and we can see how everything – the bad times when God

---

**Reflection**
- How would you define spirituality?
- What influences shape your own spirituality?
- How do you become aware of the spiritual impact of the dying process on each individual patient?
- What barriers might be created by your own spiritual perceptions when dealing with the spiritual diversity of patients and their families?

seemed to have deserted us as well as the good – was grist to the mill; and how, a bit battered, we have not only come through, but (hopefully, though not always) learned the lessons that made us more rounded people. How all in the end is part of the harvest of our lives.

(Mayne 2006: 32)

Mayne was 77 years old when he died and he had the advantage of looking back on a long and fulfilling life. When the journalist Ruth Picardie was diagnosed with breast cancer and died aged 33, she left a young husband and two-year-old twins. Her articles for *Observer Life*, titled 'Before I say goodbye', and the subsequent publication of her emails gave the public a moving insight into her deteriorating condition. What hurt most, she said, was losing the future: not being there to clap when her babies learn to write their names or to kiss their knees when they fall off their bikes (Picardie 1998: 58).

Loss is an inescapable feature of illness, highlighted by admission to a health care institution that in itself acknowledges a deteriorating lifestyle and social status (Kleinman 1988). Vanstone (1982) notes how illness results in a change in outlook, increasing isolation and transition from activity to passivity. Such losses have an impact on the dying patient, each one bearing witness to the incremental dismantling of personhood (Rose 1996).

Underpinning these losses is what may be termed 'woundedness'. Arthur Frank, a cancer survivor, notes how the wounded hip of Jacob authenticates the story of his biblical struggle with an angel (Genesis 32: 24–26). In essence, Frank regards the patient as a wounded storyteller, a raconteur whose wounds are emblematic of the story's potency. In this scenario, storytelling becomes a vehicle for recovering the voice which has been silenced by illness; a means of reclaiming power after diagnosis through the knowledge that an individual's story is both worth the telling and worthy of being heard (Frank 1995).

### Patient requirements

At the close of the twentieth century, I conducted a survey of 151 hospices and 195 hospital trusts in England and Wales to discover chaplains' perceptions of the most frequently expressed religious and non-religious requirements of patients (Wright 2001c). Eighty-nine per cent of respondents in both groups indicated that patients most frequently require somebody to listen to them; someone to 'be there' followed closely behind. Both hospital and hospice patients most frequently wish to discuss their concern for relatives and death and dying; pain also features prominently and, for hospice patients, suffering. Of the activities of the Christian faith, patients within both hospice and hospital most frequently wish to receive communion, to pray and to worship (Table 11.2).

Data from in-depth interviews with ten patients in four health settings illuminate these findings (Wright 2001a). Just one patient, Jasmine, considered herself to be religious. Although shocked by her cancer diagnosis,

**Table 11.2**  Chaplains' perceptions of the most frequent spiritual requirements of patients

|  | Hospital | | Hospice | |
| --- | --- | --- | --- | --- |
|  | *n* | *(%)* | *n* | *(%)* |
| **Non-religious requirements** | | | | |
| Someone to listen | 103 | (89) | 128 | (89) |
| Someone to 'be there' | 100 | (86) | 106 | (74) |
| **Spiritual issues** | | | | |
| – why me? | 43 | (37) | 81 | (56) |
| – pain | 81 | (71) | 81 | (57) |
| – meaning of life | 36 | (32) | 51 | (36) |
| – value of one's own life | 51 | (45) | 53 | (37) |
| – suffering | 51 | (44) | 84 | (58) |
| – forgiveness | 13 | (11) | 16 | (11) |
| – transcendence | 5 | (5) | 6 | (4) |
| – the nature of God | 15 | (13) | 26 | (18) |
| – concern for relatives | 102 | (88) | 116 | (81) |
| – death and dying | 79 | (69) | 83 | (58) |
| – afterlife | 22 | (19) | 24 | (17) |
| **Religious requirements** | | | | |
| – prayer | 49 | (43) | 88 | (61) |
| – texts | 3 | (3) | 16 | (11) |
| – worship | 25 | (22) | 51 | (36) |
| – special rituals | 9 | (8) | 39 | (28) |
| – baptism | 0 | (0) | 11 | (8) |
| – confession/absolution | 7 | (6) | 6 | (4) |
| – communion | 51 | (44) | 94 | (65) |
| – anointing | 10 | (9) | 19 | (13) |
| – last rites | 15 | (14) | 42 | (30) |

she felt uplifted by members of her family and congregation who visited frequently to pray with her. As a Jehovah's Witness, Jasmine professed a deep, personal faith and recounted a moving experience of God's presence, 'When I were praying to him, I put my hand over the trolley when I were going to theatre, and in my mind, because my faith was so strong, he was holding my hand'.

In the group of nine participants who claimed to be 'non-religious' each of them believed in God or a 'larger being'. Seven patients prayed frequently: three admitting to daily prayer and one to 'praying all the time'. Christine says, 'I pray to God every morning and every evening. Just because I don't go to Church it doesn't mean I don't believe in him, because I would say "he giveth and he taketh" '. Faith leaders played an important role for three patients and two focused on an afterlife. Hettie is a widow whose daughters live abroad, causing her to feel lonely. To her surprise, she found unexpected strength when she moved to the ward where her husband had died. She felt close to him and looked forward to joining him in another life. 'I believe there's something there, somewhere. My husband died in this hospital and I've said to him many times, "Ne'er mind lad, I'll be there with you before long, I've just this and that to see to". Then, sometimes, a day like today, I've thought: Oh I wish it were today!'

### Relative narratives

In their groundbreaking article, Rosemary and Victor Zorza (1978) tell how their daughter, Jane, developed a painful melanoma and was admitted to an Oxford hospice where she died eight days later. She was 25 years old. Surprised by the change in Jane's demeanour after admission and charged with the task of making her last days happy, the Zorzas write as follows:

> As things worked out, the time of greatest suffering was when the doctors were refusing to tell her what her chances of survival were. Once she was told . . . there was no great anguished sobbing, but a sad, resigned little sigh, almost of relief, and just a few tears. 'Now that I know, she said, I want to enjoy every day I have left and I want to be happy, and I want you to help me to be happy'.
>
> (Zorza and Zorza 1978)

Against the backdrop of cancer, a source of happiness for both Jane and her parents was her new-found ability to transcend the disease and rediscover the presence of beauty; in music, in the sunset, in the flowers she wore in her hair. Victor recalls a poignant moment. 'One morning, I had put on a Mozart tape for her, just as she was waking up. She slowly opened her eyes, listened with obvious enjoyment for a few minutes and glanced at me . . . "How beautiful you are making it for me to die," she said slowly' (Zorza and Zorza 1978).

More recently, Grinyer (2002) has provided a telling account of 28 young adults seen from their parents' perspectives as they encounter illness and, in some cases, death. Serious issues emerge such as the tension between dependence and independence and the loss of a child on the threshold of adulthood. Spiritual issues figure prominently. For example, as George's physical strength decreased his spiritual awareness increased, becoming a source of strength not only for himself but also for his mother. For those with a religious faith, having beliefs and belonging to a church can provide powerful support. Anne says: 'another lifeline for me has been my local church who have all been very supportive. I think my belief in an afterlife has got me through some very dark days' (Grinyer 2002: 158).

Yet religious beliefs may also be problematic. Karen comes from a Roman Catholic family and has lived with her partner, Arthur, for 14 years. Arthur has cancer of the bladder and has been admitted to a hospice. In the following extract, Karen indicates some pressures arising from her religious background:

I met Arthur just about 15 years ago, and I was – yes, I was divorced by that time. We never really wanted to get married because we felt that, I suppose, our relationship was OK as it was, and I'd been married, and – I'm steeped in Catholicism, that's the first thing, steeped in it – I don't practise now, although I do – well, we've just had a family party, and our family parties always start with mass – so it's still very much part of my family. How did I get on to that? So there was quite a lot of pressure to marry, and I suppose me mum still thinks that I committed adultery or something. There are loads of things I don't like about religion, but, if you say 'am I religious?' I'm not sure really, 'cos it's quite a comfort to think of God.

In the context of woundedness and loss, the narrative of illness places mortality centre stage, prompting an increase in spiritual activity for both patients and relatives. Despite the risk of a lost faith, there is also the possibility that faith may be strengthened; many patients who describe themselves as 'not religious' believe in God and pray every day. Not church-goers, they have rediscovered the language and imagery of both spirituality and the church, in some cases learnt in childhood and neglected in adult life. In effect, a familiar landscape has emerged as patients move towards the end of their lives. This 'pentimento' – or reappearance – has been likened to an overlaid painting, where shadows of previously drawn lines come to the surface with the passage of time to give a new, often surprising insight into a long obscured domain. 'Lives and their experiences are represented in stories; they are like pictures that have been painted over' (Denzin 1989: 81).

## Institutional perspectives

Historical links between caring for the sick and the work of religious orders were incorporated into the National Health Service (NHS) in 1948 when the Ministry of Health advised hospital authorities to provide spiritual care by appointing paid chaplains from different traditions. Further guidance (NHS 1948) advised authorities to establish a chapel and arrange schedules so that nurses and others could attend services of their denomination. By the close

**Reflection**
- What do you consider to be the most frequently required religious and non-religious spiritual requirements of patients?
- How would you respond to a patient who claimed to be 'not religious' but suddenly wanted to talk about God, prayer or an afterlife?
- What would you say to a patient who asked you what it is like to die?
- How would you respond to a relative who felt guilty for 'wanting it to be over'?

of the twentieth century, the religious climate had changed. Reflecting the multicultural nature of contemporary society, the Patient's Charter (DoH 1991) set a national standard concerning respect for religious and cultural beliefs. Guidance from the Department of Health (DoH 1992) advised the NHS to recognize the needs of both Christians and non-Christians, and with the changing demographics of modern Britain, managers now face the complex task of providing spiritual care across a range of diverse religious traditions and none (Cobb 2001).

Responses to my survey show that 56 (40 per cent) hospitals and 62 (57 per cent) hospices published a policy statement on spiritual care. Multi-faith guidelines were in place in 124 (86 per cent) hospitals and 64 (60 per cent) hospices. Within the hospitals 73 (29 per cent) chapels and 86 (91 per cent) multi-faith rooms opened during the 1990s. During the same period 41 (44 per cent) chapels and 16 (55 per cent) multi-faith rooms opened in hospices. Within hospitals, all chaplaincies were funded within a range of 30 to 368 hours per week; 98 per cent of these hours were allocated to Christians. Within hospices, 72 per cent of chaplaincies were funded within a range of 3 to 88 hours per week; 99.5 per cent of these hours were allocated to Christians. These figures suggest that in England and Wales:

- spiritual care is not fully integrated at the policy level of hospitals and hospices
- although multi-faith guidelines were in place in most hospitals, they were lacking in 40 per cent of hospices
- a changing religious landscape was reflected in the establishment of multi-faith rooms within both types of institution
- funded chaplaincy is almost exclusively Christian.

At the unit level, both hospitals and hospices attempt to inform patients of their spiritual care provision. Methods range from the publication of newsletters and information packs to the use of videotape played on strategically placed monitors. In a bedside leaflet, a chaplaincy department was introduced as follows:

> The name 'chaplaincy' derives from the Latin word cappella, which means 'cloak'. As human beings we are called to serve one another, to bring a touch of comfort, healing and strength. The symbol of chaplaincy in this Hospital Trust is of one person holding another by the hand, while both are enfolded, or cloaked, within the love and protection of God.

### Identification of spiritual needs

Survey responses from 97 trusts (71 per cent) and 102 hospices (88 per cent) indicate that an assessment was made of spiritual needs. Around three-quarters of hospices include items about worship, sacraments and preferences for a minister; fewer than half of the hospitals include these items. Spiritual assessments are complex, however, illustrated perhaps by their absence in 29 per cent of hospitals and 12 per cent of hospices. The NHS (E) Northern and Yorkshire Chaplains and Pastoral Care Committee (1995) suggest that a patient's spiritual needs should be assessed during an interview conducted shortly after admission. Attention would focus on the interface between religion and health care; information would be collected on the patient's religious and cultural requirements and, if appropriate, there may be an exploration of the patient's wishes in the event of death.

Questions arise about what is being assessed. A record of patient wishes surrounding worship, diet or ritual washing may be seen as a note of spirit-ual *behaviours* rather than any assessment of spiritual *needs*. Cobb (1998) suggests that Bradshaw's taxonomy of social need – normative need, com-parative need, expressed need and felt need – helps to illuminate the issues. Yet, while an institution may seek to provide for the general spiritual needs of its clients (normative need), maintain equity of service for different groups (comparative need) and encourage patients to make their own wishes known (expressed need), the deeper, more elusive 'felt needs' – the need for meaning, purpose and fulfilment in life – remain difficult to assess.

A variety of measures are used within the spiritual domain. Stoll set the scene when she published her spiritual history guide in 1979 (Stoll 1979). Using in-depth interviews, data were gathered concerning the patient's con-cept of God, sources of strength, and perceptions regarding the relationship between spiritual beliefs and health status. Other measures have come to rely heavily on interview techniques, together with the skills of discernment when being with, observing or listening to a patient (Emblem and Halstead 1993; King *et al.* 1995; Stanworth 2004). The relationship between spirituality and well-being has received increasing attention since Paloutzian and Ellison (1982) developed their Spiritual Well-Being Scale in the early 1980s. Similar measures include the JAREL Spiritual Well-Being Scale (Hungelmann *et al.* 1996) and the Spiritual Perspective Scale (Reed 1987). In the quality of life arena, existential issues have been included in the McGill Quality of Life Questionnaire (Cohen *et al.* 1996) and in Wyatt and Friedman's (1996) quality of life model for long-term survivors of breast cancer. Against the background of this activity, Speck *et al.* make a plea for 'user friendly and brief measures to assess spiritual need in the absence of religious faith' (2004: 124).

The multiple case study[1] revealed that institutions were using both for-mal and informal means to identify spiritual needs. All units encouraged patients to make their own needs known – very important in the case of the acute hospital with 1,000 beds. Common to all institutions was a formal checklist, used to gather information around admission. Supplementary assessments and patient reviews figured prominently in both settings. Informal means encompassed receptiveness to patient questions, observing the patient's demeanour and obtaining the perceptions of relatives.

### Spiritual care

Institutions deliver spiritual care in various ways. Physical resources such as chapels, quiet rooms and prayer rooms – together with facilities for viewing and handling the dead – have a part to play. Alongside these physical resources is the need for human resources: chaplains, chaplaincy volunteers and local faith leaders. In some institutions, opportunities for worship and the celebration of world-faith festivals form part of a religious calendar; so do broadcast services, guided reflection, meditation and prayer, accompanied by opportunities for the occasional baptism, marriage and funeral service.

A key factor within spiritual care provision is the expertise of staff and the creation of a spiritual ethos. Attempts to meet a broad range of spiritual needs within a caring community contribute to this ethos. In addition, good communication and notions of 'being there', 'sharing the patient's journey' and 'helping a person to find meaning' have the capacity to engage on a spiritual level. Ultimately, the activities of giving time and listening are crucial.

### Spiritual care-givers

Traditionally, chaplains have assumed a special responsibility for spiritual care. Yet a comparison of the chaplain's duties reported by the first Commission of the Hospital Chaplaincies Council (1951) and findings of the survey reported in this chapter, shows how the role has changed. Christian chaplains still retain a core responsibility for conducting services and administering the sacraments; and among the 90 per cent of hospital chaplains and 70 per cent of hospice chaplains who hold job descriptions, these mostly include the spiritual care of patients, relatives *and* staff. Gone, however, is the mid-twentieth century assumption that every patient will receive a visit on their day of admission (1951: 5). Highlighting their expanded role, more than 80 per cent of chaplains within both groups report a responsibility for spiritual care education; 98 per cent of hospital chaplains and 85 per cent of hospice chaplains liaise with religious leaders of faiths other than Christian; and around one half of hospital chaplains and one third of hospice chaplains assume a management responsibility for bereavement care.

Chaplains are not the only care-givers to acknowledge the place of spirituality. Florence Nightingale was a committed Unitarian with a strong faith that caused her to regard nursing as a religious calling, and evidence of this tradition remains today (Carson 1989; Fry 1997). Theorists like Watson (1974) advise nurses to create a supportive spiritual environment, whereas Abdella seeks to facilitate progress towards the patient's spiritual goals (Abdella *et al.* 1960). Among the grand theories, Roy's (1976) adaptation model and Neuman's (1995) systems model both identify the place of the spiritual self. Significantly, Travelbee (1971) regards suffering as a spiritual encounter. In 1984 the United Kingdom Central Council for Nursing, Midwifery and Health Visiting (UKCC) considered it a nurse's duty to take account of the customs, values and spiritual beliefs of patients. This view became incorporated into Project 2000 (UKCC 1986) and since then, the spirituality element of nurses' pre-registration courses has featured more prominently.

Despite suggestions that nurses are uncomfortable in the spiritual domain (Golberg 1998), the burgeoning literature on spirituality and nursing suggests a growing interest. Within the case studies, spiritually aware nurses were found in all institutions. Typical of nurse responses is the following: 'I always did equate spirituality with religion, you know, religious beliefs and that, until I came here [hospice]. Now my sort of thing is "What has my life been about? What is the meaning of life? Has it been worthwhile?"; those kinds of questions'.

An analysis of patient contacts showed that all patients in all units had encounters with spiritually aware personnel (Table 11.3). In this instance, 'spiritually aware personnel' is taken to mean those members of staff or volunteers who have undertaken some form of professional training, either in-depth or at a basic level. This latter form is amplified by the following comment from a spiritual care director:

> Part of my role with staff in the non-clinical areas is around helping people to understand that they actually do contribute to the well-being of patients by how they receive them in reception, by how they present

**Table 11.3**   Patient encounters with spiritually aware personnel

| | Patients | | | | | | | | | |
| --- | --- | --- | --- | --- | --- | --- | --- | --- | --- | --- |
| | Hospice 1 | | Hospice 2 | | | | Hospital 1 | | Hospital 2 | |
| | A | B | C | D | E | F | G | H | I | J |
| *Recorded religion* | *C/E* | *None* | *C/E* | *C/E* | *J* | *C/E* | *C/E* | *C/E* | *RC* | *JW* |
| *Practising/Non-practising* | *NP* | *NP* | *NP* | *NP* | *NP* | *NP* | *NP* | *NP* | *NP* | *P* |
| Chaplain (Free Church) | • | • | | | | | | • | | |
| Chaplain (Roman Catholic) | | | • | • | • | • | | | • | |
| Chaplain (Church of England) | | | | | | | • | | • | • |
| Chaplain (student) | | • | | | | | | | | |
| Chaplaincy volunteer | | | • | • | • | • | • | • | • | • |
| Visiting minister/elder | | | | | • | | | | • | • |
| Visiting believers | | | | | • | | | | | • |
| Palliative care physician | • | • | • | • | • | • | • | • | | |
| Nurse: (palliative care specialist) | • | • | • | • | • | • | • | • | | |
| Nurse: (trained care of dying) | • | • | • | • | • | • | • | • | • | • |
| Nurse: (unit trained) | • | • | • | • | • | • | | • | | |
| Health care assistant (unit trained) | • | • | • | • | • | • | • | | | |
| Social worker | • | • | • | • | • | • | | | | |
| Support staff (receptionists, domestics) | • | • | • | • | • | • | | | | |
| Care staff (personal faith) | • | • | • | • | • | • | • | • | | |

the food – the spiritual aspects of all that – and people need to be helped sometimes to see the connections.

In all cases, encounters with spiritually aware personnel included a Christian chaplain or chaplaincy volunteer whether or not patients professed the Christian faith or regarded themselves as religious. In addition, Patient E received visits from the Rabbi; Patient J from the congregation of Jehovah's Witnesses; and Patient I from her Roman Catholic parish priest.

The separation of religion from spirituality has become a marked feature of current thought. Consequently, although the care-giving of chaplains may include a unique denominational role, a broader role that relates to the spiritual activities of transcending, finding meaning and connecting has come to attract a wider ownership: an ownership that includes the psychologist, the physician, the complementary therapist and the nurse. A consequence of this wider ownership has led to a patchwork of spiritually aware personnel. Some – such as chaplaincy volunteers – have a strong religious faith. Others have no faith, yet relate easily to the spiritual personhood of the confused – or routinely create privacy and accompaniment for the dying. They include staff whose spiritual awareness has been raised through in-depth education alongside those who have spent just a little time reflecting upon how their role contributes to the spiritual ethos of the institution; all in addition to chaplains and all found in the field.

# Conclusion

The palliative care ideal is characterized by an integrated approach that accepts the inevitability of death alongside the spiritual implications of the event. In practice, the delivery of spiritual care may be problematic – due partly to the sense of mystery associated with the spiritual domain but also to the widely held belief that religion and spirituality are separate entities. Evidence suggests that as the narrative of illness centres on mortality, there is an increase in spiritual activity on the part of patients and relatives. Many who describe themselves as 'not religious' pray regularly and believe in God; and spiritual needs, both religion-based and religion-free, come to the fore. In this scenario, a key element of spiritual care provision is the expertise of staff and the creation of a spiritual ethos. The challenge for those charged with spiritual care delivery is how to blend a cohesive team of spiritually

**Reflection**
- Who are the spiritual care-givers in your institution?
- In what areas of spiritual care do you feel comfortable/uncomfortable?
- What are your training needs?
- How could spiritual assessment be further developed?

aware personnel, drawn from disparate spiritual perspectives, which owns an inclusive vision and gently meets the patient with affirmation and understanding at the point of need.

# Note

1   Some data presented in this chapter were collected during the author's doctoral study of the spiritual care of cancer patients in the acute hospital and specialist inpatient palliative care unit. The objectives of this study were to identify (a) the nature of spirituality, (b) the means whereby spiritual needs are assessed and met and (c) the perceptions of spiritual care stakeholders, patients and relatives. A multi-method, three-phase design was used, incorporating (1) a survey by postal questionnaire of the views of chaplains in 151 hospices and 195 hospital trusts in England and Wales, (2) a phenomenological enquiry into the spiritual care perceptions of palliative care stakeholders and (3) a multiple case study in four health settings (Wright 2001a).

# References

Abdella, F.G., Beland, I.L., Martin, A. and Matherny, R. (1960) *Patient-Centred Approaches to Nursing.* New York: Macmillan.
Ainsworth-Smith, I. and Speck, P. (1999) *Letting Go.* London: SPCK.
Brierley, P. (1999) *Religious Trends.* London: Marshall Pickering.
Buber, M. (1970) *I and Thou.* Edinburgh: T. & T. Clark.
Burkhardt, M.A. (1994) Becoming and connecting: elements of spirituality for women. *Holistic Nursing Practice*, 8(4): 12–21.
Butler, B. and Butler, T. (1996) *Just Spirituality in a World of Faiths.* London: Mowbray.
Carson, V.B. (1989) Spiritual development across the life span. In: V.B. Carson (ed.) *Spiritual Dimensions of Nursing Practice.* Philadelphia, PA: W.B. Saunders.
Chung, L.S.T. (1997) The hospice movement in a Chinese society – a Hong Kong experience. In: C. Saunders and R. Kastenbaum (eds) *Hospice Care on the International Scene.* New York: Springer.
Clark, D. and Wright, M. (2003) *Transitions in End of Life Care: Hospice and Related Developments in Eastern Europe and Central Asia.* Buckingham: Open University Press.
Cobb, M. (1998) Assessing spiritual need: an examination of practice. In: M. Cobb and V. Robshaw (eds) *The Spiritual Challenge of Health Care.* London: Churchill Livingstone.
Cobb, M. (2001) *The Dying Soul: Spiritual Care at the End of Life.* Buckingham: Open University Press.
Cohen, S.R., Mount, B.M., Tomas, J.J.N. and Mount, L.F. (1996) Existential well-being is an important determinant of quality of life. *Cancer*, 77: 576–86.
Davie, G. (1994) *Religion in Britain since 1945.* London: Blackwell.
Denzin, N.K. (1989) *Interpretive Biography.* London: Sage.
Department of Health (1991) *The Patient's Charter.* London: HMSO.

Department of Health (1992) *Meeting the spiritual needs of patients and staff*. HSG (92)2. London: HMSO.

Emblem, J.D. and Halstead, L. (1993) Spiritual needs and interventions: comparing the views of patients, nurses and chaplains. *Clinical Nurse Specialist*, 7(4): 175–82.

Erricker, C. and Erricker, J. (2001) *Contemporary Spiritualities: Social and Religious Contexts*. London: Continuum.

Ferrucci, P. (1993) *What We May Be: the Vision and Techniques of Psycho-synthesis*. New York: Harper Collins.

Frank, A. (1995) *The Wounded Storyteller*. London: University of Chicago Press.

Frankl, V.E. (1959) *Man's Search for Meaning*. London: Touchstone Press.

Froggatt, K. (1997) Rites of passage and the hospice culture. *Mortality*, 2(2): 123–35.

Fry, A.J. (1997) Spirituality: connectedness through being and doing. In: S. Ronaldson (ed.) *Spirituality: The Heart of Nursing*. Melbourne: Ausmed Publications.

Gallup International Millennium Survey. In: G. Sturdy, Europe 'leads world in godlessness'. *Church Times*, 17 December 1999.

Gill, J.H. (1998) *Mediated Transcendence: A Postmodern Reflection*. Macon, GA: Mercer University Press.

Golberg, B. (1998) Connection: an exploration of spirituality in nursing care. *Journal of Advanced Nursing*, 7(4): 836–42.

Gray, A., Ezzart, A. and Boyer, A. (1997) Palliative care for the terminally ill in Saudi Arabia. In: C. Saunders and R. Kastenbaum (eds) *Hospice Care on the International Scene*. New York: Springer.

Grinyer, A. (2002) *Cancer in Young Adults through Parents' Eyes*. Buckingham: Open University Press.

Hallorsdottir, S. and Hamrin, E. (1996) Experiencing existential changes: the lived experience of having cancer. *Cancer Nurse*, 19: 29–36.

Harrison, J. (1993) Spirituality and nursing practice. *Journal of Clinical Nursing*, 2: 211–17.

Hawkins, A.H. (1999) *Reconstructing Illness: Studies in Pathography*. West Lafayette, IN: Purdue University Press.

Heelas, P. and Woodhead, L. (2005) *The Spiritual Revolution. Why Religion is Giving Way to Spirituality*. Oxford: Blackwell.

Heidegger, M. (1962) *Being and Time*. Oxford: Blackwell.

Helman, C. (1990) *Culture, Health and Illness*. London: Butterworth Heinemann.

Hervieu-Léger, D. (2000) *Religion as a Chain of Memory* (translated by S. Lee). New Brunswick, NJ: Rutgers University Press. First published as *La Religion pour Mémoire*. Éditions du Cerf, Paris, 1993.

Hollins, S. (2005) Spirituality and religion: exploring the relationship. *Nursing Management*, 12(6): 22–6.

Hospital Chaplaincies Commission of the Church Assembly (1951) *C A 1003: Final Report*. London: SPCK.

Hungelmann, J.A., Kenkel-Rossi, E., Klassen, L. and Stollenwerk, R. (1996) Focus on spiritual wellbeing: harmonious interconnectedness of mind-body-spirit – use of the JAREL Spiritual Wellbeing Scale. *Geriatric Nursing*, 17: 262–6.

Husserl, E. (1962) *Ideas: General Introduction to Pure Phenomenology*. New York: Collier.

Jacobson, M. (2004) Interviewed by David Clark for the Palliative Care in Africa project, 4 June.

Jewell, A. (ed.) (2003) *Ageing, Spirituality and Well-being*. London: Jessica Kingsley Publishers.

Kellehear, A. (2000) Spirituality and palliative care: a model of needs. *Palliative Medicine*, 14: 149–55.

King, M., Speck, P. and Thomas, A. (1995) The Royal Free interview for religious and spiritual beliefs: development and standardization. *Psychological Medicine*, 25(6): 1125–34.

Kleinman, A. (1988) *The Illness Narratives: Suffering, Healing and the Human Condition*. New York: Basic Books.

Markham, I. (1998) Spirituality and the world of faiths. In: M. Cobb and V. Robshaw (eds) *The Spiritual Challenge of Health Care*. London: Churchill Livingstone.

Mayne, M. (2006) *The Enduring Melody*. London: Darton, Longman and Todd.

McGrath, P. (1998) Buddhist spirituality – a compassionate perspective on hospice care. *Mortality*, 3(3): 251–63.

McSherry, W. (2006) *Making Sense of Spirituality in Health Care Practice. An Interactive Approach*. London: Jessica Kingsley.

Merleau-Ponty, M. (1962) *Phenomenology of Perception* (translated by C. Smith). London: Routledge & Keegan Paul.

National Health Service (1948) *Appointment of chaplains*. HMC (48) 62, London: HMSO.

National Health Service Executive Northern and Yorkshire Chaplains and Pastoral Care Committee (1995) *Framework for Spiritual Faith and Related Pastoral Care*. The Institute of Nursing: University of Leeds.

Neuman, B. (1995) *The Neuman Systems Model*. Norwalk, CT: Appleton and Lange.

Otto, R. (1902) *The Idea of the Holy* (translated by J.W. Harvey, 1968). London: Oxford University Press.

Page, R. (1995) Transcendence and immanence. In: A.V. Campbell (ed.) *A Dictionary of Pastoral Care*. London: SPCK.

Paloutzian, R.D. and Ellison, C.W. (1982) Loneliness, spiritual wellbeing and the quality of life. In: L.A. Peplau and D. Perlman (eds) *Loneliness: A Sourcebook of Current Theory, Research and Therapy*. New York: Wiley.

Pattison, R. (2001) Dumbing down the spirit. In: H. Orchard (ed.) *Spirituality in Health Care Contexts*. London: Jessica Kingsley Publishers.

Picardie, S. (1998) *Before I Say Goodbye*. London: Penguin.

Reed, P.G. (1987) Spirituality and wellbeing in terminally ill hospitalised adults. *Research in Nursing and Health*, 10: 335–44.

Renetzky, L. (1979) The fourth dimension: applications to the social services. In: D.O. Moberg (ed.) *Spiritual Wellbeing: Sociological Perspectives*. Washington DC: University Press of America.

Ronaldson, S. (ed.) (1997) *Spirituality: The Heart of Nursing*. Melbourne, VIC: Ausmed Publications.

Rose, N. (1996) *Inventing Ourselves: Psychology, Power and Personhood*. Cambridge: Cambridge University Press.

Roy, C. (1976) *Introduction to Nursing: An Adaptation Model*. Engelwood Cliffs, NJ: Prentice Hall.

Saunders, C. (1986) The modern hospice. In: F. Wald (ed.) *In Quest of the Spiritual Component of Care for the Terminally Ill*. New Haven, CT: Yale School of Nursing.

Scott Peck, M. (1987) *The Different Drum*. London: Arrow Books.

Singh, K.D. (1999) *The Grace in Dying: How We Are Transformed Spiritually As We Die*. Dublin: Newleaf.

Speck, P. (1995) *Being There: Pastoral Care in Time of Illness*. London: SPCK.

Speck, P., Higginson, I. and Addington-Hall, J. (2004) Spiritual needs in health care. *British Medical Journal*, 329: 123–4.

Stanworth, R. (2004) *Recognizing Spiritual Needs in Patients Who Are Dying*. Oxford: Oxford University Press.

Stoll, R.I. (1979) Guidelines for spiritual assessment. *American Journal of Nursing*, September, pp. 1574–7.

Stoll, R.I. (1989) The essence of spirituality. In: V.B. Carson (ed.) *Spiritual Dimensions of Nursing Practice*. Philadelphia, PA: W.B. Saunders.

Styles, M.K. (1994) The shining stranger: application of the phenomenological method in the investigation of the nurse-family spiritual relationship. *Cancer Nurse*, 17(1): 18–26.

Swinton, J. (2001) *Spirituality and Mental Health Care*. London: Jessica Kingsley.

Travelbee, J. (1971) *Interpersonal Aspects of Nursing*. Philadelphia, PA: F.A. Davis.

UK Council for Nursing, Midwifery and Health Visiting (1984) *Code of Professional Conduct for the Nurse, Midwife and Health Visitor*. London: UKCC.

UK Central Council for Nursing, Midwifery and Health Visiting (UKCC) (1986) *Project 2000: A New Preparation for Practice*. London: UKCC.

Vanstone, W.H. (1982) *The Stature of Waiting*. London: Darton, Longman & Todd.

Watson, J. (1974) *Nursing: the Philosophy and Science of Caring*. Boston, MA: Little, Brown & Company.

Wilson, P. H. (1999) Memory, personhood and faith. In: A. Jewell (ed.) *Spirituality and Ageing*. London: Jessica Kingsley.

Wright, M., George, R. and Mingins, R. (2004) Exploring the meaning of spiritual care in the Indian context: findings from a survey and interviews. *Progress in Palliative Care*, 12(5): 221–6.

Wright, M.C. (2001a) Spiritual health care: an enquiry into the spiritual care of patients with cancer within the acute hospital and specialist inpatient palliative care unit in England and Wales. Unpublished PhD thesis, University of Sheffield.

Wright, M.C. (2001b) Spirituality: a developing concept within palliative care. *Progress in Palliative Care*, 9: 143–8.

Wright, M.C. (2001c) Chaplaincy in hospice and hospital: findings from a survey in England and Wales. *Palliative Medicine*, 15: 229–42.

Wright, M.C. (2002) The essence of spiritual care: a phenomenological enquiry. *Palliative Medicine*, 16: 125–32.

Wyatt, G.K.H. and Friedman, L.L. (1996) Developing and testing of a quality of life model for long-term female cancer survivors. *Quality of Life Research*, 5: 387–94.

Zorza, V. and Zorza, R. (1978) Death of a daughter. *Washington Post Outlook*, 22 January.

# 12

# Working with difficult symptoms

*Jessica Corner*

---

**Key points**

- Adopt a critical and reflective stance to understanding why particular problems are 'difficult' and to trying to understand what might need to change so that problems are addressed from a broader perspective.
- Use the person's story as the starting point for intervention or support. Hearing about the problem can in itself be therapeutic and may offer insights into how the problem may be tackled.
- Facilitating the person's own journey in learning to live with, manage or find relief from problems may be more fruitful than presenting oneself as the agent of 'control' for symptoms.
- Enabling self-management; that is, maintain activities and practices that are unique to oneself in maintaining one's sense of 'self'. Learning to master or deal with problems rather than relinquishing them to health professionals may be an important new direction for what has to date been known as 'symptom management'.

---

Rather than providing a tool kit for working with difficult symptoms as in many other palliative care texts, a critical view of symptom management is offered here, as well as some different ideas about approaches that may be adopted while working with people facing physical, emotional or practical problems as a result of life-limiting illness. I have chosen to adopt a critical and reflective stance, since this seems to be a more fruitful avenue to finding ways of working with some of the most challenging problems faced in caring practice. I have chosen not to offer a set of solutions or guidance on the management of difficult symptoms, since these are unlikely to be addressed through this kind of approach; the problems are both complex and bound up in the particular contexts in which people with life-limiting illness live. I do, however, draw out some ideas that might be used to guide the development of caring practice.

Cribb (2001), in writing about knowledge and caring, identifies two worlds, the world of science and the 'human world'; that is, there is scientific knowledge and there are 'lay beliefs'. He argues that the human world is being displaced and colonized by the natural and human sciences, so that personal and common sense knowledge is being displaced by 'expert' knowledge. Cribb argues that alongside this knowledge there is also what he calls 'real knowledge'; that is, knowledge about how to do things that cannot be gained through textbooks – how to ride a bike, conduct a conversation, be a good listener, for example. It is this real knowledge that is primary, as it provides the frame of reference on which all other knowledge rests or is made use of. Other authors have outlined ways of knowing in the context of nursing practice (see, for example, Carper 1978; Johns 1995; Nolan and Lundh 1998). Like the 'real' knowledge of Cribbs, these authors argue that there is knowledge that comes from direct involvement with situations or experiences.

Cribb (2001) argues that 'the stories that weave our domestic lives indicate a reality just as substantial as the stories which tell us about the material of which they are made' (page 17). Cribb suggests that a different relationship between expert and lay 'knower' may be needed; that instead of falling short of knowledge, the lay person, with their 'every day knowing', has knowledge that is continuous with more specialized forms of knowledge. It is understanding the relationship between expert knowledge and 'lay', or what might also be called 'embodied' knowledge (Benner and Wrubel 1989), that seems to be at the heart of how we should consider the approach to managing difficult symptoms. Valuing different kinds of knowledge, particularly the knowledge that people have about the problems of their own limiting illness, has influenced the way I set out my thoughts here.

## Symptom management as a dominant construct in palliative care

A powerful impetus for palliative care has been the goal to relieve the symptoms and problems that accompany life-limiting illness and are part of the process of dying. From the outset, hospice and palliative care services were established to tackle the particular needs of people dying from cancer. Symptom management, a core function in palliative care, has largely focused on a set of symptoms and problems commonly associated with advanced or metastatic stages of cancer, the most prevalent symptom being pain. The early success of the hospice and palliative care movement in developing effective approaches to the management of cancer pain using opioid drugs was an important driving force behind how palliative care as a speciality subsequently evolved, and has been instrumental in its success. As Robbins (1998) states: 'a large part of the impetus of setting up hospices and palliative care teams was the belief that the pain of terminal illness, especially the pain of progressive cancer, can be controlled effectively . . . relief of symptoms is largely the foundation upon which all other aspects of palliative care rest' (page 20). Thus, 'symptom management' is now seen as an essential part of the skills required in providing palliative care and, although not the exclusive form of help or intervention offered to patients and families, it is often the focus for the intervention of specialist palliative care teams.

While offering symptom management to people who are dying has become a major part of the *raison d'être* of palliative care, the way in which symptom management has become the primary focus has implications for the way care is organized and experienced. Palliative care, originating in the work of Cicely Saunders and others in the 1950s and 1960s, set out to offer a radical and alternative model of care for people who were dying to the prevailing model of increasingly institutionalized and medically managed care. Although the palliative care approach was devised as an alternative model, it has over time increasingly become embedded within the traditions, or discourses, of health care, particularly that of biomedicine. This has been a natural consequence of the professionalization of hospice services, but also means that approaches to managing the problems associated with dying have become defined and addressed in particular ways.

Palliative care as it exists in contemporary health care, defined by a dominant culture orientated to the 'management' or 'control' of symptoms, places heavy emphasis on the biomedical model of disease management, and is one aspect of the so-called 'medicalization' of death described by Field (1994). Field suggests that while the hospice movement was founded on a desire to reject the trend whereby dying was increasingly becoming the province of health workers and managed within highly technical health care institutions, palliative care is perhaps unintentionally perpetuating some aspects of the medicalization of dying. There is, for example, a trend towards the heavy use of technical procedures and medical technology. Also, palliative care becoming the overarching speciality for care in life-limiting illness has moved the emphasis away from dying and death to an unspecified time earlier in the course of illness, thereby focusing attention away from dying and death.

The point here is not to revisit a rather well-trodden path in relation to the critique of medicalization of society (see, for example, Ivan Illich's ([1976] 1990) now seminal critique *Limits to Medicine, Medical Nemesis: The Expropriation of Health*), whereby medicine is revealed and denigrated for having acquired extraordinary power and control over people's lives, or over people in medical encounters. Rather, it is to understand that the biomedical paradigm has provided a system of knowledge and practices that can, because they are dominant, define our very experience of ourselves; they become part of the way we understand and live our lives (Lupton 1997). This has not been intentional; rather, it is an effect of the very success of biomedicine. It does, however, have some consequences and in the context of palliative care and in the management of difficult symptoms these are apparent. Clark (1999), for example, traces the origins of the concept of 'total pain' in the work of Cicely Saunders. Clark notes a paradox in the concept resulting from the radical intention to move the relief of pain arising from terminal cancer into territory where wider dimensions of suffering are acknowledged, and beyond the biomedical paradigm whereby pain is seen as simply a sensation arising from largely physical causes. It nevertheless can also be seen to be an extension of medical dominion where 'pain relief' is also an instrument of power. Clark argues that the principle of giving regular analgesia and thereby constant control of pain, can be seen to extend to the 'constant control of the patient' – that is, patients offered pain control regimes in palliative care are no longer expected to articulate their needs, since these will be anticipated in advance by someone else. Thus pain relief is achieved, but at the cost of loss of personal autonomy. The concept of 'total pain' that incorporates psychological, spiritual and social aspects of the pain experience can also be seen as extending the range of medical 'gaze', which Clark argues has an imperialist feel about it. From this perspective, then, holism 'is revealed as something other than we might suppose. Paradoxically and contrary to its own claims, this is a strategy of power, one which in subjecting human suffering to a new nosology, at the same objectifies it and prescribes strategies for its relief. In this sense "total pain" becomes a nomenclature of inscription, albeit unintended by its author' (Clark 1999: 734).

The foundation for palliative care within the discourse of biomedicine has led to the belief that the problems of dying should be understood as manifestations of disease, rather than more generally how one dies. Since symptoms are considered to be disease-related problems, it is assumed that they are properly managed by health professionals within the formal structures of health care. These assumptions tend to generate a particular set of responses to problems and excludes others. One assumption, for example, is that for individuals to have a peaceful death they must, as far as is possible, be symptom-free. While this is a laudable goal for care, it also focuses the activity of those involved in providing ever more effective symptom management, even when the goal to be 'symptom-free' while dying may be unrealistic. Another consequence is that there is little room for acknowledging social, professional or individual constraints that may operate as part of the dying process and that may contribute to the experience of difficult symptoms, or that may prevent the development of supportive but also more liberating regimes of care, for example those that prioritize preservation of personal autonomy.

## The consequences of a biomedical construction for symptom management in palliative care

It is worth exploring for a moment the ways in which symptom management has become defined and practised within palliative care. The ability to manage cancer pain through a biomedical approach using morphine was a very significant discovery for the hospice movement. The approach of using powerful drugs, or combinations of drugs, for cancer pain led to the search for new and better drugs and other treatments, first for pain and then for other symptoms common in cancer. A consequence of the success in using drugs to manage symptoms is that, in many instances, not only is 'symptom management' the primary endeavour, but drug treatments have become the primary approach used in tackling problems. Frequently, drug treatment for problems reported by a person who is dying is the first approach or perhaps the only solution considered. While this may be entirely appropriate, it has also had certain consequences for the way palliative care has developed and become organized. Care constructed around the use of drug treatments for symptoms emphasizes 'relief', 'control' or 'management' of the symptoms, the object being the removal, obliteration or disguise of symptoms as manifestations of the disease people are dying from. The goal of care is 'relief' or 'control', reducing the symptom to a level such that it is in the background or absent entirely. It is arguable that in pursuing this strategy to 'relieve' or 'control' symptoms, other aspects of the experience of symptoms, such as suffering, distress, the ability to function and even personal autonomy, independently have been relegated to secondary importance. Also, the assumption that the perception of a symptom such as pain, once removed or reduced using powerful pharmacology, ceases to be of concern to the person who experienced it, overlooks the possibility that suffering or the ability to function may not be addressed by the treatment.

The dominance of symptom management as the central goal of palliative care has had other ramifications. As a pharmacological approach became dominant, the doctor as the person who prescribes treatment aimed at symptom management also became the natural leader of services, reinforcing the trend towards biomedical or pharmacological solutions to the problems people who are dying bring to the attention of palliative care services. An illustration of the dominance of this approach can be seen in the palliative care research literature; there has been a preoccupation within palliative care research to chart or map the prevalence of symptoms among people who are dying. This has been motivated no doubt by a need to record demand for palliative care and to provide information on which to make decisions in determining where to target limited resources. For example, in a historical review of palliative care research, studies of symptoms – especially symptom prevalence studies among people admitted to hospices and palliative care services – were found to be the most common form of research published in the palliative care literature (Corner 1996). These studies have commonly used retrospective case note reviews, or questionnaires in which groups of patients were asked to indicate which of a list of symptoms they were experiencing.

Symptom prevalence studies provide an indication of the common and most difficult symptoms for people who are dying and yield insights into the problems that palliative care services are most commonly attempting to alleviate. However, the symptoms identified in these studies are largely defined by palliative care clinicians or the researcher undertaking the research and, as a result, reflect biomedical categories of different manifestations of disease, rather than problems identified and defined by people with life-limiting illness themselves. It is difficult to know whether or not 'common symptoms' identified through this process would be broadly similar if there had been more room for people who are dying or family members to define for themselves the nature of their problems. If the emphasis for palliative care services is on managing symptoms as constructed through these various studies, there is a risk that palliative care is not currently addressing need more broadly. Also important is that less attention has been paid to the extent to which palliative care services have achieved 'symptom relief' for individuals who are dying. There has been relatively little work into the effectiveness of symptom control, as constructed through this model of care. We know little about the extent to which the symptoms of people with cancer are indeed 'relieved' or 'managed'; indeed, there is evidence that in many circumstances this is not the case (see, for example, Higginson and McCarthy 1989; Hinton 1994; Addington-Hall and McCarthy 1995).

Our understanding of what it is like to live with particular symptoms is benefiting from research, although there is still much that is unknown. Studies have been conducted of the frequency with which symptoms and problems occur among individuals receiving palliative care and a few have reported detailed work into how these develop over time, or are manifested in the last weeks of life. The orientation of research has been to examine a particular set of clinical problems that are deemed amenable to intervention by palliative care services. Little work has been undertaken from a more insider or user/consumer oriented perspective. It is surprising that no concerted effort has been made to determine which symptoms or problems individuals may wish to be 'managed' on their behalf by health professionals, an issue I shall return to later. Importantly, since the very word 'managing' implies a certain stance when working with people who are ill or dying, this also warrants critical exploration.

Among the various limitations of the biomedical model identified is the biomedical construction of the body. Critical accounts of biomedicine identify the term 'symptom' as a biomedical construction; that is, it has developed as part of the way in which medicine has developed systems of knowledge and understanding of the body and of illness, but that is only one way of understanding one's body and the way one feels. It belongs firmly to the territory of 'expert' or scientific knowledge identified by Cribb. Armstrong (1995), for example, drawing on the work of Michel Foucault ([1973] 1986), identifies the biomedical 'spatialization of illness', where the relationship of symptoms and illness are configured in a three-dimensional framework: symptom, sign and pathology. The symptom is understood to be a marker of illness experienced by the patient, a sign is the intimation of disease elicited by the doctor, for example through physical examination, and together these are used to infer pathology. However, this spatialization or ordering of how illness is determined is not seen to be entirely benign. To align the three elements, the body of the patient is submitted to the 'gaze' – medical investigations which the patient must submit to. The patient is only required to answer questions that are deemed relevant to the identification of biomedically defined pathology and its treatment; other issues that may be deemed important by the person who is ill are not explored.

According to Lyon and Barbalet (1994), the model whereby biomedicine regards the body as an external object assumes that the practitioner is in control of the body of the patient; the patient is subordinate to the practitioner. Biomedicine deals with malfunctioning organs or other subsystems of the body, and with symptoms, but not the 'body' that is the person:

> The medical body is passive; any active capacities it may display are regarded as internal to its physiology, and these can be revealed to external observers as external knowledge. The body is readily subordinated to the authority of medical practice. It is disciplined and made, or at least made better, through the social institution of medicine. The medical body is a partial body. It is partial in a dual sense: it is the internal body, and it is the body patients have, but not the body patients are in the full sense.
>
> (Lyon and Barbalet 1994: 53)

Lyon and Barbalet (1994) argue that 'the medical body' is but one among a number of different constructions of the body that can be identified and have variously been described in scholarly writing. For example, 'the consumerist body' – that is, the body in consumerist society as manifested in magazines or in relation to our beliefs about the health products we buy. Another construction could be described as the 'social body' – that is, the body that is subject to social and cultural norms and practices. An alternative to the biomedical view of the body, where mind or self and physical body are considered separate entities, is the notion of 'embodiment'; that is, the idea that the body is experienced and is where and how 'self' is located. From this perspective, it is argued that the body, being one with self, acts to construct its own world; it is not a discrete physical entity external to the self. It is intercommunicative and active. Within health care and more particularly palliative care, these different ways of understanding the body are largely unacknowledged. There is, however, a developing interest in exploring the implications of acknowledging these different 'bodies', as well as the potential value of incorporating such understanding into approaches to offering health care.

The notion of a 'social body' recognizes that individuals are subject to power relations at large within society, such as the influence of doctors in medical encounters, and that how the body is understood is socially determined rather than 'real'. For example, how one should 'manage' one's bodily processes to be socially acceptable is generated and passed on through history and culture; it is socially determined and not simply the province of individuals. As Taussig (1980) states: 'things such as the signs and symptoms of disease . . . are not only biological and physical, but are also signs of social relations disguised as natural things, concealing their roots in human reciprocity' (p. 3).

The notion of an 'embodied body' proposes that the 'lived body' is experienced as a fluid entity; a combination of physicality and emotionality.

It is 'a pre-objective structure of lived experience; one in which mind and body, reason and emotion, pleasure and pain are thoroughly interfused' (Williams and Bendelow 1998: 133). Williams and Bendelow (1998) explain how, in chronic illness, the taken-for-granted normal state of embodiment, experienced as a kind of bodily disappearance in which one is not conscious of one's body as distinct from oneself, can be radically disrupted. In these circumstances, one becomes suddenly very aware of one's bodily failings and one's bodily identity is undermined. As a consequence, loss of self becomes a fundamental form of suffering in illness. This process can be reinforced and exacerbated by biomedical approaches to managing and treating disease, since these tend to disregard the importance of 'self'. Where symptoms are treated as physical manifestations of disease that need to be controlled or managed, we may fail to acknowledge emotional, social or individual processes that create the very experience of the symptom.

McNamara (2001) notes that symptom relief is a medicalized, technical and pharmacologically driven response to the dying process that 'masks' the physical process of dying, and has been prioritized above psychological, spiritual or other forms of care. McNamara does not elaborate on precisely what she believes to be 'masked' through this; however, this highly technical and externally 'managed' system of symptom control may well remove the possibility of self-management, or what Williams (1996) describes as achieving a 'negotiated settlement' with illness or dying. In relation to living with chronic illness, Williams notes that over time individuals reach for themselves a kind of resolution, a realignment of body, self and society.

While the relief of physical symptoms among people who are dying is an important and legitimate goal, it is worth considering why it has become a priority and what other aspects of caring may have been excluded or neglected as a result. While in many instances pharmacological interventions and other technical treatments are of value, all too often problems are only partially alleviated or are viewed as 'intractable', since they are not readily amenable to pharmacological intervention. Once labelled as 'intractable', symptoms may be overlooked as other avenues for assisting people experiencing the problem are not pursued. Moreover, those who are thought to have 'intractable' or difficult to manage symptoms, because they do not respond to symptom control strategies as expected or who have socially unacceptable problems, may themselves be identified as 'difficult'. Intractable symptoms challenge staff members in hospice and palliative care settings, since they confront widely held beliefs about what is a 'good' death and raise questions as to whether this is being provided (McNamara 2001).

Thought needs to be given to how one might start to work with some of the themes already outlined with people experiencing difficult symptoms at the end of their lives, and some principles for working with the various highlighted problems need to be established. However, it is also important to acknowledge that the mere act of identifying a particular symptom as 'difficult' could also mean that individuals risk being designated as outsiders, beyond help, and when this occurs it may challenge the very ability of staff to care.

# What are difficult symptoms?

The term 'difficult' suggests symptoms or problems in illness that are difficult to manage, that are perhaps difficult to bear or that cannot be controlled. What becomes defined as 'difficult' in practice is interesting, since there is often a discrepancy between symptoms that one might anticipate would be understood to be 'difficult' and those that in reality are labelled as such. The term could denote illness problems that cause an individual suffering, in which case all symptoms are potentially difficult, even those that may be possible to control in physical terms. However, many problems are defined as 'difficult' because health professionals or carers may feel that they do not know what to offer or that they have failed to provide 'relief'. Symptoms may be difficult to watch; for example, extreme breathlessness can be very distressing to observe, especially if it appears that there is little effective intervention available and can leave health professionals and family members feeling extremely helpless. Problems such as loss of appetite may not be perceived as a problem for the person concerned but can be deeply distressing to family members, since eating is life sustaining and not eating is a clear manifestation of the dying process. Other problems remain unrecognized as symptoms and therefore are left unresolved, perhaps because they have not been defined within a logical symptom 'category' in biomedical terms or because the person experiencing them finds it difficult to express the nature of the problem, yet these may cause considerable distress and suffering. Finally, there may be instances where individuals have difficult symptoms or problems resulting from their illness that challenge social taboos, or result in them exhibiting demanding or highly emotional behaviour, or that are simply beyond relief; in these situations, the result may be that the person can become defined as 'difficult'. This suggests that there is a close relationship between symptoms and a person's self and identity (as described in Chapter 1).

# Difficult symptoms: some exemplars

The many complex problems that arise for people while living with life-limiting illness and while dying cannot be defined using a neat list of symptoms or strategies for dealing with each one listed, although this is typically how many textbooks on palliative care present symptom management. I have argued elsewhere that symptoms are often a constellation of states of mind and body where problems such as pain, breathlessness, fatigue, anxiety or depression are often experienced simultaneously, each problem related to and often difficult to distinguish from all the others (Corner and Dunlop 1997). They are problems that take on significant meanings when someone is knowingly facing death and although they are a result of physiological decline due to illness, they are experienced as part of that person's own social and cultural world. The person's own reactions and ways of understanding and living with problems directly influence the particular constellation of problems and needs that arise, as does the response of others. I now describe some common problems of life-limiting illness. These are used as examples of the issues already identified and also to illustrate some themes around which nurses and other health professionals might approach offering support to people who experience them.

### *Fatigue*

Fatigue is acknowledged to be a very common problem in life-limiting illness and considerable research has been undertaken into fatigue associated with cancer and cancer treatment, although relatively little work has been undertaken in the context of palliative care. Richardson and Ream (1996) define fatigue as 'a total body feeling ranging from tiredness to exhaustion creating an unrelenting overall condition which interferes with an individual's ability to function to their normal capacity' (page 527). Armes (2004) has reviewed studies of the experience of fatigue among people with cancer highlighting multidimensional physical, emotional, social and cognitive effects as well as a profound effect on how one views one's self. While tiredness is a normal and everyday experience, fatigue experienced during chronic or life-limiting illness is of a different order and strategies such as resting or sleeping are often of little help. In these circumstances, fatigue can be extremely incapacitating and distressing and yet it is often difficult to convey the extent of fatigue as a problem to others because it is such a normal and everyday experience; perhaps this is also because the language available to people when describing their fatigue draws on the same language used to express the everyday and normal experience of tiredness.

In a study of 15 patients with advanced cancer suffering from fatigue who were being cared for in a palliative care unit, Krishnasamy (2000) reveals a complex condition that patients found difficult to put into words and a limited dialogue between patients and professional carers about the condition. Medical and nursing records made very little specific reference to the problem of fatigue even when the patients reported being severely disabled by it; the patients experienced it to be of an entirely different quality and order than day-to-day tiredness. There was also no reference to intervention or help being offered. The severity of fatigue reported was not related in any way to physiological indicators such as anaemia or hypercalcaemia, but it was described as having a profound emotional impact on those who were suffering from it. The study used several standardized measures of fatigue, anxiety and depression and of functional status. What was interesting was that scores recorded using the measures did not appear to reflect the depth of distress and difficulty that patients described during interviews. Somehow the research measures seemed to miss the point. Only three of the 15 patients' scores on the Hospital Anxiety and Depression Scale, for example, indicated evidence of 'clinical depression'; when asked about this, one of the three patients who was 'apparently' depressed rejected the suggestion that the score might indicate this because he felt that low mood was a normal response to his situation. The measurement of functional status was also rejected as a useful means of assessing the impact of fatigue, as the measure tended to assume that a problem is fixed, so that scores relating to severity or impairment can be recorded as a reflection of the problem at a given point in time. Patients described their fatigue as an unpredictable and patternless problem and thus could not be neatly 'captured' in this way. Fatigue for these patients was a diffuse, inexpressible experience with no obvious cause. Yet it was also the very means by which they understood that they were deteriorating; the symptom 'told' them that they were dying. For family members and friends, watching someone become so incapacitated by fatigue was deeply distressing.

The mismatch between the experience of fatigue and it 'falling below the line of detection' for physiological parameters or quality-of-life measures partly explains why it seemed not to be recognized or addressed by health professionals. Somehow it does not fit into standard assumptions about symptoms and problems in palliative care. This was expressed by a woman who participated in Krishnasamy's study: 'He [a doctor] has no idea . . . he doesn't listen to what it's like, really like to feel like this all the time, you see, they don't take it seriously, this is taking it seriously, talking about . . . it, and listening, really listening, to me tell you this is awful.'

This important study reveals a recurrent theme in relation to how health professionals might respond to and work with people experiencing difficult symptoms. That is, listening to and making it possible for people to talk about and express their experiences of difficult symptoms and of their illness is important. Acknowledging the problem is in itself experienced as supportive and helpful.

### Eating and emaciation

Loss of appetite is commonly reported in life-limiting illness and may be associated with weight loss. Equally, weight loss may occur as a consequence of loss of appetite or as a result of disease processes. Eating has social meanings that go much further than simply being a means of obtaining sustenance; it is associated with the most deeply felt human experiences and has many symbolic meanings (Lupton 1994). The significance of not being able to participate in the rituals and social processes surrounding food preparation and consumption are profound, yet have received little attention in palliative care.

A review of studies on the weight loss and loss of appetite of patients with advanced cancer and their carers identified only 50 studies covering such issues as measurement, incidence and prevalence, the experiences of patients and carers, and interventions (Poole and Froggatt 2002). Few of these studies attempted to assess the distress associated with anorexia or weight loss. A recent study of the prevalence of weight loss and eating difficulties among people under the care of two palliative care services in England suggests that problems with eating and weight loss are experienced by most people receiving palliative care of whom over half had concerns about their weight and eating irrespective of proximity to death. In fact it seems that concern may increase rather than diminish as death approaches (Hopkinson *et al.* 2006). Problems with eating were found to be rather different from fatigue, where the symptoms appear to be uniquely experienced by individuals, since this is also profoundly difficult for those closest to the person who is ill, especially if they are responsible for preparation of meals. Weight loss in contrast to eating difficulties is a highly visible manifestation of life-limiting illness. Tate and George (2001) explored the impact of weight loss among HIV-positive gay men. Weight loss that occurred as part of illness for these men had a dramatic effect on their lives and led them to avoid social activities because they were conscious of their emaciated appearance. Emaciation in this context was an undisguisable manifestation of their disease and their sexuality. Hopkinson *et al.*'s study (2005, 2006) of the experiences of people with eating difficulties and weight loss while dying of cancer suggests that health professionals rarely ask about problems with weight loss, feeling that it might cause anxiety. There were many examples of people withdrawing from social activities because of their difficulties especially in participating in family meals. The study reveals insights into how people with advanced cancer interpret weight loss and eating difficulties as signaling proximity to death, but also how they make choices about their eating in an attempt to manage their cancer and sometimes to hasten death.

What is revealed by the little work that has been undertaken into what is difficult about weight loss or eating difficulties is not simply that they are inevitable and often irreversible manifestations of the process of dying, but that they are inextricably bound up with deeply held cultural beliefs and practices, and therefore they disrupt intimate and more public social relationships. The 'managing' of the problems associated with difficulties in eating or with emaciation, then, may more fruitfully lie in working with the interplay between self and an individual's social world rather than more direct nutritional interventions.

### *Odour and exudate*

In her important observational study, Lawton (2000) observes that many symptoms requiring 'control' in hospice settings appear to share the distinctive feature that they are associated with or a cause of the body's surfaces rupturing or breaking down. Lawton describes people as having 'unbounded bodies', meaning the literal erosion of the body's physical boundaries. Here, symptom control was observed to be directed at a range of bodily ailments such as incontinence of urine and faeces, uncontrolled vomiting including faecal vomit, fungating tumours and weeping limbs from skin breaking down in lymphoedema. Symptom 'control' was aimed at controlling the body's boundaries to minimize the effects of 'unboundedness'.

Lawton presents the case of Annie, a woman dying of cervical cancer with a recto-vaginal fistula; faecal leakage from the fistula was completely unmanageable and resulted in a severe stench that filled the hospice. Annie's problem was the profound effect this had on her sense of self, and resulted in her desire to withdraw from family life and remain in the hospice rather than return home. Her situation deteriorated and her diarrhoea became so bad that Annie, feeling such a profound fear and loss of self-esteem, asked to be sedated. Her request was granted and she was sedated until she died two weeks later. Lawton describes the use of sedation in Annie's case as a kind of imposed and orchestrated social death by hospice staff – she was, following sedation, removed to a side room and visits from her family ceased soon after. Annie's symptoms (her severe diarrhoea and odour) were profoundly difficult – practically unmanageable but also socially difficult because of the profoundly unacceptable nature of her problem. 'Control' in these circumstances meant removing Annie's consciousness of her predicament.

It seemed to Lawton that symptom 'control' in cases such as that of Annie was about imposing control on what was becoming uncontrollable, those things in normal situations that would be considered to be socially unacceptable. For patients whose bodies were becoming 'unbounded', symptom control – when it was successful – provided the function of restoring the body's 'boundedness' and enabled a return to normal life. When it fails, the consequence for patients could be a profound loss of self. Lawton theorizes that hospices have become places where people with unbounded bodies and who are undergoing 'dirty' dying may be sequestered or shut away, and symptoms are only 'managed' in the sense that the hospice permits and provides for their removal from society.

Lawton's account is shocking not because palliative care staff struggle in dealing with these enormously challenging problems, but because symptom control as a form of social control and yet relief of profound suffering in Annie's case could not have been said to have been achieved. Annie's problems were 'unmanageable', but her case challenges us to find ways of supporting people more effectively in a similar predicament.

### Breathlessness

Breathlessness is a very common problem among patients needing palliative care. Since the physical causes of breathing difficulties are irreversible, biomedical intervention often at best only offers partial relief. Breathlessness can be disabling and terrifying at the same time, so that simply addressing it as a physical problem does not assist people to deal with the intense fear of dying that the symptom often engenders, or the practical problems of managing everyday activities when these trigger breathlessness. Several carefully researched accounts have been published of the experience of breathlessness in different illness contexts; see, for example, Williams (1993) and Skilbeck *et al.* (1998) in relation to chronic respiratory illnesses, and Roberts *et al.* (1993) and O'Driscoll *et al.* (1999) in relation to advanced lung cancer. These accounts reveal the complex interplay of mind and body in the experience of breathlessness in life-limiting illness.

Breathlessness is an example of a symptom where some attempts have been made to address the issues and difficulties outlined. In trying to respond to the particular circumstances of people with lung cancer who develop difficulties with breathing, together with colleagues I have developed and evaluated an approach to working with breathlessness, describing this as a parallel model of management (Corner 2001; see Figure 12.1). The model has been developed and formally evaluated over a series of studies. These indicate that patients appear to derive benefit from the approach when compared with patients not offered it (Corner *et al.* 1996; Bredin *et al.* 1999).

An integrative model of breathlessness was adopted, in which the emotional experience of breathlessness is considered inseparable from the sensory experience and from the pathophysical mechanisms. The approach to managing breathlessness is rehabilitative in its orientation even though patients may be at the very end of their lives. Care is directed at assisting individuals to manage the problem of breathlessness themselves, rather than to find ways of eliminating it or taking charge of it as a health professional.

The relationship with the person with breathlessness is considered a reciprocal one; breathlessness is viewed as a problem about which both patient and nurse have a mutual interest. Ways of managing breathlessness are therefore discovered together. The nurse is therapist, but the object of therapy (i.e. breathlessness) is the subject of mutual enquiry by both patient and nurse. The relationship is therefore one of equality. Care is focused on agreed goals to reduce the duration and frequency of episodes of breathlessness and to improve function.

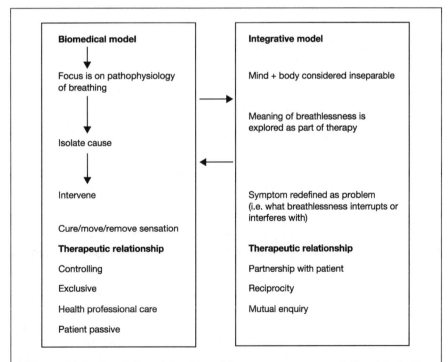

**Figure 12.1**   Parallel models of breathlessness management. Reprinted with permission from Corner (2001).

The importance of encouraging and listening to the patient's story of their illness and how breathlessness is experienced as part of this is recognized and is a central part of intervention. Intervention begins with assessment in the form of facilitating storytelling, or narration, about illness and breathlessness; this becomes an ongoing part of care. In developing this approach, we were influenced by Kleinman's (1988) notion of 'illness narratives' and the importance of working with such narratives with patients who have chronic health problems. Fundamental is the recognition that much of what is therapeutic in listening to patients' stories of their breathlessness is hearing and 'holding' the fear and distress associated with the symptom. In describing the approach as 'therapy', Bailey (1995) draws on Bion (1977) and Fabricius (1991) to explain the process of therapeutic work. The nurse as 'therapist' makes themself available, psychically, as a container for anxieties that are intolerable. This is a maternal function whereby, like a mother with an infant, intolerable stress is contained and processed and, in time, fed back in a more tolerable form. The primal link between breathing and life, ceasing to breathe and dying, is frequently central to fear of breathlessness and may itself evoke or exacerbate attacks of the symptom. Often patients fear they will die during the next attack of breathlessness, yet often have never voiced this fear. In exploring experiences of breathlessness, the aim is to assist patients to understand how and why such associations and fears arise and that these are in themselves not real. Hearing about sadness, anger or frustration may also be therapeutic.

Intervention employs a number of techniques from respiratory rehabilitation, including breathing retraining, energy conservation, life adaptation, and relaxation and distraction techniques. These are strategies that can be used by patients, often supported by close family members or carers, to manage episodes of breathlessness or situations that have become difficult or unmanageable because of breathlessness. The integrative model is realized in practice through a complex balancing of practical assistance and facilitation of adjustment to the limitations of breathlessness, with explicit and implicit recognition of the distress and fear that accompanies the symptom. What has been important to me over the years when working with people experiencing breathlessness is what I have learnt about talking with them and using their experiences within the supportive framework that I could offer as a nurse. 'Managing' symptoms using this approach is about helping people to manage the problem for themselves; this may also mean learning to live with the problem, and 'control' is about handing back control. As Bailey states:

> There is scope for developing nursing roles within a framework that makes it possible to be more accepting of patients' 'conscious and unconscious demands', to employ nursing as therapy. The order of nursing situations; the routine; the way in which 'symptoms' are dealt with at a high level of abstraction; the prevalence of models or algorithms that 'stand for' human entities without expressing them; the splitting of human experience into neatly bound categories, setting aside the

undisciplined whole; all of this stands in the way, provides a means to become detached, to leave painful things untouched. If nursing can change these things, the opportunities are unlimited.

(Bailey 1995: 189)

## Working with difficult symptoms: some ideas

It is not possible to draw up a set of definitive guiding principles for working with difficult symptoms; indeed, it would be unwise to try, especially as the intention of this chapter has been to reveal the impossibility of finding 'neat' solutions for the hugely challenging problems identified. However, it is possible to identify some themes that might at least offer a starting point for developing thinking and work with people in this area. The first and possibly most important is to adopt the kind of critical and reflective stance used here to develop understanding about why particular problems are 'difficult' and what might need to change so that care addresses the issues identified. Also, to consider whether 'symptom management' should continue to occupy the primary place it does currently.

The second is the potential importance of people's narratives in developing therapeutic approaches for difficult symptoms. The possibility of using a person's particular story as the starting point for intervention or support has been revisited throughout this chapter. Bury (2001) reminds us that it is no accident that there is an increasing interest in patients' narratives, since this reflects wider social trends, in particular the increasing emphasis on self in modern identity, the rise of chronic illness where everyday living with illness becomes paramount, and the various challenges to a single medical authority over illness. Bury also points out that illness narratives are themselves a constructed form of 'storytelling' in which the teller makes choices about the form in which the story is told and is influenced by the listener. As such, these are not 'truer' pictures of illness; they are, however, rich sources of insight into the problems of life-limiting illness that are as yet largely unexplored. Kleinman (1988), however, does promote the active facilitation of 'storytelling' as a therapeutic approach to the problems of chronic illness and this warrants further examination for its potential value in the context of palliative care.

Third, the idea of nurse or health professional as facilitator of the person's own journey in learning to live with, manage or find relief from the particular problems they are facing seems more fruitful than presenting oneself as the agent of 'control' for symptoms. Thus, the principle of fostering 'self-management' brings a fresh perspective that might usefully be explored further (Corner 2001). Self-management or 'self-care' does not necessarily mean remaining entirely self-maintaining or fully functional. It does, however, mean maintaining one's usual practices of self-care; those things that are important and unique to oneself in maintaining one's sense of self. Self-management also implies being given the means to master or deal with problems, rather than relinquishing them to others. This could be in relation to managing attacks of breathlessness for oneself or it could mean reaching some level of comfort with oneself while facing death. The important thing is that these are active strategies owned and used by people who are ill. Strategies to help people manage difficult symptoms for themselves are at the heart of the approach to managing breathlessness that I have outlined above, and have also been actively employed in the context of interventions for managing fatigue following cancer treatment (see Winingham and Barton-Burke 2000 and Armes *et al.* 2004). Assisting people to take control of the problems they are facing and manage activities around these using techniques such as breathing control and activity pacing can be powerful in enabling people to adjust to and manage the consequences of illness, even when it is very advanced.

Hopkinson *et al.*'s (2005) work also suggests that facilitating people to manage difficulties in relation to eating and weight loss through learning with them about their difficulties and working with individuals around the choices they may wish to make about eating, may also be very helpful. In the context of chronic illness, programmes designed to help people manage their own condition more effectively, as well as have greater input and control over interactions with health professionals, are advocated (Coulter and Ellins 2006; Foster in press). These approaches may readily translate into the context of palliative care and should be actively pursued. It is interesting that in Hopkinson *et al.*'s (2005) study people were actively managing their eating in very individual ways, either to optimize their body's ability to fight cancer or for some individuals to hasten death.

These very difficult subjects were not raised with health professionals caring for them but are subjects that can be shared openly as 'self-management', as even the timing of death seems, for some people, to be happening regardless of professional intervention. Opie (1997, 1998) offers a helpful critique of how the notion of 'empowerment' has been adopted within health care. She observes that too often teams inadvertently marginalize clients through pursuing professional discourses. Commonly team work by health professionals is oriented around a 'needs-related' approach which too easily leads to a focus on a technologized, physiologically oriented approach to an individual's '*mal*functioning' body divorced from social and psychological dimensions. She advocates an approach of '*thinking jointly*' with clients whereby space is made to think reflexively, foregrounding the way team members assess their performance, particularly in the way they represent clients in their discourse. Thinking jointly requires the full participation of the person, where their needs and desires are fully present and used to assess and critique team performance in relation to outcomes delivered from their input. The combination of focusing input around 'self-management' and 'thinking jointly' with people who have difficult symptoms could provide a fruitful approach.

Work is needed on the variety of problems faced by people with life-limiting illness to provide a more detailed understanding of the nature of what it is that is 'difficult' about the symptoms or problems experienced, and to examine the potential for the kind of approaches I have proposed for working with them.

# Conclusion

It may appear that more criticism than guidance has been offered here; this has not been the intention. However, I wanted to avoid glib or facile solutions to the most challenging aspects of working with people with life-limiting illness. I have chosen to explore why certain problems are difficult and why the way we construct our responses to them may also be part of the problem. I have tried to make reference to key texts that support the arguments and issues set out, so that these may be used as sources for further reading. I have also tried to adopt a critical and reflective stance, as I believe this is the route to learning about more supportive and ultimately more effective health care. As Nikolas Rose (1994) states: 'in revealing the complex contingencies that have made up the territory we inhabit and the horizons of our experience, in showing that things could have been different, such analyses encourage us to weigh up the costs as well as the benefits of the present we inhabit. They thus allow us to dream of a time in which our times could be different again' (page 71).

# References

Addington-Hall, J. and McCarthy, M. (1995) Dying from cancer: results of a national population-based investigation. *Palliative Medicine*, 9: 295–305.

Armes, J. (2004) The experience of cancer related fatigue. In: J. Armes, M. Krishnasamy and I. Higginson (eds) *Fatigue in Cancer*. Oxford: Oxford University Press.

Armstrong, D. (1995) The rise of surveillance medicine. *Sociology of Health and Illness*, 17(3): 393–404.

Bailey, C. (1995) Nursing as therapy in the management of breathlessness in lung cancer. *European Journal of Cancer Care*, 4: 184–90.

Benner, P. and Wrubel, J. (1989) *The Privacy of Care: Stress and Coping in Health and Illness*. Menlo Park, CA: Addison-Wesley.

Bion, W. (1977) Learning from experience. *Seven Servants: Four Works*. New York: Jason Aronson.

Bredin, M., Corner, J., Krishnasamy, M., Plant, H., Bailey, C. and A'Hern, R. (1999) Multicentre randomized controlled trial of nursing intervention for breathlessness in patients with lung cancer. *British Medical Journal*, 318: 901–4.

Bury, M. (2001) Illness narratives: fact or fiction? *Sociology of Health and Illness*, 23(3): 263–85.

Carper, B.A. (1978) Fundamental patterns of knowing in nursing. *Advances in Nursing Science*, 1: 13–23.

Clark, D. (1999) 'Total pain', disciplinary power and the body in the work of Cicely Saunders, 1958–1967. *Social Science and Medicine*, 49(6): 727–36.

Corner, J. (1996) Is there a research paradigm for palliative care? *Palliative Medicine*, 10: 201–8.

Corner, J. (2001) Management of breathlessness in lung cancer: new scientific evidence of developing multidisciplinary care. In: M. Muers, F. Macbeth, F.C. Wells and A. Miles (eds) *The Effective Management of Lung Cancer*. London: Aesculapius Medical Press.

Corner, J. and Dunlop, R. (1997) New approaches to care. In: D. Clark, J. Hockley and S. Ahmedzai (eds) *New Themes in Palliative Care*. Buckingham: Open University Press.

Corner, J., Plant, H., A'Hern, R. and Bailey, C. (1996) Non-pharmacological intervention for breathlessness in lung cancer. *Palliative Medicine*, 13: 375–84.

Coulter, A. and Ellins, J. (2006) *Patient focused interventions: a review of the evidence*. London: The Health Foundation.

Cribb, A. (2001) Knowledge and caring: a philosophical and personal perspective. In: J. Corner and C. Bailey (eds) *Cancer Nursing: Care in Context*. Oxford: Blackwell Science.

Fabricius, J. (1991) Running on the spot or can nursing really change. *Psychoanalytic Psychotherapy*, 5: 97–108.

Field, D. (1994) Palliative medicine and the medicalization of death. *European Journal of Cancer Care*, 3: 58–62.

Foster C (in press) Self management and self help. In: J. Corner and C. Bailey (eds) *Cancer Nursing: Care in Context* (2nd edn). Oxford: Blackwell Scientific.

Foucault, M. ([1973] 1986) *The Birth of the Clinic*. London: Routledge.

Higginson, I. and McCarthy, M. (1989) Measuring symptoms in terminal cancer: are pain and breathlessness controlled? *Journal of the Royal Society of Medicine*, 82: 264–7.

Hinton, J. (1994) Can home care maintain an acceptable quality of life for patients with terminal cancer and their relatives? *Palliative Medicine*, 8: 183–96.

Hopkinson, J., Wright, D. and Corner, J. (2005) Exploring of weight loss in people with advanced cancer. *Journal of Advanced Nursing*, 54(3): 304–12.

Hopkinson, J., Wright, D.N.M., McDonald, J.W. and Corner, J.L. (2006) *Journal of Pain and Symptom Management*, 32(4): 322–31.

Illich, I. ([1976] 1990) *Limits to Medicine, Medical Nemesis: The Expropriation of Health*. London: Penguin.

Johns, C. (1995) Framing learning through reflection within Carper's fundamental ways of knowing nursing. *Journal of Advanced Nursing*, 22: 226–34.

Kleinman, A. (1988) *The Illness Narratives: Suffering, Healing and the Human Condition*. New York: Basic Books.

Krishnasamy, M. (2000) Fatigue in advanced cancer: meaning before measurement. *International Journal of Nursing Studies*, 5: 401–14.

Lawton, J. (2000) *The Dying Process: Patients' Experiences of Palliative Care*. London: Routledge.

Lupton, D. (1994) Food, memory and meaning: the symbolic and social nature of food events. *Sociological Review*, 42: 664–85.

Lupton, D. (1997) *Medicine as Culture: Illness, Disease and the Body in Western Societies*. London: Sage.

Lyon, M.L. and Barbalet, J.M. (1994) Society's body: emotion and the 'somatization' of social theory. In: T.J. Czordas (ed.) *Embodiment and Experience*. Cambridge: Cambridge University Press.

McNamara, B. (2001) *Fragile Lives: Death, Dying and Care*. Buckingham: Open University Press.

Nolan, M. and Lundh, U. (1998) Ways of knowing in nursing and health care practice. In: P. Crookes and C. Davies (eds) *Research into Practice*. Edinburgh: Ballière Tindall.

O'Driscoll, M., Corner, J. and Bailey, C. (1999) The experience of breathlessness in lung cancer. *European Journal of Cancer Care*, 8: 37–43.

Opie, A. (1997) Thinking teams thinking clients: issues of discourse and representation in the work of health care teams. *Sociology of Health and Illness*, 19(3): 259–80.

Opie, A. (1998) 'Nobody's asked for my view': users empowerment by multidisciplinary teams. *Qualitative Health Research*. 8(2): 188–206.

Poole, K. and Froggatt, K. (2002) Loss of weight and loss of appetite in advanced cancer: a problem for the patient, the carer, or the health professional. *Palliative Medicine*, 16: 499–506.

Richardson, A. and Ream, E. (1996) Fatigue: a concept analysis. *International Journal of Nursing Studies*, 33(5): 519–25.

Robbins, M. (1998) *Evaluating Palliative Care*. Oxford: Oxford Medical Publications.

Roberts, D.K., Thorne, S.E. and Pearson, C. (1993) The experience of dyspnoea in late stage cancer. *Cancer Nursing*, 16: 234–6.

Rose, N. (1994) Medicine, history and the present. In: C. Jones and R. Porter (eds) *Reassessing Foucault: Power, Medicine and the Body*. London: Routledge.

Skilbeck, J., Mott, L., Page, H., Smith, D., Hjelmeland-Ahmedzai, S. and Clark, D. (1998) Palliative care in chronic obstructive airways disease: a needs assessment. *Palliative Medicine*, 12: 245–54.

Tate, H. and George, R. (2001) The effect of weight loss on body image in HIV-positive gay men. *AIDS Care*, 13: 163–9.

Taussig, M.T. (1980) Reification and the consciousness of the patient. *Social Science and Medicine*, 14: 3–13.

Williams, S. (1993) *Chronic Respiratory Illness*. London: Routledge.

Williams, S. (1996) The vicissitudes of embodiment across the chronic illness trajectory. *Body and Society*, 2(2): 23–47.

Williams, S. and Bendelow, G. (1998) In search of the 'missing body': pain suffering and the (post) modern condition. In: G. Scrambler and P. Higgs (eds) *Modernity, Medicine and Health*. London: Routledge.

Winningham, M.L. and Barton-Burke, M. (2000) *Fatigue in Cancer: A Multidimensional Approach*. Sudbury, MA: Jones & Bartlett Publishers.

# 13

# Pain

Theories, evaluation and management

*Silvia Paz and Jane Seymour*

---

**Key points**

- Pain is a very complex human experience.
- Over the past century, the understanding of pain has moved from con-ceptualizing a simple, specific pain pathway in the nervous system to the complexity of the multidimensional pain phenomenon.
- A classification of pain types is required to facilitate its management and study.
- Nurses have a crucial role in assessing, measuring and addressing pain experienced by patients.
- Today, the relief of cancer and chronic pain comprises pharmacological and non-pharmacological strategies that are needed at all levels in the health system.

---

It is only during the past 50 years that pain has been recognized as a condi-tion that requires specialized treatment and dedicated research. Before the availability of analgesics and anesthetics, pain was regarded as a natural and an expected part of life, and was explained primarily in terms of a religious belief system within which medicine had little part to play. During the nineteenth century, with the emergence of 'modern' medical and scientific ideas, advances in anatomy, physiology, chemistry and pharmacy heralded the discovery of analgesics and anaesthetics, together with techniques for their application. As a result, medical and research interest in the subject was generated, and by the beginning of the twentieth century physicians engaged not only in controlling pain but also in finding a scientific explanation for its occurrence. Until the 1960s, pain was considered by most clinicians as an inevitable sensory and physiological response to tissue damage: there was little recognition or understanding of the effects on pain perception of individual expectations, anxiety, past experience or genetic differences. Moreover, there was no distinction made between 'acute' and 'chronic' pain states. It is only in more recent years that the physiological, psychological and socio-cultural factors that contribute to the perception of pain have begun to be understood, and the necessary differentiation made in treatments of acute and chronic pain. This chapter aims to: provide a framework for understanding theories of pain and pain mechanisms, and how these have developed over time; describe basic principles for the management of chronic and cancer pain; and examine the role of the nurse in the assessment and measurement of pain, and in the administration of analgesics.

# What does 'pain' mean: contemporary definitions

Pain is difficult to define because of the complexity of its anatomical and physiological foundations, the individuality of its experience, and its social and cultural meanings. Pain has had different significances and meanings throughout the ages and in various societies existing at the same time. In spite of this, definitions have been developed that are widely accepted as both clinically useful and phenomenologically valid. Thus, the International Association for the Study of Pain (IASP) defines pain as 'an unpleasant sensory and emotional experience associated with actual or potential tissue damage, or described in terms of such damage' (Mersky and Bogduk 1994). In other widely accepted definitions pain is described as being 'whatever the experiencing person says it is, existing whenever he says it does' (McCaffery 1968: 95, cited in Fink and Gates 2001) or as '. . . what the patient says hurts' (Twycross and Wilcock 2002: 17). These three 'classic' definitions present pain as:

- being an individual experience
- comprising emotional and sensorial components
- having temporal characteristics
- having undefined boundaries.

In the next section, we summarize how pain has been understood across the course of the past century and we outline current concepts of acute, chronic and cancer pain. We present recognized methods for pain assessment and pharmacological and non-pharmacological approaches for adequate pain control emphasizing the role of the nurse in chronic and cancer pain relief.

# Theories of pain and pain mechanisms

For centuries, medical physicians and scientists have been engaged in establishing a theoretical explanation for questions about how the human body perceives pain, why the experience of pain is different from other sensations, and why individuals perceive pain differently in objectively similar conditions. Here we outline the following theories of pain: *specificity theory; patterning theory; gate control theory*; and the *neuromatrix theory*.

### Specificity theory

During the first half of the twentieth century, the most enduring theory of pain was the *specificity theory of pain* (Melzack and Wall 1996). This proposes that a specific 'pain pathway' in the spinal cord carries messages from pain receptors in the skin to a pain centre in the brain, and pain is evidenced by the withdrawal of the relevant body part from the noxious stimulus as a result of the action of nerves. It emphasized the mechanistic nature of pain and implied a 'linear causality', with no modulating factors acting between the stimulus, the receptor and the response (Horn and Munafo 1997: 1–2).

The greatest weakness of the specificity theory of pain is its assumption that there is a rigid and direct relationship between the physical stimulus and a sensation felt by the individual. Clinical evidence of phantom limb pain, neuralgias and causalgias in which any type of non-noxious stimuli can trigger excruciating pain constitute a strong challenge to the idea of a fixed, direct-line nervous system and thus to the simplicity of the specificity theory of pain (Melzack and Wall 1982: 156).

### Patterning theory

In an early critique of specificity theory, Goldscheider hypothesized in 1894 that pain was due to excessive peripheral stimulation that produces a pattern of nerve impulses interpreted centrally as pain (Horn and Munafo 1997: 5). He formulated the theory of pattern generation of pain, popularly known as the 'patterning theory of pain'. The important contribution made by this theory to the understanding of pain was the idea of the summation phenomenon in the spinal cord implying that '*something else*' needs to happen at the transmission level before the pain sensation would be perceived.

### An emergent critique of specificity and pattern theories: The impact of the First and Second World Wars

It could be said that the advances made on the understanding of pain during the first half of the twentieth century, resulted from: (1) the work undertaken by Rene Leriche during the First World War that introduced the concept of visceral pain and its components, and (2) the invaluable observations made in battlefields by Henry Beecher during the Second World War that highlighted that pain was a multidimensional and individual experience.

In the post-war periods the idea of a 'specific pain pathway' led to the development of numerous surgical techniques to control pain. It was believed that by sectioning the pain pathway the perception of pain would be avoided (Rey 1995: 307). The French surgeon, Rene Leriche was, arguably, a pioneer of the 'surgery of pain'. His work covered two types of surgical operations: one performed on the sensibility tracts of the central nervous system; and the other performed on the sympathetic nervous system. The latter was the area in which Leriche made his most significant contribution (Rey 1995). By performing different interventions to the sympathetic nervous system, he was able to define the two elements of 'visceral pain': 'true' and 'referred' pain; concepts hotly debated at the time (Rey 1995: 312–15).

Later, an anaesthetist, Henry Beecher, had a considerable influence based on his observations of wounded soldiers during the Second World War, when he reported that many rarely complained of pain (Beecher 1946, cited in Meldrum 1998). Beecher hypothesized that this was because of a culture of stoicism, relief among the men that they survived, or their expectation that they would now be able to return home. From these observations and his subsequent clinical work, Beecher theorized that the perception of pain was largely dependent upon a 'reaction component' which depended on variables such as age, gender, ethnicity, experience, context, culture and distraction.

Another American anaesthetist, John Bonica, built on Beecher's work, putting forward the radical view that pain was a *composite* of neurophysiologic and psychological factors that should be 'apprehended clinically as a whole' (Baszanger 1998: 27). Most notably, Bonica argued that the mental and physical effects of pain needed to be understood as catalysts of each other. This overturned a position in which the approach to pain was confined to diagnosis and cause, and in which any emotional or 'subjective' element was excluded (Baszanger 1998: 29).

In the decades after the Second World War, the study of pain gained momentum primarily for two reasons. First, the search for strong and non-addictive analgesics as alternatives to morphine and aspirin led to the study of pain under laboratory controlled conditions with the aim of detecting and measuring changes in pain perception in order to document the efficacy of the analgesics (Meldrum 1998). Until then, morphine and aspirin were the only painkillers widely used and easily accessible. While morphine and other opium derivatives had many medical uses, aspirin was the first drug purely marketed as an analgesic. Second, published observations made by physicians of their clinical practice began to provide a richer understanding of pain as a multidimensional and individual experience.

### The emergence of 'gate control' theory

By the 1960s, pain was defined by unconnected concepts of patterning, possible modulation in the dorsal horn of the spinal cord, ascending pain pathways from the periphery to the brain, and the multidimensional qualities of the *pain experience*. The spinal cord was conceived as a passive transmission station, and the brain, as a final receptive station.

In 1965, Ronald Melzack and Patrick Wall presented a new theory: the 'gate control theory of pain' (Melzack and Wall 1965), which effectively provided a comprehensive model that was, for the first time, able to account for both neurophysiological and psychological factors. They suggested that input signals from primary sensory neurons were actively modulated in the spinal cord by a neural mechanism, the 'gate'. The balance between peripheral (ascending and facilitatory) and central (descending and inhibitory) inputs would open or close the 'gate'. As a result, both the spinal cord and the brain were actively involved in the pain process. The spinal cord was presented as a controlling centre where activations, inhibitions and modulation occurred, and the brain as an active system that filters, selects and also modulates sensory inputs. The gate control theory allows us to explain: (a) the cultural, affective and emotive dimensions of pain that make severely wounded patients feel less pain than expected (Beecher 1946); (b) situations of pain without evident tissue damage, such as migraine or chronic low back pain.

After the publication of the gate control theory, an explosion in research occurred on the physiology and pharmacology of the dorsal horn of the spinal cord and the descending control systems from the brain. Psychological factors started to be seen as an integral part of the pain process and new approaches for pain control were opened, such as the Transcutaneous Electrical Nerve Stimulation (TENS) technique that later became an important modality for the treatment of chronic and acute pain (Tulder *et al.* 2002).

### The neuromatrix theory

In 1999, Ronald Melzack proposed a model to explain how the human body perceives pain in relation to itself and the outside world (Melzack 1999). He called his model *the neuromatrix* theory of pain. He proposed that the whole body is represented in a neural network in the brain, the *neuromatrix*. Melzack suggested that its structure is determined genetically and modified by experience over time. The perception of pain by the neuromatrix in the brain results from the summary of sensory inputs that arrive from the site of injury, current levels of endocrine products of stress release in response to the pain, such as cortisol, adrenaline and glucose, and emotive inputs derived from past individual experiences (Dickenson 2002).

### Neuroplasticity

Today, it is acknowledged that when tissue is damaged many different chemical inflammatory messengers form locally an 'inflammatory soup' and sensitize a network of neural structures (Dickenson 2002). These peripheral changes then alter the activity in central systems and drive central compensations and adaptations, so that the mechanisms involved in the pain are likely to be multiple and located at a number of sites. As a result of these observations, potential new targets for analgesic therapy are currently being researched and a rationale on which to base the use of opioids and other analgesics has emerged. On the other hand, it has also been suggested that sensory neurons share the ability to use information previously acquired to respond to current demands following a neuronal 'learning' process. This capacity of sensory neurons to change the pattern of transmission according to previous experience and the surrounding environment is recognized as the plasticity of the nervous system or *neuroplasticity* (Dickenson 1995).

### Pain and the brain: contemporary understandings

During recent decades, a major challenge in the study of pain mechanisms has been to understand how the brain works (Melzack and Wall 1996: 154). The development of relatively non-invasive imaging techniques has made possible the study of functional brain activity during the process of pain. There are three relevant imaging techniques currently available for the study of pain:

- Single Photon Emission Computed Tomography (SPECT)
- Positron Emission Tomography (PET)
- Functional Magnetic Resonance Imaging (fMRI).

These imaging techniques have been applied to the problem of localizing brain areas associated with a variety of experimental and clinical pain conditions (Berman 1995) They can also be used in human beings to study the distribution of brain receptors.

### Pain and the genes: current research approaches

Pain and palliative care research at the beginning of the twenty-first century emphasizes the importance of 'diversity' as a key determinant of reactions and responses to pain therapies and models of pain care. With the emergence of disciplines such as pharmacogenetics and pharmacogenomics in health research, looking into the way in which each individual responds to analgesic therapies has gained especial attention in recent years (Winslow *et al.* 2007). It is argued that much can be gained in terms of reducing side effects and improving patients' responses to analgesics if the molecular and genetic mechanisms underlying pain are better understood. In this sense, areas of particular research interest are 1) opioid and non-opioid pain related genes polymorphisms; 2) joint effects of pain related genes in the response to morphine; 3) the influence of ethnicity and gender in differences in pain perceptions, and 4) metabolic enzymes' and transporters' genes polymorphisms. The main expected outcome of these research endeavours is to identify therapeutically meaningful targets.

We now provide a brief summary of the variety of understandings of pain, and their evolution (see Box 13.1)

A variety of key concepts have been used to describe the mechanisms of pain (see Box 13.2). Knowledge about these concepts help to understand the information presented in the following sections of this chapter.

**Box 13.1**    Summary of pain understandings

| | |
|---|---|
| Before the nineteenth century | <ul><li>People expected to suffer pain as a life natural event. It had magical and religious connotations.</li><li>Raw opium was the only medicine available with analgesic properties, although alcohol was also used to dull the senses. Principles of anaesthesia were unknown.</li></ul> |
| Nineteenth century | <ul><li>Morphine was first isolated from opium in 1803 and subsequently other opioids were found.</li><li>Anaesthetic techniques started to be developed and the principles for anaesthesia became understood.</li><li>The study of pain gained more interest alongside developments in surgical procedures.</li><li>Acetylsalicylic acid (aspirin) was first discovered in 1873 and was the first medicine marketed as a painkiller or analgesic.</li><li>The *specificity theory* of pain was formulated following a mechanistic understanding of the pain process rigid, unidirectional and structured. Pain receptor (skin) → pain pathway (spinal cord) → pain centre (brain).</li></ul> |
| First half of the twentieth century | <ul><li>The specificity theory of pain further developed and dominated understandings of pain mechanisms.</li><li>Surgical techniques to 'cut' the 'pain pathway' were developed and used to control severe chronic pain.</li><li>Patients who suffered from pain of uncertain origin with no evidence of tissue damage (e.g. migraine, low back pain) were sent to psychiatrists as it was not possible to explain their painful conditions with the knowledge at the time.</li><li>Visceral pain was described and recognized as a possible variety of pain.</li><li>The need for further alternative analgesics led the study of pain in experimental and clinical conditions.</li><li>Earliest observations and documentations of the emotive, affective and cultural aspects of pain gained recognition.</li></ul> |
| Second half of the twentieth century | <ul><li>Cancer and chronic pain started to gain medical recognition as a relevant public health problem.</li><li>In 1960, the *gate control theory* of pain incorporated the physical and psychological components of pain, changing the way in which the pain process was understood and researched.</li></ul> |

- The hospice movement and the development of pain clinics emphasized the need for a multiprofessional approach to pain relief.
- Pain became to be seen as a multidimensional phenomenon with its physical, social, psychological, emotional and cultural components.
- A significant development in analgesic interventions and methods for the administration of painkillers developed.
- Imaging techniques helped to study the brain behaviour in human beings during painful events.

Twenty-first century
- Pain research moves on towards understanding molecular mechanisms and pain genes' interactions that generate and modulate pain phenomenon.
- The study of polymorphisms in genes coding for the mu-opioid receptor and the catechol-*O*-methyl transferase, for instance, becomes relevant to the pharmacogenetics and pharmacogenomics of cancer and chronic pain.
- Pain and palliative care developments are studied at a 'global level'. Comparative research between countries and regions becomes the paradigm to understand diversity and its impact worldwide.
- The 'hospice movement' and palliative care moves beyond 'cancer care' and 'care of the dying' to include non-malignant conditions and older people close to the end of their lives.

**Box 13.2**   Pain concepts

**Receptor** is a 3-D structure localized in the cell membrane with special architectural features that enables it to bind different molecules, such as drugs, to form a 'drug-receptor' complex. By binding their specific receptors, drugs and other molecular mediators have their effect in the body.

**Nociceptor** is a receptor preferentially sensitive to a noxious stimulus or to a stimulus which would become noxious if prolonged.

**Noxious stimulus** is one which is damaging to normal tissues.

**Nociception** is the physiological process necessary for pain to occur. It is a sensory process that involves three steps:

a)   nociceptor activation in the periphery (transduction)
b)   relay of the information from the periphery to the central nervous system (transmission)

c)   neural activity that leads to control of the pain transmission pathway (modulation).

**Pain perception** is the awareness of pain frequently initiated by a noxious stimulus, such as an injury or a disease, or by lesions in the peripheral or central nervous system, such as diabetic neuropathy, spinal cord compression and stroke. Pain is a perceptual phenomenon that involves higher central nervous system mechanisms.

**Pain behaviours** are the things somebody does or does not do that can be described as a result of the presence of pain and the menace of tissue damage or disease that it represents. Examples of pain behaviours are grimacing, anger, lying down, stop working, crying, recourse to medical advice.

# Different types of pain: classifications

Two main types of pain can be identified according to the reaction they generate:

- functional or physiological pain
- clinical pain.

The *functional or physiological* pain has a primary protective role: it warns us of imminent or actual tissue damage and elicits coordinated reflex and behavioural responses to keep such damage to a minimum. It does not require medical intervention. Examples of physiological pain are present in everyday life, such as the way we quickly remove our hand when touching a hot plate. By contrast, *clinical pain* comprises persistent pain syndromes that offer no biological advantage and cause suffering and distress. Types of clinical pain are summarized in Box 13.3. People presenting with any type of clinical pain may seek medical advice and frequently need regular assessment and supervision.

As Box 13.3 indicates, clinical pain can be described in a temporal sense as either *transient, acute* or *chronic*. It can also be described in terms of the type of tissue damage with which they are associated. *Inflammatory pain* is associated with visceral or somatic tissue damage or inflammation. *Neuropathic pain* results from damage to the peripheral or central nervous systems.

### Transient pain

This can appear in the absence of any tissue damage and is elicited by the activation of sensitive receptors in the skin or other tissues. It has been suggested that this type of pain probably develops *to protect people from physical damage* due to an adverse surrounding or due to over stress of the

| | Inflammatory | | Neuropathic |
|---|---|---|---|
| | *Visceral* | *Somatic* | *Neuropathic* |
| **Transient** | Painful endoscopy | Intramuscular injection | Shooting pain elicited by knocking the elbow |
| **Acute** | Inflamed appendix | Broken bone | Trigeminal neuralgia |
| **Chronic** | Metastatic enlargement of the liver | Low back pain | Diabetic neuropathy |

**Box 13.3**    Clinical pain

body tissues (Loeser and Melzack 2001). In the clinical setting, transient pain is seen in procedural manoeuvres, such as during an endoscopy or an intramuscular injection.

### Acute pain

This has been defined as 'the normal, predicted physiological response to an adverse chemical, thermal or mechanical stimulus associated with surgery, trauma and acute illness' (Federation of State Medical Boards of the United States 1998). It typically results from tissue injury or inflammation, and it can be considered *to have a biologically reparative function*. Because tissue damage has already occurred and cannot be prevented, the presence of acute pain enables healing and repairs to occur undisturbed, making the injured or inflamed area and surrounding tissue hypersensitive to all stimuli so that contact with any external stimulus is avoided. Usually, the local injury does not overwhelm the body's reparative mechanisms and 'healing' occurs without medical intervention (Carr and Goudas 2001). However, medical interventions may be useful in preventing or reducing pain and speeding up the healing process by shortening the duration of the injury (Loeser and Melzack 2001). Because clinical observations have indicated that the biological and psychological foundation for chronic pain is in place within hours of an acute injury, early control of acute pain can shape its subsequent evolution, prevent it from transforming to persistent and long-term pain and, for many patients, minimization of pain can improve clinical outcomes (Carr 1998). Patients' attitudes, personalities and previous experiences will strongly influence their immediate reaction to acute pain, a typical example of which is post-operative pain.

### Chronic pain

Chronic pain persists long after the tissue damage that initially triggered its onset has resolved, and in some people, chronic pain presents without any identified ongoing tissue damage or antecedent injury, such as chronic low back pain or migraine (Bonica 1990, cited by Ashburn and Staats 2001). The inability of the body to restore its physiological functions to normal homoeostatic levels distinguishes acute from chronic pain (Niv and Devor 1998). In some cases chronic pain exists because the injury exceeds the body's capability for healing. This occurs in cases of extensive trauma and subsequent scarring, loss of a body part, or when the nervous system is affected by the injury itself (Loeser and Melzack 2001). For other chronic pain syndromes, such as chronic low back pain, headache, neuropathic pain and phantom limb pain, the available knowledge about their underlying pathophysiology is limited. These chronic pain syndromes are usually diagnosed and treated on the basis of clinical criteria alone without existing definitive scientific evidence or confirmatory studies (Ashburn and Staats 2001). The traditional classification, based on the duration of pain, that describes acute pain as the pain of recent onset and short duration and chronic pain as persistent after an injury has healed, is increasingly questionable (Carr and Goudas 2001). A 1994 report of the International Association for the Study of Pain Task Force on Taxonomy (Merskey and Bogduk 1994) has acknowledged that acute pain associated with new tissue injury might last for less than one month, but at times for longer than six months. However, since the healing process usually takes a few days or a few weeks, pain that persists for several months or years tends not to be classified as acute. Chronic pain tends to have a more profound impact on a patient's general state than acute pain: it often affects the patient's mood, personality and social relationships. People with chronic pain usually experience concomitant depression, sleep disturbance, fatigue and decreased overall physical and mental functioning (Ashburn and Staats 2001).

### Approaches to managing chronic pain

In the 1950s, John Bonica developed an interdisciplinary approach designed to integrate the efforts of health care providers from several disciplines, each of whom specializes in different features of the pain experience (Baszanger 1998). Bonica's legacy has been the concept of the *pain clinic*: a model for managing chronic pain that has been adopted across the world. Bonica's work in the USA was mirrored in many respects by the pioneering work on cancer pain of Cicely Saunders in the UK during the 1960s (Clark 1999).

It is now widely understood that the management of chronic pain should be an interdisciplinary endeavour, with a core team typically comprising a pain management physician, a psychologist, a nurse specialist, a physical therapist and a pharmacist. The team tailors the care plan according to the individual needs of the patient, with a focus on achieving measurable treatment goals in reasonable periods of time established with the patient. Cognitive and behavioural therapies are used in the management of chronic pain to alter the effect of the pain on the individual's life (see Box 13.4).

**Box 13.4** Roles of members of an interdisciplinary pain management team (adapted from Ashburn and Staats 2001: 4)

| Physician | Nurse | Psychologist | Physical and occupational therapist | Pharmacist |
|---|---|---|---|---|
| Regular assessment and neurological and musculoeskeletal examination<br><br>Review of preview interventions<br><br>New therapy considerations<br><br>Specialist referral<br><br>Education | Coordination of care<br><br>Education to medical and non-medical staff<br><br>Regular assessment of patient's and relatives' needs<br><br>Continuous support<br><br>Consideration and provision of non-pharmacological interventions | Comprehensive psychological support<br><br>Regular psychological assessment<br><br>Coping skills reinforcement<br><br>Cognitive behaviour therapies<br><br>Education on the use of self-management techniques | Regular assessment of physical endurance<br><br>Regular assessment of the work site and home<br><br>Management of physical rehabilitation techniques | Regular review of past and current pharmacological interventions<br><br>Education with regard to adequate use of pharmacological interventions<br><br>Regular update on available alternative pharmacological interventions |

### Nociceptive and neuropathic pain

The term nociceptive is applied to pains that are presumed to be maintained by continual tissue injury (Twycross and Wilcock 2002). *Nociceptive pain* is called *somatic* when it is produced by damage of structural tissues, such as skin, bone, muscle or joint (Woolf 1995). Pain of somatic origin is usually focal and well localized, dull or stabbing. It usually responds well to conventional analgesics, such as non-steroidal anti-inflammatory and opioid drugs. Nociceptive pain is known as *visceral pain* when it is produced by an injury of internal organs, such as lung, heart, gut. *Visceral pain* has five important clinical characteristics (Cervero and Laird 2001):

- It is not evoked from all viscera (organs such as liver, kidney, most solid viscera, and lung parenchyma, are not sensitive to pain). Pain in the area of these organs is usually due to inflammation, distention or irritation of the surrounding tissues (e.g. pain due to distention of the liver capsule due to hepatic malignant infiltration).
- It is not always linked to visceral injury (cutting the intestine causes no pain, whereas stretching the bladder is painful).
- It is diffuse and poorly localized.
- It is referred to other locations.
- It is accompanied with motor and autonomic reflexes, such as nausea,

vomiting, and local muscle tension such as the lower back muscle tension that occurs in renal colic.

There are two distinct types of localization of visceral pain: deep, 'true' visceral pain, and superficial, 'referred' visceral pain. The pain that is perceived as being deep within the body is often called 'true' visceral pain. It is usually perceived as arising in the midline, and perceived as anterior or posterior. 'True' visceral pain is usually extensive rather than focal and with diffuse boundaries. It is frequently associated with a sense of nausea and being ill. Autonomic and motor reflexes are often extreme and prolonged. 'Referred' visceral pain appears in distant structures from the affected organ. The area of referral is often superficial and segmental, that is to muscle, skin or both, innervated by the same spinal nerves as the affected viscus. The site of referral may additionally show hyperalgesia and it might be tender when touching. 'True' and 'referred' visceral pain may be present at the same or different times (Cervero and Laird 2001).

Tissue damage provokes a local inflammatory response that alters the sensitivity of sensory fibres in the periphery. The inflammatory response is characterized by the local release of many different chemical messengers, such as growth factors; histamine, bradykinin, cytokines, substance 'P', which are responsible for the sensitization of the peripheral sensory fibres. They tend to act synergistically together rather than individually, by producing a 'soup' or 'cocktail', usually called the 'inflammatory soup' (Loeser and Melzack 2001). Non-steroid anti-inflammatory drugs, such as aspirin and ibuprofen, act by modifying this inflammatory soup. For this reason, they are of particular benefit for pain in which inflammation is a major component, such as bone metastasis and tissue infiltration (Twycross and Wilcock 2002). Figure 13.1 depicts this process.

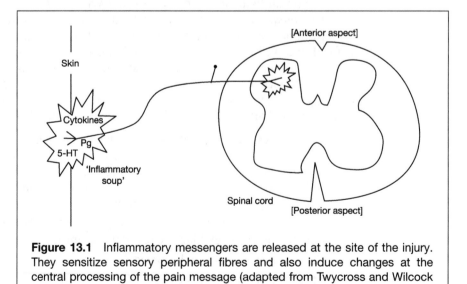

**Figure 13.1** Inflammatory messengers are released at the site of the injury. They sensitize sensory peripheral fibres and also induce changes at the central processing of the pain message (adapted from Twycross and Wilcock 2002: 33).

The term *neuropathic pain* is used when the pain results from damage to the nervous system, such as peripheral nerve, the dorsal root ganglion or dorsal root, or the central nervous system (Woolf and Mannion 2001). It is sustained by an aberrant somatosensory processing in either the peripheral or the central nervous system. In cancer patients, for instance, neuropathic pain appears when a peripheral nerve is trapped by the growth of the tumour. Other more complex syndromes are also labelled as neuropathic pain, namely central pain; neuropathies, either mononeuropathies or polyneuropathies; and complex regional pain syndromes (see Box 13.5).

Many patients with neuropathic pain exhibit persistent or paroxysmal pain that is independent of a stimulus (Woolf and Mannion 2001). This pain appears without any identified stimulus and it can be shooting, stabbing or burning. It may depend on activity in the sympathetic nervous system. Stimulus-evoked pain is a common component of peripheral nerve injury and has two key features: hyperalgesia and allodynia. Although neuropathic pain can respond well to conventional analgesics, in many patients it does not respond to non-steroidal anti-inflammatory drugs and it is resistant or insensible to opioid drugs. Patients are usually treated with combinations of drugs that may include opioid analgesics, such as morphine; non-steroids anti-inflammatory drugs, such as diclofenac; tricyclic antidepressants, such as amitriptiline; serotonin uptake inhibitors, such as sertraline; and anti-convulsants, such as carbamazepine or gabapentin. Local anaesthetic blocks targeted at trigger points, peripheral nerves, plexi, dorsal roots, and the sympathetic nervous system have useful but short-lived effects. Chronic epidural administration of drugs such as clonidine, steroids, opioids or midazolam has also been used with variable results (Woolf and Mannion 2001). Overall, the diagnosis of neuropathic pain indicates the need for a combination of therapies and the aim of the treatment is often to help the patient to cope by means of psychological, complementary or occupational therapies, rather to eliminate the pain completely (see Figure 13.2).

---

**Box 13.5**  Neuropathic pain syndromes associated with an injury of a nervous system structure

- *Central pain* is the pain initiated or caused by a primary lesion or dysfunction in the central nervous system, such as post stroke pain and spinal cord compression pain.
- *Neuropathies* represent a disturbance of function or pathological change in a peripheral nerve:

    – in one nerve, *mononeuropathy*;
    – if diffuse and bilateral affecting several nerves, *polyneuropathy*.

- *Complex regional pain syndromes*, such as

    – *causalgia* is a syndrome of sustained burning pain and allodynia after a traumatic nerve lesion, often combined with vasomotor and sudomotor dysfunction and later trophic changes.

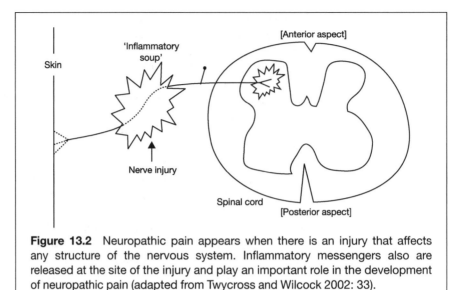

**Figure 13.2** Neuropathic pain appears when there is an injury that affects any structure of the nervous system. Inflammatory messengers also are released at the site of the injury and play an important role in the development of neuropathic pain (adapted from Twycross and Wilcock 2002: 33).

The ability to clinically differentiate inflammatory, either visceral or somatic, from neuropathic pain has relevant therapeutic implications since different analgesics are better at controlling different types of clinical pain.

Box 13.6 presents a summary of this section of the chapter:

**Box 13.6**　A summary of types of pain

- *Somatic pain* is the pain elicited when the body's structural elements, such as bone or muscle, are damaged.
- *Visceral pain* is the pain caused by the injury of internal organs or their surrounding tissues, such as liver, heart and appendix.
- *Neuropathic pain* is the pain initiated or caused by a primary lesion or dysfunction in the nervous system.
- *Referred pain* is a feature of visceral pain. The area of referral is generally localized to distant structures, segmental and superficial, that are muscle, skin or both, innervated by the same spinal nerves as the affected internal organ.
- *Breakthrough (unpredictable) pain* is an intermittent exacerbation of pain that can occur spontaneously, usually not related with a specific activity or weight-bearing.
- *Incident (predictable) pain* is a type of intermittent pain that is related to a specific activity, such as eating, defecation, weight-bearing or walking. Also referred to as 'movement-related pain'.
- *End of dose failure pain* occurs shortly before the next dose of regular analgesics is due. It is usually controlled with an increase in the regular dose of analgesics.
- *Hyperalgesia* is an increased response to a stimulus, which is normally

painful. It appears when a noxious stimulus applied on the skin caused more pain than that expected in a normal tissue.

- *Allodinya* is the pain caused by a stimulus that would not normally produce pain.
- *Dysesthesia* is an abnormal painful sensation, such as burning, caused by a non-noxious stimulus.

# Cancer pain

The prevalence of chronic pain in cancer patients has been estimated to be 30–50 per cent among patients with cancer who are undergoing active treatment for a solid tumour and 70–90 per cent among those patients with advanced disease (Portenoy and Lesage 2001).

Prospective surveys indicate that as many as 90 per cent of patients could attain adequate relief with simple drug therapies, but this success rate is not achieved in routine practice (Pargeon and Hailey 1999). Inadequate management of pain is the result of various factors, such as deficiency in proper education of physicians and other health professionals on pain control and palliative care; fear among health professionals of drug dependence and addiction that results in under-prescription and under-use of analgesics; lack of general awareness that pain can be adequately controlled; misguided drug legislation and inappropriate availability of suitable drugs (The World Health Organization, Expert Committee Report 1990). The World Health Organization (WHO) advocates a strategy to respond to these issues (WHO 1996). It relies on three key components:

- *Government policies*, emphasizing the need to alleviate chronic cancer pain.
- *Drug availability*, improving the prescription, distribution, dispensation and administration of drugs (especially opioids).
- *Education* of the public, health care professionals, drug regulators, policy-makers.

Based on more than 15 years' experience with the WHO strategy, it has recently been suggested that to effectively be capable of changing the experience of patients in pain and their families, palliative care should be widely integrated in society (Stjernswärd *et al.* 2007). In doing this, all three previously mentioned components of the WHO strategy together with implementing public palliative care services at all levels in the health system should be considered.

Cancer pain management has had several implications in public health initiatives and policies and has been suggested as a possible indicator of adequate health service provision (Breivik 2002).

### Pain syndromes in cancer

A cancer patient might present acute and chronic pain syndromes, due to or associated with the tumour or another painful condition unrelated to it (Pargeon and Hailey 1999). Chronic pain syndromes in cancer patients may result from a direct effect of the neoplasm; and may be related to therapies administered to manage the disease or to disorders unrelated to the disease or its treatment (Portenoy and Lesage 2001). Although, most acute pain syndromes are caused by common diagnostic or therapeutic interventions, acute flare-ups of pain are common among patients with chronic pain (see Box 13.7). Many patients with well-controlled chronic pain have transitory 'breakthrough' pain. Recognition of cancer pain syndromes helps to identify the specific aetiology responsible for the pain, guide the need for additional evaluation, suggest specific therapies, or assist in assessment of patients' outcome.

---

**Box 13.7**   Acute pain syndromes in cancer patients (adapted from Portenoy and Lesage 2001: 3–4)

**Acute pain may be associated with:**

- Diagnostic procedures:

    - Lumbar puncture headache
    - Bone marrow biopsy
    - Venepuncture
    - Paracentesis
    - Thoracentesis
- Analgesic techniques

    - Acute pain after strontium therapy of metastatic bone pain

- Therapeutic procedures

    - Pleurodesis
    - Tumour embolization
    - Nephrostomy insertion

- Chemotherapy

    - Intravenous or intraperitoneal infusions
    - Painful peripheral neuropathy (platins and taxanes)
    - Diffuse bone or muscle pain from colony-stimulating factors
    - Oral pain due to chemotherapy induced mucositis

- Hormonal therapy

    - Painful gynaecomastia

- Immunotherapy

    - Arthralgia and myalgia from interferon and interleukin (flu-like syndrome)

---

- Radiation therapy

    - Headache after brain metastasis irradiation
    - Acute post-radiation proctocolitis or enteritis

**Acute pain can be due to:**

- Tumour-related pathology:

    - Vertebral collapse
    - Pathological fracture
    - Headache from intracranial hypertension

- Intercurrent infection

    - Pain associated with wound infection or abscesses

- Intercurrent pathology

    - Cardiac angina
    - Ureteral colic pain

*Tumour-related somatic pain syndromes* might be due to neoplastic invasion of bone, joint, muscle or connective tissue causing persistent somatic pain. The spine is the most common site of bone metastases and many patients with cancer have back pain. Extension of a malignant tumour from the vertebra has the potential to damage the spinal cord causing devastating neurological disorders. With early diagnosis and treatment the neurological complication can be prevented. For this reason, a high level of suspicion of this complication is extremely important to prevent it and to ask for immediate medical assessment is mandatory. Different visceral and somatic pain syndromes can be caused by obstruction, infiltration or compression of visceral structures, and connective supporting tissues. Tumour infiltration or compression of nerve, plexus or dorsal roots ganglion can be the reason for neuropathic pain syndromes. These can also be a consequence of the remote effect of malignant disease on peripheral nerves. The syndromes are highly variable. Patients react differently to each situation and they may refer aching pain or dysesthesias (abnormal pain sensations, such as burning) anywhere innervated by the damaged neural structure (Portenoy and Lesage 2001).

*Iatrogenic pain syndromes* may emerge after chemotherapy or radiotherapy or a combination of both. However, in general, specific somatic pain syndromes related to chemotherapy, radiation therapy or surgery are rare (e.g. radiation-induced or corticosteroid-induced necrosis of femoral or humeral head). More frequently, patients may complain of general malaise and aching, a flu-like syndrome, after these interventions have been preformed. Visceral pain can follow intraperitoneal chemotherapy or abdominal radiation therapy. These syndromes can mimic tumour-related pain and in the assessment it is important to exclude recurrence. Most pain syndromes that appear some time after the treatment has been completed are neuro-pathic. Radiation induced fibrosis can damage a peripheral nerve or nerves and cause neuropathic pain; symptoms usually occur months to years after treatment. The neuropathic pain can be associated with slowly progressive weakness, sensory disturbances, radiation changes of the skin, and lymphoedema (Portenoy and Lesage 2001).

## The patient with pain due to cancer: the nurse's role in pain assessment and pain measurement

Patients with cancer are likely to experience a range of psychological, social and spiritual problems which extend far beyond the experience of physical pain. The concept of 'total pain', first coined by Cicely Saunders (Clark 1998), and subsequently developed by Twycross (see, for example, Twycross 1997), captures the range of issues with which nurses and other members of the multidisciplinary team need to be concerned when caring for patients suffering from pain due to cancer (see Figure 13.3).

The concept of 'total pain' alerts us to the fact that pain is a deeply personal experience which cannot be understood as merely a biological phenomenon. One of the nurse's greatest challenges and contributions to pain management is to facilitate the expression of each individual's encounter with pain (Krishnasamy 2001: 340), and to begin to understand through this what factors, beyond the purely physical and physiological, impinge upon this. Although exploring what pain means to the person experiencing it can be very difficult, Krishnasamy (2001: 341) identifies a range of questions

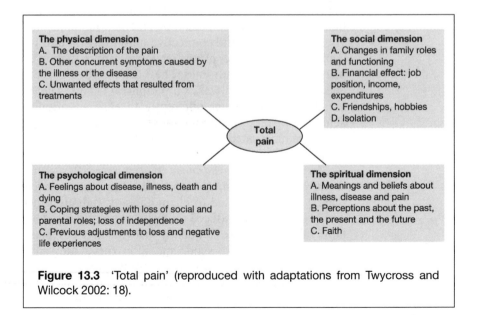

**Figure 13.3** 'Total pain' (reproduced with adaptations from Twycross and Wilcock 2002: 18).

that can be used to begin to evaluate and assess the experience of pain for a person with cancer and thus inform an effective care strategy (Box 13.8).

While these questions are invaluable for understanding the personal experience of pain and the impact that pain has on the lives of patients and their family carers, nurses will also be responsible for contributing to *measuring* the severity of pain such that the effectiveness of therapeutic interventions can be evaluated. Pain measurement refers to a quantified measure of one aspect of the pain experience: its severity. The measurement of pain relies on patient's self-reports, or the inference that health professionals make on the basis of the patient's behaviour. Several methods are used to measure pain severity: numeric scales, descriptive rating scales, visual analogues scales, box scales.

One of the most frequently used instruments to measure pain is the McGill Pain Questionnaire (Turk and Okifuji 2001). It has three parts:

1   The first part includes a descriptive scale that rates the intensity of the present pain; numbers are assigned to each of five adjectives: 1 (mild), 2 (discomforting), 3 (distressing), 4 (horrible), 5 (excruciating).

2   In the second part, patients mark the location of their pain on ventral and dorsal views of a human figure.

3   The third part explores the sensory, affective and cognitive components of pain. It comprises 20 categories grouped in a pain-rating index.

Although this questionnaire provides a great deal of information, it requires a long time to complete. A shorter version has been produced (Wright *et al.* 2001).

Categorical verbal rating scales have been used to assess the effectiveness of a given analgesic. The patient is asked to rate the pain and the analgesic effect and the observer documents the patient's ratings. They are one of the

---

**Box 13.8**   Suggested questions to comprehensively assess the experience of cancer pain

- When did you first notice you were ill?
- How have things been with your family and friends?
- What was happening in your life when the cancer was diagnosed?
- Did you experience any pain when you were first ill?
- What makes it better?
- Is the pain the same now or has it changed?
- What are your fears for the future?

- How have things been since you were told about the cancer?
- How have things been for your family and friends?
- What plans in your life has it disrupted or stopped?
- When did you first experience any pain?
- What makes it worse?
- What are your expectations and hopes for the future?
- What does the pain mean to you?

(from Krishnasamy 2001: 341)

most reliable, sensitive and reproducible tools, although the information they provide about other pain characteristics is very limited (Carroll and Bowsher 1993). The Oxford Pain Chart (McQuay 1990), for instance, incorporates categorical scales into a pain diary. During seven days, the patient is asked to fill in a pain diary before going to bed and is asked to estimate at the end of the week the overall effectiveness of the pain treatment over the seven days (Carroll and Bowsher 1993: 24).

The Edmonton Staging System (ESS) for cancer pain is an instrument developed to characterize pain in advanced cancer patients and to predict its possible response to analgesic therapies according to certain prognostic factors (Bruera *et al.* 1995). Patients are asked to determine the intensity of pain using visual analogue scales (VAS, 0 = no pain; 10 = worst possible pain) while the analgesic treatment is decided by an experienced palliative care physician. Pain intensity is measured on a daily basis until a stable control of pain is achieved. The original version of the ESS has recently been revised (rESS) to improve the inter-rater reliability and the predictive value of the scale (Fainsinger *et al.* 2005). The ESS takes into account four pain and patient features, such as the pain mechanism (presence or not of neuropathic pain either alone or in combination with nociceptive pain), incidental pain (present or absent), cognitive function, psychological distress and past history of addictive behaviour to alcohol or drugs. It is assumed that patients with less complex pain features should require a shorter time to achieve stable pain control, require more simple analgesic regimens, be more responsive to opioid treatments, and use lower opioid doses. The rESS appears to be especially useful to compare cancer pain populations in research studies.

There are many other tools for pain measurement. There are no rules as to which pain measurement tool should be used or which is the best one. It may be useful to find out what tools are used by other colleagues and what their perceptions about available tools are. Functional scales are useful in measuring patients' ability to engage in functional activities, such as walking up stairs, sitting or resting for a specific time, performing activities of daily living. They are self-report measures that require no more than 5–10 minutes to complete. Another approach would be to ask the patient to keep a diary of the activities performed during the day, the pain related with them and the actions taken to control it.

It is important to note that pain reports provide useful information in well-defined and homogeneous patient groups. There seems not to be an optimal cut-off point for mild, moderate or severe pain based on patients' ratings nor a linear relationship between cancer pain severity and interference with function. Furthermore, little is known about the influence that cultural and ethnic differences may have in how individuals interpret pain intensity ratings (Paul *et al.* 2005).

In patients who are unable to communicate, autonomic reactions to pain and distress can be measured, such as high heart rate, perspiration and nausea. Similarly, *pain behaviours* (such as grimacing, restlessness or protection of a painful limb) can be observed and quantified (Turk and Okifuji 2001).

Special attention should be given to older adults with dementia who may suffer unrecognized pain. Several tools for pain assessment in adults who have lost the ability to verbalize have been developed and are based on the direct observation of behaviour and on surrogate reporting of pain (Herr *et al.* 2006). Most pain behaviours and indicators of pain relate to changes in facial expressions, verbalizations and vocalizations, mental status changes, changes in interpersonal interactions, and changes in activity patterns and routines. However, a standardized tool of this type for broad adoption in clinical practice and research does not yet exist.

*Pain assessment* is distinguished from *pain measurement* by denoting a combination of an attempt to understand the experience, quality and duration of pain, to quantify its severity through measurement and to contribute to a clinical diagnosis of its cause. As such, pain assessment requires that nurses consider the interrelationship between pain and the experience of suffering in terms of the degree of spiritual or existential distress that someone may be experiencing (Brant 2003), and that they are aware of issues that relate to the particular characteristics of the patient for whose care they are responsible (Aranda 1999). For example, nurses should be aware that pain and clinical depression are frequently found together in patients with chronic pain, and that therefore it is extremely important to assess depression in this group of patients.

Pain assessment should be carried out at regular intervals and well documented so that all members of the multidisciplinary team have access to an understanding of the patient's pain problem (Fink and Gates 2001: 55) and in order that a comprehensive pain management strategy can be developed.

## Pain management: pharmacological and non-pharmacological interventions

In 1982 a panel of experts were invited by the World Health Organization (WHO) to create an easily applicable approach for the management of pain: this is known as *the WHO three-step analgesic ladder* (see Box 13.9).

The three-step ladder is the method most widely accepted and recognized as the basis for adequate pain control. Its methodology involves a stepwise approach to the use of analgesic drugs, going from the first to the third step in analgesic strength. It recommends that analgesics should be used:

- *By the mouth*: the mouth is the standard route for the administration of opioids including morphine and other opioids.
- *By the clock*: emphasizing the importance of a preventive attitude towards pain control. Analgesics should be given regularly and prophylactically.
- *By the ladder*: using the three-step analgesic ladder, moving always up the ladder and not sideways in the same efficacy group (Twycross and Wilcock 2002: 30–1).

**Box 13.9**   The WHO three-step analgesic ladder (adapted from Twycross and Wilcock 2002: 31)

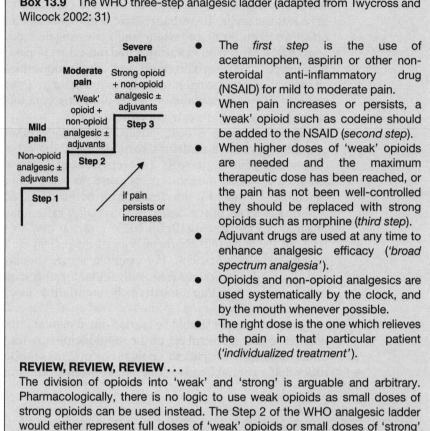

- The *first step* is the use of acetaminophen, aspirin or other non-steroidal anti-inflammatory drug (NSAID) for mild to moderate pain.
- When pain increases or persists, a 'weak' opioid such as codeine should be added to the NSAID (*second step*).
- When higher doses of 'weak' opioids are needed and the maximum therapeutic dose has been reached, or the pain has not been well-controlled they should be replaced with strong opioids such as morphine (*third step*).
- Adjuvant drugs are used at any time to enhance analgesic efficacy (*'broad spectrum analgesia'*).
- Opioids and non-opioid analgesics are used systematically by the clock, and by the mouth whenever possible.
- The right dose is the one which relieves the pain in that particular patient (*'individualized treatment'*).

REVIEW, REVIEW, REVIEW . . .
The division of opioids into 'weak' and 'strong' is arguable and arbitrary. Pharmacologically, there is no logic to use weak opioids as small doses of strong opioids can be used instead. The Step 2 of the WHO analgesic ladder would either represent full doses of 'weak' opioids or small doses of 'strong' opioids. However, due to reasons of non-availability or restricted supplies of morphine and other strong opioids in many countries worldwide Step 2 has been placed for practical reasons with an international perspective (Twycross *et al.* 2002: 159).

- *Review*: in a regular basis to assess response to analgesics, to adjust doses and to identify different sources of pain and possible aggravating factors.

The emphasis on the use of oral opioids for moderate to severe pain has been recognized as the most important reason for the success of the three-step ladder. It is not a rigid protocol; it allows considerable flexibility in the choice of specific drugs. Pain treatment can be started at the first, second or third step in the ladder according to the pain intensity, and in many circumstances, the second step may need to be ignored. The mainstay approach for the management of cancer pain is opioid-based pharmaco-therapy, using opioids (such as morphine, methadone, fentanyl) usually in combination with non-opioid analgesics, such as acetaminophen (para-cetamol), NSAIDS (non-selective COX-2 inhibitors, such as aspirin and selective COX-2 inhibitors, such as celecoxib), and analgesic adjuvants, such as cortiscoteroids (e.g. dexamethasone), tricyclic antidepressants (e.g. amitryptiline) and anticonvulsants (e.g. gabapentin) (see Box 13.10).

In 2001, an expert working group of the research network of the European Association for Palliative Care (EAPC) published a series of 20 recommendations for the use of morphine and alternative opioids in cancer pain control (Hanks *et al.* 2001).

The WHO and the EAPC thus recommend morphine as the opioid of first choice to be considered for cancer pain relief. The oral route is the preferred one and it should always be considered in the first instance. If morphine is given orally it should be titrated upward in gradually increasing doses until a dose is found which maintains continuous pain relief. The goal is to obtain a result in which the patient is pain free at all times (Melzack and Wall 1996: 277). The attitude towards cancer pain control should be preventive and proactive without waiting until the patient is in pain to administer the required dose of opioid. Doses of painkillers and adjuvant medications need to be given regularly and extra doses should be advised and available to be taken 'as required' by the patient in order to relieve episodes of 'breakthrough' and 'incidental' pain.

*Adjuvant analgesics* are a miscellaneous group of drugs; their primary indication is not for pain control but they can relieve pain in specific circumstances. They include:

- *corticosteroids*, such as dexamethasone and prednisolone, which are especially helpful for the reduction of pain associated with nerve root or spinal cord compression. Their general anti-inflammatory effect reduces the oedema surrounding the tumoural mass
- *antidepressants*, such as amitriptiline
- *anticonvulsants*, such as sodium valproate and gabapentin.

---

**Box 13.10**   Commonly used analgesics

| Acetaminophen (paracetamol) | NSAIDS | 'Weak' opioids | 'Strong' opioids | Adjuvants |
|---|---|---|---|---|
| | Acetyl salicylic acid (aspirin) | Codeine | Morphine | Corticosteroids |
| | Diclofenac Ibuprofen | Hydrocodone Tramadol | Hydromorphone Fentanyl | Anticonvulsants Tricycle antidepressants |
| | Selective COX-2 inhibitors | Buprenorphine | Diacetylmorphine | Biphosphonates |
| | | Propoxyphene | Oxicodone Methadone | |

Antidepressants and anticonvulsants are specially used in cases of nerve compression due to malignant invasion or compression.

- *NMDA-receptor-channel blockers* are usually used when neuropathic pain does not respond well to standard analgesics together with an antidepressant and an anti-epileptic. Ketamine, which is the NMDA-receptor-channel blocker most widely used, is an anaesthetic induction agent. Methadone, a synthetic opioid, also seems to act in the NMDA-receptor-channel. It represents a very good opioid alternative in these circumstances. It has a comparatively lower cost. However, due to its long half life, it may remain in the bloodstream for a long time leading to higher risk for accumulation and side effects.

- *Antispasmodics*, such as hyoscine butylbromide and glycopyrronium are used to relieve visceral distension pain and colic pain.

- *Muscle relaxants*, such as diazepam (which is a benzodiazepine), are used in cases of painful muscle spasm (cramps). Relaxation therapies are recommended as complementary therapies in these situations.

Generally, adjuvant analgesics should be given in combination with morphine, or another opioid, and a NSAID. The relief of pain will be obtained gradually: the first step is to help the patient obtain a good night's sleep; the second step is to reduce the intensity of pain during the day to a bearable level, and the third step is to obtain sustained and adequate pain control around the clock. The patient needs to be informed that a week or so might be necessary to obtain major benefits (Twycross and Wilcock 2002: 51–8).

A range of potential strategies can also be considered to complement pharmacological treatment, such as palliative radiation therapy and chemotherapy, behavioural therapies, lifestyle therapies, complementary therapies and local anaesthetic techniques. The main aim remains always to provide adequate pain control in order to help patients to improve their functioning despite the pain and, at more advanced stages, to ensure comfort and the best possible quality of life at the end of their life (see Box 13.11).

---

**Box 13.11**    The principles of cancer pain management (based on Krishnasamy 2001: 339)

- Recognize and promptly assess pain in cancer patients.
- Identify psychological and spiritual influences on pain perception and management.
- Aim to alleviate pain first, at night; second, at rest; and finally, on movement.
- Maximize independence and best possible quality of life.
- Address and relief current fears about pain.
- Anticipate and discuss possible concerns about future painful episodes and therapeutic options.
- Provide support and encouragement for family members, friends and professional care-givers.
- Invite participation of the patient, family and other informal carers.

- Adopt a collaborative, multidisciplinary approach.
- Design analgesic regiments tailored to each patient's needs and tolerance.
- Regular outcome follow up.
- Refer early to pain specialist services if pain control is not achieved.

# Routes of analgesic administration

Many options are available for the delivery of analgesics in the management of acute, chronic and cancer pain. It is essential to consider that the relief of chronic and cancer pain requires a long-term therapeutic strategy which is dynamic and individually tailored. The decision of using one preparation or delivery system over another should take into consideration the ability of the patient to use a specific type of delivery system, the efficacy of that system to deliver acceptable analgesia, the ease of use by the patient and his or her carers, the potential complications associated with that system, and costs attached to its use (Stevens and Ghazi 2000). For nursing practice, it is particularly important to be familiar with different routes for the administration of analgesics, especially opioids, and with the formulations available in each individual place of work. This knowledge allows the confident use of several options for appropriate pain control when it is necessary.

### The oral route

The oral route is the easiest, least invasive, cheapest and most common route used for the administration of analgesics in patients with chronic and cancer pain. There are no major complications associated with its use. There are usually two types of formulations: 'normal release' and 'slow (or modified) release' formulations. Slow release formulations have been designed to provide long-lasting analgesia. Morphine, oxycodone and hydromorphone are the opioids currently available in slow release formulations. They are usually given twice a day. Normal release formulations are used to titrate opioid requirements against pain and should always be available for breakthrough pain relief.

Some patients may find it difficult or impossible to take oral medications. For instance, in patients with head and neck cancer or esophageal or gastric cancer, the malignant growth might obstruct the anatomical passages and make it impossible to swallow. In the case of severely ill, debilitated or very confused patients, the oral route might be better avoided. In all these circumstances, other routes for the administration of analgesics need to be considered.

### The intravenous route

The intravenous route for the administration of analgesics should only be considered when using other less invasive routes does not control a patient's pain. This route represents several disadvantages: it requires an in-dwelling intravenous central or peripheral catheter; the preparation of the opioid solution by a pharmacist; the use of an external infusion pump; and out-patient and inpatient skilled nursing support. All these aspects significantly increase costs. On the other hand, any in-dwelling intravenous catheter can serve as an entry port for infection and for this reason it requires regular and skilled nursing attention. Intravenous infusions of opioids can be given as continuous infusions, or they can be used in conjunction with a patient-controlled analgesia (PCA) device, which provides continuous infusion plus on-demand boluses that the patient self-administers. PCA devices are not recommended in confused patients (Stevens and Ghazi 2000).

### The subcutaneous route

When the oral route is not appropriate, the subcutaneous route is a simple method of parental administration of analgesics (Stevens and Ghazi 2000). There is no need for vascular access and problems associated with in-dwelling intravenous catheters are avoided. The subcutaneous route can be used to give medications by bolus or for continuous infusions. An area on the chest, abdomen, upper arms or thighs is shaved and cleaned with anti-septic and a butterfly needle is inserted. When continuous infusion of analgesics is considered, the tubing is attached to an infusion pump or a syringe driver. If not, a loop of tubing is secured with adhesive tape and used to give subcutaneous bolus injections. A clear plastic occlusive dressing is applied to cover the needle. The injection site should be changed weekly or as needed, and allergies to metal needles should always be assessed. The volume of fluid that can be injected per hour represents the main limiting factor. It has been suggested that infusion rates of 2ml to 4ml per hour can be administered safely without causing pain at the site of injection (Bruera *et al.* 1987). If adequate precautions of cleaning and rotating the sites for injection are taken, the rate of skin infection is very low (1 in 117 patients in one study) (Swanson *et al.* 1989, cited by Stevens and Ghazi 2000).

### The transdermal route

The transdermal route is a non-invasive option for continuous administration of opioids for patients unable, or unwilling, to take oral medications (Stevens and Ghazi 2000). Fentanyl has been available to be given through the skin for several years. The delivery system consists of a reservoir of fentanyl and alcohol that holds a three-day supply of fentanyl in the form of a patch, similar to the better known nitroglycerine or oestrogen patches. A permeable membrane separates the drug reservoir from the skin and controls the release of fentanyl from the reservoir. An adhesive layer saturated with fentanyl holds the system in place. After the patch is applied, a bolus of fentanyl is delivered to the bloodstream through the skin. Fentanyl saturates the subcutaneous fat beneath the patch to form a subcutaneous 'depot'. Steady-state plasma fentanyl concentrations are reached after approximately 12 hours and these concentrations are maintained for about 72 hours. Once it has been placed, the patch releases fentanyl at a constant rate until the reservoir is depleted. Multiple patches may be placed if higher doses than that in one patch are needed. In case of opioid toxicity, the patch should be removed. It takes many hours to resolve opioids' side effects after the removal of a patch due to a prolonged elimination of the drug from the body. However, adverse effects of the fentanyl patch, such as dermatological reactions, are rare and usually easily treated. The transdermal route is best suited for patients with stable pain in whom the 24-hour opioid requirement has already been determined. It is not suitable for rapid titration of opioid requirements in patients with uncontrolled pain. Some sort of breakthrough pain coverage is usually needed (e.g. immediate-release oral morphine). In patients unable to take oral medications, the transmucosal (e.g. fentanyl lozenge), rectal (e.g. morphine suppository) and the subcutaneous (e.g. subcutaneous diamorphine) routes are available for 'breakthrough' administration of fast-acting opioids. More recently, buprenorphine patches have also been introduced on the market.

### The transmucosal and the sublingual routes

These routes for analgesic administration are useful as an alternative in patients who cannot tolerate the oral route because of nausea, vomiting or dysphagia and in those that cannot receive parental opioids due to emaciation, coagulation defects or lack of venous access (Stevens and Ghazi 2000).

Compared with the oral route, the sublingual region guarantees rapid absorption and entry of medications to the system and a quicker onset of action due to its rich venous drainage. It is very simple; it requires little expertise, preparation or supervision. More lipophilic drugs, such as methadone, fentanyl or buprenorphine, are better absorbed sublingually than hydrophilic ones. The transmucosal route is similar to the sublingual route. It differs from the sublingual route in that the absorption of the medication takes place mainly through the oral mucosa of the cheek. A fentanyl lozenge has been specially formulated for transmucosal absorption for the treatment of breakthrough pain. The lozenge needs to be rubbed against the mucosa of the cheek, rather than sucked. Side effects associated with the use of the sublingual and the transmucosal routes are bitter taste and a burning sensation when the formulation is first applied in contact with the mouth (Stevens and Ghazi 2000). Sublingual formulations are much cheaper options compared against the fentanyl lozenge.

### The rectal route

This route constitutes an alternative to the oral route specially in an emergency situation when the oral route is not suitable due to altered consciousness, severe nausea or vomiting, or gastrointestinal tract obstruction. It is also useful when the motility of the gastrointestinal tract is compromised or the gastric emptying is severely compromised. The most suitable form for the rectal route is the suppository, although if necessary, any tablet or capsule of any opioid that is used for oral administration can be used rectally (Stevens and Ghazi 2000). The disadvantage of the rectal route is the great deal of anatomical variations among individuals that requires titration and individualization of doses. Due to the small surface area of the rectum, drugs' absorption may be delayed or limited. It can also be interrupted by defecation and the small amount of fluid available in the rectum may slow down the dissolution of tablets or capsules. In situations of constipation, medications may be absorbed into faeces. The rectal route should not be used if the patient finds it unpleasant or if the patient has painful anal conditions, such as fissures, anal tumour or inflamed haemorrhoids.

### 'Interventional' approaches to pain control

Although the vast majority of patients with chronic and cancer pain can be relieved appropriately by the administration of analgesics via the oral, subcutaneous, rectal or transmucosal routes, a small proportion of patients may fail to obtain adequate analgesia despite the use of large systemic doses of analgesics, or they may suffer from uncontrollable side effects, such as nausea, vomiting, constipation, confusion or over-sedation while still in pain. These patients may benefit from the administration of opioids, local anaesthetics and other medications via the perispinal route and from the use of nerve blockade procedures and surgical interventions. The latter procedures are indicated only in patients with severe, intractable pain in whom less aggressive manoeuvres are ineffective or intolerable either because of poor physical condition or the development of intolerable side effects (Stevens and Ghazi 2000).

### The perispinal (epidural or intrathecal) route

The goal of perispinal opioid therapy is to place a small dose of an opioid and/or local anaesthetic close to the spinal opioid receptors situated in the dorsal horn of the spinal cord to enhance analgesia and reduce systemic side effects by decreasing the total daily opioid dose. An in-dwelling catheter is placed into the epidural or intrathecal space and the medications are delivered by using an external or implantable pump. By using this route, smaller doses of opioids can be effectively administered to act locally and directly at the opioid receptor level, and only small amounts of drugs reach the systemic circulation causing fewer side effects. The various perispinal approaches for opioid delivery include epidural bolus, continuous epidural infusion, intrathecal injection and continuous intrathecal infusion. Deciding between epidural versus intrathecal placement or external versus implantable pumps to deliver the opioid is based on multiple factors including duration of therapy, type and location of the pain, disease extent and central nervous system involvement, opioid requirement and individual preference and expertise. The complications and side effects associated with the use of this route can be divided into three categories: procedural and surgical complications – infection, bleeding at various sites, postdural puncture headache; complications related to a system malfunction – kinking, obstruction, disconnection, tearing or migration of the catheter; and pharmacological complications that include possible overdoses and pump-filling errors. In general, with the exception of constipation, side effects of perispinal opioids in patients already tolerant to opioids are rare (Stevens and Ghazi 2000).

### Sympathetic blockade

The sympathetic chain exists along the vertebral column and carries nociceptive information mainly of visceral origin (Miguel 2000). It is suitable for intervention at various levels (see Figure 13.4) for respective pain complaints and the blockade of sympathetic ganglia may improve visceral pain. It can also be considered an option for the diagnosis of pain and possible long-term pain relief. For instance, this procedure has been most commonly used

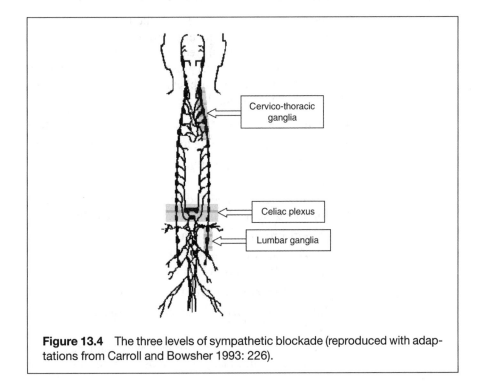

**Figure 13.4** The three levels of sympathetic blockade (reproduced with adaptations from Carroll and Bowsher 1993: 226).

for the control of abdominal pain due to pancreatic cancer and pelvic pain from cervical cancer (Leon-Casasola 2000).

### Neurolysis

Neurolysis implies the use of neurolytic agents or techniques to destroy nerves and interrupt the conduction of pain. It can be: chemical, using alcohol in concentrations of 50 per cent or 100 per cent or 7 per cent to 12 per cent phenol; thermal, applying cryoanalgesia or radiofrequency lesioning; or surgical, by surgically interrupting the nerve pathway. Chemical neurolysis is the most commonly used modality. The results of the injection of alcohol or phenol are similar to those obtained by sectioning the nerve, although the effect is usually seen for only three to six months. An example in which a trial injection is useful is in areas where pain is limited to a very circumscribed section, such as a tumoural rib invasion, or rib metastases treated with intercostals neurolysis. Its effect is not permanent, and pain returns either from a regrowth of neural structures or by progression of the underlying disease beyond the treated area. A risk/benefit ratio should be considered and properly addressed prior to implementing any invasive analgesic method and an accurate identification of the situations where these pain therapies are justified.

### The nurse's role and responsibility in analgesic administration

The nurse spends more time with the patient than any other health profes-sional and is thus in an ideal position to constantly assess and evaluate the effectiveness of their pain treatments (McCaffrey and Beebe 1994). For these reasons, nurses play a very active role in assuring good pain control in patients suffering from unrelieved pain. McCaffrey and Beebe (1994: 54–8) identify that nurses should:

- Determine whether the analgesic is to be given and, if so, when.
- Choose the appropriate analgesic(s) when more than one is prescribed.
- Be alert to the possibility of certain side effects as a result of the analgesic.
- Evaluate effectiveness of the analgesic at regular frequent intervals following each administration, but especially the initial doses.
- Report promptly and accurately to the doctor when a change is needed.
- Make suggestions for specific changes, such as route of administration, interval, formulations.
- Advise the patient about the use of analgesics.
- Inform the patient about non-pharmacological interventions for pain relief.
- Develop a preventive approach with analgesics by teaching the patient to request painkillers as soon as pain occurs or before it increases, and

by regularly assessing the patient and enquiring about the pain. A preventive attitude towards pain relief have several benefits:

- the patient spends less time in pain
- doses of analgesics can be lower than if pain is allowed to increase or become severe
- fewer side effects due to lower doses
- decreased concerns about obtaining relief when needed
- overall increase in activities
- decreased anxiety about the returning of pain.

Productive interactions between the practice team and the patient would warrant high-quality care (Wagner *et al.* 2001). Experienced nurses are crucial to guarantee the effective management of cases across settings, to ensure support for self-management in patients and families and to provide timely follow-up to achieve meaningful outcomes. These interactions do not necessarily require face-to-face visits. Regular telephone contacts, for instance, have proved to be of great value (Teunissen *et al.* 2007).

# Non-pharmacological interventions

Although drug therapy is one of the major modalities used in managing chronic and cancer pain, it represents only one of many methods available. Pharmacological interventions are most effective when used in combination with other non-pharmacological approaches and psychosocial support.

### Cognitive behavioural therapy

Cognitive behavioural therapy (CBT) involves changing people's thoughts and behaviour and enhancing their coping skills. In the context of chronic pain, CBT aims to teach patients the skills they need to cope better with the pain in order to reduce their suffering and enhance their overall quality of life. The therapeutic work is structured and planned according to patients' own set of relevant and achievable goals. The activity level is increased by small steady steps at a rate set jointly by therapist and patient towards the long-term purpose. Instead of a reduction in the pain level, goals achieved and improvements in quality of life and mood represent the successful outcomes of an adequate treatment (Carroll and Bowsher 1993: 60–2).

### Relaxation techniques

These have been used as therapeutic tools for the treatment of pain because pain is associated frequently with muscular tension, and stress and anxiety are usually associated with the onset and maintenance of pain (Horn and Mufano 1997: 115). Techniques involve the progressive relaxation of skeletal muscle groups over a period of 20 to 40 minutes. Relaxation needs to take place in a quiet environment, and in a comfortable posture on a bed or a couch. Some schedules include some sort of calming mental exercise or a period of controlled breathing after the muscular relaxation. It has been reported that successful relaxation is associated with decreased autonomic stimulation and decreased skeletal muscle tension (Horn and Mufano 1997: 116). It may also act as a distracter because it involves focused attention to instructions, and it can also have a positive impact on the management of pain because it is essentially a self-management technique, which may enforce a sense of self-control and self-efficacy (Horn and Mufano 1997: 116).

### Biofeedback

This comprises the use of instruments to enhance and transform information from the body, such as temperature of the skin or the amount of tension in skeletal muscles, into a vivid form like a flashing light or oscilloscope readout, a tone or a series of clicks (Horn and Mufano 1997: 118). In this way, physiological responses associated with stress or tension and not normally under voluntary control are measured and displayed to the patient (Carroll and Bowsher 1993: 110). Operant conditioning is the learning paradigm, and the knowledge of results acts as a reinforcer as it signals success. In the treatment of pain, physiological parameters subjected to biofeedback conditioning include muscle tone, finger temperature, temporal pulse and alpha EEG activity (Horn and Mufano 1997: 118). It is often used with a relaxation procedure, with the measurement providing the patient with an objective appreciation of the extent to which relaxation has been achieved.

*Physiotherapy* may be applied either to help cure, or alleviate, the tissue source of pain, or to reduce the severity of the pain the patient is experiencing. Physical therapies can be grouped into four categories:

- electrical therapy
- massage and manipulative procedures
- exercise therapy, including hydrotherapy
- relaxation procedures.

In the four categories the patient subjectively assesses the degree of pain relief. These categories differ in the amount of cooperation required by the patient. While electrical therapy, massage and other manipulative procedures are applied to patients who passively receive them, the last two categories require active cooperation from the patient (Carroll and Bowsher 1993: 147).

### Transcutaneous Electrical Nerve Stimulation (TENS)

This is an example of electrical therapy. Sensory cutaneous nerve endings in the skin are stimulated by an electrical current generated by the TENS unit. These electrical impulses feel like a buzzing, vibratory sensation on the skin under the electrodes. It has been suggested that as the brain selectively concentrates upon skin sensation rather than on deeper sensations, TENS helps to close the conscious gate experience of pain (Carroll and Bowsher 1993: 148). TENS has been used to relieve the pain of rheumatoid arthritis, neck and back pain, labour pain, metastatic pain, acute unpleasant pain due to peripheral nerve injuries.

### Complementary therapies

Several complementary therapies have gained popularity in the treatment of chronic and cancer pain, such as massage, aromatherapy, reflexology, hypnosis, guided imagery, visualization and shiatsu. Their aim is usually to add another source for comfort and relief to pharmacological approaches.

### Conclusion

Pain is a complex subject. Interventions for its relief have become established over the past 50 years and, for cancer pain, promoted under the auspices of the World Health Organization. The rationale for, and popularity of, particular interventions over time can be related to changing understandings of the relationship between the perception of pain and the reaction to pain: gate control theory and the developments of techniques for the use and administration of opioids are perhaps the most notable scientific advances that influence contemporary understandings of pain, cancer pain and pain control. Less well charted is the role of charismatic figures such as John Bonica in the pain field, and Cicely Saunders in the hospice and palliative care field. Their attempts resulted, arguably, in a movement from a narrow biomedical focus in the management and assessment of pain, towards a broader frame of reference in which understanding the individual experience of pain and suffering and valuing the collaborative contributions of the multidisciplinary team in measuring, assessing and relieving pain are understood to be crucially important. Pain is now understood as the 'fifth vital sign': this chapter has elucidated the historical developments which have led to this reformulation and has attempted to distil from contemporary sources the information necessary to underpin evidence-based care for persons in pain. We provide a range of sources below which we hope can aid further enquiry into this important subject.

## ▌References

Aranda, S. (1999) A pain assessment approach to nursing the person with complex pain. In: M. O'Connor and S. Aranda (eds) *Palliative Care Nursing: A Guide to Practice*, 1st edn. Melbourne: Ausmed.

Ashburn, M.A. and Staats, P.S. (2001) Management of chronic pain. *The Pain Series*, available at www.thelancet.com/journal/vol357/isss1/full/llan.357.s1.pain_series.15831.1 (accessed 1 September 2002).

Baszanger, I. (1998) *Inventing Pain Medicine. From the Laboratory to the Clinic.* New Brunswick: Rutgers University Press.

Beecher, H.K. (1946) Pain in men wounded in battle. *Annals of Surgery*, 123(1): 96–105.

Berman, J. (1995) Imaging pain in humans. *British Journal of Anaesthesia*, 75: 209–16.

Bonica, J. (1990) Definition and taxonomy of pain. In: *The Management of Pain*, 2nd edn. Philadelphia: Lea and Febiger.

Brant, J. (2003) Pain management. In: M. O'Connor and S. Aranda (eds) *Palliative Care Nursing: A Guide to Practice*, 2nd edn. Melbourne: Ausmed.

Breivik, H. (2002) International Association for the Study of Pain: Update on WHO-IASP Activities. *Journal of Pain and Symptom Management*, 24(2): 97–101.

Bruera, E., Brenneis, C. and MacDonald, R.N. (1987) Continuous sc infusion of narcotics for the treatment of cancer pain: an update. *Cancer Treatment Reports*, 71(10): 953–8.

Bruera, E., Schoeller, T., Wenk, R., MacEachern, T., Marcelino, S., Hanson, J. and Suarez-Almazor, M. (1995) A prospective multicenter assessment of the Edmonton Staging System for cancer pain. *Journal of Pain and Symptom Management*, 10(5): 348–55.

Carr, D.B. (1998) Preempting the memory of pain. *Journal of the American Medical Association*, 279(14): 1114–15.

Carr, D.B. and Goudas, L.C. (2001) Acute Pain. *The Pain Series*, available at www.thelancet.com/journal/vol357/isss1/full/llan.357.s1.pain_series.15828.1 (accessed September 2002).

Carroll, D. and Bowsher, D. (1993) *Pain Management and Nursing Care.* Oxford: Butterworth-Heinemann.

Cervero, F. and Laird, J.M.A. (2001) Visceral Pain. *The Pain Series*, available at www.thelancet.com/journal/vol357/isss1/full/llan.357.s1.pain_series.15834.1 (accessed September 2002).

Clark, D. (1998) Originating a movement: Cicely Saunders and the development of St Christopher's Hospice, 1957–67. *Mortality*, 3(1): 43–63.

Clark, D. (1999) 'Total pain', disciplinary power and the body in the work of Cicely Saunders, 1958–1967. *Social Science and Medicine*, 49(6): 727–36.

Dickenson, A.H. (1995) Spinal cord pharmacology of pain. *British Journal of Anaesthesia*, 75: 193–200.

Dickenson, A.H. (2002) Editorial I. Gate control theory of pain stands the test of time. *British Journal of Anaesthesia*, (88)6: 755–7.

Fainsinger, R., Nekolaichuk, C., Lawlor, P., Neumann, C., Hanson, J. and Vigano, A. (2005) A multicenter study of the revised Edmonton Staging System for classifying cancer pain in advanced cancer patients. *Journal of Pain and Symptom Management*, 29(3): 224–37.

Federation of State Medical Boards of the United States (1998) *Model guidelines for the use of controlled substances for the treatment of pain.* Euless, TX: The Federation. Cited in: D.B. Carr and L.C. Goudas (2001) Acute Pain. *The Pain Series*, available at www.thelancet.com/journal/vol357/isss1/full/llan.357 .s1.pain_series.15828.1 (accessed September 2002).

Fink, R. and Gates, R. (2001) Pain assessment. In: B.R. Ferrell and N. Coyle (eds) *Textbook of Palliative Nursing.* Oxford: Oxford University Press.

Hanks, G.W., de Conno, F., Cherney, N., Hanna, M., Kalso, E., McQuay, H.J., Mercadante, S., Meynadler, J., Poulain, P., Ripamontl, C., Radbruch, L., Roca i

Casas, J., Sawe, J., Twycross, R.G. and Ventafridda, V. (2001) Expert Working Group of the Research Network of the European Association for Palliative Care Morphine and alternative opioids in cancer pain: the EAPC recommendations. *British Journal of Cancer*, 84(5): 587–93.

Herr, K., Bjoro, K. and Decker, S. (2006) Tools for assessment of pain in nonverbal older adults with dementia: a state-of-the-science review. *Journal of Pain and Symptom Management*, 31(2): 170–92.

Horn, S. and Munafo, M. (1997) *Pain: Theory, research and intervention.* Buckingham, Open University Press.

Krishnasamy, M. (2001) Pain. In: J. Corner and C. Bailey (eds) *Cancer Nursing Care in Context.* Oxford: Blackwell Science.

Leon-Casasola, O.A. (2000) Critical Evaluation of Chemical Neurolisis of the Sympathetic Axis for Cancer Pain. *Cancer Control*, 7(2): 142–8.

Loeser, J.D. and Melzack, R. (2001) Pain: an overview. *The Pain Series*, available at www.thelancet.com/journal/vol357/isss1/full/llan.357.s1.pain_series.15830.1 (accessed September 2002).

McCaffery, M. (1968) *Nursing practice theories related to cognition, bodily pain, and man–environment interactions.* Los Angeles, CA: University of Los Angeles Students' store.

McCaffrey, M. and Beebe, A. (1994) Assessment. In: J. Latham (ed.) *Pain: A Clinical Manual for Nursing Practice.* London: Mosby.

McQuay, H.J. (1990) Assessment of pain and effectiveness of treatment. In: A. Hopkins and D. Costain (eds) *Measuring the Outcomes of Medical Care.* Cited in: D. Carroll and D. Bowsher (1993) *Pain Management and Nursing Care.* Oxford: Butterworth-Heinemann.

Meldrum, M.L. (1998) 'Tell me if this hurts': the problem of pain and analgesic measurement, 1940–1960. Paper presented to the History of Pain Symposium, *Pain and Suffering in History. Narratives of Science, Medicine and Culture.* University of California, Los Angeles, 13–14 March.

Melzack, R. (1999) From the gate to the neuromatrix. *Pain*, (suppl. 6): S121–S126.

Melzack, R. and Wall, P.D. (1965) Pain mechanisms: A new theory. *Science*, 3699(150): 971–9.

Melzack, R. and Wall, P.D. (1982) *The Challenge of Pain.* London: Penguin.

Melzack, R. and Wall, P.D. (1996) *The Challenge of Pain*, 2nd edn. Middlesex: Penguin Books, pp. 149–93.

Merskey, H. and Bogduk, N. (eds) (1994) *Classification of chronic pain: descriptions of chronic pain syndromes and definitions of pain terms.* Report by the International Association for the Study of Pain Task Force on Taxonomy, 2nd edn. Seattle, WA: IASP Press.

Miguel, R. (2000) Interventional Treatment of Cancer Pain: The fourth step in the World Health Organization Analgesic Ladder? *Cancer Control*, 7(2): 149–56.

Niv, D. and Devor, M. (1998) Transition from acute to chronic pain. In: D.B. Carr and L.C. Goudas (2001) Acute Pain. *The Pain Series*, available at www.thelancet.com/journal/vol357/isss1/full/llan.357.s1.pain_series.15828.1 (accessed September 2002).

Pargeon, K.L. and Hailey, B.J. (1999) Barriers to effective cancer pain management: a review of the literature. *Journal of Pain and Symptom Management*, 18(5): 358–68.

Paul, S., Zelman, D., Smith, M. and Miaskowski, C. (2005) Categorizing the severity of cancer pain: further exploration of the establishment of cutpoints. *Pain*, 113: 37–44.

Portenoy, R.K. and Lesage, P. (2001) Management of cancer pain. *The Pain Series*, available at www.thelancet.com/journal/vol357/isss1/full/llan.357.s1.pain_series.15835.1 (accessed September 2002).

Rey, R. (1995) *The History of Pain*. Cambridge, MA: Harvard University Press.

Stevens, R.A. and Ghazi, S.M. (2000) Routes of Opioid Analgesic Therapy in the Management of Cancer Pain. *Cancer Control*, 7(2): 131–41.

Stjernswärd, J., Foley, K. and Ferris, F. (2007) The Public Health Strategy for Palliative Care. *Journal of Pain and Symptom Management*, 33(5): 486–93.

Swanson, G., Smith, J., Bulich, R., New, P. and Shiffman, R. (1989) Patient controlled analgesia for chronic cancer pain in the ambulatory setting: a report of 117 patients. *Journal of Clinical Oncology*, 7: 1903–8.

Teunissen, S.C., Verhagen, E.H., Brink, M., van der Linden, B.A., Vost, E.E. and de Graeff, A. (2007) Telephone consultation in palliative care for cancer patients: 5 years of experience in The Netherlands. *Supportive Care in Cancer*, 15(6): 577–82.

Tulder, M.W., Cherkin, D.C., Berman, B., Lao, L. and Koes, B.W. (2002) Acupuncture for low back pain (systematic review). *Cochrane Database of Systematic Reviews*, 2: CD001351.

Turk, D.C. and Okifuji, A. (2001) Assessment of patients' reporting of pain: an integrated perspective. *The Pain Series*, available at www.thelancet.com/journal/vol357/isss1/full/llan.357.s1.pain_series.15829.1 (accessed September 2002).

Twycross, R. (1997) *Oral Morphine in Advanced Cancer*, 3rd edn. Beaconsfield: Beaconsfield Publishers.

Twycross, R., Wilcock, A., Charlesworth, S. and Dickman, A. (2002) *Palliative Care Formulary*, 2nd edn. Oxford: Radcliffe Medical Press.

Twycross, R. and Wilcock, A. (2002) *Symptom management in advanced cancer*, 3rd edn. Oxford: Radcliffe Medical Press.

Wagner, E., Austin, B., Davis, C., Hindmarsh, M., Schaefer, J. and Bonomi, A. (2001) Improving chronic illness care: translating evidence into action. *Health Affairs*, 20(6): 64–78.

Winslow, M., Paz, S., Clark, D., Seymour, J. and Noble, B. (2007) Pharmacogenetics and the relief of cancer pain. *International Journal of technology, knowledge and society*, 2(7): 129–34.

Woolf, C.F. (1995) Somatic pain-pathogenesis and prevention. *British Journal of Anaesthesia*, 75: 169–76.

Woolf, C.J. and Mannion, R.J. (2001) Neuropathic pain: aetiology, symptoms, mechanisms, and management. *The Pain Series*, available at www.thelancet.com/journal/vol357/isss1/full/llan.357.s1.pain_series.15833.1 (accessed September 2002).

World Health Organization (WHO) Expert Committee Report (1990) *Cancer Pain Relief and Palliative Care*: Technical Report Series 804. Geneva: World Health Organization.

World Health Organization (WHO) (1996) *Cancer Pain Relief, Second Edition, with a guide to opioid availability*. Geneva: World Health Organization.

Wright, K., Asmundson, G. and McCreary, D. (2001) Factorial validity of the short-form McGill Pain Questionnaire (SF-MPQ). *European Journal of Pain*, 5(3): 279–84.

# Suggested reading list

Beecher, H.K. (1946) Pain in men wounded in battle. *Annals of Surgery*, pp. 96–105.

Carroll, D. and Bowsher, D. (1995) *Pain: Management and nursing care*. Oxford, Butterworth Heinemann.

Horn, S. and Munafo, M. (1997) *Pain: theory, research and intervention*. Buckingham: Open University Press.

Melzack, R. and Wall, P.D. (1996) *The Challenge of Pain*, 2nd edn. Middlesex: Penguin Books, Chapter 8 'The Evolution of Pain Theories' and Chapter 9 'Gate control and other mechanisms' for a full description of the pain theories.

Twycross, R. and Wilcock, A. (2002) *Symptom management in advanced cancer*, 3rd edn. Oxford: Radcliffe Medical Press.

World Health Organization (WHO) Expert Committee Report (1990) *Cancer Pain Relief and Palliative Care*. Technical Report Series 804. Geneva: World Health Organization.

## Useful websites

http://www.library.ucla.edu/libraries
*The Pain Series* available at http://www.thelancet.com/

# 14

# Balancing feelings and cognitions

*Mari Lloyd-Williams and John Hughes*

---

**Key points**

- Terminally ill patients frequently experience psychiatric morbidity which often goes undiagnosed.
- Patients may be reluctant to inform health professionals that they are experiencing symptoms of psychiatric morbidity.
- Nurses have a vital role to play in identifying patients with psychiatric symptoms.
- A number of effective pharmacological, self-management and non-pharmacological treatment options exist for terminal patients with anxiety and/or depression.

---

# Introduction

The presence of psychiatric morbidity in terminally ill patients and the fact that it is often not diagnosed has been well recognized and reported (Rodin and Voshart 1986; Kathol *et al.* 1990; Pirl and Roth 1999; Murray *et al.* 2002). Nursing staff have an important role in identifying patients who may have psychiatric symptoms (McVey 1998). Nurses spend more time in direct patient contact enabling them to observe behaviour more closely and the nature of intimate nursing tasks may give an opportunity for patients to express any psychological distress. Sadness and depression exist along a continuum. This chapter will explore how patients can be supported in coping with their feelings when confronted with a terminal illness and will focus on depression and anxiety in particular and the difficulties involved in diagnosis.

Two brief case histories will be used to illustrate the issues discussed – all names and details have been changed to protect anonymity.

---

**Case history 14.1**

Andrew was 46 years old, worked in an office and was the proud father of three small children. He noticed he was passing some blood mixed with the stool and after presenting to the GP was referred for barium enema and colonoscopy that revealed a cancer of the rectum. Andrew was told his diagnosis at the outpatient clinic with, as he recounted later, 'the world and his wife also there'. He was told that the surgery would probably mean a stoma and was admitted a week later for surgery. This was followed by 20 fractions of radiotherapy and chemotherapy. He found the stoma difficult to accept, but returned to work after finishing his treatment. Eighteen months later he developed a series of chest infections, which were resistant to antibiotic treatment. An x-ray revealed that he had multiple pulmonary metastases and an abdominal ultrasound revealed liver metastases. This was devastating to Andrew who believed he had 'beaten' the cancer. He withdrew from family and friends and said he was no longer any use to them and they had better get used to life without him. He stayed in bed for most of the day and could not tolerate the chatter of his small sons when they returned from school. His wife found his withdrawn behaviour difficult to handle and they were now having frequent rows during which Andrew would often say, 'If I had a gun I would just end it all.' Andrew was referred to the palliative care outpatient clinic and asked to talk about how he felt. 'What's the point of you talking to me? I'm no use to anybody', was his response.

---

# The support of patients

All of us will have met patients like Andrew and the case reflects how patients perceive and remember the way in which bad news is communicated. When a patient is told that their disease is incurable they tend to show what can be called a characteristic emotional response. There is a period of shock and disbelief followed by a period of turmoil with anxiety, irritability and disturbance in appetite and sleep pattern. Concentration on daily tasks is impaired and thoughts regarding the diagnosis and fears for the future may intrude. There is also the sense of grief that life will be shortened and at the loss of future hopes and dreams. These symptoms usually resolve within seven to ten days with support from family and friends (Massie and Holland 1992). There is wide acknowledgement that all patients with a terminal illness should be given honest information and patients with terminal cancer are usually given such information – in other diseases this may not be the case and there is considerable cultural variation (Higginson and Costantini 2002). Recent research has shown, for example, that medical students' attitudes and expectations of caring for terminally ill patients is influenced by their age (Lloyd-Williams *et al.* 2004a) and country of origin (Lloyd-Williams 2003). Further research has shown that, although the majority of relatives wished to be told if they themselves developed dementia, they did not wish this information to be conveyed to the patient (Maguire *et al.* 1996). This can be compared to the communication of a cancer diagnosis and the similar reasons given 30 years ago for withholding information; that is, that being truthful with patients would precipitate anxiety and depression. In reality many patients in the early stages of dementia are fully aware of their cognitive impairment and withholding such information is likely to do more harm. Sensitive communication of the diagnosis can have benefits as patients may be able to participate in decisions regarding their future health care and also decisions regarding life-sustaining treatment before their condition deteriorates and they are rendered incapable of making such decisions themselves (Meyers 1997). The emergence of new therapies for patients with dementia, although palliative (Mechatie 1997), further supports the need for patients to be conveyed their diagnosis so that they may opt for treatment.

When conveying a diagnosis, medical and nursing staff can help by providing information and more importantly reassuring the patient that they will not be abandoned or die in pain or distress. For a significant number of patients, however good and appropriate this support, their distress escalates and these are the patients who present with anxiety or develop a depressive illness. Research suggests that patients who perceive they have little social support are more likely to go on to develop psychiatric morbidity than those who perceive they have more support (Hipkins *et al.* 2004), but the existence of excellent family and social support by no means precludes patients from developing anxiety or a depressive illness – which is illustrated by Andrew's case history.

In order to provide patients with terminal illness with optimum psychological care, as well as palliation of physical symptoms, health care professionals should have excellent communication and interpersonal skills. Clinical experience suggests the presence of a caring, empathic professional who is able to give honest information sensitively might be adequate. Such a professional may, for example, be a member of the primary care team or nurse specialist.

To summarize therefore, all nursing and medical staff require excellent communication skills but also need to be aware of the patients who may benefit from referral to another professional either from within their team itself, or outside the team to a psychologist or liaison psychiatrist, for example. The remainder of this chapter will focus on those patients who develop anxiety or depression and the strategies that can be employed to support these patients and their families.

# Aetiology of psychological distress

The exact aetiology of psychological morbidity in cancer and other terminal illness is unknown, but theories have been put forward. Goldberg and Cullen (1986) believed that the five psychosocial factors leading to significant psychological symptoms were: disruption of key relationships; dependence; disability; disfigurement; and approaching death. Patients referred to palliative care, for example, will normally have undergone a considerable part of their 'cancer journey' and already have experienced a range of emotions. The shock and disbelief of diagnosis, the acceptance of treatment and the fact that something can be done, is followed by the uncertainty of radiotherapy and chemotherapy. The detection of metastases, and sometimes the hope that further treatment may help, and the final referral to a palliative care team is the 'emotional cancer journey' for the majority of patients referred for palliative care. Some of the earliest work looking at the physical and mental distress of dying patients was undertaken by Hinton (1963). He studied 102 patients who were dying in hospital and used hospital inpatients that were not terminally ill as controls in a study looking at psychological distress. Thirty-minute informal, structured interviews were conducted with patients and Hinton found that terminally ill patients had higher levels of both physical and emotional distress and 24 per cent were depressed and 37 per cent were suffering from anxiety. Hinton concluded that both depression and anxiety had significant associations with the degree and duration of the terminal illness, with patients under 50 years of age having greater physical and mental distress. Addington-Hall and McCarthy (1995) explored the care-givers' perception of symptoms in the last year and week of life and found that perceptions of feeling low and miserable were reported by 69 per cent during the last year and 52 per cent during the last week of life.

Age appears to be an important factor in adjustment to cancer – younger patients reacting more acutely and dramatically than older patients, but having a greater capacity to adapt and develop new interests than older patients (Novotony *et al.* 1984). Younger patients with cancer are at a greater risk of developing depression and other psychiatric morbidity; Harrison *et al.* (1995) found in their study that cases of anxiety and depression were found in a significantly younger population. Ethnicity and culture also appear to affect the way in which patients respond to a cancer diagnosis, how they deal with the disease, and adjust to it (Johnson 1998). For example, a study by Formenti *et al.* (1995) found a substantial number of Latino women discontinued their radiotherapy treatment without a medical reason. During interviews to explore their reasons for discontinuing treatment, they found cultural linguistic factors influenced their decision, with patients expressing a preference for Spanish-speaking Latino physicians. Formenti *et al.* (1995) also found patients were unsure of their aetiology and prognosis, despite information being provided to them in their native Spanish. This finding is concordant with earlier work by Perez-Stable *et al.* (1992) which found a cultural belief of 'fatalismo' among some members of the Latino community, where a diagnosis of cancer is equated with certain death (Johnson 1998).

A sense of hope is vital to all patients and even in the terminal stages of illness, hope can still be fostered ensuring that patients feel supported and cared for. There is a need for psychosocial interventions to be an integral part of every palliative care patient's management plan (Fallowfield *et al.* 1995). In cancer, where the majority of research has been carried out, it is recognized that psychiatric disorders occur more frequently in cancer patients than in the general population. It is estimated that 50 per cent of patients will have no significant psychiatric symptoms, 30 per cent will have what is defined as an adjustment reaction and 20 per cent will have a formal psychiatric diagnosis, the most common being depression. It is estimated that for a quarter of all patients admitted to a palliative care unit, depression will be a significant symptom (Barraclough 1994). Bergevin and Bergevin (1995) in a review paper highlight the fact that as the prevalence of depression in the general population is 6–10 per cent, a number of patients with advanced cancer may have a pre-existing psychiatric disorder and the advancing cancer will place these patients at greater risk of developing further episodes. Research in renal disease (Kimmel 2002) and end-stage pulmonary disease (Singer *et al.* 2001) has also identified that many patients have unidentified psychological morbidity and that nursing, medical and paramedical staff have a role in identifying patients who may have psychiatric symptoms (Fincannon 1995; McVey 1998).

In a questionnaire study of 100 oncology nurses caring for 475 patients in the USA on one particular day, Pasacreta and Massie (1990) found that nurses perceived that 55 per cent of patients had symptoms requiring further psychiatric evaluation – a higher figure than would be expected, which included 13 per cent already under psychiatric care. They concluded that although nurses may not be able to identify specific psychiatric disorders, they are skilful in recognizing significant psychological distress.

# Anxiety

Anxiety is a normal emotion experienced by everybody at some time in their lives. Patients with any form of terminal illness will almost universally experience some degree of anxiety especially at the time of diagnosis, and at times when their disease status changes. This 'normal' anxiety often dispels when patients adjust to their new situation but in a proportion of patients anxiety can become severe and disabling. Anxiety can result in both physical and psychological symptoms which nurses may observe in some of their patients. Physical symptoms of anxiety can be explained by increased autonomic activity and include palpitations, sweating, headaches, breathlessness, gastrointestinal symptoms and feelings of inability to swallow – 'lump in the throat'. Psychological expression of a patient's anxiety can be more difficult to detect as patients can frequently react to anxiety in different ways.

However, psychological signs to look out for include apprehension, irritability, difficulty concentrating, an inability to relax, and disturbed sleep. Anxiety can be present most of the time – the so-called free-floating anxiety – or present in certain situations such as when waiting for test results (Boini *et al.* 2004). A generalized anxiety disorder can be defined as an unrealistic or exaggerated anxiety in regard to life events which has a duration of more than six months (Steifel and Razavi 1994). Anxiety and depression are often present in the same patient (McCarthy *et al.* 1996). Risk factors include previous anxious predisposition, poor social support and social isolation. Often the anxiety is related to fear of illness and death, but anxiety itself causes physical symptoms, which leads to a vicious circle of thought processes. Anxious patients tend to selectively remember the more 'threatening' information given to them and often the process of explanation of their diagnosis, treatment plan, and so on, by a knowledgeable professional, can be therapeutic in itself.

When caring for a patient for whom anxiety is a major problem, the patient may be reluctant to give a true history of how they feel and the history may need to be obtained from friends or relatives. The history often reveals that the patient has been tearful, completely preoccupied and unable to think of anything other than their illness. They will invariably have a disturbance of sleep and be experiencing autonomic disturbance, for example bowel disturbance.

Prevention of some anxiety is possible – much could be prevented by better organization of services for patients. Informing patients of the results of investigations as soon as possible, ensuring that all information is communicated between primary and secondary care and that those caring for patients possess good communication skills can all minimize morbidity. Often a patient may require medication to remove the feelings of anxiety and a short-acting benzodiazepine, e.g. Lorazepam or Diazepam or a beta blocker, is helpful. It is important that fears are addressed and that they are discussed with the patient and their main carer if appropriate.

A number of self-management and non-pharmacological options are also available to palliative patients experiencing symptoms of anxiety. Anxiety management groups have produced encouraging clinical outcomes, and are often offered under the supervision of a liaison psychiatry or psychology service (Prior 1998; Ormrod and Leadhead 1999). Referral to a palliative care day centre can similarly reduce the sense of isolation for a patient and also offer support for their family (Goodwin *et al.* 2002). There has also been considerable interest in self-management programmes which emphasize patients' central role in managing their long-term illness. Two areas of self-management which have been investigated with palliative care patients is cognitive behavioural therapy (CBT) and relaxation training, both of which have been found to be effective interventions for anxiety. A recent meta-analysis of the effects of CBT on commonly reported symptoms in adult cancer survivors concluded that CBT is associated with short-term effects on anxiety and depression (Osborn *et al.* 2006). A number of randomized trials have investigated the effects of relaxation therapy on anxiety, depression or mood in cancer patients. Bindemann *et al.* (1991), for example, randomly assigned patients with newly diagnosed cancer to relaxation training or control groups. They found that anxiety and psychiatric morbidity increased more significantly in control groups than with patients receiving relaxation training. They additionally found relaxation training had a positive effect on depression scores in women. Relaxation training and hypnosis have also been shown to elicit an effect on anxiety during treatment procedures such as chemotherapy or bone-marrow aspiration, in some (Olmsted *et al.* 1982; Kazak *et al.* 1996) but not all (Wall and Womack 1989) randomized trials.

A number of complementary therapies may also be useful adjunctive interventions for palliative care patients experiencing anxiety. A number of randomized controlled trials have evaluated the impact of massage, largely concluding that it can be an effective treatment at relieving anxiety in palliative care patients. Ahles *et al.* (1999), for example, conducted a trial of massage for patients undergoing autologous bone-marrow transplantation and found clinically significant improvements in anxiety compared to controls.

There is evidence that massage combined with aromatherapy also provides relief from anxiety. A systematic review of aromatherapy and massage identified four randomized controlled trials that evaluated impact on anxiety, with these trials reporting a reduction in anxiety of between 19 per cent and 32 per cent (Fellowes *et al.* 2006). Music therapy has also been found to have an effect on the anxiety level of palliative care patients. An early study by Bailey (1983) explored the effects of music therapy on the mood of patients with cancer, with 50 hospital inpatients being randomly assigned to either a live music session or tape-recorded music. Patients who received live music reported significantly lower anxiety scores than those listening to taped music. A recent review also found a benefit from music therapy on anxiety and cancer pain, although the number of controlled clinical trials was small (Hilliard 2005). There is also limited evidence that reflexology may be a useful complementary technique for reducing anxiety in patients with cancer (Stephenson *et al.* 2000; Quattrin *et al.* 2006); however, other researchers have failed to find any such benefit (Ross *et al.* 2002).

# Depression

Depression can present in a variety of ways, for example agitation, retardation and withdrawal. Patients are often reluctant to disclose their feelings of being low for fear of being thought a 'bad' or 'difficult' patient or because they may fear troubling or upsetting their doctor. It is important therefore that depression is acknowledged and thought about in palliative care as much as the assessment of pain or nausea. One of the main difficulties is distinguishing between depression and sadness – all patients can be expected to be sad at the end of life but how can we distinguish between what can be called 'appropriate sadness' from a treatable depressive illness? What may be useful indicators that a patient is depressed? Feelings of overwhelming hopelessness and helplessness, guilt and thoughts of self-harm are all thought to be useful indicators of depression (Casey 1994).

A very wise psychiatrist when asked how he was able to distinguish sadness from depression in patients with advanced cancer, stated that patients who are depressed blame themselves for how they feel whereas patients who are sad blame their illness for how they feel – and from clinical experience this is invariably the case. Patients who are depressed frequently look more unwell than they really are. There may also be difficulties with symptom management – depression should be considered in the patient for whom no analgesia appears to work and whose symptoms are never fully resolved (Lloyd-Williams *et al.* 2004b). Research in patients with end-stage renal disease has suggested that psychological distress can contribute to greater morbidity and earlier mortality in this population (Christensen and Ehlers 2002); while the need for psychological care has been found to be as great among those dying of non-malignant disease as it is in cancer patients (Luddington *et al.* 2001).

## How much of a problem is depression for palliative care patients?

The prevalence of depressive spectrum syndromes differs widely from 3 per cent to 58 per cent depending on the conceptualization of depression; the criteria used to define depression; the methodological approach employed within the study; and the population of patients surveyed (Grassi *et al.* 1996; Minagawa *et al.* 1996; Hotopf *et al.* 2002). As the prevalence of depression in the general population is 6–10 per cent, a number of patients who present with advanced disease may have a pre-existing psychiatric disorder and the advancing disease will place these patients at greater risk of developing further episodes (Bergevin and Bergevin 1995). Grassi *et al.* (1996), studying 86 terminally ill patients being cared for at home and using the HAD scale and quality of life tool EORTC QLQ-C30, found that 45 per cent of patients were depressed and reported correlations between quality of life and depression. Ramsay (1992) evaluated all referrals to a liaison psychiatry service during one year: 26 patients were referred – 10 per cent of the total number of patients admitted to the unit during the year. Of these 26 patients, 50 per cent had a diagnosis of depression. More recent work comparing patients with lung cancer and end-stage chronic pulmonary obstructive disease (COPD) has suggested that 90 per cent of patients with COPD suffered clinically relevant anxiety and depression compared with 52 per cent of patients with terminal lung cancer (Gore *et al.* 2000). The psychosocial needs of patients with cancer are frequently inadequately addressed by the services they receive, with depression often going unrecognized (Lloyd-Williams 2000; Sharpe *et al.* 2004). An early study by Maguire (1985) found up to

80 per cent of the psychological and psychiatric morbidity which develops in cancer patients goes unrecognized and untreated. More recently, Fallowfield *et al.* (2001) conducted a study to assess the sensitivity and specificity of oncologists' identification of clinical distress in cancer outpatients; finding that only 29 per cent of patients were correctly identified as having psychiatric morbidity.

A reason for this low rate of detection is thought to be due to nondisclosure by patients who may either feel they are wasting the doctors' time or that they are in some way to blame for their distress and therefore choose to hide it (Maguire and Howell 1995). There are no universally accepted criteria for diagnosing depression in the medically ill. In the physically healthy population, depression is diagnosed if patients have a persistent low mood and at least four of the following symptoms which are present most of the day for the preceding two weeks:

- diminished interest or pleasure in all or almost all activities
- psychomotor retardation or agitation
- feelings of worthlessness or excessive and inappropriate guilt
- diminished ability to concentrate and think
- recurrent thoughts of death and suicide
- fatigue and loss of energy
- significant weight loss or gain
- insomnia or hypersomnia.

Many of the symptoms of depression, however, exhibit communality with symptoms of cancer or the side effects of its treatment (Tavio *et al.* 2002). These include disturbances of sleep and appetite, neurovegetative arousal or sedation. Patient concerns relating to death may reflect contemplation of illness issues, as opposed to morbid depressive preoccupation or suicidal thinking (Reuter and Harter 2004). Consequently, the overlap between symptoms of depression and somatic symptoms of cancer and its treatment make diagnosing depression among cancer patients more difficult than with the general population (Akechi *et al.* 2003). Buckberg *et al.* (1984) believed that anorexia, with loss of appetite and low energy were such common symptoms in the medically ill and proposed eliminating these somatic symptoms as a criteria for diagnosis of depression. They also found that the point prevalence of major depression dropped from 42 per cent to 24 per cent when all somatic symptoms were eliminated as criteria. Such criteria therefore need to be used with caution in palliative care.

Assessing for depression is difficult when a patient has a terminal illness – asking patients how they have felt in their mood or their spirits over the last week or a general 'How are you feeling in yourself' may be the opening the patient needs. Asking about previous history of depression and also establishing the patient's fears should also be part of the examination. Rating scales are widely used – the Hospital Anxiety and Depression scale (Zigmond and Snaith 1983) being the most frequently used. This scale, however, has poor validity in terminally ill patients and can be difficult to use (Lloyd-Williams *et al.* 2001). The Edinburgh depression scale has been found to have a sensitivity and specificity of over 80 per cent at a cut-off threshold of 13 and may be worth considering as an appropriate screening tool for palliative care (Lloyd-Williams *et al.* 2000, 2004c). Although developed for the use with mothers in the post-natal period, it contains symptoms such as hopelessness, worthlessness, guilt and thoughts of self-harm which are thought to be particularly discriminating symptoms in the palliative care population (Casey 1994). Further work on this tool has revealed that the Brief Edinburgh Scale (BEDS) is a sensitive tool when used in the palliative care setting (Lloyd-Williams *et al.* 2007). Researchers have suggested asking patients if they were depressed would be a useful indicator as to whether patients may be depressed (Chochinov *et al.* 1997) and reported a sensitivity and specificity of 100 per cent for this item making it almost a diagnostic tool. Further research in the UK population using the single question 'Are you depressed?' has found that this item does not perform so well (Lloyd-Williams *et al.* 2003). Additionally, patients under-report their psychological and psychiatric symptoms and may be reluctant to respond truthfully to such questions if asked in isolation (Maguire 1985). Visual analogue scales have been used in patients with cancer (Lees and Lloyd-Williams 1999), but the subjective experience of the patient may lead to either under- or overscoring and many patients experience difficulty in understanding the concept of a visual analogue scale. It must be stressed, however, that screening is not a solution in itself and that patients who are screened and score above a pre-determined and validated cut-off threshold require further assessment.

## Management of depression

The management of depression in palliative care patients is similar for all other patients but time is frequently shorter. Explaining to the patients and their relatives that depression is common in cancer can itself be part of the healing process, as many patients believe they are somehow not coping as they should. Trying to uncover what is really bothering the patient, that is in terms of their families, their disease or mode of death, can also help to lessen the feelings of isolation associated with depression. While psychological support is of course vital, there is no evidence to suggest that counselling alone is effective for these patients, indeed a recent study suggested that in patients for whom time is limited counselling alone should not be recommended (Chilvers *et al.* 2001).

Antidepressants are not prescribed as frequently as they should be (Lloyd-Williams *et al.* 1998; Maguire 2000). There is considerable debate as to which antidepressant to choose. Clinical evidence suggests that the Selective Serotonine Reuptake Inhibitors (SSRIs) cause fewer side effects in the terminally ill and are also safer in overdose. The main reason antidepressant therapy is ineffective is that it is commenced too late in the patient's illness or due to difficulties with compliance; considerable encouragement may be required to enable a patient to persevere with medication while waiting for a therapeutic benefit. It is suggested that, if possible, treatment should be maintained for at least three months. Patients may benefit from support from community nurses or palliative care specialist nurses. Complementary therapies, such as aromatherapy or relaxation, can also enhance a feeling of well-being and be of benefit to the patient. Seventy per cent of cancer patients treated with antidepressants had a full therapeutic response in one prospective study (Chaturvedi *et al.* 1994), but some patients may be very resistant to taking medication. A trial of one antidepressant for four to five weeks with no therapeutic benefit and proven compliance may require the intervention of a psychiatrist to assess the patient and suggest further strategies for management. Patients with long-standing mental health problems also develop life threatening illnesses and there may be particular issues surrounding medication, which may require specialist intervention from a psychiatrist.

Friends and relatives may require considerable support in knowing how to help the depressed patient who may have withdrawn from them. Again, like anxiety, there has been a number of studies conducted which have evaluated the use and effectiveness of self-management and non-pharmacological interventions for depression in palliative care patients. The mindfulness-based stress reduction programme, which consists of sitting meditation, body scan and mindful movements, appears to decrease depression and anxiety in patients with cancer (Speca *et al.* 2000; Carlson *et al.* 2001, 2003). A recent pragmatic two-armed randomized controlled trial based across four cancer centres and a hospice in the UK evaluated the effectiveness of supplementing usual supportive care with aromatherapy massage in the management of depression and anxiety in cancer patients, finding it confers clinically important benefit up to two weeks after implementing the intervention. However, it should be noted that no long-term benefits were identified (Wilkinson *et al.* 2007). In a recent uncontrolled clinical trial of homoeopathy for symptom relief in 100 cancer patients, of which 20 had been diagnosed with depression and 17 were judged as being borderline depressed (Thompson and Reilly 2002), 75 per cent of those patients taking part rated the homoeopathic treatment as having been helpful or better, with treatment producing a significant improvement in depression scores. St John's Wort has also frequently been shown to be an effective treatment option in depression, with effects comparable to the antidepressants sertraline and fluoxetine (Brenner *et al.* 2000; Schrader 2000; Fava *et al.* 2005; Linde *et al.* 2005). However, considerable care needs to be taken when using St John's Wort for patients with cancer, as it has been found to interact with the mechanism of action for a number of pharmaceutical interventions commonly used by patients with cancer including cyclosporine, hormones, antibiotics and chemotherapeutic agents (Quimby 2007).

# When things go wrong

Anecdotally, suicide is thought to be a rare event in terminally ill patients but a survey of palliative care units found 21 suicides and 37 attempted suicides within a five-year period in the UK (Grzybowska and Finlay 1997). Other studies have also found an increased suicide risk in both male and female terminally ill patients, although some have found a higher risk in men (Levi *et al.* 1991; Storm *et al.* 1992), while others report a higher risk among women (Crocetti *et al.* 1998; Tanaka *et al.* 1999). A recent population-based analysis of cancer patients concluded that the cancer patient most at risk of suicide was male, with head and neck cancer or myeloma, advanced disease, little social or cultural support, and with limited treatment options (Kendal 2007). When suicide does occur, support may be required not only for the family but also for other members of the team who may feel they have failed the patient.

# Supporting the staff

Some patients are very depressed at the end of life when little can be done therapeutically and occasionally all measures fail.

---

**Case history 14.2**

Penny was 42 and the mother of two children aged five and three when she presented with suicidal ideas and was admitted to the hospice with metastatic melanoma at the GP's request. She was withdrawn, agreed she was depressed and refused to get out of bed. Over a five-week period, staff spent a large amount of time encouraging her; she was offered several interventions including relaxation, aromatherapy, etc. all of which she declined. She was seen by a psychiatrist and agreed to take antidepressant medication but declined it two days later and remained withdrawn and uncommunicative until her death four weeks later.

After her death members of staff from all disciplines were left with feelings of despondency that they had done nothing to help her. During a discussion of the case it was realized that Penny had always remained in control during her life and by her actions remained in control during her dying – true holistic palliative care is all about acceptance and the knowledge that, despite combined best efforts, we won't always in our own view 'get it right', but it is staying alongside the patient whatever they are going through that is most important.

# Conclusion

Terminally ill patients frequently have concomitant psychiatric morbidity which is often not diagnosed (Rodin and Voshart 1986; Kathol *et al.* 1990; Pirl and Roth 1999; Murray *et al.* 2002). For example, it is estimated that depression will be a major symptom for a quarter of all patients admitted to a palliative care unit (Barraclough 1994), with many of these patients also exhibiting symptoms of anxiety as well (McCarthy *et al.* 1996). A number of patients exhibiting psychiatric morbidity may be reluctant to inform their treating health professionals that they are experiencing these symptoms. In addition, ethnocultural factors appear to influence both the ways in which patients respond to a terminal illness diagnosis, how they deal with the disease, and adjust to it; as well as the views and attitudes of those health professionals caring for them (Johnson 1998; Higginson and Costantini 2002; Lloyd-Williams 2003; Lloyd-Williams *et al.* 2004a).

Due to the amount of time nurses spend with terminally ill patients, and the intimate nature of the care they provide, nurses have an important role to play in the identification of patients who have psychiatric symptoms. An appreciation for the ways in which symptoms of psychiatric morbidity are expressed in terminally ill patients, and possessing the necessary communication and interpersonal skills to deal effectively with these patients, are both essential if patients are to receive optimal psychological care. When detected, depression and anxiety in terminally ill patients have been shown to respond to various pharmacological, self-management and non-pharmacological interventions. The recognition of psychological distress and the assessment and treatment of anxiety and depression are vital to ensure that patients are able to use and enjoy what remaining time they have left effectively.

# References

Addington-Hall, J. and McCarthy, M. (1995) Dying from cancer: Results of a national population-based investigation. *Palliative Medicine*, 9(4): 295–305.

Ahles, T.A., Tope, D.M., Pinkson, B., Walch, S., Hann, D., Whedon, M., Dain, B., Weiss, J.E., Mills, L. and Silberfarb, P.M. (1999) Massage therapy for patients undergoing autologous bone marrow transplantation. *Journal of Pain and Symptom Management*, 18(3): 157–63.

Akechi, T., Makano, T., Akizuki, N., Okamura, M., Sakuma, K., Nakanishi, T., Yoshikawa, E. and Uchitomi, Y. (2003) Somatic symptoms for diagnosing major depression in cancer patients. *Psychosomatics*, 44(3): 244–8.

Bailey, L.M. (1983) The effects of live music versus tape-recorded music on hospitalised cancer patients. *Music Therapy*, 3(1): 17–28.

Barraclough, J. (1994) *Cancer and Emotion.* Chichester: Wiley.

Bergevin, P. and Bergevin, R. (1995) Recognising Depression. *American Journal of Hospice and Palliative Care*, 12(5): 22–3.

Bindemann, S., Soukop, M. and Kaye, S.B. (1991) Randomised controlled study of relaxation training. *European Journal of Cancer*, 27: 170–4.

Boini, S., Briancon, S., Guillemin, F., Galan, P. and Hercberg, S. (2004) Impact of cancer occurrence on health-related quality of life: A longitudinal pre-post assessment. *Health and Quality of Life Outcomes*, 2(1): 4.

Brenner, R., Azbel, V., Madhusoodanan, S. and Pawlowska, M. (2000) Comparison of an extract of hypericum (LI 160) and sertraline in the treatment of depression: A double-blind, randomized pilot study. *Clinical Therapeutics*, 22(4): 411–19.

Buckberg, J., Penman, D. and Holland, J. (1984) Depression in hospitalised cancer patents. *Psychosomatic Medicine*, 46(3): 199–211.

Carlson, L.E., Speca, M., Patel, K.D. and Goodey, E. (2003) Mindfulness-based stress reduction in relation to quality of life, mood, symptoms of stress, and immune parameters in breast and prostate cancer outpatients. *Psychosomatic Medicine*, 65(4): 571–81.

Carlson, L.E., Ursuliak, Z., Goodey, E., Angen, M. and Speca, M. (2001) The effects of a mindfulness meditation-based stress reduction program on mood and symptoms of stress in cancer outpatients: 6-month follow-up. *Supportive Care Cancer*, 9(2): 112–23.

Casey, P. (1994) Depression in the dying – disorder or distress? *Progress in Palliative Care*, 2(1): 1–3.

Chaturvedi, S., Maguire, P. and Hopwood, P. (1994) Antidepressant medications in cancer patients. *Psycho-Oncology*, 3(1): 57–60.

Chilvers, C., Dewey, M., Fielding, K., Gretton, V., Miller, P., Palmer, B., Weller, D., Churchill, R., Williams, I., Bedi, N., Duggan, C., Lee, A. and Harrison, G. (2001) Antidepressant drugs and generic counselling for treatment of major depression in primary care: Randomised trial with patient preference arms. *British Medical Journal*, 322: 772–5.

Chochinov, H., Wilson, K., Enns, M. and Lander, S. (1997) Are you depressed? Screening for depression in the terminally ill. *American Journal of Psychiatry*, 154(5): 674–6.

Christensen, A. and Ehlers, S. (2002) Psychological factors in end-stage renal disease: An emerging context for behavioural medicine research. *Journal of Consulting and Clinical Psychology*, 70(3): 712–24.

Crocetti, E., Arniani, S., Acciai, S., Barchelli, A. and Buiatti, E. (1998) High suicide mortality soon after diagnosis among cancer patients in central Italy. *British Journal of Cancer*, 77: 1194–6.

Fallowfield, L., Ford, S. and Lewis, S. (1995) No news is not good news: Information preferences of patients with cancer. *Psycho-Oncology*, 4(3): 197–202.

Fallowfield, L., Ratcliffe, D., Jenkins, V. and Saul, J. (2001) Psychiatric morbidity and its recognition by doctors in patients with cancer. *British Journal of Cancer*, 84: 1011–15.

Fava, M., Alpert, J., Nierenberg, A.A., Mischoulon, D., Otto, M.W., Zajecka, J., Murck, H. and Rosenbaum, J.F. (2005) A double-blind, randomized trial of St John's Wort, fluoxetine, and placebo in major depressive disorder. *Journal of Clinical Psychopharmacology*, 25(5): 441–7.

Fellowes, D., Barnes, K. and Wilkinson, S. (2006) Aromatherapy and massage for symptom relief in patients with cancer. *Cochrane Database Systematic Reviews*, 4: CD002287.

Fincannon, J. (1995) Analysis of psychiatric referrals and interventions in an oncology population. *Oncology Nurses Forum*, 22(1): 87–92.

Formenti, S., Meyerowitx, B., Ell, K., Muderspach, L., Groshen, S., Leedham, B., Klement, V. and Morrow, P.C. (1995) Inadequate adherence to radiotherapy in Latino immigrants with carcinoma of the cervix. *Cancer*, 75(5): 1135–40.

Goldberg, R. and Cullen, L. (1986) Depression in geriatric cancer patients: Guide to assessment and treatment. *The Hospice Journal*, 2(2): 79–98.

Goodwin, D., Higginson, I., Myers, K., Douglas, H. and Normand, C. (2002) What is palliative day care? A patient perspective of five UK services. *Supportive Care Cancer*, 10(10): 556–62.

Gore, J., Brophy, C. and Greenstone, M. (2000) How well do we care for patients with end stage chronic pulmonary disease (COPD)? A comparison of palliative care and quality of life in COPD and lung cancer. *Thorax*, 55(12): 1000–6.

Grassi, L., Indelli, M., Marzalo, M., Maestri, A., Piva, E. and Boccalon, M. (1996) Depressive symptoms and quality of life in home-care assisted cancer patients. *Journal of Pain and Symptom Management*, 12(5): 300–7.

Grzybowska, P. and Finlay, I. (1997) The incidence of suicide in palliative care patients. *Palliative Medicine*, 11(4): 313–16.

Harrison, J., Maguire, P. and Pitceathly, C. (1995) Confiding in crisis: Gender differences in patterns of confiding among cancer patients. *Social Science and Medicine*, 41(9): 1255–60.

Higginson, I. and Costantini, M. (2002) Communication in end of life cancer care: A comparison of team assessments in three European countries. *Journal of Clinical Oncology*, 20(17): 3674–82.

Hilliard, R.E. (2005) Music therapy in hospice and palliative care: A review of the empirical data. *Evidence Based Complementary and Alternative Medicine*, 2(2): 173–8.

Hinton, J. (1963) The physical and mental distress of the dying. *Quarterly Journal of Medicine*, 32(1): 1–21.

Hipkins, J., Whitworth, M., Tarrier, N. and Jayson, G. (2004) Social support, anxiety and depression after chemotherapy for ovarian cancer: A prospective study. *British Journal of Health Psychology*, 9: 569–81.

Hotopf, M., Chidgey, J., Addington-Hall, J. and Lan, L.K. (2002) Depression in advanced disease: A systematic review. Part 1: Prevalence and case finding. *Palliative Medicine*, 16(2): 81–97.

Johnson, K.R.S. (1998) Ethnocultural influences in cancer. *Journal of Clinical Psychology in Medical Settings*, 5(3): 357–64.

Kathol, R., Noyes, R., Williams, J., Mutgi, A., Carroll, B. and Perry, P. (1990) Diagnosing depression in patients with medical illness. *Psychosomatics*, 31(4): 434–40.

Kazak, A.E., Penati, B., Boyer, B.A., Himelstein, B., Brophy, P., Waibel, M.K., Blackall, G.F., Daller, R. and Johnson, K. (1996) A randomized controlled prospective outcome study of a psychological and pharmacological intervention protocol for procedural distress in pediatric leukaemia. *Journal of Pediatric Psychology*, 21(5): 615–31.

Kendal, W.S. (2007) Suicide and cancer: A gender-comparative study. *Annals of Oncology*, 18(2): 381–7.

Kimmel, P. (2002) Depression in patients with chronic renal disease: What we know and what we need to know. *Journal of Psychosomatic Research*, 53(4): 951–6.

Lees, N. and Lloyd-Williams, M. (1999) Assessing depression in palliative care patients using the Visual Analogue Scale: A pilot study. *European Journal of Cancer Care*, 8(4): 220–3.

Levi, F., Bulliard, J.L. and la Vecchia, C. (1991) Suicide risk among incident cases of cancer in the Swiss national canton of Vaud. *Oncology*, 48: 44–7.

Linde, K., Mulrow, C.D., Berner, M. and Egger, M. (2005) St John's Wort for depression. *Cochrane Database of Systematic Reviews*, 2: CD000448.

Lloyd-Williams, M. (2000) Difficulties in diagnosing and treating depression in the terminally ill cancer patient. *Postgraduate Medical Journal*, 76(899): 555–8.

Lloyd-Williams, M. (2003) A comparison of attitudes of medical students in England and in South Africa towards patients with life-limiting illness. *Journal of Palliative Care*, 19(3): 188–91.

Lloyd-Williams, M., Dennis, M., Taylor, F. and Baker, I. (2003) A prospective study to determine whether it is appropriate to ask palliative care patients 'are you depressed?' *British Medical Journal*, 327: 372–3.

Lloyd-Williams, M., Dogra, N. and Petersen, S. (2004a) First year medical students' attitudes towards patients with life-limiting illness: Does age make a difference? *Palliative Medicine*, 18(2): 137–8.

Lloyd-Williams, M., Dennis, M. and Taylor, F. (2004b) A prospective study to determine the association between physical symptoms and depression in patients with advanced cancer. *Palliative Medicine*, 18(6): 558–63.

Lloyd-Williams, M., Dennis, M. and Taylor, F. (2004c) A prospective study to compare three depression screening tools in patients who are terminally ill. *General Hospital Psychiatry*, 26: 384–9.

Lloyd-Williams, M., Friedman, T. and Rudd, N. (1998) A survey of antidepressant prescribing in hospices. *Palliative Medicine*, 13(3): 293–8.

Lloyd-Williams, M., Friedman, T. and Rudd, N. (2000) The validation of the Edinburgh Postnatal Depression Scale in the terminally ill population. *Journal of Pain and Symptom Management*, 20(4): 259–65.

Lloyd-Williams, M., Friedman, T. and Rudd, N. (2001) The validation of the Hospital Anxiety and Depression scale in terminally ill patients. *Journal of Pain and Symptom Management*, 22(6): 990–6.

Lloyd-Williams, M., Shiels, C. and Dowrick, C. (2007) The development of the Brief Edinburgh Depression Scale (BEDS) to screen for depression in patients with advanced cancer. *Journal of Affective Disorders*, 99: 259–64.

Luddington, L., Cox, S., Higginson, I. and Livesley, B. (2001) The need for palliative care for patients with non-cancer diseases: A review of the evidence. *International Journal of Palliative Nursing*, 7(5): 221–6.

Maguire, C., Kirby, M. and Cohen, R. (1996) Family members' attitudes toward telling the patient with Alzheimer's disease their diagnosis. *British Medical Journal*, 313: 529–30.

Maguire, P. (1985) Improving the detection of psychiatric problems in cancer patients. *Social Science and Medicine*, 20(8): 819–23.

Maguire, P. (2000) The use of antidepressants in patients with advanced cancer. *Supportive Care and Cancer*, 8(4): 265–7.

Maguire, P. and Howell, A. (1995) Improving the psychological care of cancer patients. In: A. Houses, R. Mayou and C. Mallinson (eds) *Psychiatric Aspects of Physical Disease*. London: Royal College of Physicians and Royal College of Psychiatrists.

Massie, M. and Holland, J. (1992) The cancer patient with pain: Psychiatric complications and their management. *Journal of Pain and Symptom Management*, 7(2): 99–109.

McCarthy, M., Lay, M. and Addington-Hall, J. (1996) Dying from heart disease. *Journal of the Royal College of Physicians of London*, 30(4): 325–8.

McVey, P. (1998) Depression among the palliative care oncology population. *International Journal of Palliative Nursing*, 4(2): 86–93.

Mechatie, E. (1997) New Alzheimer's drug delays sentence. *Clinical Psychiatric News*, 25(1): 28.

Meyers, B. (1997) Telling patients they have Alzheimer's disease. *British Medical Journal*, 314: 321–2.

Minagawa, H., Uchitomi, Y., Yamawaki, S. and Ishitani, K. (1996) Psychiatric morbidity in terminally ill cancer patients: A prospective study. *Cancer*, 78(5): 1131–7.

Murray, S.A., Boyd, K., Kendall, M., Worth, A., Benton, T.F. and Clausen, H. (2002) Dying of lung cancer or cardiac failure: Prospective qualitative interview study of patients and their carers in the community. *British Medical Journal*, 325: 929.

Novotony, E., Hyland, J., Coyne, L., Travis, J. and Pruyser, H. (1984) Factors affecting adjustment to cancer. *Bulletin of the Menninger Clinic*, 48(4): 318–28.

Olmsted, R.W., Zeltzer, L. and LeBaron, S. (1982) Hypnosis and nonhypnotic techniques for reduction of pain and anxiety during painful procedures in children and adolescents with cancer. *Journal of Pediatrics*, 101(6): 1032–5.

Ormrod, J. and Leadhead, E., (1999) Anxiety management in groups: An evaluation. *Mental Health Nursing*, 19(2): 8–10.

Osborn, R.L., Demoncade, A.C. and Feuerstein, M. (2006) Psychosocial interventions for depression, anxiety, and quality of life in cancer survivors: Meta-analyses. *International Journal of Psychiatry in Medicine*, 36(1): 13–34.

Pasacreta, J. and Massie, M. (1990) Nurses reports of psychiatric complications in patients with cancer. *Oncology Nurses Forum*, 17(3): 347–53.

Perez-Stable, E.J., Sabogal, F., Otero-Sabogal, R., Hiatt, R.A. and McPhee, S.J. (1992) Misconceptions about cancer among Latinos and Anglos. *Journal of the American Medical Association*, 268(22): 3219–23.

Pirl, W. and Roth, A. (1999) Diagnosis and treatment of depression in cancer patients. *Oncology*, 13(9): 1293–302.

Prior, S. (1998) Determining the effectiveness of a short-term anxiety management course. *British Journal of Occupational Therapy*, 61(5): 207–13.

Quattrin, R., Zanini, A., Buchini, S., Turello, D., Annunziata, M.A., Vidotti, C., Colombatti, A. and Brusaferro, S. (2006) Use of reflexology foot massage to reduce anxiety in hospitalised cancer patients in chemotherapy treatment: Methodology and outcomes. *Journal of Nursing Management*, 14(2): 96–105.

Quimby, E.L. (2007) The use of herbal therapies in pediatric oncology patients: treating symptoms of cancer and side effects of standard therapies. *Journal of Pediatric Oncology Nursing*, 24(1): 35–40.

Ramsay, N. (1992) Referral to a liaison psychiatrist from a palliative care unit. *Palliative Medicine*, 6(1): 54–60.

Reuter, K. and Harter, M. (2004) The concepts of fatigue and depression in cancer. *European Journal of Cancer Care*, 13(2): 127–34.

Rodin, G. and Voshart, K. (1986) Depression in the medically ill: An overview. *American Journal of Psychiatry*, 143(6): 696–705.

Ross, C.S.K., Hamilton, J., Macrae, G., Docherty, C., Gould, A. and Cornbleet, M.A. (2002) A pilot study to evaluate the effect of reflexology on mood and symptom rating of advanced cancer patients. *Palliative Medicine*, 16(6): 544–5.

Schrader, E. (2000) Equivalence of St John's Wort extract (Ze 117) and fluoxetine: A randomized, controlled study in mild-moderate depression. *International Clinical Psychopharmacology*, 15(2): 61–8.

Sharpe, M., Strong, V., Allen, K., Rush, R., Postma, K., Tulloh, A., Maguire, P., House, A., Ramirez, A. and Cull, A. (2004) Major depression in outpatients attending a regional cancer centre: Screening and unmet treatment needs. *British Journal of Cancer*, 90(2): 314–20.

Singer, H., Ruchinskas, R., Riley, K., Broshek, D. and Barth, J. (2001) The psychological impact of end-stage lung disease. *Chest*, 120(4): 1246–52.

Speca, M., Carlson, L.E., Goodey, E. and Angen, M. (2000) A randomized, wait-list controlled clinical trial: The effect of a mindfulness meditation-based stress reduction program on mood and symptoms of stress in cancer outpatients. *Psychosomatic Medicine*, 62(5): 613–22.

Steifel, F. and Razavi, D. (1994) Common psychiatric disorders in cancer patients: Anxiety and acute confusional states. *Supportive Care in Cancer*, 2(4): 233–7.

Stephenson, N.L., Weinrich, S.P. and Tavakoli, A.S. (2000) The effects of foot reflexology on anxiety and pain in patients with breast and lung cancer. *Oncology Nursing Forum*, 27(1): 67–72.

Storm, H.H., Christensen, N. and Jensen, O.M. (1992) Suicides among Danish patients with cancer: 1971 to 1986. *Cancer*, 69: 1507–12.

Tanaka, H., Tsukuma, H., Masaoka, T., Ajiki, W., Koyama, Y., Kinoshita, N., Hasuo, S. and Oshima, A. (1999) Suicide risk among cancer patients: Experience at one medical center in Japan, 1978–1994. *Japanese Journal of Cancer Research*, 90(8): 812–17.

Tavio, M., Milan, I. and Tirelli, V. (2002) Cancer related fatigue (review). *International Journal of Oncology*, 21(5): 1093–9.

Thompson, E.A. and Reilly, D. (2002) The homeopathic approach to symptom control in the cancer patient: A prospective observational study. *Palliative Medicine*, 16(3): 227–33.

Wall, V.J. and Womack, W. (1989) Hypnotic versus active cognitive strategies for alleviation of procedural distress in pediatric oncology patients. *American Journal of Clinical Hypnosis*, 31: 181–91.

Wilkinson, S.M., Love, S.B., Westcombe, A.M., Gambles, M.A., Burgess, C.C., Cargill, A., Young, T., Maher, E.J. and Ramirez, A.J. (2007) Effectiveness of aromatherapy massage in the management of anxiety and depression in patients with cancer: A multicenter randomized controlled trial. *Journal of Clinical Oncology*, 25(5): 532–9.

Zigmond, A.S. and Snaith, R.P. (1983) The Hospital Anxiety and Depression Scale. *Acta Psychiatry Scandinavia*, 67(6): 361–70.

# 15

# Psychiatric aspects of palliative care

*William Lee and Matthew Hotopf*

---

**Key points**

- Psychiatric disorders are common, frequently missed, and adversely affect the quality of life of patients.
- Precise diagnosis is important because organic disorders can mimic psychiatric disorders.
- The best management of psychiatric disorders in palliative care is multidisciplinary, with pharmacological, psychotherapeutic and team approaches recommended.
- Nurses are uniquely placed to detect mental health problems and to instigate discussion with or referral to mental health services.

---

## Introduction

This chapter provides an overview of psychiatry in palliative care. We start by introducing some concepts fundamental to psychiatry, including definitions of health and illness and the psychiatric assessment. We then describe some of the key psychiatric problems as they present to us in palliative care. The most common such presentation – anxiety, depression and adjustment to illness – is dealt with in Chapter 14 and will not be covered here. However, we focus instead on:

- delirium
- dementia
- psychotic illness
- 'difficult' cases

- psychiatric services
- when to refer to psychiatry.

# What is psychiatry?

Psychiatry is the branch of medicine which concerns disorders of the 'higher' human functions such as beliefs, mood and perception: mental disorders. Mental disorders are common and are a major cause of disability in all populations, including individuals with advanced disease. Mental disorders are also strongly associated with disability in individuals with physical disease: having advanced disease is bad enough – but it is often the presence of a mental disorder which really affects the person's ability to go about their normal day-to-day life. In palliative care there is also a wider impact – on the families and carers of patients, and on staff.

# Normal and abnormal states

In psychiatry we do not rely on physical investigations to make diagnosis – instead diagnosis is based on groups of symptoms. In order to ensure psychiatrists around the world speak the same language, diagnostic systems such as DSM-IV and the ICD-10 (World Health Organization 1992; American Psychiatric Association 1994) set out diagnostic criteria for each disorder. As symptoms are subjective, the division between health and disease is particularly difficult in psychiatry. Some psychiatric symptoms such as command auditory hallucinations (where a patient hears voices telling him or her what to do) are clearly abnormal. Other symptoms are ordinary experiences which most people recognize; low mood is a good example. Not everyone who experiences episodes of sadness is suffering from a mental disorder. Several factors distinguish the psychiatric disorder (depression) from normal low mood: the duration of the symptom (in depression, low mood has to have been present for at least two weeks); the form of the symptom (normal sadness waxes and wanes, low mood in depression is stable); associated symptoms (the diagnosis of depression requires the presence of other psychological and biological symptoms such as guilty ideas and poor sleep); and most importantly whether the symptom has an impact on the person's ability to function. Function can be considered in many domains, for example occupational, domestic and social. For medically well adults missing work is a key indicator, but among palliative care patients, where many are retired or too physically unwell to be working, disability is best assessed by looking at the person's ability to enjoy hobbies, carry out day-to-day activities and, crucially, to engage in social relationships.

# The psychiatric assessment

Psychiatric assessment is the process by which a psychiatric diagnosis is arrived at and a plan of action made. At a minimum this consists of a thorough case-note review and an interview with the patient, though it can also be important to gain collateral histories from carers, family members and other professionals.

### Referral

Not many palliative care providers have access to specialized mental health services (Price *et al.* 2006) and referral may be a delicate process. Patients are often reluctant to see a mental health professional, particularly if services involve a trip to another hospital or community clinic. However, the fear that a patient may be upset by the idea of a psychiatric referral should not prevent it from happening. In our experience, patients are usually receptive to the idea that having suffered with a severe physical disease it is understandable that this has had an impact on their mental health, and it can be useful to discuss this with a specialist.

### Interview

Psychiatry and palliative care both place great emphasis on a patient-centred approach and listening is key to this. The first interview usually lasts at least an hour, and although there are cases when the time is reduced because the person is too frail, it is surprising how long many patients want to talk. We usually start the interview by giving the patient an opportunity to talk freely and without interruption for several minutes, where necessary using open questions. During this time the primary concerns of the patient often surface, and these will guide the remainder of the interview. A crucial part of psychiatric history taking in palliative care is asking the person to describe the disease journey, from symptoms, to going to the doctor, to having a diagnosis made, and so on. Distress is often focused on self-blame for not presenting early, or blame at doctors for not taking symptoms seriously.

Although the interview will cover the familiar elements of medical history taking, including the presenting complaint, past medical history and drug history, greater emphasis is placed on the personal history (see Box 15.1) and the mental state examination.

Another key aspect of the psychiatric assessment is gaining an informant's view of the patient. Patients may often downplay symptoms, while relatives are increasingly worried, and this happens particularly when there is a lack of insight or denial.

> **Box 15.1** Personal history
>
> The personal history is a chronology of the patient's life from birth to the present, including developmental milestones, childhood experiences, education, relationships, training, occupations, children, illnesses, forensic history and anything else the patient reveals when asked about their life. It is important to strike a balance between covering all the domains of the patient's life and allowing unexpected themes to develop.
>
> This allows the interviewer to place the current situation in the context of the whole life of the patient, and to better understand how the patient has dealt with past difficulties. Gaining a good personal history contextualizes the patient's distress, helps the patient engage, and can be therapeutic in its own right, helping the patient and the psychiatrist identify key strengths or resources.

### Mental state examination

The mental state examination is the psychiatrist's equivalent to the physical examination of medical consultations. It is a structured assessment of the patient's current mental state, broken down into sections. Many of the key parts of the mental state may be revealed as the interview progresses rather than during a separate part of the interview, as in a physical examination.

#### Appearance and behaviour

This is a short description of the patient's presentation including indications of self-care, eye contact, demeanour, ability to build rapport during the interview as well as a description of any abnormal activities such as responding to hallucinations.

#### Speech

This section describes the form of the speech (rate, rhythm, spontaneity and volume). It is important to determine whether the speech is understandable – it may not be because of dysarthria (usually a problem with the motor components of speech); expressive dysphasia (a higher neurological problem which affects the patient's ability to find certain words or form meaningful sentences); or 'formal thought disorder', which occurs in schizophrenia and other psychotic illness, where the speech superficially appears understandable, but is in fact unintelligible.

#### Mood

This section records a patient's mood (as described by the patient) and affect (the mood as observed by the interviewer). It is important to observe whether the affect fluctuates during the interview (i.e. is reactive), or whether the patient appears low throughout. Mood may also be elated as in mania or intoxication. Also recorded are the indicators of depression such as biological symptoms, including poor sleep, diurnal variation of mood (in depression of the mood to be worse in the morning and improve later in the day), anhedonia (inability to be happy) and suicidal ideas. Asking about suicidal ideas is a core skill (see Box 15.2).

## Thoughts

This section attempts to describe the patient's main preoccupations. The anxious or obsessional patient may have repetitive, unpleasant or violent thoughts which are experienced as intrusive and distressing. The depressed patient may have guilty preoccupations or believe they are impoverished.

---

**Box 15.2**  Suicidality

Asking about suicidality does not increase prevalence of suicidal ideas (Gould *et al.* 2005), and so is not thought to increase the risk of completed suicide. Asking about suicidality is central to good mental health care.

Suicide is a big killer of the young and is the biggest killer of young men under the age of 35 in the UK. The biggest personal risk factor for completed suicide is a previous attempt. That noted, it is still a rare event, occurring in approximately eight people per 100,000 population per year.

Suicidal feelings are very common, occurring in 10 per cent of the whole population every week, so mild and transient suicidal feelings are not in themselves a need for intensive intervention.

Psychiatrists divide suicidality into three levels of severity: suicidal ideation, suicidal intent and suicidal plans. All of these need to be asked about when assessing suicidality. Suicidal ideation is having ideas of suicide, or even having ideas that life is not worth living, which is called passive suicidal ideation. Suicidal intent is having an intention to commit suicide at some time. A suicidal plan is having made a plan to commit suicide, which includes having decided on a method, made preparations, and 'final acts' such as giving away property or putting affairs in order. This represents a highly significant risk.

Open questions such as 'When you're feeling depressed, have you ever felt that there is no hope or that you will never feel better?' make a good beginning. Questions such as 'Do you find yourself feeling desperate with your current situation?' or 'Do you feel that life is worth living?' build up to the key 'screening question' similar to 'Have you thought about harming yourself?' If this is answered in the affirmative, then more closed questions should be asked to ensure that all the levels of suicidality are covered including questions about intent, timing, methods and final acts.

Management will depend on the results of the assessment of suicidality and factors including the history and home situation. For example, someone who lives alone and has a history of previous attempts is more likely to need admission for his or her own safety than someone who has no history and lives with someone who is prepared to stay with him or her.

The manic patient may, by contrast, have grandiose ideas that they are in some way gifted, wealthy or in touch with a higher power.

### Abnormal beliefs and experiences

This section records the symptoms of psychotic disorders such as schizophrenia. This includes delusions and hallucinations, as well as the other symptoms of psychosis such as thought broadcast, insertion and withdrawal.

### Cognitive state

This primarily assesses orientation in time, place and person, and includes computational tasks and tasks requiring attention and concentration. Cognitive impairment is the primary indicator of organic disorders such as delirium and dementia, which are described later.

### Insight

Insight describes how well the person understands both the physical disease and any mental disorder. It is useful to describe three areas: whether the patient is aware that he or she has a mental disorder; whether he or she is able to label psychic experiences as resulting from a mental disorder; and whether he or she understands the need for treatment. Thus a depressed patient will typically agree that they are depressed, but may not recognize their guilty preoccupations as a sign of depression and may disagree to taking medication, perhaps because they think they deserve to be depressed, or are not worthy of medical care.

### Formulation

At the end of a psychiatric assessment a synthesis or 'formulation' of the problem is made, which may contain a psychiatric diagnosis. A plan of action is also decided upon after consultation with the patient, carers, family and other members of the clinical team. This will concentrate on the changeable elements of the problem.

Causative factors for mental health problems are conventionally divided up into the three 'Ps': *predisposing*, *precipitating* and *perpetuating* factors. Each of these can be *biological*, *psychological* or *social* in nature. This is known as the biopsychosocial approach, and provides the framework for the formulation and the plan of action.

# Psychiatric disorders

Psychiatric disorders are diagnosed on the basis of several symptoms being present at the same time. This means that a single individual symptom is rarely diagnostic. A person may be agitated because they are very anxious, or suffering from a psychotic illness, or because they are withdrawing from alcohol. Since these diagnoses lead to different management plans, each with a different urgency, psychiatrists place disorders in a hierarchy from organic states at the top to personality disorders at the bottom (see Figure 15.1). The purpose of this hierarchy is that the consequences of missing organic disorders are more severe than of missing – say – an anxiety disorder.

### Organic states

In disorders such as delirium and dementia, direct physical processes cause changes in behaviour and functioning which are important to recognize because identifying the problem may lead to a radically different management plan. Any psychiatric symptom can appear in an organic state, so it is important always to consider organic disorders.

### Cognitive impairment

This is a reduction in the higher cognitive functions of the brain, and is the central sign that a psychiatrist will assess to determine probability of an organic cause of a problem. Disorientation in time (confusing the time of day or date) and place (e.g. not knowing where one is) are key clinical features which suggest an organic disorder. Other key cognitive functions are memory (does the person remember simple bits of information?); language function (e.g. receptive and expressive dysphasias); concentration and attention; gnosis (the ability to interpret sensory input, e.g. recognize a face); and praxis (the ability to carry out planned actions).

Cognitive assessment can range from very simple observations which identify that a patient is 'confused', to detailed clinical and neuro-psychological assessments. There are numerous clinical tools to identify problems. One of the best known is the Mini-Mental State Examination (Folstein *et al.* 1975), which covers a range of cognitive functions including orientation, memory and attention. This is scored out of 30 and a score of less than 24 indicates significant cognitive impairment. A problem with such

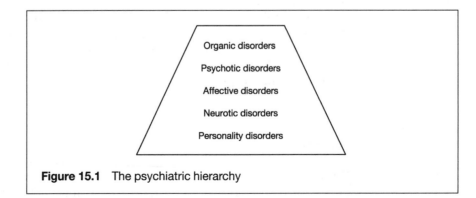

Organic disorders

Psychotic disorders

Affective disorders

Neurotic disorders

Personality disorders

**Figure 15.1**   The psychiatric hierarchy

tests is that they often lack acceptability to patients, who may dislike being asked directly if they know the date or where they are. An alternative screen for cognitive impairment is the clock drawing test (Sunderland *et al.* 1989). The patient is asked to draw a clock showing a particular time, and this drawing is assessed and scored out of ten by the assessor. It has greater acceptability to patients, carers and staff and performs as well as other tests (Henderson *et al.* 2007).

Below are some images of the clock drawing test carried out by a patient as she recovers from delirium caused by a urine infection (Shulman 2000):

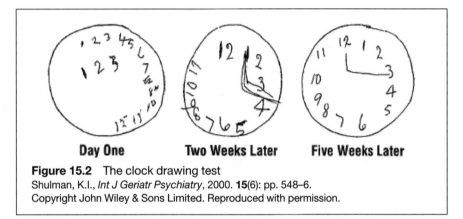

**Day One**          **Two Weeks Later**          **Five Weeks Later**

**Figure 15.2**   The clock drawing test
Shulman, K.I., *Int J Geriatr Psychiatry*, 2000. **15**(6): pp. 548–6.
Copyright John Wiley & Sons Limited. Reproduced with permission.

## Delirium

**Case history 15.1**

Maureen is 78 and has pancreatic cancer which is advanced with liver metastases. She lives in her own home with her husband. She is admitted to hospital because of a sudden deterioration in her condition, with a pyrexia, cough and shortness of breath. A chest infection is diagnosed. While in hospital she becomes very agitated thinking that she has been evacuated in the Second World War, and seeing those around her as being in some general way threatening. She describes seeing several large dogs in her room. Her agitation fluctuates – some of the time she is restless, irritable and trying to leave the ward, and at other times, she appears drowsy.

Delirium is a state of acute and potentially reversible cognitive impairment. The most important distinguishing features of delirium are an acute onset; a fluctuating course of the cognitive impairment; and a varying level of consciousness. There is usually a recent and obvious change in behaviour, and patients may fluctuate between being agitated, confused and fearful – possibly experiencing visual hallucinations – to being withdrawn or drowsy.

Some patients predominantly show a hypoactive form of delirium which may be confused with depression.

The list of causes of delirium is practically endless. Nearly all physical diseases can cause it, but the most likely causes are infection (chest, as in Maureen's case, or urinary), metabolic (hypoxia, uraemia), drugs and dehydration. The most common reversible cause of delirium in advanced disease is drug treatment (Lawlor *et al.* 2000). Although these are acute precipitants, it is better to consider the cause of delirium as a two-stage process: some individuals are more vulnerable to get it (predisposed) and require a less severe problem (precipitant) to cause it. The predisposing factors which reduce the delirium threshold are: age, having dementia, having poor nutrition or hydration status, having sensory impairments (visual or auditory), suffering from multiple physical diseases and taking multiple medicines. People with these frailties are particularly prone to become delirious when ill and placed in an unfamiliar environment (as in the case history). If predisposing factors can be identified and reversed, and if patients can be nursed in an environment where sleep/wake cycles are enhanced and noise and other confusing stimuli are minimized, then delirium can potentially be avoided (Inouye 2000).

In the general medical setting the management of delirium usually involves identifying and treating the cause, as well as providing appropriate nursing care. In palliative care there may be less focus on managing the cause, and more on providing the right nursing environment: this should be in a single room, with attention paid to each patient's own likes and dislikes. There is a role for using medication, such as low dose antipsychotics, to manage symptoms of delirium if they are very distressing, but only after other avenues have been exhausted.

### Dementia

---

**Case history 15.2**

Gerald is an 83-year-old man with lung cancer, diagnosed four months ago. He has been admitted to a hospice because his pain has been difficult to manage. He lives alone. He has told the hospice he is suspicious of his niece (the nearest relative) of stealing his money. The team talk to her and she says he has been forgetful for the past two years and has at times accused her of stealing his money, usually when he has lost his wallet. When admitted, he has difficulties finding his way around the ward, and when started on his usual dose of opiates, appears drowsy. It transpires that he has not been taking his analgesia at home.

---

Dementia is a chronic and progressive impairment of cognitive function, which is increasingly common due to the ageing population. As in the case history, a collateral history usually reveals a progressive course. Dementia has many underlying pathologies, the most common of which is Alzheimer's disease. Risk factors include age, vascular risk factors (hypertension, diabetes, smoking) and family history. Rarely, dementia is caused by a reversible problem (for example, a brain tumour or subdural haemorrhage). Dementia and delirium frequently co-exist – patients with dementia have less reserve against an acute illness and so readily develop delirium.

Typically the first symptoms of dementia are memory impairments, usually for short-term memory, with sparing of biographical information until later in the disease. Memory changes are often accompanied by mood disorder (depression), changes in personality, and frequently psychotic symptoms like hallucinations or delusions. The patient may accuse others of stealing personal belongings which have been lost. As the disorder progresses patients often find it difficult to recognize common objects (agnosia), or to carry out simple commands (apraxia), and later still the person loses language skills, develops incontinence and develops focal motor impairments.

In palliative care, the management of dementia is likely to be strongly influenced by the stage a patient is in their disease process. Dementia may cause difficulties for families, clinicians and patients if the person is unable to understand the nature of their illness, or treatment decisions relating to this.

### Psychosis

Psychosis is the term used for the mental state of a person disconnected from reality, often suffering with delusions and/or hallucinations. Psychosis is caused by a number of factors and can be part of organic states, but this section concerns functional mental illnesses associated with psychosis with no organic element.

#### Delusions

These are fixed, false beliefs that are held against societal norms, and despite evidence to the contrary. They may take many forms including being grandiose ('I am King of Lesotho'), persecutory ('the police are trying to kill me') or bizarre ('there is a microchip in my abdomen communicating with the clouds'). What makes a delusion is not so much the nature of the belief (many people hold irrational beliefs which are not delusions) but the form of the belief – the belief is typically formed with no credible evidence and is held with complete conviction. While religious beliefs might be said to share some of these characteristics, the belief in a delusion is usually not shared by other people within society. It is important therefore to gain an understanding of a person's cultural background when assessing delusions.

#### Hallucinations

A hallucination is a perception without an object. Typically the patient hears a voice which no one else can hear. The hallucination is experienced in external space – as if someone has spoken. Hallucinations can be in any sensory modality, including sound, sight, smell, touch, taste and internal sensations. Visual hallucinations strongly suggest an organic disorder.

### Illusions

Illusions occur when an existing object is in some way distorted. This can be a normal experience, particularly when tired, but illusions are frequently experienced both in delirium and opiate use. Typically a patient will complain that a familiar object has taken a more sinister form, and will usually recognize that this is 'my mind playing tricks on me'.

Other symptoms of psychosis include the symptoms of *thought insertion*, where the sensation is of thoughts being placed in the mind and *thought withdrawal*, where there is a feeling of thoughts being removed and *thought broadcasting*, where a person feels their own thoughts are available to other people.

## Schizophrenia

---

**Case history 15.3**

Paul is a 41-year-old man who has been diagnosed with malignant melanoma, which at the time of diagnosis was widely disseminated. He has a long history of schizophrenia and has had several admissions to psychiatric hospital, usually because he has been suicidal in response to auditory hallucinations. He lives in a hostel and is known to be somewhat reclusive. Although he has always disagreed that he has schizophrenia, and is sometimes reluctant to take medication, he seemed very accepting of the diagnosis of malignancy, understands the implications and is always highly cooperative with staff.

---

Schizophrenia is a chronic mental illness characterized by a decline in general functioning and capability with occasional episodes of psychosis, sometimes requiring admission to psychiatric hospital for treatment. The illness usually appears in late teens or 20s and affects women and men equally. There is no cure but there is a large variation in outcome from high-functioning individuals with one or two psychotic episodes in the past to the so-called 'defect state' of poor self-care, social withdrawal and difficulty maintaining employment.

Although there is an association between schizophrenia and violence, most patients with schizophrenia are not violent, and most of the violence encountered in the palliative care setting will not be due to schizophrenia. It is important to note that while patients with schizophrenia may lack insight about their mental illness, they will – like Paul – often have a good understanding of their physical disease, and be perfectly well able to make decisions.

### Treatment of schizophrenia

The mainstay of treatment for schizophrenia is antipsychotic medication, though an increasing role for talking treatments is now being recognized. Medication is effective at shortening and preventing episodes of psychosis. It is needed both during and for at least six months after episodes of psychosis, though many patients need to take them long term to prevent relapses. Antipsychotic medication is usually taken by mouth, but in cases where patients find taking tablets difficult a weekly or monthly injection can be used. When a patient suffers with a psychotic relapse, inpatient treatment is often necessary, sometimes involuntarily using the Mental Health Act to detain a patient in hospital. Treatment at home is also possible. The key to palliative care success in this patient group is close liaison between the palliative care team and the mental health team.

# 'Difficult' cases

The hospice setting can appear to be solely a place where expertise in the care of dying people is dispensed; however, this is not the only thing that defines a hospice: there is a set of conventions with which most people comply most of the time regarding inpatient health care: Staff are courteous and thoughtful. Patients are obedient and grateful. Domestic routines are regular and rigorous. Relatives, carers and other visitors cooperate with the team. Voices are hushed. When these conventions are not respected, difficulties can arise, even if the deviations from the norms do not affect patient care at all. Some individuals have difficulties with complying with these conventions and this can affect their care. Recognizing that not all behaviour should be interpreted at face value, and that unconscious mechanisms may be at work, can be helpful (Speck 1994). When patients or their families deviate from these norms they are often said to be 'difficult'.

---

**Case history 15.4**

---

Francesca is a 49-year-old woman with breast cancer, who is married to Mark with three children aged 10, 14 and 17. Francesca was diagnosed three years before. She admitted that she had not gone to the doctor for some time with a lump in her breast. Despite the delay, she was given an 'all clear' after treatment. There was a local recurrence three months earlier and since then she has undergone further surgery. She is withdrawn and has been suicidal. Mark has responded to the situation with anger – he has accused the surgeon and oncologist who first treated her of negligence, and has written numerous letters of complaint to various figures in authority about this. The couple were very angry when palliative care input was suggested and nurses visiting have felt threatened by Mark's presence. Francesca has fallen out with two nurses because they were 'rude', and Mark has made further complaints to the hospice. Francesca now has a nurse whom she likes but calls her repeatedly throughout the day usually because of worsening symptoms.

Every palliative care clinician will have experienced difficult cases. Occasionally even first-class delivery of care results in acrimony, complaints, shouting, tears, disagreements within the team, and worse. For apparently mysterious reasons, constructive communications between the clinical team and a patient, carer or whole family breaks down. The ordinary functioning of a team, or even a whole organization, can fail. Colleagues may find themselves divided along lines of allegiance to one side or the other. Emotions predominate and the atmosphere is unpleasant for all involved.

### Psychodynamic theory

The strong emotions experienced in such cases can be bewildering and it is here that psychodynamic theory can be helpful. Core ideas developed by Freud and subsequent theorists emphasize several important themes. The first is the way in which unconscious desires and motives can be expressed in behaviours or interactions which are not immediately recognized for what they are. The second is the way in which development – particularly early experiences of relationships – may impact upon the way in which later experiences are interpreted.

### The unconscious and defence mechanisms

The unconscious mind is seen as having many unacceptable desires and goals. The defence mechanisms are theorized as methods by which unconscious motives are prevented from overwhelming the conscious mind, which describe problematic responses to circumstances which seem to defy straightforward explanation.

*Projection*

This is when a person's own unacceptable unconscious feelings are perceived to be coming from someone else. For example, a carer of a frail elderly person make many unjustified complaints that health care staff are wanting to kill that person, with no credible evidence. This can be understood as the carer's own unconscious, unacceptable desire for the death of the person they care for as being 'projected' onto the health care workers. In Mark's case (above) it may be that his anger at the clinicians is a projection of (unacceptable) anger he feels towards Francesca for presenting late and being ill, possibly leaving him with three children.

### Splitting

Here objects are perceived as either 'all good' or 'all bad'. It is thought to represent a normal early state of development for an infant but is frequently seen in clinical settings with adults. In the health care setting individuals may express wishes to be cared for only by certain members of staff, idealizing them and demonizing others. Abruptly, due to some perceived slight or deficit, the situation may switch around and different members of the team may find themselves denigrated or idolized. This can be distressing and disorientating for the team and may even affect relationships between team members. Staff who have been denigrated in this way may find themselves angry with the patient, disappointed with other team members who have had no difficulties, and may even be affected by the flattery that is part of being idealized. It is clear in Francesca's case that the experience of the previous two nurses will make the present one feel uncomfortable – she may remain favoured but if she does not live up to these expectations she may find herself denigrated.

## Managing a 'difficult' case

Like every other case, each 'difficult' case is different, but there are some techniques which may help the clinical team continue to deliver a high standard of care.

### Recognize you have a 'difficult' case

Sometimes this is very clear, but often the recognition that a difficulty is arising happens later than would be optimal, causing problems later on. Key elements to be aware of are flattery of individual members of the team, and criticizing absent individuals or organizations, especially previous health care providers. This is not to suggest that such criticisms are invalid but if the patient is praising the hospice while denigrating every other service, or making escalating demands which seem to serve little purpose, there may be difficulties ahead.

### Stick together

In the prelude to the recognition of a 'difficult' case, team members can become isolated from each other as they learn of each other's alleged misdemeanours from a patient, carer or family. Once the recognition is made that it is a difficult case, then the team needs to meet to discuss this, and preferably tell each other what they have each been told about the others. It is important that management understand the situation as well, and a policy is agreed for commonly occurring circumstances.

### Behave defensibly

When working under difficult circumstances, a complaint is more likely to result. In extremes it can be a good idea to only visit in pairs to reduce the probability of claims of misconduct, and their likely success. Thorough record keeping is vital as it is this contemporaneous record which is the team's protection from claims or malpractice or worse. Needless to say, the behaviour of the team needs to be above realistic reproach so there should be no 'corner cutting' when it comes to prescriptions or any other part of care.

### Avoid being punitive

The purpose of the unusual activities recommended when dealing with a difficult case is not to 'win' any kind of 'competition' but to keep the clinical team functioning under difficult circumstances to provide good care to the patient. Understandably, team members can wish to punish the difficult patient, and this may not be apparent to the team at the time. For example, a difficult patient may reject life-prolonging treatments and the team may, because of an unconscious desire to punish the individual, take this rejection at face value when in other circumstances they would have responded differently. What is recommended is consistent, rigorous teamwork to provide a stable environment for all concerned.

### Place boundaries

It is widely thought that it is the perceived lack of boundaries which is part of the difficulties patients in this circumstance face. Placing boundaries on a patient's behaviour to send a consistent message of what is acceptable behaviour and what is not can calm a highly emotionally charged situation very quickly. For example, explaining that violence towards staff is not acceptable and calling the police every time this occurs provides everyone, the patient or carer included, with more of a feeling of security.

### Manage expectations

When managing a difficult case it is important to be aware that even the best clinical team cannot meet every unreasonable demand placed upon it. Some people will be disappointed with the team and these disappointments should be taken seriously but this should not reduce the overall morale of the team, which strives to meet every patient's reasonable expectation.

### Have a plan

A meeting to discuss actions in the event of likely events, and a 'catch all' action for the team to carry out in the event of anything else happening, is vital. Support from senior management helps the team continue to function under the great pressure experienced in these circumstances.

### Learning from a 'difficult' case

After a 'difficult' case is over, a meeting with as many of the professionals involved often helps to crystallize learning points, and rebuild professional relationships which may have been under strain.

## Psychiatric services and when to refer

In most industrialized societies, most mental health care is provided in the community by teams organized into geographical sectors. The majority of patients with a serious mental health problem, such as schizophrenia, will be cared for by these Community Mental Health Teams (CMHT) at some time. Each CMHT has access to inpatient services when required, though the teams are not usually based at a psychiatric hospital. The staff will consist of psychiatrists, nurses, occupational therapists, physiotherapists and psychologists. Care for each patient is usually organized through a named individual, variously known as the key worker, care coordinator, or similar. In the UK and many other countries there are separate services for older adults (aged over 65) and children (aged less than 18).

CMHTs vary considerably in terms of the range of disorders they will see and treat, though most would see their primary role as providing treatment for patients with severe and pervasive mental disorders – such as schizophrenia. This means that they may lack resources to treat patients with less severe forms of depression or anxiety. Community services may also not be familiar with issues peculiar to palliative care. In some settings liaison psychiatry services exist to bridge the gap between the general hospital or hospice and psychiatric services.

It is difficult to generalize about when a palliative care team should refer a patient to a psychiatric team. The most straightforward situation is when the psychiatric disorder is associated with risk – harm to the patient or violence to others, for example. Other situations include where treatments have been attempted (for example, antidepressants for depression) with no effect. Another common reason is where there is a question about the person's ability to make a decision – when mental capacity is questioned. Often it is a question of the help that is required rather than of diagnosis, prognosis, severity, behaviour or other factors intrinsic to the patient. For example, a patient with complex mental health needs due to a serious mental health problem may not require psychiatric input at the hospice because this is well managed by the CMHT, whereas an apparently well person who seems to be exhibiting some new unusual ideas may warrant a referral, even though the problems may be small. Of course, a well-integrated psychiatric team will always be open to 'informal' approaches by members of the clinical team to ask if a referral is appropriate, so concerns of over- or under-referring can be dealt with at that stage. In addition to the above, it is usual for the patient to be asked if they are agreeable to the involvement of the psychiatric team before a formal referral is made.

# Conclusion

Mental health problems are of relevance to nurses working in palliative care. Mental health problems are common, under-diagnosed, readily treatable and have a detrimental effect on the quality of life of patients. The nurse is the closest professional to the patient, and so is as well placed to make a personal rapport with a distressed person needing time to come to terms with bad news, as he or she is in calling on and working with psychiatric services to help a patient suffering with a complex and severe mental health problem such as schizophrenia. Good psychological care is a vital part of good palliative care.

# References

American Psychiatric Association (1994) *Diagnostic and statistical manual of mental disorders: DSM-IV.* Washington, D.C.: American Psychiatric Association.

Folstein, M.F., Folstein, S.E. and McHugh, P.R. (1975) 'Mini-mental state'. A practical method for grading the cognitive state of patients for the clinician. *Journal of Psychiatric Research*, 12(3): 189–98.

Gould, M.S., Marrocco, F.A., Kleinman, M., Thomas, J.G., Mostkoff, K., Cote, J. and Davies, M. (2005) Evaluating iatrogenic risk of youth suicide screening programs: a randomized controlled trial. *Journal of the American Medical Association*, 293(13): 1635–43.

Henderson, M., Scott, S. and Hotopf, M. (2007) Use of the clock-drawing test in a hospice population. *Palliative Medicine*, 21(7): 559–65.

Inouye, S.K. (2000) Prevention of delirium in hospitalized older patients: risk factors and targeted intervention strategies. *Annals of Medicine*, 32(4): 257–63.

Lawlor, P.G., Gagnon, B., Mancini, I.L., Pereira, J.L., Hanson, J., Suarez-Almazor, M.E. and Bruera, E.D. (2000) Occurrence, causes, and outcome of delirium in patients with advanced cancer: a prospective study. *Archives of Internal Medicine*, 160(6): 786–94.

Price, A., Hotopf, M., Higginson, I.J., Monroe, B. and Henderson, M. (2006) Psychological services in hospices in the UK and Republic of Ireland. *Journal of the Royal Society of Medicine*, 99(12): 637–9.

Shulman, K.I. (2000) Clock-drawing: is it the ideal cognitive screening test? *International Journal of Geriatric Psychiatry*, 15(6): 548–61.

Speck, P. (1994) Working with dying people: on being good enough. In: A. Obholzer and V.Z. Roberts (eds) *The unconscious at work: individual and organizational stress in the human services*. London: Routledge.

Sunderland, T., Hill, J.L., Mellow, A.M., Lawlor, B.A., Gundersheimer, J., Newhouse, P.A. and Grafman, J.H. (1989) Clock drawing in Alzheimer's disease. A novel measure of dementia severity. *Journal of the American Geriatric Society*, 37(8): 725–9.

World Health Organization (1992) *The ICD-10 classification of mental and behavioural disorders: clinical descriptions and diagnostic guidelines*. Geneva: World Health Organization.

# 16

# Working with family care-givers in a palliative care setting

*Paula Smith and Julie Skilbeck*

---

**Key points**

- Enhancing the mutually beneficial relationship between the family care-giver and health and social care practitioners in order to develop more appropriate supportive strategies.
- Acknowledging the carer's own needs within the triadic relationship in the context of whether or not they consider themselves to be carers.
- Assessment and reassessment of family care-givers' needs to ensure that they are provided with adequate and appropriate information and support at appropriate time points in the disease trajectory. This will then help to reduce speculative anticipation in the caring role and enable family care-givers to focus on actual problems and needs rather than imagined needs.
- Further work needs to be considered to explore the effectiveness and usefulness of any interventions with family care-givers from their perspective, across a range of activities and care settings.

---

It is now acknowledged that ageing populations are characteristic of many countries in Europe, North America and in some parts of Asia (World Health Organization 2007). Also, the pattern of disease at the end of life is changing and more people are living with serious long-term conditions and co-morbidity and experiencing complex problems. It is likely, therefore, that more people will need help at the end of life. Many individuals spend their last year of life at home and prefer to die in familiar surroundings supported by family and friends (Lancashire and South Cumbria Cancer Network 2004). It is now widely accepted that family carers provide the majority of that care across the globe (Howe *et al.* 1997; Payne and Ellis-Hill 2001; Hudson *et al.* 2004; Williams *et al.* 2006). Working with family care-givers can be a rewarding and challenging process, particularly within the field of palliative care. Carers hold the position of both giving and needing support. It has been suggested that it is not always clear who is the 'patient'

(Neale *et al.* 1993). Despite a rapid increase in the general care-giving literature over the past 20 years, contemporary changes in family structures, migration patterns, employment and the age cohorts of potential care-givers results in a continuing need to understand the nature and context of family care-giving. Within this chapter we will begin to address some of the issues that are emerging in the literature as being particularly relevant to the family care-giver in palliative or end-of-life care. By reflecting on the construction of caring, as well as individual family care-givers' perceptions of their role, it is anticipated that health and social care professionals will be able to consider their own interactions and support of this group of people in a more systematic way.

The chapter will be divided into three sections. The first section will begin by discussing the current health and social policy and practice context relating to family care-givers in the United Kingdom (UK). Although we are focusing on the health and social care policy context in the UK, we will draw on the international caring literature to illuminate care-giving issues in different contexts. Second, the chapter will consider the development and understanding of the family care-giver role, drawing upon models of family care-giving. We will also use examples from two research studies in palliative care settings (see Box 16.1). Finally, in the last section, implications for the assessment of family care-giver needs, and the appropriateness and usefulness of supportive strategies will be explored.

# Family care-giving and current UK social policy

Changing health and social care policies in the UK have recently been developed that reflect the changing demographics and ageing population,

---

**Box 16.1**   Research study 1

This study explored the dynamic and changing nature of caring for a family member in a palliative care setting. The study was based on a case study approach similar to that described by Yin (1994), which acknowledged important background and situational information as part of the data collection and analysis within the research. One of the aims was to identify how the family care-giver's situation might change over time. Sixteen family care-givers (eight husbands, six wives and two adult daughters) from two areas in the south of England were interviewed a number of times over a four-month period. The age range of the family care-givers was 33–77 with a mean of 56.8 years. All were recruited through the visiting specialist palliative care services with whom they had contact, and all were caring for someone with a cancer diagnosis with a prognosis of six months or less.

(Smith 2000)

improving treatment regimes and changes within the National Health Service (DoH 2001, 2004; NICE 2004). There is also an increasing acknowledgement and expectation of family participation in long-term and end-of-life care-giving within the UK. Family care-givers are increasingly being relied on to provide the majority of daily care, and the management of physical, emotional and psychological consequences of advanced life-threatening illnesses (Kennedy *et al.* 1999; Weitzner and McMillan 1999). The impact on family care-givers of policy changes such as those in the UK, which have resulted in an emphasis on community care and a movement away from care delivered in institutions, remains unclear. It is important therefore that professional service providers are aware and understand the complex nature of the caring role assumed by family care-givers in order that they can adequately and appropriately meet their information and support needs (Kennedy *et al.* 1999).

In the past there have been ambiguities in relation to understanding and conceptualizing the role of 'carer' within palliative care (Smith 2000). It is not within the remit of this chapter to discuss the historical development of the terminology surrounding informal carers (for a more detailed discussion, see Twigg and Atkin 1994; Heaton 1999; Nolan *et al.* 2003). More recently in the general care-giving literature there has been an acknowledgement that family care-givers acquire experience and expertise over time, resulting in the development of an alternative typology which views informal carers as 'experts' in caring (Nolan *et al.* 1996a; DoH 2007b). Within this framework the family care-givers' expertise may be supplemented or enhanced by professional carers. Services in this scenario work with the family care-giver to provide optimum care and support to the cared-for person, while acknowledging the developing expertise that these individuals acquire. The family care-givers' expertise may have developed over a prolonged period of time, particularly in the case of long-term conditions.

Within palliative care there is increasing recognition that some family carers do not readily identify with the term 'carer', possibly as a result of the relatively short time before the death of the family member. However, development of such expertise is also increasingly true for family care-givers who are caring for a family member with cancer. For some the duration and periods of symptoms may extend over a number of years and phases throughout the disease trajectory, including periods of recurrence, active treatment and remission (Thomas *et al.* 2002). This may result in some family care-givers adopting the role of representative of the ill person (Friedrichsen *et al.* 2001), or becoming the coordinator of care between the visiting health and social care professionals and the patient (Smith 2000). Thus, being sensitive to the individual needs of each person and being able to provide an all encompassing policy in relation to family care-givers may be difficult. Rather, there is a need to be aware of the differences each family care-giver may bring to a situation in order to work most effectively with them. For example, to ensure the safety and well-being of both the family care-giver and the person they are caring for. This raises challenges in the development of supportive working relationships by health and social care professionals. First, if the individual does not recognize themselves to be a carer, then it may influence how health and social care professionals interact and support the person. For example, a study by Armes and Addington-Hall (2003) found that health and social care professionals relied on carers to assess and manage symptoms, although carers themselves did not always know whether to or what they should monitor. Second, the expectations of the involvement of the family carer may be incompatible with the carer's own expectations and this will inevitably influence the level and type of support they can access (Smith 2001).

## Understanding the family care-giver role

In order for health and social care professionals to work in partnership with family care-givers it is important to consider the following:

- Who are the family care-givers in palliative care and what do they do?
- What may influence the caring role, and what impact may this have on the family care-giver?
- What types of supportive interventions may family care-givers find useful?

### Who are the family care-givers?

The general care-giving literature, from the gerontological and dementia fields in particular, suggests that this role may be fulfilled by a number of the ill person's friends and relations working together to provide individual and holistic care (Linkewich *et al.* 1999). In practice, what usually happens is that one person, usually co-resident with the ill person, takes the predominant care-giving role and is supported in this by more extended family and friendship networks (Smith 2000; Thomas *et al.* 2002). Keating *et al.* (1994) argue that the view of one family care-giver providing all care fails to explore or take account of the wider social dynamics involved in this type of caring. Studies within the field of palliative care have demonstrated that the majority of family care-givers providing care to terminally ill relatives are women, caring predominantly for a spouse or partner (Aldred *et al.* 2005; Hudson 2006). What is not known, however, is the extent to which the wider social network is involved within the care-giving dynamic. On the whole, as would be expected, these family care-givers tend to be younger than their relative. In a study by Skilbeck *et al.* (2005) two-thirds of the patients recruited were over the age of 65, whereas two-thirds of the carers were under the age of 65. These figures reflect the age and gender distributions found between family carers generally in the literature relating to carers and older people (ONS 2004). In relation to gender, this in part possibly reflects the assumptions in many cultures that care-giving is part of a woman's role (Neale and Clark 1992). Despite this, men do participate in caring, particularly if they are the spouse of the cared-for person (Carers UK 2007), and in the older generation will engage in equal amounts of co-resident care (Arber and Ginn 1990). In the future it is likely that the age of carers, and those they care for, will increase. It is now widely acknowledged that the proportion of older people living in the UK is growing. Currently, 16 per cent of the total population are over the age of 65; of these almost half are over the age of 75 (ONS 2007). It is expected that by 2041 the numbers of people aged at least 85 are expected to double from 1.1 million to 2.3 million. It is likely, therefore, that those adopting a caring role will be older themselves and may experience multiple health problems and co-morbidity, situational constraints, and increased dependency themselves (Manfred and Pickett 1987); thus influencing their ability to provide supportive care.

### Identification with the family care-giver role

When considering who is providing family care at the end of life there is an assumption that the individual concerned has made a conscious decision to take up the caring role, or in fact wishes to take up that role. A far more holistic view of care-giving support has emerged and supportive interventions should assist the carer to take up or not take up the caring role (Askham 1998). Identification with the role of 'carer' is sometimes unclear, particularly when the role has been adopted for kinship and obligation reasons in a gradual and progressive way. The caring activities undertaken as a result therefore are not identified as being part of a particular role or job as the term 'carer' might imply. In the study by Skilbeck *et al.* (2005) exploring the experiences of individuals caring for a relative with a life-limiting illness, several participants identified that the activities that they undertook were part of their 'duty' towards their relative, and that although at times they found it hard work it was something that they would carry on doing. Smith (2000) found that it was family care-givers who had been involved in caring for a prolonged period of time who would often identify strongly with the term 'carer'. Conversely, those that had only recently undertaken such role changes strongly resisted being called a carer (see Case study 16.1).

**Case study 16.1**

Mrs Vaughan was a lady in her mid-50s who had a life-long history of caring and strongly identified with this role. She was an active member of her local carers' support group and was currently caring for both her husband, who had cancer, and her mother who had Parkinson's disease.

'I've been a carer all my life. I've always done something for somebody. I've never had nursing training, but it's a natural instinct, it's born in me.'

Due, in part, to her strong allegiance to the carer role, Mrs Vaughan's greatest concern was what she would do if both her husband and mother should die at the same time. She posed the question.

'What do the carers do when the caring ends?'

Mr Lloyd, on the other hand, did not identify with the term carer and saw his involvement as much more related to marital obligations and reciprocity for care received by his wife in the past. Mr Lloyd was in his late 30s and had never been involved in caring before.

''Cos when you're actually married to someone you're there through thick and thin any way aren't you? If I was ill she'd look after me, and if she was ill I'd look after her. Um, I remember when I was in hospital, I had two bad injuries playing rugby where I was put in hospital and I had an operation. When I came out I couldn't, I was on crutches. She always looked after me then. I mean it's just this is, I don't know, a bit longer that's all.'

Mr Lloyd admitted that he had found the caring role, which included looking after their three young children and taking on additional household responsibilities, a shock.

'I do everything around the house. Do the cleaning, cooking, looking after the kids, washing. Just got used to it now (laughs) . . . when she was well I just used to come home and have my dinner ready made for me. Big shock this!'

### How is caring constructed?

Definitions of informal caring often revolve around the overt, instrumental or tangible aspects of care. This view is reflected in the literature and in social policy in the UK. The Carers Act (HMSO 1995) sought to raise the profile of family care-givers and their support needs. However, it has been only partially effective as it emphasized the physical burden of caring (Nolan *et al.* 1996b) and the implicit assumptions underlying the role. The Carers Act (HMSO 1995) did result in the launch of the Carers National Strategy (DoH 1999), which highlighted some of the key issues in being a carer. These include a desire to maintain the well-being of the cared-for person, having a life of their own outside of caring, maintaining their own health, having confidence in the services they receive, and having a say in service provision. Furthermore, the Carers National Strategy (DoH 1999) emphasized the importance of shared responsibility for care and included in this a respect and acknowledgement of the family care-giver's knowledge within the situation. Although this strategy recognizes certain features relating to caring, it does still assume that the individual will identify with the term carer and is able and willing to undertake these roles and activities.

For health and social care professionals then, family care-giving may be constructed as negative, unwelcome and burdensome. Perhaps for this reason much of the care-giving literature views overt care-giving as having a negative impact on the family care-giver's quality of life. Indeed family care-givers within palliative care have been found to suffer from greater levels of anxiety than the ill person (Hinton 1994a). The negative impact on quality of life that may be found as a result of adopting the role of carer is often referred to in the general care-giving literature as a sense of burden. Some studies have attempted to explore what factors might constitute identification of care-givers who might be 'at risk' of a sense of burden. For example, Meyers and Gray (2001) found that the care-giving role negatively affected care-givers' quality of life and this was particularly noticeable for long-term care-givers who lived in a rural locality. They suggest that care-givers falling into this category would benefit from additional support from hospice or palliative care services.

There is now criticism of this negative approach with the recognition that within the care-giving dynamic, family care-givers also experience satisfaction in relation to caring. Indeed many family care-givers describe mixed emotions regarding their role and highlight both positive and negative aspects (Scott 2001; Hudson 2004). Nolan *et al.* (1996a) have highlighted the importance of reciprocity, as a driving force behind much of 'normal' family life, the purpose of which is to maintain a sense of balance and interdependence in relationships. Within this context, the importance of the relationship is considered to influence the nature of satisfaction experienced, as well as the meaning that is given to care-giving within the relationship. Often family care-givers recall a sense of satisfaction to feelings of reciprocity and being able to return care received in the past, or as a way of demonstrating their love for the ill person (Grbich *et al.* 2001). For others there may be social or moral obligations to participation in care-giving that negates the difficulties encountered. Recognizing the potential positive outcome of family care-giving is now being acknowledged in the literature and studies are beginning to emerge which suggest satisfaction with the care-giving role despite the difficulties this might cause (Nolan *et al.* 1996a; Grbich *et al.* 2001). Enabling carers to articulate the positive aspects of caring may influence their ability to provide care over longer periods of time.

Care-giving occurs over time; however, there has been a dearth of literature relating to the temporal and longitudinal aspects. Expectations of potential time frames from diagnosis to death are particularly common with certain diseases such as cancer. However, while this may be true in some cases, lung cancer, for example, generally has a poor prognosis, this is not the case for other cancers particularly if they are diagnosed and treated at an early stage. If caring continues beyond the anticipated time frame, the level and intensity of support may become unsustainable. Smith (2000) found that some people who had become involved in family care-giving at the point of diagnosis with cancer found it increasingly difficult to maintain their involvement at the original level when the caring was extended over a prolonged period of time. This was particularly noticeable for the younger and middle-aged care-givers who were juggling other roles such as partner, parent, adult, child and worker. Similarly, with a non-cancer diagnosis the potential time frame for which caring will be required may not be realistically considered at the beginning of the caring journey, as this is often perceived to be unpredictable. It is likely that some individuals may provide care to a relative with long-term conditions for up to 20 years before the end of life, which may impact on their ability to provide specific support at the very end of life (Skilbeck *et al.* 2005). This is clearly articulated in Case study 16.2.

---

**Case study 16.2**

Mrs Gray was a 61-year-old woman who had been caring for her husband with multiple sclerosis for 15 years. His condition was deteriorating and she was finding it increasingly difficult to manage his care at home; she was at the point of considering alternative care provision at a time when she felt she should be caring for him herself at home:

'At the moment I'm finding it increasingly difficult, I'm wondering whether I should be, we're at a cross roads, where I'm considering whether it should be nursing home care full-time. His bowels aren't functioning properly and I'm finding that to be the hardest time for moving him about and pulling him about and we keep getting bouts of him being sick as well, so that's another day where you are constantly changing him and the bed and I find that increasingly hard.'

---

### What do family care-givers do?

The amount and type of care given by family care-givers is not generally static and may change and develop throughout the disease trajectory. Nolan *et al.* (1995) suggest that throughout the care-giving experience, family care-givers are likely to engage in 'anticipatory care'. This involves anticipating what they will do should the ill person suffer from a real or imagined deterioration. Anticipatory care does not necessarily involve direct or instrumental care-giving, although it may well be as time consuming and worrying for the family care-giver as more direct involvement in supporting the ill person. Furthermore, Nolan *et al.* (1995) suggest that the level of information and knowledge the family care-giver has in relation to the disease trajectory can become important in reducing what they term 'speculative anticipation', which is characterized by a lack of information or knowledge about the situation. This can result in over or under anticipating future needs that may consequently have a detrimental effect on the family care-giver. Informed anticipation, on the other hand, can result in greater shared care and planning. By recognizing and acknowledging anticipatory care, health and social care professionals can reduce the invisibility of speculative anticipation. The difficulty arises within palliative care when the very uncertainty of the disease trajectory and potential deterioration in the cared-for person's condition make anticipating future needs difficult. Increasingly within cancer care family care-givers are faced with responding to the cyclical nature of the disease trajectory including periods of remission, recurrence and active treatment that can have a negative impact on their ability to cope with the situation (Smith 2000; Hudson *et al.* 2004).

Within the palliative care literature family carers have been described as predominantly engaging in a range of instrumental care practices. Often becoming involved in family care-giving can result in a number of role changes and routines (Denham 1999). This can range from simply providing companionship and undertaking household tasks, to assisting with personal care, transport and for some quite complex nursing care (Payne *et al.* 1999; Aranda and Hayman-White 2001; Thomas *et al.* 2002). Wyatt *et al.* (1999), in a large scale post-bereavement study, found family care-givers had been highly involved in assisting the cared-for person with activities of daily living, often averaging 10.8 hours a day of direct care-giving and 8.9 hours of providing companionship. The level of involvement that the family care-giver has in these activities will be dependent upon a number of factors such as the ill person's condition, their previous relationship with the ill person, their own health and ability to undertake such care, the level and type of support they receive from professional and social networks. Case study 16.3 highlights the range of activities that were undertaken by carers.

---

**Case study 16.3**

For some family carers personal and intimate care was provided on a regular basis. This is clearly articulated by a 67-year-old woman who cared for her husband with cerebral ataxia:

'Well I get him up in a morning with a cup of tea and pills and get him to the toilet, and wash his hair, shave him and see to him from the waist downwards, and then I get him back into the bedroom and a carer comes and sort of does from the waist up and dresses him, and then sort of lunch time I get him downstairs, I've got a stair rail and we sort of manage and then he stays down all day, he can't walk, he can stand up but he can't walk.'

For others caring involved a range of activities.

Mrs Page was in her late 50s and worked full-time. She had been 'keeping an eye' on her mother since the death of her father four years previously. This involved daily visits to her mother either before or after going to work, in order to check that her mother was well and had no immediate needs. Although her mother had a number of paid carers who heated a meal at lunch time and assisted with dressing, it was Mrs Page who took on responsibility for ensuring that the shopping was done, finances organized, bills paid, tablets sorted

and numerous other jobs around the house attended to. Mrs Page also anticipated her mother's current and future needs by instigating and organizing
appropriate services as required. She would sometimes do things herself and
sometimes call in professional services to deliver this care. After her mother
was diagnosed with cancer, Mrs Page increased the time and attention she gave
to visiting and supporting her mother.

For many family care-givers the most significant aspect of the care-
giving role is to provide emotional support to the cared-for person, as
observed in their desire to maintain a positive outlook and a sense of normality (Thomas *et al.* 2002). This creates a particular difficulty for family
care-givers within palliative care when it is known and openly acknowledged
that the cared-for person is going to deteriorate and will not recover to their
pre-illness status. Juggling both of these positions at the same time can result
in a state of tension for the family care-giver between wanting to remain
positive, on the one hand, and yet having a need to acknowledge that the
situation is not going to improve, on the other. For some, one way of dealing
with this conflict is to ignore it and focus only on the present, especially
when with the cared-for person. Often significant family events or outings
will be planned as something to look forward to (Smith 2000; Hudson 2004;
Skilbeck *et al.* 2005).

Sometimes activities that are undertaken become increasingly complex,
particularly during the terminal phase of the illness (Cameron *et al.* 2002).
For example, Aranda and Hayman-White (2001) found that family care-
givers were significantly involved in the symptom management of the ill
person and undertook assessment, monitoring and delivery of complex
therapeutic interventions such as pain and symptom control. In addition,
they took on almost total responsibility for routine household tasks. They
concluded that there is therefore a need to move towards the development of
care-giver-focused nursing interventions. Providing practical, emotional and
informational support to enable family care-givers to undertake this role
may be particularly important. This may then enable them to participate
fully in this activity (Rose 1999; Bakas *et al.* 2001) if that is the wish of both
the family care-giver and the cared-for person. While it is commendable to
provide adequate and appropriate support to family care-givers who wish
to undertake additional caring roles and responsibilities, it is important to
acknowledge that there may well be certain caring tasks that both the family
care-giver and the cared-for person feel uncomfortable participating in. For
example, provision of intimate personal care or specific nursing roles such as
catheter care. This may be particularly important if there are gender differences and/or generational issues (such as a daughter caring for her father)
that the health professional should be aware of and take into account when
negotiating and providing information and support in undertaking these
roles and responsibilities.

### *What is the impact of caring?*

Within the general care-giving literature caring has been described as burdensome and negatively affecting health, social, psychological and financial circumstances. This has also been reflected in the palliative care literature (Kinsella *et al.* 1998; Perreault *et al.* 2004). For example, in Hudson's (2004) study of cancer patients carers reported difficulties such as their own health problems, limited time for themselves and an anxiety about insufficient skills to manage their relatives' symptoms. While family care-givers are often happy to undertake additional roles and responsibilities in support of the cared-for person, they may face a number of restrictions and losses to their own valued activities and interests (Duke 1998). If this is perceived to be for a limited period of time, such as is often assumed on being given a cancer diagnosis, family care-givers may be happy to put their own needs and activities on hold. In contrast, Skilbeck *et al.* (2005) found that those caring for relatives over a long period of time found it to be physically demanding and tiring work as well as emotionally demanding. Furthermore, in addition to the general care-giving demands within palliative care there is the further distress and emotional consequences of having someone close to you die (Aranda 2004). This creates a tension for the family care-giver whereby, on the one hand, they want to prolong the life of the cared-for person and enjoy their company and shared experiences for as long as possible but, on the other, they do not wish them to suffer or become distressed. The tension is therefore one of conflict between attempting to prolong the life and quality of the cared-for person and at the same time preparing for their death and mourning the anticipated loss of shared experiences (Smith 2000).

However, there is now increasing evidence that there are also positive rewards for carers' participation in care-giving in both the general and palliative care fields (Hudson 2004). The rewards of being able to care for someone during their last days often outweigh the difficulties. Individuals report becoming closer to the dying person, being able to give something back for previous caring and knowing that they had done a good job and there was nothing to feel guilty about (Smith 2000; Hudson 2004). Further work is required to explore the extent to which positive experiences influence the more negative aspects of the role.

## Implications for practice

What then are the implications for practice, given the increasing awareness of the family care-giver role and perception of their needs? The following sections begin to highlight some of the key principles that nurses need to consider when assessing, planning, implementing and evaluating care for family care-givers.

### Understanding the family care-giver role

Although family care-givers are acknowledged within palliative care, and are generally considered integral to the care of the ill person, a clear understanding of the nature of their role and relationship with health and social care professionals remains elusive. The difficulty lies in determining how joint care with family care-givers may be organized so that equity of support can be delivered to both the ill person and their associated family care-givers. If health professionals are unclear about the extent of their responsibility towards the family there is likely to be a privileging of the patient's needs and wishes over the family care-giver, despite the rhetoric of concern for the whole family. Privileging the patient's needs and concerns in this way fails to take account of the rights of the family care-giver, even though some decisions may have a direct consequence on their health and well-being. For example, if the patient wishes to die at home and the family care-giver feels unable to provide this level of care, to what extent should services be provided in order for the patient's wishes to be met? If the time before death is fraught with anxiety and worry about how the situation can be managed, the family care-giver may feel let down and could remember the cared-for person's death in a negative light which may have implications for their own well-being post-bereavement.

By developing a clearer definition of what the role of family care-giver within palliative care involves, there is less likelihood of family care-givers being unexpectedly placed in the position of accepting a role or level of responsibility that they may feel uncomfortable with. In addition, understanding the role that the family care-giver themselves associate with their involvement may be important in tailoring the appropriate level and type of information and support required by the individual (Friedrichsen *et al.* 2001). Explicit recognition of the role would also result in an open acknowledgement of the family care-giver position, which in turn would have the benefit of highlighting the rights and needs of this group. This would help health and social care professionals to identify clear areas of responsibility and priority towards the family care-giver.

### Adequate assessment of need

Family care-giving is a complex and dynamic process, and will often involve a substantial amount of effort and commitment by the family care-giver. Over a prolonged period of time such an investment in the situation may not be viable for several reasons. First, the emotional roller coaster that this type of uncertainty produces may be one reason that family care-givers exhibit increased anxiety and negative psychological consequences (Hinton 1994b). Second, if the family care-giver is able and willing to give up, or reduce, other social contacts there is a possibility that the very mechanisms that may support them during the care-giving experience and following the death of the cared-for person will be unavailable when they are most needed. This is particularly important if the care-giving experience is conducted over a prolonged period of time. For example, research has shown the negative effect the period of care-giving can have on care-givers' own interactions with their spouses and children. Similarly, those family care-givers who are still in employment can experience a range of consequences from their employers regarding the need to take time off work to care for the ill person. This can range from full and active support of the family care-giver in undertaking this role, to open hostility and sanctions regarding the necessity of this course of action. If the supportive social relationships with extended family members or active employment roles are damaged during the care-giving experience, this may result in difficulties for the family care-giver following bereavement when there is an expectation that people will reintegrate into society. In this situation an ongoing assessment of the family care-giver's perceived level of responsibility and resources to support the ill person may help to highlight the need for additional information, or educational or counselling needs of the family care-giver, which could then be addressed.

### Supporting the family care-giver

Within palliative care there has always been a strong emphasis on supporting the family of the terminally ill person (Seale 1989), although there is little guidance as to what such support involves or indeed how to achieve this. It is clear, however, that should the family care-giver's ability to maintain the care required by the ill person be compromised there may be additional and sometimes distressing admissions to hospital or hospice (Addington-Hall *et al.* 1991; Hinton 1994a; Armes and Addington-Hall 2003). This, in turn, can result in dissatisfaction for both the cared-for person, the family care-giver and a sense of frustration and failure on the part of the health or social care professional. The discussion so far has highlighted that the range of carers' needs are vast, and include domestic support; personal assistance with the family member; informal support; coping with fatigue, financial difficulties, anxiety and depression and isolation (Payne and Ellis-Hill 2001; Scott 2001; Smith 2001; Hudson *et al.* 2004).

There is still a dearth of literature, however, in relation to interventions and their evaluation which are aimed at supporting family care-givers caring for a relative at the end of life. A systematic review by Harding and Higginson (2003) identified that there have been a number of interventions that have aimed to provide a range of support services in a variety of service configurations. In the review home care services are generally rated highly by family care-givers, and are found to be useful in terms of carer support such as information giving and providing a specific point of contact. Where studies focused on reducing unmet need and psychological morbidity, however, home care nursing services in both cancer and palliative care were unable to meet all the carer's needs. It may be that these services focus on the 'instrumental' aspects of care-giving and do not explore the meaning attributed to the caring relationship, the care-giver attributes or the wider social dynamics involved in this type of caring.

The review highlighted that more focused studies, using either one-to-one or group work interventions, have been undertaken to provide support, education, information and to build problem solving/coping skills. However, in many of these studies carer outcomes are not clearly evaluated, and the sample sizes often limit the interpretation of the findings. The one-to-one intervention studies appeared to show significant improvements in relation to how family care-givers dealt with pressing problems, knowledge and attitudes towards pain, encouraging patient communication and mutual expression of feelings. It is likely, however, that these interventions are time-consuming and costly and it is also unclear whether individual based services are acceptable to many carers (Harding and Higginson 2003). In relation to the group work interventions, although not appropriate for all family carers, it is likely that the benefits of information requesting and giving, sharing practical and coping skills, and comparing social situations may be of great benefit (Harding and Higginson 2003), therefore further studies are required to evaluate more specific outcomes. Although whether carers are able to attend such groups is another issue. Many carers find it difficult to find time and space for themselves as the care-giving role is all consuming (Skilbeck *et al.* 2005). Many may not want to leave the care-giving situation (Strang *et al.* 2002). Currently Help the Hospices have a five-year programme which aims to facilitate the development of innovative carer support programmes, using a variety of strategies. This is currently being evaluated by Payne *et al.* (2007) and will hopefully provide some further indication of appropriate supportive strategies.

Another strategy in the support of family care-givers at the end of life is the provision of respite services, which include: planned and unplanned inpatient admissions; day care services; and in-home support such as 'night-sitters' (Ingleton *et al.* 2003). There is some evidence for the efficacy of inpatient specialist palliative care services for patients and carers, however, there is less for day care or hospice at home schemes. Moreover, a systematic review revealed that there was lack of efficacy of most respite services in promoting carers' well-being (McNally *et al.* 1999). It does demonstrate, however, that inpatient respite care was more effective in improving care-givers' psychological well-being and relieving stress more than home care. In relation to specialist day care, although anecdotal reports of the benefits of day care for family carers are numerous (Ingleton *et al.* 2003), there is little evidence to suggest that it achieves positive outcomes for family carers (Hearn and Myers 2001). Most hospices offer inpatient respite services (Payne *et al.* 2004). In a recent study (Skilbeck *et al.* 2005) inpatient respite care seems to serve two user groups: family carers of relatives with a long-term chronic illness, and family carers whose relative is in the last six months of life. Although the service was well evaluated by carers the question was raised as to whether this model of respite service provision was appropriate for patients who do not necessarily require specialist palliative care, or for those who were in the terminal phase. In a study by Strang *et al.* (2002), family carers who were at the end of life wanted to remain in the care-giving environment with their relative. It may be more appropriate, therefore, to offer home respite care for certain patients in the last few months; especially at night to enable the family care-giver to rest (Kristjansson *et al.* 2001). Certainly, the provision of respite services in the current economic climate appears to be based on ritual and habit rather than on an approach which enables family care-givers to make informed choices about the types of respite that may most appropriately meet their needs at different time points along their relative's illness trajectory.

An area that warrants further exploration is when to introduce specialist palliative care supportive interventions. Where there is a known disease trajectory of limited duration specialist palliative care services are often introduced at an early stage. However, where there is a less clear disease progression and a potentially long illness it is often difficult to determine when specialist palliative care services should be introduced. This can potentially result in family care-givers being the only person involved in caring for a long period of time. For example, the cared-for person may experience a number of distressing symptoms and adaptations to various losses during the course of their illness. This may also impact on the family care-giver in a negative way. Such symptoms and adaptations have been linked to a sense of burden and anxiety in the family care-giver (Andrews 2001). Doyle-Brown (2000) found that the transitional phase of a person's illness between active participation in daily activities and being bed bound was a time of increased anxiety for family care-givers. Being able to identify factors associated with this time and educate the family regarding this process could potentially help the family care-giver to continue with end-of-life care without the need for admission to hospice or hospital (Doyle-Brown 2000).

Furthermore, for some family care-givers there may be particular time points throughout the disease trajectory when additional support or information needs may be required (McKay *et al.* 2002). The point of diagnosis can often have a significant and profound effect on the family care-giver. If this time is addressed sensitively and information is given at an appropriate level, the family care-giver may be assisted to cope with this situation. Alternatively, if the communication between the family care-giver and health profession is poor at the commencement of an illness this may well impact on the family care-giver's ability to negotiate and interact with other health professionals later in the disease trajectory. Also as the family care-giver becomes increasingly involved in instrumental or 'doing for' caring, they may have specific practical and information needs relating to providing such care that the health and social care practitioner may be able to provide.

### Information and education for family care-givers

There is a continued importance placed on the practical and burdensome aspects of caring within the literature, which fails to acknowledge the positive aspects that many family care-givers in palliative care report (Hudson 2004). However, while it is important to recognize that not everyone involved in family care-giving will be burdened by this role, some may. For those that are burdened by this role there is an implicit assumption that there will be consequences for the individual's own health and well-being either during or after bereavement. While there is little evidence available in the literature to link inadequate support for family care-givers with post-bereavement difficulties, a study by Kurtz *et al.* (1997) found that care-giver optimism, pre-bereavement depressive symptomatology and level of social support were critical in determining post-bereavement depressive symptomatology. They concluded that understanding these factors could help health professionals to identify those family care-givers who may be at increased risk of exhibiting depressive symptoms following bereavement.

Adequate preparation for care-giving may be one way of preventing the family care-giver from becoming overburdened with their role. In a UK study Scott (2001) found that insufficient preparation for care-giving significantly contributed to the negative effects on the mental health of the family care-giver. A lack of information and acknowledgement by staff may increase the sense of isolation and difficulty that family care-givers experience. Andershed and Ternestedt (2001) describe this situation as 'involvement in the dark', whereby relatives report 'groping around in the dark' in their attempts to support the patient. Alternatively, when relatives are well informed and develop a sound working relationship with staff based on trust, then a more meaningful experience of caring may result (Andershed and Ternestedt 2001; Mok *et al.* 2002). Clearly early intervention and informational support to new family care-givers is important in this process (Scott 2001). In the longer term, regular respite and opportunities to maintain social contacts may be important factors in supporting the family care-giver in palliative care (Scott 2001).

Families of those with cancer frequently report that their information and support needs are not being met to their satisfaction (Lewis *et al.* 1997; Rose 1999; Flanagan 2001). Some studies have therefore explored the effectiveness of educational training for family care-givers and health professionals who are supporting them (Pickett *et al.* 2001). However, the evidence supporting these interventions as being effective is less clear. In a US study Robinson *et al.* (1998) described a combined educational programme for both care-givers and health and social care workers. At the end of the programme care-givers reported feeling less overwhelmed and better able to cope with the care-giver experience. However, McCorkle and Pasacreta (2001) found that data supporting the effectiveness of care-giver interventions has been limited.

Education of course involves more than just the family care-giver, and we need to consider the training needs of health and social care professionals. Over the past few years there has been an increasing awareness of palliative care needs for patients with both malignant and other life-limiting illness. This is reflected in the myriad of palliative care educational programmes at undergraduate through to postgraduate levels. Many of these programmes attempt to address some of the issues relevant to family care-giving, and the role of health and social care professionals in supporting carers throughout the care-giving trajectory. However, we feel that more can be done and that there is scope to involve carers themselves in professional education, particularly of nurses, as they generally have the greatest contact from the health care perspective.

# Conclusion

This chapter has begun to explore some of the issues arising for family care-givers within a palliative care setting, focusing particularly on the relationship between family care-givers and health and social care professionals in relation to partnership working. Throughout this chapter we have drawn on the gerontological literature around family care-giving. It is important to highlight that while much of this literature is appropriate to palliative care settings, there are some significant differences in the perceptions and nature of the caring role which are unique to end-of-life care. For example, the time limited duration of caring and the knowledge that the cared-for person is going to die, which may influence the desire to be fully involved in caring. This has highlighted the need for acknowledgement and appropriate support for the family care-giver role, which is explicitly acknowledged within the palliative care philosophy. However, implementing such support remains difficult due to the complex and individual nature of the situations arising in this setting. Despite this there are clearly some areas that are worthy of consideration by health and social care practitioners. These include having an awareness of the type of support needs of the family care-givers at various points along the disease trajectory. There need to be developments in educational programmes for both professionals and family care-givers to support both the practical and emotional aspects of managing a caring role in a palliative care situation. Finally, it is clear that any such initiative should be adequately researched in order to determine the effectiveness of such interventions and, if possible, the effect they might have on subsequent bereavement outcomes for family care-givers.

# References

Addington-Hall, J., MacDonald, L., Anderson, H. and Freeling, P. (1991) Dying from cancer: the views of bereaved family and friends about the experiences of terminally ill patients. *Palliative Medicine*, 5: 207–14.

Aldred, H., Gott, M. and Gariballa, S. (2005) Advanced heart failure: impact on older patients and informal carers. *Journal of Advanced Nursing*, 49: 116–24.

Andershed, B. and Ternesedt, B.M. (2001) Development of a theoretical framework describing relatives' involvement in palliative care. *Journal of Advanced Nursing*, 34(4): 544–62.

Andrews, S.C. (2001) Care-giver burden and symptom distress in people with cancer receiving hospice care. *Oncology Nursing Forum*, 28(9): 1469–74.

Aranda, S. (2004) Palliative care and the family. *International Journal of Palliative Nursing*, 10(2): 56.

Aranda, S.K. and Hayman-White, K. (2001) Home caregivers of the person with advanced cancer: an Australian perspective. *Cancer Nursing*, 24(4): 300–7.

Arber, S. and Ginn, J. (1990) The meaning of informal care: gender and the contribution of elderly people. *Aging and Society*, 10: 429–54.

Armes, P.J. and Addington-Hall, J. (2003) Perspectives on symptom control in patients receiving community palliative care. *Palliative Medicine*, 17: 608–15.

Askam, J. (1998) Supporting caregivers of older people: an overview of problems and priorities. *Australian Journal on Ageing*, 17(1): 5–7.

Bakas, T., Lewis, R.R. and Parsons, J.E. (2001) Caregiving tasks among family caregivers of patients with lung cancer. *Oncology Nursing Forum*, 28(5): 847–54.

Cameron, J.I., Franche, R.L., Cheung, A.M. and Stewart, D.E. (2002) Lifestyle interference and emotional distress in family caregivers of advanced cancer patients. *Cancer*, 94(2): 521–7.

Carers UK (2007) The facts about carers. www.Carersuk.org/Employersforcarers/ The businesscase/Thefactsaboutcarers (accessed June 2007).

Denham, S.A. (1999) Part 2: family health during and after death of a family member. *Journal of Family Nursing*, 5(2): 160–83.

Department of Health (DoH) (1999) *Caring about carers: a National Strategy for Carers*. London: Department of Health.

Department of Health (DoH) (2001) *National Service Framework for Older People*. London: Department of Health.

Department of Health (DoH) (2004) *Health and Social Care Standards and Planning Framework 2005/06–2007/08*. London: Department of Health.

Department of Health (DoH) (2006) *Preferred place of care*. London: Department of Health.

Department of Health (DoH) (2007a) *End of life care initiative*. London: Department of Health.

Department of Health (DoH) (2007b) *Expert Carers programme*. London: Department of Health.

Doyle-Brown, M. (2000) The transitional phase: the closing journey for patients and family caregivers. *American Journal of Hospice and Palliative Care*, 17(5): 354–7.

Duke, S. (1998) An exploration of anticipatory grief: the lived experience of people during their spouses' terminal illness and in bereavement. *Journal of Advanced Nursing*, 28(4): 829–39.

Flanagan, J. (2001) Clinically effective cancer care: working with families. *European Journal of Oncology Nursing*, 5(3): 174–9.

Friedrichsen, M.J., Strang, P.M. and Carlsson, M.E. (2001) Receiving bad news: experiences of family members. *Journal of Palliative Care*, 17(4): 241–7.

Grbich, C., Parker, D. and Maddocks, I. (2001) The emotions and coping strategies of caregivers of family members with a terminal cancer. *Journal of Palliative Care*, 17(1): 30–6.

Harding, R. and Higginson, I.J. (2003) What is the best way to help caregivers in cancer and palliative care? A systematic literature review of interventions and their effectiveness. *Palliative Medicine*, 17: 63–74.

Hearn, J. and Myers, K. (2001) *Palliative day care in practice*. Oxford: Oxford University Press.

Heaton, J. (1999) The gauze and visibility of the carer: a Foucauldian analysis of the discourse of informal care. *Sociology of Health and Illness*, 21(6): 759–77.

Hinton, J. (1994a) Which patients with terminal cancer are admitted from home care? *Palliative Medicine*, 8: 197–210.

Hinton, J. (1994b) Can home care maintain an acceptable quality of life for patients with terminal cancer and their relatives? *Palliative Medicine*, 8: 183–96.

HMSO (1995) *Carers (Recognition and Services) Act 1995*. London: HMSO.

Howe, A.L., Schofield, H. and Herman, H. (1997) Caregiving: A common or uncommon experience? *Social Science and Medicine*, 45(7): 1017–29.

Hudson, P. (2004) Positive aspects and challenges associated with caring for a dying relative. *International Journal of Palliative Nursing*, 10: 58–65.

Hudson, P., Aranda, A. and Kristjanson, L.J. (2004) Meeting the supportive care needs of family caregivers in palliative care. *Journal of Palliative Medicine*, 7(1): 19–25.

Hudson, P.L. (2006) How well do family caregivers cope after caring for a relative with advanced disease and how can health professionals enhance their support? *Journal of Palliative Medicine*, 9(3): 694–703.

Ingleton, C., Payne, S., Nolan, M. and Carey, I. (2003) Respite in palliative care: a review and discussion of the literature. *Palliative Medicine*, 17(7): 567–75.

Keating, N., Kerr, K., Warren, S., Grace, M. and Wertenberger, D. (1994) Who's the family in family caregiving? *Canadian Journal on Aging*, 13(2): 268–87.

Kennedy, C., Lockhart-Wood, K. and Fielding, H. (1999) Involving the family in the use of the syringe driver in the community setting. *British Journal of Community Nursing*, 4(5): 250–7.

Kinsella, G., Cooper, B., Picton, C. and Murtagh, D. (1998) A review of the measurement of caregiver and family burden in palliative care. *Journal of Palliative Care*, 14(2): 37–45.

Kristjanson, L.J., Cousines, K., White, K., Andrews, L.L., Lewin, G., Tinnelly, C., Asphar, D. and Greene, R. (2001) Evaluation of a night respite community palliative care service. *International Journal of Palliative Nursing*, 10: 84–90.

Kurtz, M.E., Kurtz, J.C., Given, C.W. and Given, B. (1997) Predictors of post-bereavement depressive symptomatology among family caregivers of cancer patients. *Supportive Care in Cancer*, 5(1): 53–60.

Lancashire and South Cumbria Cancer Network (2004) *The Preferred Place of Care*. http://www.cancerlancashire.org.uk (accessed June 2007).

Lewis, M., Pearson, V., Corcoran-Perry, S. and Narayan, S. (1997) Decision making by elderly patients with cancer and their caregivers. *Cancer*, 20(6): 389–97.

Linkewich, B., Setliff, A.E., Poling, M., Bailey, S., Sellick, S. and Kelly, M.L. (1999) Communicating at life's end. *The Canadian Nurse*, 95(5): 41–4.

Manfred, C. and Pickett, M. (1987) Perceived stressful situations and coping strategies utilised by the elderly. *Journal of Community Health Nursing*, 4(2): 99–110.

McCorkle, R. and Pasacreta, J.V. (2001) Enhancing caregiver outcomes in palliative care. *Cancer Control*, 8(1): 36–45.

McKay, P., Rajacich, D. and Rosenbaum, J. (2002) Enhancing palliative care through Watson's carative factors. *Canadian Oncology Nursing Journal*, 12(1): 34–8.

McNally, S., Ben-Shlomo, Y. and Newman, S. (1999) The effect of respite care on informal carers' wellbeing: a systematic review. *Disability Rehabilitation*, 21: 1–14.

Meyers, J.L. and Gray, L.N. (2001) The relationships between family primary caregiver characteristics and satisfaction with hospice care, quality of life, and burden. *Oncology Nursing Forum*, 28(1): 73–82.

Mok, E., Chan, F., Chan, V. and Yeung, E. (2002) Perception of empowerment by family caregivers of patients with a terminal illness in Hong Kong. *International Journal of Palliative Nursing*, 8(3): 137–45.

Neale, B. and Clark, D. (1992) Informal palliative care. *Journal of Cancer Care*, 3: 85–9.

Neale, B., Clark, D. and Heather, P. (1993) *Purchasing palliative care: A review of the policy literature*. Sheffield: Trent Palliative Care Centre.

National Institute for Clinical Excellence (2004) *Supportive and Palliative Care Guidance*. London: NICE.

Nolan, M., Grant, G. and Keady, J. (1996a) *Understanding Family Care: A Multidimensional Model of Caring and Coping*. Buckingham: Open University Press.

Nolan, M., Grant, G. and Keady, J. (1996b) The carers act: realising the potential. *British Journal of Community Health Nursing*, 1(6): 317–22.

Nolan, M., Keady, J. and Grant, G. (1995) Developing a typology of family care: implications for nurses and other service providers. *Journal of Advanced Nursing*, 21: 256–65.

Nolan, M., Lundh, U., Grant, G. and Keady, J. (2003) *Partnerships in Family Care: understanding the caregiving career*. Maidenhead: Open University Press.

Office for National Statistics (2004) *Older people*. www.statistics.gov.uk (accessed June 2007).

Office for National Statistics (2007) www.statistics.gov.uk/default.asp.

Payne, S. and Ellis-Hill, C. (2001) *Chronic and terminal illness: new perspectives on caring and carers*. Oxford: Oxford University Press.

Payne, S., Smith, P. and Dean, S. (1999) Identifying the concerns of family carers in palliative care. *Palliative Medicine*, 13(1): 37–44.

Payne, S., Ingleton, C., Scott, G., Steele, K. and Nolan, M. (2004) A survey of the perspectives of specialist palliative care providers in the UK of inpatient respite. *Palliative Medicine*, 18: 692–7.

Payne, S., O'Brien, T. and Ingleton, C. (2007) Help the Hospices Carers Project. Oral paper presented at Help the Hospices: the heart of end-of-life care conference, Harrogate, October 2007.

Perreault, A., Fothergill-Bourbonnais, F. and Fiset, V. (2004) The experience of family members caring for a dying loved one. *International Journal of Palliative Nursing*, 10(3): 133–43.

Pickett, M., Barg, F.K. and Lynch, M.P. (2001) Development of a home-based family caregiver cancer education program. *The Hospice Journal*, 15(4): 19–40.

Robinson, K.D., Angeletti, K.A., Barg, F.K., Pasacreta, J.V., McCorkle, R. and Yasko, J.M. (1998) The development of a family caregiver cancer education program. *Journal of Cancer Education*, 13(2): 116–21.

Rose, K.E. (1999) A qualitative analysis of the information needs of informal carers of terminally ill cancer patients. *Journal of Clinical Nursing*, 8(1): 81–8.

Seale, C. (1989) What happens in hospices: A review of research evidence. *Social Science Medicine*, 28(6): 551–9.

Scott, G. (2001) A study of family carers of people with a life-threatening illness 2: implications of the needs assessment. *International Journal of Palliative Nursing*, 7(7): 323–30.

Smith, P.C. (2000) *Family caregivers in palliative care: perception of their role and sources of support*. Unpublished PhD thesis, University of Southampton.

Smith, P.C. (2001) Who is a Carer? Experiences of Family Caregivers in Palliative Care. In: S. Payne and C. Ellis-Hill (eds) *Chronic and Terminal Illness*. Oxford: Oxford University Press.

Skilbeck, J., Payne, S., Ingleton, M.C., Nolan, M., Carey, I. and Hanson, A. (2005) An exploration of family carers' experience of respite services in one specialist palliative care unit. *Palliative Medicine*, 19: 610–18.

Strang, V.R., Koop, P.M. and Peden, J. (2002) The experience of respite during home-based family caregiving for persons with advanced cancer. *Journal of Palliative Care*, 18: 97–114.

Thomas, C., Morris, S.M. and Harman, J.C. (2002) Companions through cancer: the care given by informal carers in cancer contexts. *Social Science Medicine*, 54(4): 529–44.

Twigg, J. and Atkin, K. (1994) *Carers perceived: policy and practice in informal care.* Buckingham: Open University Press.

Weitzner, M.A. and McMillan, S.C. (1999) The Caregiver Quality of Life Index-Cancer (CQOLC) Scale: revalidation in a home hospice setting. *Journal of Palliative Care*, 15(2): 13–20.

Williams, A., Crooks, V.A., Stajduhar, K.I., Allan, D. and Cohen, R. (2006) Canada's compassionate care benefit: Views of family caregivers in chronic illness. *International Journal of Palliative Nursing*, 12(9): 438–45.

Wyatt, G.K., Friedman, L., Given, C.W. and Given, B.A. (1999) A profile of bereaved caregivers following provision of terminal care. *Journal of Palliative Care*, 15(1): 13–25.

World Health Organization (WHO) (2007) *Ageing and Life Course.* http://www.who.int/ageing/en/ (accessed June 2007).

Yin, R.B. (1994) *Case study research: design and methods* (2nd edn). London: Sage Publications.

# 17

# Personhood and identity in palliative care

*Jenny Hockey*

---

**Key points**

- Identity can be seen as an active process, rather than a 'thing'.
- Identity arises out of the interaction between the patient's view of themselves and other people's perceptions.
- Western models of the self stress its independence through images or metaphors of the body 'containing' the self.
- Some non-Western models of the self involve a more interconnected or collective sense of identity.
- In the overlap between Western and non-Western models of the self, there is scope for practice which reduces the occurrence of stigma or even social death during life-limiting illness.

---

He's getting thinner by the minute,
his snapshot face is fading from colour
to black and white.
This morning I meet him on the drive,
his role taken by an actor
who looks remotely familiar
but who hasn't quite caught
the essence of the man
(from *The Man Next Door* by James Caruth, 2007)[1]

Kneeling there by the basin, I felt I was adapting already, like a creature moving from the sea to the land, evolving a new identity. And I was sealing myself away. My sense of time and space was shrinking. The invisible thread that had been tying me to home and the desperate desire to get out had slackened.

(Watt 1996: 18)

These two extracts introduce the issue of identity, our understandings of that term, and the implications of these understandings for practice among people with life-limiting illnesses. The first is from a poem written by the next-door neighbour of a man diagnosed with such an illness. The second is from the autobiographical account of a 29-year-old man who had developed Churg-Strauss syndrome, a rare and painful condition which few survived until the late 1970s. Both suggest that life-limiting illnesses can disturb, transform or erase something we call our identity. The poet uses the metaphor of acting a role to convey the disjuncture between the neighbour he remembers and the dying man on the adjoining drive. The second extract includes the term 'identity' in a description of personal disorientation which employs the powerful metaphor of a sea creature evolving into a very different beast.

The implications of such experiences for identity – and personhood – have been a focus for palliative care research.[2] Yet little consensus unites authors as to the nature of the threats and the promises they represent. Some describe the disintegration of the self in conditions which breach the body's boundaries (Lawton 2000); others argue that 'death can cause a human being to become what he or she was called to become' (Hennezel, cited in Nelson 2000). Such differences at the level of interpretation partly reflect the diversity of experiences encompassed even within a 'single' condition such as cancer. Regardless of the belief system through which a life-limiting illness is *appraised*, the body itself 'speaks', manifesting very different symptoms, depending on the type and trajectory of the illness. Yet, as Lawton argues, 'the (death studies) literature tends to build its theoretical paradigms upon assumptions of homogeneous categories such as "the dying patient" and "the dying process"' (2000: 145). This chapter therefore seeks to acknowledge the variety of experiences undergone by patients.

## Identity or personhood?

In defining his terms in an account of social identity, Jenkins (2004) differentiates between the self and the person. While the notion of the self generally refers to an individual's private, inner world, the term person describes their public persona, the individual as they appear to others. In the extracts which begin this chapter, the neighbour's point of view accompanies that of the patient, yet as Jenkins observes, 'I want to insist that selfhood and personhood are completely and utterly implicated in each other' (2004: 28). How the individual understands themselves, and how others see them, cannot, therefore, be read in isolation from one another. This is not to say that outsiders can mind-read our private thoughts and feelings, or that we inevitably take on the views of others when reflecting upon ourselves. But, rather, that we do need to get at the interaction between these two sides to issues of identity.

The notion of an *interaction* between the private self and a public persona highlights the nature of identity as a process, rather than a fixed entity such as an internal plumbing system or a label stitched to someone's clothing. Any interaction involves some kind of back and forth and so unfolds across time. While Ben Watt, cited above, describes his identity evolving, the change he perceives exists within an overall process that makes up his life course, however short or long. As Jenkins says, 'identity can *only* be understood as process, as "being" or "becoming" ' (original emphasis, 2004: 5). And if identity is an unfolding and therefore inevitably incomplete process, we can envisage it as something 'done', an *active* process involving different kinds of agency. The term 'identification' therefore usefully denotes something which the individual participates in. As argued below, such perspectives have implications for how patients and their carers/families might respond to their feelings of despair, loss and self-abnegation.

What, however, does one participate *in* during the interactive process of identification? How does the mingling of private thoughts and external responses produce something called identity? Here questions of similarity and difference highlight what is at stake, as different framings of the individual are weighed against one another. Who are we like and who are we different from are issues with considerable relevance for the experience of a life-limiting illness. One of *The Oxford English Dictionary*'s definitions of identity raises the related question of the stability of our identities *vis-à-vis* other people: 'the consistency or continuity over time that is the basis for establishing and grasping the definiteness and distinctiveness of something' (cited in Jenkins 2004: 4). Yet this emphasis on continuity appears to be at odds with the notion of identification as *change*, process, agency and participation.

Here, a parallel argument offered in Leder's (1990) phenomenology of bodily *absence* during periods of good health is helpful. In his view, the body is the site from which we perceive the surrounding world, the vehicle through which we sense and make sense of our surroundings. Constant bodily-self awareness therefore potentially undermines the body's capacity to engage with its environment. When we stroke the cat, we focus on the cat's fur, not the bodily process of stroking. Injury or illness, however, can cause the body to obtrude into consciousness, to become *present* – and the difficulty of concentrating on the task in hand with backache is a familiar example. So, just as a malfunctioning body assumes a dominant position within our consciousness, change in our everyday lives may precipitate more explicit concern with who we are and who others might understand us to be. By contrast, during periods of personal and social stability, it may take a sociologist to remind us that our identity is negotiated! Changes with implications for identity include: a new ethnic mix within our neighbourhood; a new job; the recent politicization of sexuality; moving to a new town or country; becoming seriously ill.

Establishing similarity and difference through processes of negotiation is not, however, simply a matter of being clear that I am English and you are Welsh. It encompasses the difference between who I 'know' I am and who my diagnosis suggests I might become. The ways in which patients might negotiate and experience their identities is therefore an aspect of a life-long process of identification, albeit one with potential unevenness across time and events. As Jenkins says: 'levels of concern about identity may wax and wane' (2004: 7).

# Who do we think we are?

Theories of identity can therefore usefully draw practitioners' attention to connections between the rupture which the onset of a life-limiting illness might represent and the *ongoing* processes of negotiation and change which all identification entails. That said, the kind of 'selfhood' which we negotiate does reflect a particular model of what it means to be human. Ideas about the very nature of the self as an embodied entity are culturally and historically specific. So, while we may be aware that life-limiting illness can threaten identity, what exactly is under threat is worth some consideration. As the examples explored later in the chapter will demonstrate, it can be the notion of the self which is specific to Western societies which is most vulnerable to potential changes brought about by the dying process, as Lawton (2000) argues.

This model of the self, arguably, stems from a long history of individualism, particularly within Great Britain (see McFarlane 1978), one which has resulted in the framing of selfhood in terms of the autonomy and independence of the individual. As someone who is free to make their way in the world, the Western individual is someone who is politically unfettered by governmental constraints, and socially and emotionally unconstrained by difficult relations of kinship, marriage or friendship (Dalley 1988; Giddens 1991; Battersby 1993; Lawton 2000).

This model of the self has been represented by the image or root metaphor of a container which divides one individual from another – and has been a focus for recent attention within the social sciences. Lawton (2000) draws on it when arguing that hospices are in part a site at which bodies which can no longer conform to the image or metaphor of a container are removed from everyday life, or sequestered. This institutional containment of the unbounded body, however, cannot repair breaches at the level of identity. Nonetheless, as Lawton's (2000) data indicate, the removal of the patient from their home potentially restores the 'container' selves of *carers* who can otherwise experience the patient's body as a distressing, barely manageable extension of their own. In sum, then, conditions such as a complete loss of continence, the emergence of fungating tumours through the body's surfaces, and faecal vomiting, so disrupt the body's boundaries that personhood disintegrates and patients quite literally turn their faces to the wall. In Lawton's data they close their eyes and refuse all communication; demand heavy sedation; call for euthanasia. As Lawton says, 'it could be argued that patients with unbounded bodies lost one of the criteria for personhood by virtue of their lacking the corporeal capacity for "self-containment" ' (2000: 142). The outside of their body, she suggests, no longer acts as a boundary between themselves and other people.

## Diversity and selfhood

The container self can be compared with evidence of different ways of conceptualizing and so negotiating identity. While apparently 'exotic', they do provide some critical distance from the taken-for-granted ideas of Westerners as to what is, or is not, a threat to personhood. In addition, as the examples below suggest, they can alert us to different dimensions of the container self and raise the possibility that there is more flexibility within Western thinking than might be apparent.

What unites the non-Western examples which anthropologists have described is a more diffuse sense of embodied human identity. Thus, the Hau people of the Highlands of Papua New Guinea (see Meigs 1984, cited in Lawton 2000: 140) define identity in terms of those fluids and scents which escape the body. Thus, a man will smear his sweat, oil and vomit over relatives' bodies to facilitate their growth, via the ingestation of such substances through the skin. Among 'Rwandan' people (see Taylor, n.d., cited in Lawton 2000: 140), the social incorporation of a newborn baby is achieved through a ritual meal containing some of the baby's faeces. These notions of selfhood are more intersubjective; they are about fluid connections between people. As such, they undermine the possibility of a clear-cut inner/outer division between selfhood and personhood. Becker's Fijian ethnography similarly describes a social context where 'bodily experience transcends the individual body, is diffused to other bodies, and is even manifest in the environment' (1995: 127). This is expressed in the belief that nurture and food exchange generate a valued intersubjective identity which connects, rather than being contained within individual bodies. Similarly, Leenhardt's account of the New Caledonian peoples describes the body as 'diffused with other persons and things in a unitary sociomythic domain' (cited in Csordas 1994: 7). In sum, as Csordas argues, embodied experience is 'contingent on how the self is situated in a relational matrix' (1994: 127).

For Westerners, however, life-limiting illness can generate dependencies previously experienced only during childhood. For them, 'growing up' involves learning bodily independence and containment if they are to 'stand on their own two feet' (see Hockey and James 1993). Yet Western history reminds us that prior to the mid-nineteenth century, notions of personal and bodily 'privacy' were largely unrecognized (see Lupton 1998). Instead excretion, defaecation, spitting, belching, eating and sexual intercourse could be witnessed in public places. Sociality did not require the strict control of the body's boundaries but instead was understood in terms of connectedness and flow, as epitomized by shared bodily activities (see Elias 1994).

# Reappraising Western identities

These examples remind us that our embodied sense of who we are is specific to our time and our social context. How might we think differently, either about who we imagine ourselves to be, *or* about how best to manage the implications of the Western container self during life-limiting illness? Willmott (2000), a sociologist, draws on Buddhist philosophy to question some of the assumptions made by death studies about the nature of being human. Bauman's (1992) argument that death equates to chaos, that anomic terror is a universal human response to mortality, underpins the view that only the fragile constructions of human society and culture can stave off this threat. However, Willmott suggests that, 'ontological and existential anxieties . . . are not universal, or endemic, to the human condition but, instead, are expressions of the socially organized privileging of a separation between wo/man and world' (2000: 657). It is the system of order, the rules and roles we live by, which sociologists such as Bauman (1992) describe as our defence against mortality, that is precisely what Willmott (2000) sees as the problem. *They* are what we fear losing. Death, he suggests, can also be an advisor, enabling us to think about social identity and social institutions in more fluid or even playful ways which do not assume their *defensive* function. To what extent, then, can this view inform the practicalities of addressing emotional and bodily distress in the UK today?

Arnold's (2006) ethnography of a Thai Buddhist hospice describes this philosophy's apparently very different outcomes for practice. Working in this setting profoundly disrupted his Western assumptions about the embodied experience of dying: 'As I stood or sat next to the dying person I expected something, something unique and powerful, to occur. The person stopped breathing; there was no explosion of emotion or drama of any kind from anyone' (2006: 34). Instead, he observed the 'calm "waiting" stance exhibited by the elderly (patients)', and a lack of tension between paid and volunteer staff, all of which he understood as 'a product of their Buddhist spiritual ontology' (2006: 32); that is, their beliefs about the transitory, even illusory nature of human life. Dying was thus viewed as integral to life, a process which manifested the temporary nature of the self. 'These behaviours', he argues, 'can therefore be seen as an extension of the cultural emphasis on interdependence, which is usually an inevitable and salient circumstance at the end of life, as opposed to the tensions and distress among the elderly in western societies who struggle from positions of independence to ones of dependence during the latter stages of their lives' (Arnold 2006: 31).

Can Arnold's work (2006) contribute practical guidance for practitioners and patients from other cultural traditions? McGrath's (1998) study of the community-based Karuna Hospice Service, a Buddhist organization in Brisbane, demonstrates that while the central tenets of Buddhist philosophy – practical, outward-focused compassion; tolerance; a duty to do no harm; and a view of death as life's most significant moment – reflect specific cultural roots, they are entirely compatible with the ethos of the Hospice Movement. Practices and attitudes observed in health care settings which reflect Buddhist philosophy may not, therefore, be inappropriate models for the development of good practice within Western environments.

## Stigma and social death

So far, identity has been described as a process, unfolding over time and ever open to change. It involves personal reflection *and* the perceptions of an external world, and concerns differences and similarities between self and others, and between the individual's remembered, present and imagined identities. In addition, as argued, models or metaphors of the self are both culturally-specific and heavily implicated in such processes. These features of identity have relevance for issues surrounding practice within palliative care. However, in addition to identity's fluidity and contingency, its capacity to be multilayered also needs to be recognized. As Jenkins says, 'who we are is always singular *and* plural' (2004: 5).

Being diagnosed with a life-limiting illness can profoundly undermine what has previously been a more pluralistic sense of oneself. Payne and Seymour (2004: 20), for example, describe the resonance of diagnostic labels within health care settings, citing studies undertaken on hospital wards for older adults where initial diagnosis (along with name, age and resuscitation status) constituted the hospital-based identity of individuals receiving care. The resilience of such an identity is evidenced by its persistence, despite amended diagnoses and the presence of co-morbidities. In light of patients' dependency upon the care of nursing staff, such an identity can acquire a 'master status' (Glaser and Strauss 1971), taking precedence over other, parallel and contextually-located identities.

Alongside, the resonance of diagnostic *labels*, which emanate from the patient's external social world, the bodily changes brought about by illness also have implications for the patient's sense of self. As Jenkins stresses, identity 'always begins – literally or figuratively – from the body. There is nowhere else to begin' (2004: 46). Thus, unwelcome bodily changes associated with life-limiting illness can seriously undermine a sense of oneself as both the person one was *and* as someone who possesses or represents social value (see Price 2000). This stigmatizing process links powerfully with the concept of a master status. As Price suggests: 'Terminal illness undermines body image, not only because it produces changes in the look, sound or smell of the human body, but because it stigmatizes the individual' (2000: 180).

Goffman's (1963) account of how stigma can 'spoil' the individual's identity emphasizes the importance of both the body and an institutional setting. Describing how 'the abominations of the body' can produce 'undesired differentness' (1968: 14–15), he details the ways in which the loss or removal of markers of identity can reduce the multiple nature of identity to a single, dominant 'master' status. During life-limiting illness, both the bodily changes which Price (2000) identifies and the settings within which diagnosis is made and treatment offered can be potent threats to a sense of personal continuity or stability. Goffman (1968) demonstrated the impact of a shrinking personal world most powerfully in his work on the total institutions of his time – for example, the military services and mental hospitals. While the holistic approach of palliative care was developed in settings designed to be as homely or home-like as possible, as an antidote to potentially de-humanizing hospital regimes, it remains important to recognize the implications for identity of a setting where medical and bureaucratic practices and procedures retain a place.

Stigma links with another helpful sociological concept, that of social death (Glaser and Strauss 1965; Sudnow 1967; Mulkay 1993; Johnston 2004). Rather than an irrevocable moment of social erasure, Mulkay talks of 'social death sequences' (1993: 33) extending over time and potentially transcending death itself. Thus, he suggests that, 'it is entirely possible for people to sustain a lasting, personal relationship which the course of their daily lives with an individual whom they know to be dead' (1993: 33). Prior to death, however, personal relationships can become attenuated or erased. Sweet and Gilhooly's (1997, cited in Johnston, 2004: 354–5) work among the carers of elderly relatives with dementia gets at the negotiated nature of both social life and social death in that carers' responses were not uniform. Rather they could be divided into those who believed that, and behaved as if, their relative was socially dead; those who believed that social death had occurred but treated their relative *as if* socially alive; those (few) who treated their relative as if socially dead yet failed to acknowledge this; and those who drew on their memories of the individual's previous social identity in sustaining their social life, in both belief and practice.

These data concern external sources of identification, such as carers, and how they might construct identity, in the case of dementia. With respect to life-limiting illness, Lawton's data reveal the patient's own embodied sense of who they are – and the suffering of those who elected to 'switch themselves off' (2000: 132) once their body's boundaries had irretrievably broken down. By contrast, however, 'social death' can be seen as a positive and strategic withdrawal. For example, patients may seek to manage their own dying trajectory through fasting, a practice which resonates with spiritual and cultural traditions where death is more openly embraced (see Ahronheim 1995).

As already noted, then, questions of stigma and social death can divide authors, a reflection of the diversity of depredations which a life-limiting illness might involve, as well as the social milieu within which care is provided. Johnston, for example, describes 'social deadness' as something which 'evolves', and which can be 'self-imposed or enforced by others' (2004: 355).

# Rethinking identity: some implications for practice

The concept of stigma highlights the stripping away of many markers of identity. Altered body image (Price 2000), diminished competencies, faculties and functions, and loss of active engagement in social institutions such as paid work, family life and leisure, can all eradicate particular modes or sites of identification. Drawing on the theoretical perspectives detailed above, the ways in which patients and their carers might respond to such changes is the focus for the remainder of this chapter.

Kabel and Roberts (2003) take up Lawton's (2000) argument that, in a Western cultural context, the breakdown of the body's boundaries seriously threatens the integrity of personhood. While their study acknowledges differences in the ways in which personhood is conceived of, the scope within palliative care for sustaining personhood that they identify is largely framed within a Western model. Using ethnographic interviewing and participant observation among 30 staff in two inpatient hospices in north west England, they identified a range of body-focused and more social practices which addressed this problem. In terms of the body, then, established palliative approaches were important: controlling pain, masking foul odours through the use of essential oils and an ozone machine, and maintaining patients' personal grooming. In addition, Western cultural models of autonomous selfhood are acknowledged in practices designed to foster independence among patients. 'Total care' of patients, while an important value within hospice nursing, was something which staff sought to deliver 'at their pace': 'I'm a firm believer that if a patient turns round and says, "I don't want a wash today" then that patient doesn't have to have a wash that day. It's totally up to them', one nurse said. From the patient's perspective, another study presents the statement: 'to start with they helped me have a bath, and as I got better I said "I can manage this, but can you just help me with this". They were quite happy not to do the whole thing but to come in and do parts I couldn't do, you know, let me do what I could do, which I don't know whether it might sound funny, but I think you need that . . .' (Seymour *et al.* 2003: 29).

Kabel and Roberts (2003) also reveal staff's recognition of the *interactive* nature of personhood as a social phenomenon. For example, they deliberately maintained eye contact with patients experiencing distressing or embarrassing symptoms. If, as argued, identification is a process, then ensuring that processes of social recognition continue to take place is important. If patients lost consciousness, staff continued to talk to them as they worked and to provide expressive rather than simply instrumental touch, by holding their hands. Through example, staff encouraged families to do the same, so helping sustain long-standing sites of identification.

This evidence exposes one of the paradoxes of the Western container self. Personal autonomy or integrity is not simply a matter of maintaining interpersonal boundaries. Connectedness and social interaction do play an important role within Western notions of personhood. This brings up the implications of Kabel and Roberts's (2003) evidence for staff and families, as well as patients. Discussing the notion that staff commit more resources to 'special cases' in fruitless attempts to sustain the (social) life of what are often young people (see Lawton 2000; Kabel and Roberts 2003) contest the argument that resources devoted to such patients undermine provision for others. In their view, the more intense social interaction which a 'special case' can involve potentially sustains the personhood of *staff*: 'you reaffirm . . . that it is a worthwhile job you are doing . . .', said a hospice therapist.

Unpacking the paradoxes implicit within the container metaphor of the Western self can thus have implications for practice. In the cross-cultural and historical examples presented earlier, embodiment is seen to transcend what Westerners understand as an individualized 'container' of the self. Yet the Western connection between the individual body and the self which can result in stigma or social death when bodily integrity is lost has other implications. If self and body can *diverge*, for example, when bodily 'life' persists despite seriously impaired brain function, the possibility of social life *despite* bodily death also has to be recognized (see Hallam *et al.* 1999). Thus, for example, Copp (1999, cited in Kabel and Roberts 2003: 288) describes nurses separating the dying patient's body from the person that they are, in a social sense. In this way they guard against the complete erasure of not only the body but also the person and the self. They thereby establish conditions within which survivors may choose to maintain 'continuing bonds' with the individual who has died (see Klass *et al.* 1996).

This practice resonates with other devices for asserting the identity of the individual at or soon after the time of death: for example, families who show hospice staff photographs of the dead individual prior to the onset of illness and the use of photographs which reflect previous roles within public life in obituaries (see Bytheway and Johnson 1996). The 'container' self is therefore not only a product of social interaction; it also encompasses greater fluidity than might be assumed, here in terms of its scope for being sustained across time – and beyond the confines of embodied life (Hockey and Draper 2005).

In conditions where an illness has unravelled the mind, rather than simply the body, the integrity of identity may be preserved not by retaining and projecting forwards a sense of self outwith the body – but through strategies which relocate a former identity in the present. Gillies and Johnston, for example, describe the comments made by the carers of people who have become heavily dependent as a result of cancer: 'he's no' my man', said one woman (2004: 439). Such examples are set alongside similar statements made by carers of people with Alzheimers: 'That's not my mother any more. That's another pleasant wee woman who looks like her' (2004: 440). In this way, the person previously known and loved is withheld from the stigmatizing circumstances of the present and more safely relocated in the past.

# Intercorporeal personhood

Alongside the role of social interaction in sustaining personal integrity, then, we can identify the scope for social life outwith or beyond embodied life. What cross-cultural and historical comparison also suggests is the possibility of intersubjective or intercorporeal personhood. In other words, identity can derive from a combination of more than one person's body and/or mind. To what extent might this too be a less 'exotic' dimension of everyday life and death than we imagine? Orona (1990, cited in Gillies and Johnston 2004: 441) describes carers supplying missing dimensions of someone with Alzheimers, suggesting the possibility of a more composite self which is, in part, located in the past. In drawing on their memories of who the patient once was, carers can sometimes 'work both sides of a relationship' (1990, cited in Gillies and Johnston 2004: 441). Gillies and Johnston's (2004) comparative account of studies among patients with cancer and with Alzheimers, and their carers, bears this out; a patient with dementia said of her husband, 'he's more or less my memory now' (2004: 438). These authors conclude by saying that despite the mental and physical depredations of Alzheimers and cancer:

> a self can be preserved and made manifest both explicitly and implicitly and can further be maintained by perpetuating in the present, attributes from the past which confirm current ideas of the self (2004: 441).

> In order to support identities grounded in the past, but made 'live' through more composite forms of selfhood, practitioners are urged to take full account of personal details 'as presented by the care recipient and to provide care which nurtures and maintains that self' (2004: 441).

Reiterating the centrality of social interaction to the maintenance of personal integrity, the importance of *collective* identity is evidenced in Seymour *et al.*'s (2003) study. This describes patients' use of the terms 'family' and 'home' to express, metaphorically, the precise quality of intimacy they enjoyed with staff, both at the level of 'chatting' and 'having a laugh', as well as in the expression of concern for more deep-seated issues. Here a shared, familial identity, rather than a composite self, is used to sustain a sense of the self which transcends any diagnostic master status (Glaser and Strauss 1971). 'Home', as these authors argue, can be understood as 'a quality of service provision rather than a physical location' (2003: 31). Lawton's (2000) data remind us, however, that the scope of more collective sites of personal identification may be restricted to the earlier stages of a life-limiting illness: 'the absence of autonomous aspects of patients' selves, for example, was masked and negated within day care through the formation of pseudo-surrogate family relationships which enabled exterior components of the self to be emphasised' (2000: 183).

While 'family' and 'home' can figure within a patient's environment as metaphoric terms, these metaphors can also be materialized. Kabel and Roberts's (2003) data describe photos and other items from home being used to personalize hospice space. Indeed notions of privacy, expressed most profoundly in the notion of 'home', are given form in, for example, a quiet room for family gatherings and a glass conservatory converted by staff into a honeymoon suite for a patient who married in the hospice chapel.

# Agency revisited

This final section critically revisits the Western container self to suggest that alongside strategies geared towards strengthening its integrity – for example, through delivering 'total care' at the patient's self-determined pace – a more intersubjective or intercorporeal notion of the self admits the possibility of reframing dependency as a form of shared agency. As shown in Exley's (1999) account of women with life-limiting illnesses negotiating their after-death identities, patients themselves can exercise agency in ways which sustain their personhood in both the present and in a future beyond their own embodied lives. Thus, Exley's data describe not only the provisions women make for their families and children, in terms of funeral plans and memory boxes; but also the humorous or 'light' manner in which such plans are laid. This, Exley argues, 'served a dual purpose of "protecting" both themselves and significant others, while at the same time enabling conversations about difficult topics to take place' (1999: 261). In opting for this style, women thereby sustained their identity as a caring 'partner' and 'parent'.

Such activities cannot, however, be undertaken by all patients, given variation in their particular condition and its stage of development. Here Price's (2000) work on strategies through which practitioners can address the stigmatizing implications of altered body image is helpful. While the women Exley (1999) describes seem able to take charge of social interactions with family members, the case study of a 46-year-old woman with a fungating breast carcinoma presented by Price (2000) shows someone managing the stigmatizing conditions of her life-limiting illness through reluctant social withdrawal. What Price (2000) describes, in response, is a strategy whereby the skills of the practitioner enable agency on the part of the patient. Via the shared efforts of the practitioner and the patient, a review of social reactions to the patient's bodily condition was achieved. Such responses included avoidance, over-involvement, protectiveness and social boundary management. The practitioner then worked to co-produce strategies which the patient could enact. Thus, avoidance of the patient's fungating tumour could either be challenged or colluded with. The patient would decide at the time. Over-involvement could either be challenged or dissipated by drawing attention to other aspects of (shared) identity. Again the patient decides which to opt for, at the time. Over-protectiveness at the boundaries of the patient's social relationships was dealt with by rewarding the good intentions of the relative concerned and expressing the non-threatening view that the patient was still deciding what she wished others to know about her circumstances. Such strategies, Price suggests, are 'designed to help the patient feel in control, not only of the body but also of social encounters with others (2000: 184).

# Conclusion

This chapter has drawn upon theoretical perspectives which are current within the social sciences to explore the ways in which life-limiting illness might undermine identity and personhood. Key features of identity were its processual, participative nature; its ongoing emergence out of interactions between the individual and those around them; its multilayered, contextual nature; and the importance of establishing degrees of similarity and difference with other people, and with previous or projected images of the self. The specificity of the Western self was evidenced through cross-cultural and historical comparison and the implications of these data for practice involved; considering the ways in which threats to a container self might be repaired; and exploring convergences between Western and non-Western conceptions of the self. While life-limiting illness can result in stigma and indeed social death, reflection upon the nature of the self and the co-production of identity not only helps make sense of patients' emotional and social distress, but also informs the development of practices which can support a more welcome sense of self during and indeed after the dying process.

# Notes

1   I am grateful to James Caruth for permission to reproduce part of his poem.
2   Many thanks to Julie Ellis, University of Sheffield, for help in preparing material for this chapter.

# References

Ahronheim, J. (1995) Refusal of artificial feeding as a natural part of dying. In: N. Albery, M. Mezey, M. McHugh and M. Papworth (eds) *Before and After*. London: The Natural Death Centre.

Arnold, B.L. (2006) Anticipatory Dying: Reflections Upon End of Life Experiences in a Thai Buddhist Hospice, *Qualitative Sociology Review*, II(2): 21–41.

Battersby, C. (1993) Her body/her boundaries: gender and the metaphysics of containment. In: A.E. Benjamin (ed.) *The Body*, Special Issue of *Journal of Philosophy and the Visual Arts*, 4: 30–9.

Bauman, Z. (1992) *Mortality, Immortality and other Life Strategies*. Cambridge: Polity.

Becker, A. (1995) *Body, Self and Society. A View from Fiji*. Philadelphia: University of Philadelphia Press.

Bytheway, B. and Johnson, J. (1996) Valuing lives? Obituaries and the life course, *Mortality*, 1(2): 219–34.

Caruth, J. (2007) *A Stone's Throw*. Nottingham: Staple Press.

Csordas, T. (1994) *Embodiment and Experience*. Cambridge: Cambridge University Press.

Dalley, G. (1988) *Ideologies of Caring: Rethinking Community and Collectivism*. London: Macmillan.

Elias, N. (1994) *The Civilizing Process: the History of Manners and State Formation and Civilization*. Oxford: Blackwell.

Exley, C. (1999) Testaments and memories: negotiating after-death identities, *Mortality*, 4(3): 249–68.

Giddens, A. (1991) *Modernity and Self-Identity*. Cambridge: Polity Press.

Gillies, B. and Johnston, G. (2004) Identity loss and maintenance: commonality of experiences in cancer and dementia, *European Journal of Cancer Care*, 13: 436–42.

Glaser, B. and Strauss, A. (1965) *Awareness of Dying*. Chicago: Aldine.

Glaser, B. and Strauss, A. (1971) *Status Passage*. London: Routledge and Kegan Paul.

Goffman, E. (1963) *Stigma: Notes on the Management of Spoiled Identity*. Englewood Cliffs, N.J.: Prentice Hall.

Goffman, E. (1968) *Asylums: Essays on the Social Situation of Mental Patients and Other Inmates*. Harmondsworth: Pelican.

Hallam, E., Hockey, J. and Howarth, G. (1999) *Beyond the Body. Death and Social Identity*. London: Routledge.

Hockey, J. and Draper, J. (2005) 'Beyond the Womb and the Tomb: Identity, (Dis)-Embodiment and the Life Course', *Body and Society*, 11(2): 41–58.

Hockey, J. and James, A. (1993) *Growing Up and Growing Old. Ageing and Dependency in the Life Course*. London: Sage.

Jenkins, R. (2004) *Social Identity*, 2nd edition. London: Routledge.

Johnston, G. (2004) Social Death. The impact of protracted dying. In: S. Payne, J. Seymour and C. Ingleton (eds) *Palliative Care Nursing. Principles and Evidence for Practice*, 1st edition. Buckingham: Open University Press.

Kabel, A. and Roberts, D. (2003) 'Professionals perceptions of maintaining personhood in hospice care', *International Journal of Palliative Nursing*, 9(7): 283–9.

Klass, D., Silverman, P. and Nickman, S. (1996) *Continuing Bonds. New Understandings of Grief*. Washington: Taylor and Francis.

Lawton, J. (2000) *The Dying Process. Patients' experiences of palliative care*. London: Routledge.

Leder, D. (1990) *The Absent Body*. Chicago: University of Chicago Press.

Lupton, D. (1998) *The Emotional Self*. London: Sage.

Macfarlane, A. (1978) *The Origins of English Individualism*. Oxford: Basil Blackwell.

McGrath, P. (1998) 'Buddhist spirituality – a compassionate perspective on hospice care', *Mortality*, 3(3): 251–64.

Mulkay, M. (1993) 'Social death in Britain'. In: D. Clark (ed.) *The Sociology of Death*. Oxford: Blackwell.

Nelson, G. (2000) 'Maintaining the integrity of personhood in palliative care', *Scottish Journal of Healthcare Chaplaincy*, 3(2): 34–9.

Payne, S. and Seymour, J. (2004) Overview. In: S. Payne, J. Seymour and C. Ingleton (eds) *Palliative Care Nursing. Principles and Evidence for Practice*, 1st edition. Buckingham: Open University Press.

Price, B. (2000) 'Altered Body Image: managing social encounters', *International Journal of Palliative Nursing*, 6(4): 179–85.

Seymour, J.E., Ingleton, C., Payne, S. and Beddow, V. (2003) 'Specialist palliative care: patients' experiences', *Journal of Advanced Nursing*, 44(1): 24–33.

Sudnow, D. (1967) *Passing On: the social organisation of dying*. Englewood Cliffs: Prentice Hall.

Watt, B. (1996) *Patient. The true story of a rare illness*. London: Penguin.

Willmott, H. (2000) 'Death. So What? Sociology, sequestration and emancipation', *The Sociological Review*, 48(4): 649–65.

# 18

# No way in

## Including disadvantaged population and patient groups at the end of life

*Jonathan Koffman and Margaret Camps*

---

**Key points**

- Certain groups of people with advanced disease are excluded from specialist health care near the end of life.
- Access to good quality care towards the end of life is a basic human right.
- Those most likely to be socially excluded are the poor, older people, people with learning disabilities and mental health problems.

---

> We emerge deserving of little credit; we who are capable of ignoring the conditions that make muted people suffer. The dissatisfied dead cannot noise abroad the negligence they have experienced.
>
> (Hinton 1967)

## Introduction: the universal right to care at the end of life and during bereavement

Forty years ago in this statement John Hinton drew attention to the deficiencies evident in the care offered to many patients with advanced disease and their families. While we have witnessed a dramatic growth in the provision of palliative care and a greater understanding of the palliative care needs of patients and their families, actual access to services has been wholly inequitable. In recent years, both in the United Kingdom, the USA and Australia, questions are being asked about the extent to which palliative care and related services are available to all who can benefit from them given that accessible and good quality care towards the end of life must be recognized as a basic human right:

Everyone has the right to . . . security in the event of sickness, disability, widowhood, old age or other lack of livelihood in circumstances beyond his [or her] control. Article 25, United Nations Universal Declaration of Human Rights 2001.

(Office of the High Commissioner for Human Rights 2005).

## The growth of palliative care and demands on services in the United Kingdom: Is there a problem?

Palliative care now encompasses a wide range of specialist services. The number of hospices and specialist palliative care services has increased rapidly since the 1960s. In 1980, there were less than 80 inpatient hospices and 100 home support teams in the United Kingdom and the Republic of Ireland. By 2006 this had increased to 221 inpatient hospices comprising approximately 2,500 beds, 356 home care and extended home care support teams, and 257 day care centres. In addition, there are more than 350 hospital support teams (Hospice Information 2006). While the actual supply of specialist palliative care plays a role in determining which patients with progressive disease and their families receive care, concerns have been raised about other factors that influence the accessibility of care at the end of life for those who might benefit from it.

This chapter critically appraises the evidence, principally from the United Kingdom and the USA, to determine in what ways the 'socially excluded' – the poor, older people, people with learning disabilities and mental health problems, black and minority ethnic groups, asylum seekers and refugees, the homeless, the mentally ill, those within the penal system, and drug users – fare with respect to accessing specialist palliative care and related services during their advanced disease and at the end of life. While the chapter has limited itself to these population groups, other socially excluded sectors of the population are not immune. They include travelling communities and those who abuse alcohol. To date, however, little attention and therefore published research has focused on either their met or unmet palliative care needs, a testimony to their social distance from the mainstream. This chapter then makes suggestions how those involved in the planning and delivery of palliative care and related services can extend care to include these disadvantaged population groups.

## What is social exclusion?

The concept of equity of access to health care is a central objective of many health care systems throughout the world and has been an important buttress of the United Kingdom National Health Service since its inception in 1948. In the early 1970s, Julian Tudor Hart coined the phrase 'inverse care law' to describe the observation that those who were in the greatest apparent need of care often had the worst access to health care provision (Hart 1971). Although this is not true of the whole health system (Haynes 1991; Goddard and Smith 2001), a growing body of research evidence has accumulated demonstrating that socially disenfranchised sections of society fare poorly with regard to secondary and tertiary medical care (Townsend and Davison 1982; Whitehead 1992; Department of Health 1998; Goddard and Smith 2001). This is true for care for patients with advanced disease and their families (Ahmed *et al.* 2004; Higginson and Koffman 2005). Renewed commitment to tackle health inequalities has recently been harnessed under the wing of 'social exclusion', a relatively new term in the United Kingdom policy debate to describe an old problem (Barratt 2001). It includes poverty and low income but is broader and addresses some of the wider causes and consequences of social deprivation. The United Kingdom Government has defined social exclusion as:

> a shorthand term for what can happen when people or areas suffer from a combination of linked problems such as unemployment, poor skills, low incomes, poor housing, high crime, bad health and family breakdown.
>
> (Social Exclusion Unit 2001)

This is a deliberately flexible definition, and the factors they suggest are only examples. Simply put, an individual is socially excluded if he or she cannot participate in the normal activities of citizens in that society, and he or she would like to so participate but is prevented from doing so by factors beyond his or her control. Many other dimensions of exclusion could also be added. The most important characteristic is that these problems are linked and mutually reinforcing, and can combine to create a complex and fast-moving vicious cycle. The result is hugely expensive for society, not only in human but also in economic terms. Importantly, it can also lead to a society that is unpleasant for so many.

## Who are at risk of social exclusion?

Social exclusion is something that can happen to anyone. Some people, however, from certain backgrounds and experiences are more likely to suffer. Older people are particularly at risk of social exclusion. Many are at disproportionate risk of falling into poverty. People from black and minority ethnic communities are disproportionately exposed to risk of social exclusion. For example, they are more likely than others to live in deprived areas and in unpopular and overcrowded housing; they are also more likely to be poor and to be unemployed, regardless of age, sex, qualifications and place of residence. Pakistani, Bangladeshi and black Caribbean people living in the United Kingdom are more likely to report suffering ill health than white people (Acheson 1998). None of these risk categories are mutually exclusive and may operate in combination with others at any point in time. The key risk factors are presented in Box 18.1.

> **Box 18.1**   The socially excluded
>
> • The economically disadvantaged
> • Those living in a deprived neighbourhood in either urban or rural areas
> • Those with mental health problems
> • Older people
> • People with disabilities
> • Black and ethnic minority groups

## The causes of social exclusion

According to the Social Exclusion Unit, past United Kingdom government policies and structures have not coped well with helping socially excluded elements of society. Some of the reasons for this failure are specific to the nature of social exclusion. Others are more general difficulties in public services. Many social exclusion issues cut across the boundaries between services and departments. Box 18.2 illustrates some of the causes and their consequences.

Attempts to tackle social exclusion in the past have also suffered from some of the more general difficulties that can affect any government programme. They include: little emphasis on working in partnership with businesses, local government, service providers, communities, and voluntary and faith groups; focus on processes rather than on outcomes; tendency to look at averages which can mask the worsening position of those at the bottom; weaknesses in the collection and use of evidence; and relying on short-term programmes, rather than sustained investment.

## Social exclusion: the concept in question

It has been suggested that the concept 'social exclusion' is misleading since it denotes being deliberately 'shut out'. Groups within society are only shut out as a result of the normal social processes society unconsciously subscribes to and abides by, but not as an act of deliberate social exclusion directed solely at them (Rose 1996). It has therefore been suggest that it might be more productive to refer to these population groups as 'marginalized' or 'disenfranchised' groups (Morrell 2001). Isolated and marginalized people do not enjoy the same opportunities as the rest of society. They lack fulfillment of personal potential, and dwell in a social space where there is a perceived distance between them and others. They also lack participation in social institutions which springs from commonality in interests and a social sense of belonging.

| **Box 18.2**    Causes and consequences of social exclusion | |
|---|---|
| **'Orphan' issues** | Problems currently tackled by the Social Exclusion Unit exacerbated in the past because no one was in charge of solving them, either in government or on the ground. |
| **Lack of 'joining up'** | Some services have not effective in tackling inequality because they are dealing with problems whose causes are outside their remit of responsibility. |
| **Duplication** | With many organizations and departments involved in an issue, efforts sometimes end up being duplicated. |

# Who are the 'excluded' at the end of life?

Palliative care, free at the point of delivery from the NHS and the independent charitable sector, has become more prominent within the United Kingdom. Nevertheless, it has still been slow to reach certain patients and population groups who could benefit from it. Below we have focused on the available evidence on access to palliative care to poor and other disenfranchised population groups. Our list of groups is restricted – other vulnerable sectors of the society may fare as badly.

## The poor

Poverty means going short materially, socially and emotionally. It means spending less on food, on heating, and on clothing than someone on average income ... Above all, poverty takes away the tools to build the blocks of the future and steals away the opportunity to have a life unmarked by sickness, a decent education, a secure home and a long retirement.

(Oppenheim 1990: 3)

Britain leads Western Europe in its poverty, with twice as many poor households as Belgium, Denmark, Italy, Holland or Sweden (Shaw *et al.* 2005). While overall personal income rose substantially in the 1980s and 1990s, the gap between the richest and the poorest has grown dramatically (Office for National Statistics 2000b). Evidence from studies suggests that poverty influences the experience of those at the end of life in a number of ways. First, dying has great potential to be a financially 'greedy' experience involving frequent trips to hospital, hospital clinics, GPs, pharmacies, in addition to purchasing aids, loss of income, and loss of future income if the dependant or loved one was employed. The legacy of poverty extends beyond death causing financial worries which have been shown to lead to psychological distress (Koffman *et al.* 2005).

Second, poverty influences place of care and death. Studies have shown that between 50 and 70 per cent of patients would prefer to be cared for at home for as long as possible, and to die at home given the choice (Gomes and Higginson 2004). But in poorer areas, however, fewer people die at home. Further, they are more likely to die in a hospital and less likely to die in a hospice compared to other groups (Sims *et al.* 1997; Kessler *et al.* 2005). If specialist palliative care services are available in these areas they tend to require more resources to achieve the same level of care than in areas where deprivation is lower (Clark 1997).

Third, poverty contributes to shaping patients' and their families' know-ledge base and expectations about palliative care and related services. This may have consequences for the up-take of services at the end of life and during bereavement. Recent research conducted among oncology patients who lived in materially and socially deprived areas were more that eight times less likely not to understand what palliative care was compared to patients who lived in more affluent areas and seven times less likely not to understand the role of Macmillan nurses compared to patients who lived in affluent neighbourhoods (Koffman *et al.* 2007).

### Older people

Populations in European and other developed countries are ageing. This presents a growing challenge to health and social care services in developed countries. It is therefore no surprise that most deaths in European and other developed countries occur in people aged over 65 years. Despite the fact that older people have varied needs for health and social care at the end of life, there is evidence that many of their needs are not met. A body of evidence is mounting to show that older people suffer unnecessarily because of wide-spread under-assessment and under-treatment of their problems. One important cause of individual suffering is pain. Community surveys have consistently shown that pain is an important symptom in around one-third of older people (AGS Panel on Persistent Pain in Older Persons 2002; Teunissen *et al.* 2006).

Pain makes people feel less positive about their health, and in around one-fifth of people it is bad enough to limit their everyday activity (Allard *et al.* 2001). However, older people tend to under-report their symptoms, and health care professionals, in turn, tend to under-treat pain in older people, particularly in non-malignant disease, but also in patients being treated for cancer. A large US study of over 4,000 cancer patients in nurs-ing homes who reported daily pain found that a quarter received no pain-killers of any type. As age increased a greater proportion of people in pain received no pain relief, and judged according to the World Health Organiza-tion's (WHO) pain ladder, those over 85 years of age were least likely to receive drugs such as opiates (see Figure 18.1).

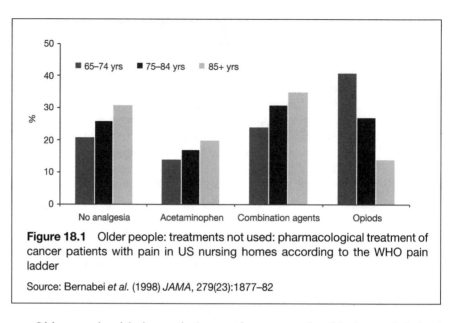

**Figure 18.1**   Older people: treatments not used: pharmacological treatment of cancer patients with pain in US nursing homes according to the WHO pain ladder

Source: Bernabei *et al.* (1998) *JAMA*, 279(23):1877–82

Older people with dementia (see section on people with dementia below) are at particular risk of poor pain control, because their communication problems make them less able to report distressing symptoms and it is more difficult for their attendants to assess it properly. There is also evidence that older people do not receive palliative care to the same extent as younger people as they experience many more chronic illnesses such as heart failure and dementia, which have not traditionally been the focus of specialist palliative care and where models of palliative care are only just beginning to be applied (National Council for Palliative Care 2006). Nevertheless, even older people with cancer may not have access to specialist palliative care. In England and Wales, for example, older people are underrepresented in settings such as inpatient hospices, where high-quality end-of-life care can be offered (Addington-Hall *et al.* 1998; Office for National Statistics 2000a). With increasing age they are less likely to receive care for their final illness in an inpatient hospice.

A study in Australia found that 73 per cent of cancer patients under 60 years of age were referred to palliative care services compared to only 58 per cent of those aged over 80 years (Hunt *et al.* 2002). Specialist palliative care services in the United States reach more non-cancer patients than many other services, but overall only 17 per cent of all dying people are reached by federally funded hospice services (Haupt 1998). In one analysis in Australia, 30 per cent of patients cared for by inpatient hospice services suffered from non-cancer illnesses, most commonly cardiac failure, chronic obstructive pulmonary disease, stroke, dementia and renal failure (Hunt *et al.* 2002). By comparison, figures for the United Kingdom are far lower (Eve and Higginson 2000).

There is relatively little information on the needs of very old people receiving specialist palliative care in hospital. One American study found that patients aged 80 who were referred to the specialist palliative care service in one hospital were more likely to be women living in nursing homes. They were less likely to have cancer and more likely to have dementia, and this factor was the major influence on their ability to take part in decisions about their care and treatment (Evers *et al.* 2002).

Between 2 per cent and 5 per cent of people aged 65 or older live in nursing homes. Mainly, however, these are older people who are frail or with chronic physical or mental disability, and diagnoses commonly include stroke, cardiac failure, chronic pulmonary disease, Parkinson's disease and dementia. Many people recognize a move to a nursing home as a 'last resting place' before death, and many people living in these homes will clearly have palliative care needs (Hockley and Clark 2002). In many countries, nursing homes already play an increasing role in caring for frail older people at the end of life. In the United States, for example, the proportion of people dying in nursing homes increased from just under one in five in 1989 to one in four in 1997 (WHO 2004). About half spend some time in a nursing home in the last month of life. People dying in nursing homes are more likely to endure a prolonged period of disability before death than those dying at home. Most residents complain of pain, and data suggest that pain is not well treated and sometimes not treated at all (Gambassi 1999). Up to two-thirds of people living in nursing homes are affected by cognitive impairment and this complicates the assessment and recognition of pain (WHO 2004).

### *The serious and persistently mentally ill*

In the United Kingdom and the USA, there is currently no consistent system in place for people who are dying and who also experience serious and persistent mental illness (SPMI). Few articles have been published that specifically discuss the needs of this complex, and at times challenging, patient population (Baker 2005; Fotti 2007). The lack of research is not surprising as the socially and materially deprived, which includes people with SPMI, has historically been a neglected area in society. However, physical health-related issues are common among those with SPMI. Felker and colleagues found that half of psychiatric patients experienced known medical disorders and 35 per cent had an undiagnosed medical disorder (Felker *et al.* 1996).

When a patient is dying and has a mental illness, there is some evidence that health care professionals do not possess the core skills to manage their behaviour and their associated palliative care needs. Patients with SPMI may express their distress in a manner that is challenging for health care professionals to diagnose (Felker *et al.* 1996). Under-diagnosis and under-treatment may lead to an illness not being detected until it is already in its advanced stages. Given a late referral, it is often difficult for the palliative care provider to make a difference in the dying experience. Research in the late 1970s found that patients who suffered from schizophrenia did not willingly verbalize their disease-related pain and were more likely than the general population to tolerate advanced and non-healing lesions and tumours on their bodies (Talbott and Linn 1978). Some believe that the pain that would ordinarily bring mentally healthy people to seek medical attention is either muted or highly tolerated in many people with schizophrenia. As a result, symptoms and behaviours associated with schizophrenia often are the cause of a significant delay in both diagnosis and treatment of medical illness, making palliative care the first line of treatment in these individuals (Goldenberg *et al.* 2000). Patients with SPMI have emotional and behavioural problems that may make them unwelcome in the health care community and may influence the care they receive (Felker *et al.* 1996). These patients may lack the skills and knowledge of how to use the health care system, have difficulty keeping appointments, and may be dependent on unreliable care-givers (McConnell *et al.* 1992).

### The homeless mentally ill

It is well known that the environments of homelessness are hazardous and contribute to higher levels of physical and mental health morbidity and mortality (Koffman and Fulop 1999). The homeless comprise those who lack customary and regular access to conventional housing and include people living in shelters, on streets, in abandoned buildings, in subways, or in other places not intended as dwellings (Kushel and Miaskowski 2006). As much as a third of the homeless population may suffer from SPMI (Hughes 2001). Providing palliative and end-of-life care to a homeless seriously mentally ill person is particularly challenging because continuity and follow-up are extremely difficult if the patient is not living in a stable environment. For persons with SPMI living on the streets or in prison with a terminal illness, their bleak life circumstances also may contribute to their rapid decline. Hopelessness may be associated with the early stages of severe physical illness: there is a correlation between adverse life events and the onset of serious illness and death (Sims 1987). Many homeless people are cut off from their families of origin. The effect of this is that providing home hospice care in which family members may offer considerable help becomes highly challenging if not impossible.

### People with dementia

Dementia is a term used to describe various different brain disorders that have in common a loss of brain function that is usually progressive and eventually severe. In recent years dementia has become a major concern for all developed countries (Koffman *et al.* 1996) and the number of people with this condition has increased steadily. In 2005, there were an estimated 684,000 people with dementia in the United Kingdom (Bayer 2006).

About 100,000 people with dementia die each year in the UK (Bayer 2006). Dementia can legitimately be seen as a terminal illness and patients die with this mental illness (Addington-Hall 2000; National Council for Palliative Care 2006). Further, new variant CJD may also become a significant cause of dementia in younger people in the future. Research has indicated that many patients with dementia have symptoms and health needs comparable with those who have cancer but for longer periods of time (McCarthy *et al.* 1997). Despite the wish of most patients and their families that loved ones or dependants with dementia should die in their own home, most people currently die in hospital, on acute wards, where staff are inadequately trained to recognize and address their special needs. Families typically describe poor advance care planning and inadequate symptom control, with distress associated with pain, pressure sores, constipation, restlessness and shortness of breath. It is exceptional for these patients to spend their last days in a hospice, and any involvement of formal palliative care services is still unusual (Bayer 2006). Recent research has indicated that older people with dementia dying on an acute medical ward in a London hospital were less likely to be referred to palliative care teams compared to patients who are cognitively intact and were prescribed fewer palliative medications. Further, few patients had their spiritual needs assessed or addressed while they were dying. Further, few patients with dementia had information documented regarding their religious beliefs (Sampson *et al.* 2006).

### People with learning disabilities

In the early 1990s the Department of Health in the United Kingdom adopted the term 'learning disability' as the successor to other terms such as 'learning difficulty' (which is still used with regard to the education of children), 'mental handicap', 'mental sub normality', 'mental retardation' (used in the USA). 'Learning disability', the term used within this chapter, is preferable because it describes the effect of lower than average intelligence in a manner consistent with the World Health Organization definitions of impairment, disability and handicap (World Health Organization 1980).

Producing precise information on the number of people with learning disabilities in the population is difficult. The United Kingdom's government's White Paper, *Valuing People*, suggests that there may be approximately 210,000 people described as having severe and profound learning disabilities, and approximately 1.2 million people with mild or moderate learning disabilities in England (Secretary of State for Health 2001).

In recent years, knowledge of the general health needs of people with learning disabilities has increased. Research indicates that this client group have more demanding health needs than the general population and are also experiencing increased life expectancy, especially among people with Down's syndrome (NHS Executive 1998). Increased life expectancy has in part been due to advances in medical treatments that are now available to this group of people. This, however, has resulted in the increased incidence of progressive disease, for example, myocardial and vascular disease, cancer, and Alzheimer's disease (Jancar 1993). Surveys have shown that many people with learning disabilities have undetected conditions that cause unnecessary suffering or reduce the quality or length of their lives (Howells 1986;Tuffrey-Wijne 1998; Keenan and McIntosh 2000).

Failure to diagnose advanced disease for this population group may mean that not only are treatment options limited but also that the window for accessing palliative care becomes truncated. This prevents both patients and their care-givers from adequately planning and preparing for the final stages of their advanced illness (Brown 2000). Once the opportunity for palliative care presents, problems continue. Little is known about how people with learning disabilities experience pain and evidence suggests they may experience difficulties communicating its presence (Beirsdorff 1991). Other symptoms, for example, nausea, fatigue or dysphagia are similarly poorly communicated by individuals or poorly understood by health care professionals, and this may result in their sub-optimal assessment and management (Tuffrey-Wijne 1997, 1998).

### People from black and minority ethnic (BME) groups

Ethnicity is difficult to define but most definitions reflect self-identification with cultural traditions that provide both a meaningful social identity and boundaries between groups (Koffman 2006). The size of the minority ethnic population was 4.6 million in 2001 or 7.9 per cent of the total population of the United Kingdom (Office for National Statistics 2004). The majority of minority ethnic populations live in England (approximately 90 per cent), although nationally there is significant variations in the geographical distribution of populations, with minority ethnic groups being concentrated in urban areas (Office for National Statistics 2004). Although there is a significant lack of data about people from minority ethnic communities, the available data from the United Kingdom, the USA and Australia, confirm that some BME groups experience high levels of social and economic disadvantage.

People from minority ethnic communities also suffer the consequences of overt and inadvertent racial discrimination – individual and institutional – and an inadequate recognition and understanding of other complexities they may experience, for example barriers like language, cultural and religious differences (Anonymous 2000; Coker 2001). They also experience 'social invisibility' where routinely collected data from a number of sources is partially or completely inadequate. For example, death registration certificates only record country of origin or country of birth, not ethnicity. Hospital minimum data set (MDS) information and cancer registration data frequently omits self-assigned ethnicity, or classifications of ethnic difference are outdated or applied incorrectly (Koffman and Higginson 2000; Thames Cancer Registry 2006).

Health system level factors such as poor access to health care services have been reported among BME groups in the United Kingdom and the USA (Harding and Maxwell 1997; Department of Health 1998; O'Neill and Marconi 2001; Blendon *et al.* 2002; Dyer 2005). This is also an issue for end-of-life care where the impact of ageing on BME groups now means larger numbers of older members within these communities will require health services for advanced disease. A limited number of reports have levelled criticism of care at the end of life for these communities and poor access to appropriate care. Low rates of cancer were seen as one explanation to account for low uptake of service provision (Hill and Penso 1995), but the figures were likely to have been inaccurate because of inadequate ethnic monitoring (Aspinall 1999). A study in an inner London health authority demonstrated that black Caribbean patients with advanced disease experienced restricted access to some specialist palliative care services compared to white British patients (Koffman and Higginson 2001), yet an analysis of local provision revealed no lack of palliative care services (Eve *et al.* 1997). This example of under-utilization of palliative care services by the black Caribbean community at the end of life supports other recent research among minority ethnic communities (Farrell 2000; Skilbeck *et al.* 2002).

Two recent qualitative studies have alluded to inadequate knowledge about end-of-life care among BME communities living in the USA and United Kingdom. Participants in Born *et al.*'s study of African Americans and Latinos revealed 'an overwhelming lack of awareness of hospice, and what it had to offer' (Born *et al.* 2004). Randhawa and Owens' focus groups of Sikh women living in Luton in the United Kingdom were aware of hospice, but none were familiar with the term 'palliative care' or Macmillan nursing care (Randhawa and Owens 2004). Other reasons are highlighted in Box 18.3.

---

**Box 18.3**  Black and minority ethnic social exclusion at the end of life: why does it occur?

| | |
|---|---|
| **Social and economic deprivation** Low socio-economic status has been positively linked to an increased likelihood of hospital deaths, although this would apply equally to all population groups (Higginson *et al.* 1998, 1999; Koffman *et al.* 2007). | **Attitudes to palliative care** Barriers to health care that the poor and the disenfranchised have traditionally encountered may influence their receptivity to palliative (Gibson 2001). |
| **Cultural mistrust** Evidence from USA supports the contention that black and minority ethnic groups are less likely than white patients to trust the motivations of doctors who discuss end-of-life care with them (Caralis *et al.* 1993). | **Dissatisfaction with health care** Uptake of health and social services among certain minority ethnic communities has revealed lower utilization of services due to dissatisfaction of services (Lindsay *et al.* 1997). |
| **Ethno-centralism** Demand for services may be influenced by the 'ethnocentric' outlook of palliative care services, discouraging black and minority ethnic groups from making use of relevant provision (Smaje and Field 1997). | **Gatekeepers** Some health care professional 'gatekeepers' to services experienced by minority ethnic groups contribute to lower referral rates (Smaje and Field 1997). |

### Refugees and asylum seekers

Estimating the total number of refugees and asylum seekers worldwide is extremely difficult, as definitions differ widely. In the United Kingdom, refugees are defined as those who have been granted permission to stay in the United Kingdom under the terms of the 1951 Refugee Convention because of a well-founded fear of persecution due to race, religion, nationality, political opinion or membership of a social group (Office of the High Commissioner for Human Rights 1951). Asylum seekers are those who have submitted an application for protection under the Geneva Convention and are waiting for the claim to be decided by the Home Office. There were in the region of 27,500 new applications for asylum in 2005 (Heath *et al.* 2006) and between 350,000 and 420,000 located in London alone (Greater London Authority 2001).

Refugees and asylum seekers form significant minority populations in many United Kingdom towns and cities. It is extremely difficult to obtain demographic information on refugees and asylum seekers at the local level in the UK and this lack of information represents one of the difficulties in developing services that are accessible for these groups (Bardsley *et al.* 2000).

Although refugees and asylum seekers are often grouped together they are not necessarily a homogenous group, and have varying experiences and needs (Burnett and Fassil 2002). Many refugees have health problems, for example parasitic or nutritional diseases (Jones and Gill 1998), and diseases such as hepatitis, tuberculosis and HIV and AIDS, which frequently overlap with problems of social deprivation. Their health problems are also amplified by family separation, hostility and racism from the host population, poverty and social isolation (Jones and Gill 1998; Bardsley and Storkey 2000; Kisely *et al.* 2002).

Individuals from sub-Saharan Africa, many of whom may be refugees and asylum seekers, make up the second largest group of people affected by HIV in the UK (Brogan and George 1999). They are more likely to be socially disadvantaged and isolated, be much less aware of the health care to which they are entitled, and be more likely to present only when symptomatic. Experience has demonstrated that this patient group continues to require palliative care despite the advances made with highly active anti-retroviral therapy (HAART) because they tend to present late with AIDS-related illnesses and have higher rates of tuberculosis, both of which are linked to a poorer prognosis. For many patients, who do not have a GP and are reluctant to register with one, lack of a stable home environment and reluctance to access local services may mean that dying at home is not an option (Easterbrook and Meadway 2001).

### Drug users

In England, during the year 2000–2001, the number of drug misusers reported as receiving treatment from both drug misuse agencies and GPs was approximately 33,200 (Department of Health 2002). There is very little literature on how drug misusers utilize specialist palliative care services.

Researchers who have examined the problem of pain population have mostly conducted studies on how pain is managed among patients with cancer or AIDS where pain reports and adequacy of analgesic therapy were compared in patients with AIDS with and without a history of substance abuse (Breitbart *et al.* 1997; Cox 1999; Morgan 2006). A single exploratory study in the USA explored the experiences of hospices providing care to intravenous HIV/AIDs drug users (Cox 1999). The survey revealed that the provision of community palliative care for these patients was frequently problematic because of patients' poor living conditions, many of which were considered unsafe to visit. Differences have also been found in psychological distress and adequacy of pain treatment. Patients with substance abuse also had higher levels of depression and psychological distress, fewer sources of support, and significantly lower quality of life, and were less likely to receive adequate pain medication (Breitbart *et al.* 1997).

It has been suggested that drug users require a modified health care system, which understands and considers the problems of drug users; but that the initiation and maintenance of contact may require a variety of initiatives (Brettle 2001). Morrison and Ruben (1995) similarly argue that services need to deliver care to these groups in imaginative and innovative ways, which are not judgemental and encourage contact without reinforcing traditional stereotypes. Without appropriate services, they argue, high levels of mortality among drug users will continue.

### *Prisoners*

In 2007 there were an estimated 80,000 prisoners in England and Wales of whom 9,120 were indeterminate sentences (National Offender Management Service 2007). Historically, prison health care has been organized outside the NHS. This has given rise to questions about equity, standards, professional isolation and whether the Prison Service has the capacity to carry out its health care function (Joint Prison Service & National Health Service Executive Working Group 1999). The government is now committed to developing a range of proposals aimed at improving health care for prisoners. The aims include ensuring that prisoners have access to the same quality and range of health care services as the general public receives from the NHS by promoting a closer partnership between the NHS and the Prison Service at local, regional and national levels.

To date, very little United Kingdom literature has focused on the palliative care needs of prisoners and that available is largely descriptive or relates to single case histories (Oliver and Cook 1998; Wilford 2001). More research has taken place in the USA where a number of palliative care programmes have been developed for prisoners; for example, the Louisiana State Penitentiary at Angola (Project on Death in America 1998). This has been largely because in Louisiana, where the sentencing laws are tougher than of any state in the USA, the courts hand out a large number of life sentences where parole is rarely granted. As a result an estimated 85 per cent of Angola's 5,200 inmates will grow old and will die there (Project on Death in America 1998).

There are a number of problems in introducing palliative care into prisons, not least the mutual distrust between staff and prisoners. Effective symptom control, particularly adequate pain control, can be difficult under these circumstances. Drugs to manage pain control may be used for other illicit purposes. In addition, visiting by family and friends can be restricted, not least because the prison may be located at some distance from them.

## Conclusion: The magnitude of the problem: implications for palliative care policy and service development

Since the introduction of the National Health Service in the United Kingdom and other countries where social welfare has become common place, health care has been widely extended across many sections of the population. However, universal access to care and treatment has remained elusive. Palliative care provided by the modern hospice movement, with laudable aspirations to extending the right to care as widely as possible, has been shown to be inequitable on a number of fronts. This chapter has explored evidence that population and patients' groups silent in life remain so during death. Potential solutions to the problems come in many forms, none of which will be successful in isolation. First, health and social care professionals' knowledge and attitudes about engaging socially excluded populations must be improved (O'Neill and Marconi 2001). This concern can be addressed, in part, through the conduct of a comprehensive needs assessment be it epidemiological (including a deeper understanding of demographic and economic factors that impact on the experience of advanced disease and providing informal care), comparative, or corporate including the meaningful collation and interpretation of experiences and views from a variety of sources. These include the views of patients and informal carers, providers of care, as well as purchasers and planners.

A number of regional implementation groups have successfully undertaken similar exercises in order to plan palliative care services in their own areas, offering the potential to explore strategy at an epidemiological and corporate level, for example in London (Higginson 2001) and Wales (Welsh Office 1996). Both established a framework for the development of local policies and recommended closer links between agencies involved in the provision of care. Significantly, they have recommended devoting more resources to research that explore the unmet palliative care needs of the socially excluded, given the paucity of evidence in certain areas. Without more comprehensive information, moving these complex agendas forward remains challenging.

Second, there is an urgent need to raise public awareness of palliative care services and to provide public education about the care provided to reduce any misconceptions about services that may be influencing access. Innovative approaches to disseminating relevant information about patient-

and care-related issues and local palliative care services may also offer scope to raise awareness of relevant services. NHS Direct, the national nurse-led telephone helpline represents an example (Department of Health 1997). However, current evidence indicates it has been underused by older people, ethnic minorities and other disadvantaged groups (George 2002). Widening the user base of the helpline requires a deeper understanding of appropriate and acceptable methods of sharing information.

Last, the charitable sector is uniquely suited to support new ideas that extend care to the point where they can be accepted and integrated in society and become the social norm rather than the exception. Despite differences in the funding arrangements of care in the USA, the Robert Wood Johnson Foundation has been successful in pump-priming pilot projects that have increased awareness of, and access to, palliative care among socially deprived communities (Gibson 2001). In recent years the UK has followed suit with two noteworthy examples. At a national level, Help the Hospices is working with representatives from local hospices and other key organizations on a widening access project (WAP). The project aims to work with local adult and children's hospices to reduce the barriers to hospice and palliative care that people face as a result of social exclusion. At a local level, the Brent and Harrow Palliative Care Pathways Project, funded through the New Opportunities Fund, has attempted to understand what previously 'hard-to-reach' groups perceive about end-of-life care services in order to develop more accessible palliative care services (St Luke's Hospice 2006). The outcomes of this project are yet to be reported. Both these ventures are to be applauded, but only if the momentum they create can be sustained over the long term.

# References

Acheson, D. (1998) *Independent Inquiry into Inequalities in Health Report*. London: The Stationery Office.

Addington-Hall, J. (2000) *Positive Partnerships: palliative care for adults with severe mental health problems*. London: National Council for Hospices and Specialist Palliative Care Services.

Addington-Hall, J.M., Altman, D. and McCarthy, M. (1998) Who gets hospice in-patient care?, *Social Science and Medicine*, 46: 1011–16.

AGS Panel on Persistent Pain in Older Persons (2002) The management of persistent pain in older persons, *Journal of the American Geriatrics Society*, 50: S205–S224.

Ahmed, N., Bestall, J.C., Ahmedzai, S.H., Payne, S.A., Clark, D., and Noble, B. (2004) Systematic review of the problems and issues of accessing specialist palliative care by patients, carers and health and social care professionals, *Palliative Medicine*, 18(6): 525–42.

Allard, P., Maunsell, P., Labbe, J. and Dorval, M. (2001) Educational interventions to improve cancer pain control: a systematic review, *Journal of Palliative Medicine*, 4: 191–203.

Anonymous (2000) Personal view: Trying to overcome racism in the NHS, *British Medical Journal*, 320: 357.

Aspinall, P.J. (1999) Ethnic groups and *Our healthier nation*: whither the information base?, *Journal of Public Health Medicine*, 21: 125–32.

Baker, A. (2005) Palliative and end-of-life care in the serious and persistently mentally ill population, *Journal of the American Psychiatric Nurses Association*, 11(11): 298–303.

Bardsley, M. and Storkey, M. (2000) Estimating the numbers of refugees in London, *Journal of Public Health Medicine*, 22(3): 406–12.

Bardsley, M., Hamm, J., Lowdell, C. and Morgan, M. (2000) *Developing health assessment for black and minority ethnic groups: analysing routine health information*, London: Health of Londoners Project.

Barratt, H. (2001) The health of the excluded, *British Medical Journal*, 323: 240.

Bayer, A. (2006) Death with dementia: the need for better care, *Age and Ageing*, 35(2): 101–2.

Beirsdorff, K. (1991) Pain intensity and indifference: alternative explanations for some medical catastrophes, *Mental Retardation*, 29(6): 359–62.

Bernabei, R., Gambassi, G., Lapane, K., Landi, F., Gatsonis, C., Dunlop, R., Lipsitz, L., Steel, K. and Mor, V. (1998) Management of pain in elderly patients with cancer. *The Journal of the American Medical Association*, 279(23): 1877–82.

Blendon, R.J., Schoen, C., DesRoches, C.M., Osborn, R., Scoles, K.L. and Zapert, K. (2002) Inequities in health care: a five-country survey, *Health Affairs*, 21(3): 182–91.

Born, W., Allen Greiner, K., Sylvia, E., Butler, J. and Ahluwalia, J. (2004) Knowledge, attitudes, and beliefs about end-of-life care among inner-city African Americans and Latinos, *Journal of Palliative Medicine*, 7(2): 247–56.

Breitbart, W., Rosenfeld, B., Passik, M. and Kaim, M. (1997) A comparison of pain report and adequacy of analgesic therapy in ambulatory AIDS patients with and without a history of substance abuse, *Pain*, 72: 235–43.

Brettle, R.P. (2001) Injection drug use-related HIV infection. In: M.W. Adler (ed.) *ABC of AIDS*, 5th edn. London: British Medical Journal Publishing.

Brogan, G. and George, R. (1999) HIV/AIDS: symptoms and the impact of new treatments, *Palliative Medicine*, 1(4): 104–10.

Brown, H. (2000) The service needs of people with learning disabilities who are dying, *Psychology Research*, 10(2): 39–47.

Burnett, A. and Fassil, Y. (2002) *Meeting the Health Needs of Refugees and Asylum Seekers in the UK: An Information and Resource Pack for Health Workers*. London: Department of Health.

Caralis, P.V., Davis, B., Wright, K. and Marcial, E. (1993) The influence of ethnicity and race on attitudes toward advanced directives, life-prolonging treatments, and euthanasia, *Journal of Clinical Ethics*, 4: 155–65.

Clark, C. (1997) Social deprivation increases workload in palliative care of terminally ill patients, *British Medical Journal*, 314: 1202.

Coker, N. (2001) Understanding race and racism. In: N. Coker (ed.) *Racism in Medicine: An Agenda for Change*. London: King's Fund Publishing, pp. 1–22.

Cox, C. (1999) Hospice care for injection drug using AIDS patients, *The Hospice Journal*, 14(1): 13–24.

Department of Health (1997) *The New NHS: modern, dependable*. Cmd 3807. London: The Stationery Office.

Department of Health (1998) *Inequalities in Health: Report of an Independent Inquiry Chaired by Sir Donald Acheson*. London: The Stationery Office.

Department of Health (2002) *Statistics from the Regional Drug Misuse Databases for six months ending March 2001*. Bulletin 2002/07: London: Department of Health.

Dyer, O. (2005) Disparities in health widen between rich and poor in England, *British Medical Journal*, 331: 419.

Easterbrook, P. and Meadway, J. (2001) The changing epidemiology of HIV infection: new challenges for HIV palliative care, *Journal of the Royal Society of Medicine*, 94(442): 448.

Eve, A. and Higginson, I.J. (2000) Minimum dataset activity for hospice and hospital palliative care services in the UK 1997/98, *Palliative Medicine*, 14: 395–404.

Eve, A., Smith, A.M. and Tebbit, P. (1997) Hospice and palliative care in the UK 1994–5, including a summary of trends 1990–5, *Palliative Medicine*, 11(1): 31–43.

Evers, M.M., Meier, D.E. and Morrison, R.S. (2002) Assessing differences in care needs and service utilization in geriatric palliative care patients, *Journal of Pain and Symptom Management*, 23: 424–32.

Farrell, J. (2000) *Do disadvantaged and minority ethnic groups receive adequate access to palliative care services?* Glasgow University.

Felker, B., Yazel, J.J. and Short, D. (1996) Mortality and medical comorbidity among psychiatric patients: a review, *Psychiatric Services*, 47: 1356–63.

Fotti, M.E. (2007) 'Do It Your Way': a demonstration project on end-of-life care for persons with serious mental illness, *Journal of Palliative Medicine*, 6: 661–9.

Gambassi, G. (1999) Cross-national comparison of predictors of pain in elderly in long-term care, in *Annual Meeting of the American Geriatrics Society – American Federation for Aging Research, Philadelphia, PA, May 19–23*, American Geriatrics Society, New York, 159.

George, S. (2002) NHS Direct audited, *British Medical Journal*, 324: 558–9.

Gibson, R. (2001) Palliative care for the poor and disenfranchised: a view from the Robert Wood Johnson Foundation, *Journal of the Royal Society of Medicine*, 94: 486–9.

Goddard, M. and Smith, P. (2001) Equity of access to health care services: Theory and evidence from the UK, *Social Science and Medicine*, 53: 1149–62.

Goldenberg, D., Holland, J. and Schachter, S. (2000) Palliative care in the chronically mentally ill. In: H.M. Chochinov and W.W. Breitbart (eds) *Handbook of Psychiatry in Palliative Medicine*. New York: Oxford University Press, pp. 91–6.

Gomes, B. and Higginson, I.J. (2004) Home or hospital: choices at the end of life, *Journal of the Royal Society of Medicine*, 97(9): 413–14.

Greater London Authority (2001) *Refugees and asylum seekers in London: A GLA perspective*. London: Greater London Authority (GLA).

Harding, S. and Maxwell, R. (1997) Difference in mortality of migrants. In: F. Drever and M. Whitehead (eds) *Health Inequalities: Decennial supplement Series DS no.15*. London: The Stationery Office.

Hart, J.T. (1971) The inverse care law, *Lancet*, 1: 405–12.

Haupt, B.J. (1998) Characteristics of hospice care users: data from the 1996 National Home and Hospice Care Survey, *Advance Data*, 28: 1–16.

Haynes, R. (1991) Inequalities in health and health service use: evidence from the General Household Survey, *Social Science & Medicine*, 33: 361–8.

Heath, T., Jeffries, R. and Pearce, S. (2006) *Asylum Statistics United Kingdom 2005*. London: Home Office.

Higginson, I.J. (2001) *The Palliative Care for Londoners: Needs, Experience,*

*Outcomes and Future Strategy*. London: London Regional Strategy Group for Palliative Care.

Higginson, I.J., Astin, P. and Dolan, S. (1998) Where do cancer patients die? Ten-year trends in the place of death of cancer patients in England, *Palliative Medicine*, 12: 353–63.

Higginson, I.J., Jarman, B., Astin, P. and Dolan, S. (1999) Do social factors affect where patients die: an analysis of 10 years of cancer deaths in England, *Journal of Public Health Medicine*; 21: 22–8.

Higginson, I.J. and Koffman, J. (2005) Public health and palliative care, *Clinics in Geriatric Medicine*, 21: 41–5.

Hill, D. and Penso, D. (1995) *Opening doors: Improving access to hospice and specialist palliative care services by members of the black and minority ethnic communities*. Occasional Paper 7. London: National Council for Hospice and Specialist Palliative Care Services.

Hinton, J. (1967) *Dying*. London: Penguin.

Hockley, J. and Clark, D. (2002) *Palliative Care for Older People in Care Homes*. Buckingham: Open University Press.

Hospice Information (2006) *Hospice and Palliative Care Directory: United Kingdom and Ireland*. London: Help the Hospices.

Howells, G. (1986) Are the medical needs of mentally handicapped adults being met?, *British Journal of General Practice*, 36(449): 453.

Hughes, A. (2001) The poor and underserved. In: B.R. Ferrell and N. Coyle (eds) *Textbook of Palliative Nursing*. New York: Oxford University Press, pp. 461–6.

Hunt, R.W., Fazekas, B.S., Luke, C.G., Priest, K.R. and Roder, D.M. (2002) The coverage of cancer patients by designated palliative services: a population-based study, South Australia, 1999, *Palliative Medicine*, 16(5): 403–9.

Jancar, J. (1993) Consequences of a longer life for the mentally handicapped, *American Journal of Mental Retardation*, 93(2): 285–92.

Joint Prison Service & National Health Service Executive Working Group (1999) *The future organisation of prison health care*. London: Department of Health.

Jones, D. and Gill, P.S. (1998) Refugees and primary care: tackling the inequalities, *British Medical Journal*, 317: 1444–6.

Keenan, P. and McIntosh, P. (2000) Learning disabilities and palliative care, *Palliative Care Today*, pp. 11–13.

Kessler, D., Peters, T.J., Lee, L. and Parr, S. (2005) Social class and access to specialist palliative care services, *Palliative Medicine*, 19: 105–10.

Kisely, S., Stevens, M., Hart, B. and Douglas, C. (2002) Health issues of asylum seekers and refugees, *Australian and New Zealand Journal of Public Health*, 26(1): 8–10.

Koffman, J. (2006) The language of diversity: controversies relevant to palliative care research, *European Journal of Palliative Care*, 11(1): 18–21.

Koffman, J., Burke, G., Dias, A., Ravel, B., Byrne, J., Gonzales, J. and Daniels, C. (2007) Demographic factors and awareness of palliative care and related services, *Palliative Medicine*, 21(2): 145–53.

Koffman, J., Donaldson, N., Hotopf, M. and Higginson, I.J. (2005) Does ethnicity matter? Bereavement outcomes in two ethnic groups living in the United Kingdom, *Palliative and Supportive Care*, 3: 183–90.

Koffman, J., Fulop, N.J., Pashley, D. and Coleman, K. (1996) No way out: the use of elderly mentally ill acute and assessment psychiatric beds in north and south Thames regions, *Age & Ageing*, 25: 268–72.

Koffman, J. and Fulop, N.J. (1999) Homelessness and the use of acute psychiatric beds: findings from a one-day survey of adult acute and low-level secure psychiatric beds in north and south Thames regions. *Health and Social Care in the Community*, 7(2): 140–8.

Koffman, J. and Higginson, I.J. (2000) Minority ethnic groups and our healthier nation, *Journal of Public Health Medicine*, 22(2): 245.

Koffman, J. and Higginson, I.J. (2001) Accounts of carers' satisfaction with health care at the end of life: a comparison of first generation black Caribbeans and white patients with advanced disease, *Palliative Medicine*, 15(4): 337–45.

Kushel, M.B. and Miaskowski, C. (2006) End-of-life care for homeless patients: 'She says she is there to help me in any situation', *Journal of the American Medical Association*, 296: 2959–66.

Lindsay, J., Jagger, C., Hibbert, M., Peet, S. and Moledina, F. (1997) Knowledge, uptake and the availability of health and social services among Asian Gujarati and white persons, *Ethnicity and Health*, 2: 59–69.

McCarthy, M., Addington-Hall, J.M. and Altmann, D. (1997) The experience of dying with dementia: a retrospective survey, *International Journal of Geriatric Psychiatry*, 12: 404–9.

McConnell, S.D., Inderbitzen, L.B. and Pollard, W.E. (1992) Primary health care in the CMHC: a role for the nurse practitioner, *Hospital and Community Psychiatry*, 43: 724–7.

Morgan, B. (2006) Knowing how to play the game: hospitalized substance abusers' strategies for obtaining pain relief, *Pain Management Nursing*, 7(1): 31–41.

Morrell, P. (2001) Social exclusion (electronic letter), *British Medical Journal*, p. 323.

Morrison, C.L. and Ruben, S.M. (1995) The development of health care services for drug misusers and prostitutes, *Postgraduate Medical Journal*, 71: 593–7.

National Council for Palliative Care (2006) *Exploring Palliative Care for People with Dementia: A Discussion Document – August 2006*. London: National Council for Palliative Care.

National Offender Management Service (2007) *Population in Custody: Monthly Tables England and Wales April 2007*, Ministry of Justice.

NHS Executive (1998) *Signpost for successful commissioning and providing health services for people with learning difficulties*. London: HMSO.

O'Neill, J. and Marconi, K. (2001) Access to palliative care in the USA: why emphasize vulnerable populations?, *Journal of the Royal Society of Medicine*, 94(9): 452–4.

Office for National Statistics (2000a) *Mortality statistics, general*. Series DH1 No. 33, Table 17. London: Office for National Statistics.

Office for National Statistics (2000b) *Social Trends*. London: HMSO.

Office for National Statistics (2004) *Ethnicity and Identity*. http://www.statistics.gov.uk/cci/nugget.asp?id=455 (accessed 20 August 2007).

Office of the High Commissioner for Human Rights (1951) *Convention relating to the Status of Refugees*. Geneva: Office of the High Commissioner for Human Rights.

Office of the High Commissioner for Human Rights (2005) *Universal Declaration of Human Rights*. United Nations Department of Public Information.

Oliver, D. and Cook, L. (1998) The specialist palliative care of prisoners, *European Journal of Palliative Care*, 5(3): 70–80.

Oppenheim, C. (1990) *Poverty: The Facts*. London: Child Poverty Action Group.

Project on Death in America (1998) Dying in prison: a growing problem emerges from behind bars, *PDIA Newsletter*, 3: 1–3.

Randhawa, G. and Owens, A. (2004) The meanings of cancer and perceptions of cancer services among South Asians in Luton, UK, *British Journal of Cancer*, 91: 62–8.

Rose, G. (1996) *The strategy of preventative medicine.* Oxford: Oxford Medical Publications.

Sampson, E.L., Gould, V., Lee, D. and Blanchard, M.R. (2006) Differences in care received by patients with and without dementia who died during acute hospital admission: a retrospective case note study, *Age and Ageing*, 35: 187–9.

Secretary of State for Health (2001) *Valuing People: A New Strategy for Learning Disability for the 21st Century.* CM 5086. London: HMSO.

Shaw, M., Davey Smith, G. and Dorling, D. (2005) Health inequalities and New Labour: how the promises compare with real progress, *British Medical Journal*, 330: 1016–21.

Sims, A. (1987) Why the excess mortality from psychiatric illness?, *British Medical Journal*, 294: 986–7.

Sims, A., Radford, J., Doran, K. and Page, H. (1997) Social class variation in place of death, *Palliative Medicine*, 11(5): 369–73.

Skilbeck, J., Corner, J., Beech, N., Clark, D., Hughes, P., Douglas, H.R., Halliday, D., Haviland, J., Marples, R., Normand, C., Seymour, J. and Webb, T. (2002) Clinical nurse specialists in palliative care. Part 1. A description of the Macmillan Nurse caseload, *Palliative Medicine*, 16(4): 285–6.

Smaje, C. and Field, D. (1997) Absent minorities? Ethnicity and the use of palliative care services. In: J. Hockey and N. Small (eds) *Death, gender and ethnicity.* London: Routledge, pp. 142–65.

Social Exclusion Unit (2001) *Preventing Social Exclusion.* London: HMSO.

St Luke's Hospice (2006) *Palliative Care Pathways Project Brent and Harrow 2001–2006.* London: St Luke's Hospice.

Talbott, J.A. and Linn, L. (1978) 'Reactions of schizophrenics to life threatening disease', *Psychiatric Quarterly*, 50: 218–27.

Teunissen, S.C.C.M., Wesker, W., Kruitwagen, C., de Haes, H.C.J.M., Voest, E.E. and de Graeff, A. (2006) Symptom prevalence in patients with incurable cancer: a systematic review, *Journal of Pain and Symptom Management*, 34(1): 94–104.

Thames Cancer Registry (2006) *Cancer in South East England 2004: Cancer Incidence, Prevalence, Survival and Treatment of Residents of South East England.* London: Thames Cancer Registry, King's College London.

Townsend, P. and Davison, N. (1982) *Inequalities in Health: The Black Report.* Harmondsworth: Penguin.

Tuffrey-Wijne, I. (1997) Palliative care and learning disabilities, *Nursing Times*, 93(31): 50–1.

Tuffrey-Wijne, I. (1998) Care of the terminally ill, *Learning Disability Practice*, 1(1): 8–11.

Welsh Office (1996) *Palliative Care in Wales: Towards Evidence Based Purchasing.* Cardiff: Welsh Office.

Whitehead, M. (1992) *Inequalities in Health: The Black Report and The Health Divide.* Harmondsworth: Penguin.

Wilford, T. (2001) Developing effective palliative care within a prison setting, *International Journal of Palliative Nursing*, 7(11): 528–30.

World Health Organization (1980) *International Classification of Impairments, Disabilities, and Handicaps. A Manual Relating to the Consequences of Diseases.* Geneva: World Health Organization.

World Health Organization (2004) *Better Palliative Care for Older People: the Solid Facts.* Milan: The World Health Organization Regional Office for Europe.

# 19

# Palliative care in institutions

*Jeanne Samson Katz*

---

**Key points**

- Palliative care remains accessible mostly to those in Western societies, and less relevant to those dying of infectious diseases in other countries.
- Despite growth in hospice provision most people still die in general hospitals in Western countries.
- Palliative care services in hospitals are developing and working with services in the community; community hospitals need to be recognized as a legitimate place for end-of-life care for older people.
- Long-term care for older people is growing as a major consumer of end-of-life care and different models are being explored in Western societies to promote better care for residents as well as addressing the diverse requirements of care-givers.
- As the prison population ages, end-of-life care for this and other excluded populations needs to be adapted, ensuring protection for all parties.

---

## Introduction

In some countries, palliative or hospice care is often seen as synonymous with hospice buildings, where people with cancer go to die in their last weeks of life. However, end-of-life care takes place in many different situations and settings, the longest period of the terminal phase is usually spent in one's own home. Unlike the nineteenth century where most people were cared for and actually died at home, changes in family structure and household composition have impacted on the site of care for dying people. In the UK, while health and social care policies have resulted in a reduction in long-stay hospital beds for older people, almost 60 per cent of deaths still occur in hospitals (Office of National Statistics 2004).

Previous chapters have described the development of palliative care in different parts of the world. This process remains dynamic, spawning a variety of organizations to meet local needs. It is sanguine to acknowledge that the bulk of the world's population lives in developing countries where the predominant health problems relate to sheer survival: famine, malnutrition, poverty, paucity of health services and so forth (Clemens *et al.* 2007). Where palliative services do exist, for example in Kerala, India, where there is a Neighbourhood Network in Palliative Care, this care does not take place in institutions but through community services (*ibid.*). Even in countries such as Canada where palliative care is believed to be widely available only 15 per cent of adult Canadians have access to hospice palliative care.

The early development of palliative care services in the UK focused on 'buildings with inpatient provision' the prototype of which was St. Christopher's with an 'institutional' base, although the intention was to ensure that the environment was uninstitutional in a conventional sense. This meant that 'wards' were to be as home-like as possible, hospice staff would often refrain from wearing uniform and hospice personnel took an informal approach to relationships with dying people (not patients) and their families.

Following the founding of St. Christopher's, other palliative care services began in the UK and, partly for funding reasons, many of these services began as home care services, while funding was being sought to create a 'proper hospice'. So although this chapter focuses primarily on palliative care in institutions, the history, philosophy and practice of the kind of palliative care that takes place in institutions such as hospices and hospitals are intertwined with those in the community. This is less the case in prisons and care homes.

The way in which the services in inpatient hospices have developed has had a 'ripple effect' on all other palliative care services in the UK and elsewhere (Hockley 1997). For this reason this chapter first explores hospices followed by hospitals, and then looks in more depth at two other institutional settings which to date are not firmly within the palliative care net: long-term care homes and prisons.

Much has been researched and written about the efficacy of treatments as well as services available to people with palliative care needs (e.g. Doyle *et al.* 2005). For example, studies have explored the extent to which, for example, volunteers have contributed to the running of hospice and palliative care services and their training requirements (Cummings 1999). Surprisingly, however, there is relatively little evidence which evaluates the provision of palliative care services according to type of service. This chapter will review the secondary evidence currently available about the types of services provided for dying people and their care workers in selected countries by statutory and voluntary health services and suggest areas for future enquiry.

# Palliative care in hospices

The development of hospice and palliative care services in the UK was spearheaded initially by a push from voluntary groups to imitate the St. Christopher's model; in other words, establish a 'hospice', a purpose-built or adapted building, housing inpatient beds. The funding for the establishment of hospices and the running thereof varies even today; for example, finance may come exclusively from voluntary or independent organizations (registered charities) or with some support from statutory health services, such as the National Health Service (NHS) in the UK. The provision in England, Wales and Northern Ireland in January 2006 included 193 specialist inpatient units providing 2,774 beds, 20 per cent of which were NHS beds, 295 home care services, 234 day care services and 314 bereavement support services (www.hospiceinformation.info/hospicesworldwide.asp). Inpatient units, due to their unplanned nature, are spread rather unevenly in the UK with the highest concentration in the south east of England (Clark and Seymour 1999).

In 2005, 29 per cent of adult inpatient units in the UK were managed by the NHS. Even where statutory provision is not available, many people in the UK requiring inpatient hospice care are admitted to voluntary hospices (often independent charities) through contractual funding arrangements with health authorities. Organizations delivering inpatient care for terminally ill people call themselves by a variety of names, the most common of which are hospices, hospice wards or dedicated specialist palliative care units. They may be: wards within a general or specialist hospital; freestanding buildings within the grounds of a hospital (general or specialist); and not attached to any other particular hospital or medical/health setting (Doyle 1999). At the beginning of the twenty-first century, 80 per cent of inpatient provision in the UK was in the form of free-standing, geographically separate, independently funded hospices (Doyle 1999).

Hospice and palliative care services in the UK continue to serve primarily people dying from cancer and, in many ways, their needs determined the nature of the services ultimately developed. Some hospice foundations explicitly state that they serve people with cancer exclusively; thus providing services for people with other diseases who also have palliative care needs has proven difficult. The focus on cancer has persisted – in 2005 of 41,000 new patients admitted to inpatient units only 5 per cent did not have a cancer diagnosis. Those diagnoses include HIV/AIDS, motor neurone disease, heart disease and stroke. The average hospice unit in the UK accommodates 15 inpatients; three of every seven patients are discharged to another setting; and an average stay in a hospice is 13 days.

Inpatient hospices are designed with dying people in mind; planning includes facilitating easy access to beds and facilities for care workers as well as dying people themselves; in addition, where possible, the environment is warm and home-like. The physical location of a hospice building can influence the ways in which it operates; for example, a hospice on a hospital site might benefit from the advice of hospital personnel and yet might also have conflicts with hospital management (Doyle 1999). Hospices away from hospitals do not have the on-site availability of diagnostic facilities nor easy access to consultant advice. The composition of hospice staff is far from standard and this may influence the ethos as well as hospice services.

Dying people are usually admitted to an inpatient unit for one of three reasons: in order to achieve symptom control, to give them or their carers respite (a few days relief with assured quality of care) or for terminal care. The population served by palliative care services in the UK is predominantly white (96 per cent) and over 68 per cent are aged over 65 (Hospice Information 2007a, 2007b). As pointed out by Koffman in this volume, ethnic minorities have been under-represented in hospice admissions and a number of explanations have been proposed to explain this anomaly – from assumptions by GPs that people from ethnic minorities would not want admission to hospices, to assumptions that people from ethnic minorities are not offered this facility to the same extent as the host population.

Hospices provide a range of services for dying people in addition to conventional inpatient services – for example, day care services and bereavement care. Day care services are an integral part of hospice provision in the UK, the first such service was established in 1975 at St. Luke's Hospice in Sheffield. Current figures suggest that day care services in the UK on average cater for 15 patients per day: 32,000 patients are cared for annually by day care (excluding Scotland). Hospice palliative day care provides support in a variety of ways for dying people and ranges from advice on clinical problems (i.e. assessing appropriate drug dosage) and physical care to social, emotional and practical support (Doyle 2004). In addition to symptom review and some physical care such as bathing, activities include physiotherapy, beauty therapy, hairdressing and complementary therapies. Supervised care of dying people also provides respite for home carers. As with other services these are usually free.

Is inpatient hospice care in the UK justified? Anecdotal evidence has suggested for the past 20 years that the quality of life while dying in a hospice is considerably better than in other settings. After all that is what the hospice sets out to do. In the UK, information about palliative care services is collected annually in order to understand what is available and to improve care. Attempts to demonstrate the value of inpatient hospice care usually compares hospice with other forms of care. Clark and Seymour (1999) observed that 'All the evidence so far reviewed suggests that those who receive hospice care value it particularly for the "human" approach it can offer, for the reductions in anxiety and improvements in communication it can achieve and for the standards and style of nursing care which it delivers' (p. 167). But Salisbury *et al.* (1999) note that measuring the impact of palliative care on patients' quality of life is not an easy task. Reviewing relevant studies they found some, albeit dated, evidence that dying people in inpatient palliative care facilities received better pain control than those receiving palliative care at home or in hospital.

In the UK, the hospice building itself personifies palliative care and is seen as an ideal type. James and Field (1992) courageously identified how 'routinization and medicalization' had crept into hospice care and indeed reflected some of the concerns about conventional medical care in relation to caring for dying people. These critiques were sustained throughout the 1990s, with suggestions regarding the extent to which hospice care had been absorbed into mainstream health care and had lost its potential to lead and innovate (Corner and Dunlop 1997). Lawton (2000) argues that 'contemporary inpatient hospices are increasingly becoming enclaves in which a particular type of bodily deterioration and decay is set apart from mainstream society' (pp. 123–4). She demonstrates how inpatient hospice care has become super-specialized and in many ways has moved away from providing a setting for those with a variety of malignancies to die; instead inpatient hospice care is now primarily for those with the most extreme physical symptoms or social conditions. Critiques such as those already cited emphasize the need for further research to demonstrate the value of inpatient hospice care and compare this with palliative care in other institutional settings as well as other approaches to caring for dying people.

## Palliative care in hospitals

The section first explores palliative care in general hospitals (both teaching and district) and then concludes with a short overview of community hospitals, which exist in the UK, Ireland and Australia.

In Western countries, most people die in hospitals. Although dying people spend most of their last months in their own homes, they may be admitted to hospital on a regular basis or attend as outpatients or day patients. Those with cancer may be referred or admitted to teaching or district hospitals under the medical supervision of an oncology or radiotherapy team who may have treated them during acute phases of their illness. Dying people may also be under the care of a number of other specialists, particularly general physicians or surgeons.

In 2006 there were 314 hospital based palliative care services in the UK, whereas in the USA only 15 per cent of hospitals reported any end-of-life services and only 36 per cent pain management services (Pan *et al.* 2001). Hospital palliative care teams may include all or any of the following staff members – doctors (oncologists, specialist palliative care or general physicians), social workers, nurses and clergy. In addition support nurses work on their own in some hospitals. The International Association for Hospice and Palliative Care promotes the concept of palliative care delivery in acute hospitals (www.hospicecare.com/gs/page3.html), viewing it as multifunctional, providing the glue between acute hospital care and community palliative care, as well as undertaking an important teaching function.

Many hospital teams (in Western countries) operate in much the same way as support teams working out of hospices or other settings. They spend much of their time in the community, in patients' homes, where they provide symptom control, pain relief and emotional and other support to dying people, who are managed by a hospital consultant, as well as supporting carers, such as relatives and friends. They extend the same kind of support to inpatients and people attending outpatient appointments. These teams also play a particular role in the institution providing expertise, information, support and advice to medical, nursing and paramedical colleagues. While home care teams and individual Macmillan nurses in the UK see part of their role as educating primary health care teams and other providers of health and social care in the community, providing palliative care services and undertaking an educational role in a hospital setting is particularly challenging (Seymour *et al.* 2002).

Although there has been considerable movement towards embracing a concept of care in tertiary health care settings, the primary goal remains cure, and this is the target towards which the health care team works, particularly in specialist cancer wards. The death of a patient is often seen as a medical failure and therefore the presence of a group of people dedicated to a good death can be experienced as an irritant. This may be a partial explanation why these teams may feel marginalized, as evidenced by their siting in inaccessible or inadequate accommodation.

In describing the demise of an early hospital based support team Herxheimer *et al.* (1985) illustrate some of the conflicts inherent in establishing the first teams, some of which may still be seen as irreconcilable with working in acute settings striving for 'cure'. They concluded that in order for such a team to function adequately, in addition to substantial and realistic funding, leadership was essential, preferably from a hospital clinician (i.e. a physician) to give it the required status in the setting. Additionally, Herxheimer *et al.* noted that good communication between team members was essential. Many of these factors identified more than 20 years ago still hamper the effective functioning of hospital palliative care teams (www.hospicecare.com/gs/page3.html) and there is still little robust evidence about the effectiveness of these teams in relation to the tasks performed. McQuillan *et al.* (1996) demonstrated that symptoms experienced by patients with cancer and HIV were indeed alleviated following the introduction of a palliative care service. A modified support team assessment schedule (STAS: Higginson 1993), used in a variety of forms in community palliative care teams to measure change in symptoms and functioning of patients, was used by Edmonds *et al.* (1998) to ascertain whether hospital palliative care teams improve symptom control. Their findings suggested that other than depression, patients assessed three or more times using the STAS demonstrated improvement (in descending order) in psychological distress, anorexia, pain, mouth discomfort, constipation, breathlessness, nausea and vomiting. Another study in the hospital setting undertaken by the same research team (Edmonds *et al.* 2000) explored the palliative care needs of hospital inpatients. In addition to establishing that 12 per cent of the hospitals' medical and surgical patient population suffered from advanced disease, the study identified communication issues about discharge, and described relationships with community palliative team teams and primary care teams as problematic. They concluded that hospital palliative care teams can make a significant difference to patients' overall well-being including pain and symptom control, relationships with family and other professional care workers.

Higginson *et al.* (2002) searched databases to ascertain whether hospital-based palliative teams improved care for dying patients and their families. The outcome measures included quality of life, number of days spent in hospital and time allocated to a palliative care team. Many of the studies examined did not demonstrate strength in research methods, and none looked at different models of hospital teams. However, the skills and services that hospital palliative care teams provide do indicate some benefits (Higginson *et al.* 2002) but further research using similar and comparable tools is necessary to provide definitive evidence.

The impact of hospital palliative care teams, or specialist nurses, on the rest of the hospital community is a relatively new research area. To date, there has been an assumption that: hospital medical staff might resent the intrusion of these specialists; or they might discount their 'skills' (www.hospicecare.com/gs/page3.htm accessed 14 August 2007). Research by Jack *et al.* (2002) exploring the impact of a team in one large acute hospital suggests that general nursing and medical staff might feel deskilled by this service while empowering junior staff. The introduction in the UK of specialist nurses operationalizing the Gold Standards Framework as well as the Liverpool Care Pathway (adapting care plans developed in the UK, see Chapter 27) in hospitals (e.g. Seymour *et al.* 2005; McNicholl *et al.* 2006) should provide evidence in the next few years about the effectiveness of intervention of palliative care practitioners in the acute sector as well as an increased understanding of their interrelationships with their host (acute settings) and palliative care teams operating in the community.

### Community hospitals

Research undertaken by Payne *et al.* (2007a, 2007b) over a number of years has explored how community hospitals address the needs of dying people. Community hospitals serve smaller populations than the conventional district general hospital in the UK, Australia and Ireland, and find themselves with a large percentage of older people approaching death. Unlike teaching and district general hospitals, staff in community hospitals 'mainstream' the care of dying patients; managers believed that general palliative care could be delivered by staff as they possessed adequate expertise, equipment, resources and facilities although they acknowledged less expertise in psychosocial aspects of care (Payne *et al.* 2007b).

For patients in rural communities, community hospitals are suitably located and provide them with continuity of medical care. The surveys of staff, patients and relatives undertaken by Payne *et al.* noted that uncomplicated deaths could be well managed by staff in community hospitals. But predicting deaths and particularly changing status to 'go palliative' was often last minute and therefore not entirely satisfactory, resembling some of the difficulties encountered in long-term care (Katz and Peace 2003).

Payne's studies have demonstrated that for many older people, ending their lives in community hospitals is preferable to the large sterile atmosphere of district hospitals. They recommend that, in the UK, where choice is perceived as paramount, community hospitals should be seen as part of the resource package available for older people. We now move on to consider the setting where larger numbers of older people live and also die – long-term care.

# Palliative care in long-term care

The demographic profile of Western industrialized societies in the twenty-first century reflects an ageing population. For example, it is projected that by 2026 20 per cent of the population of Canada will be over 65; already currently 75 per cent of Canadian deaths occur in 'seniors' (Carstairs 2005). Similarly in the UK, there are almost as many people over 65 as there are under 16 years of age (ONS 2004 population statistics census). Thus dying in old age is now the norm in developed Western societies, with 77 the median age at death in the USA where most deaths occur at 65 and older (Kapo *et al.* 2007). Despite the introduction of many programmes (most notably the PACE programme in the USA) which endeavour to keep dying older people at home by providing day care, substantial percentages of older people in Western societies reside and die in assisted living facilities (known as care homes in the UK) (Zerzan *et al.* 2000; Zinn 2002). Twenty per cent of all deaths of people over 65 in the UK and in the USA occur in nursing homes and 30 per cent of hospital deaths occur within five days following an admission from a nursing home in the USA (Kapo *et al.* 2007). In England alone the resident population of care homes is 400,000 of whom 100,000 die annually (www.endoflifecare.nhs.uk). Nursing homes in the USA tend to accommodate large numbers of residents (over 100) whereas the average size of care homes in the UK is much smaller, usually ranging from 20 to 40 beds.

Only in recent years has research in the USA, Canada, Australia and the UK specifically investigated the quality of dying and management of death in care home settings (e.g. Katz *et al.* 1999, 2000a, 2000b; Froggatt 2000, 2001a, 2001b; Katz and Peace 2003; Seymour *et al.* 2005; Froggatt *et al.* 2006). Official and semi-official documents in the UK and in other countries have consistently observed the poor quality of dying in care settings and more recently have identified the urgency of improving terminal care in these settings and set targets for doing so (Palliative Care Australia www.pallcare.org.au; My Home Life 2006; SCIE 2005; www.endoflifecare. nhs.uk). In the UK, a number of palliative care programmes deemed successful in other settings have been trialled in care homes. These include modified versions of the Liverpool Care Pathway (e.g. Duffy and Woodland 2006), the Preferred Priorities for Care Plan and the Gold Standards

Framework in Care Homes. Initial results suggest that the number of crisis hospital admissions could be reduced by 12 per cent and hospitals deaths by 8 per cent (National Council for Palliative Care 2007; Thomas and GSF central team 2007). The appropriateness of these tools, albeit perceived as successful in other settings, has however been questioned (Partington 2006), as well as the wisdom of government organizations in endorsing them without proof of effectiveness (My Home Life 2006).

Crisis admissions to hospital of nursing home residents remain a factor which has forced a re-evaluation of policy and practice (Katz and Peace 2003; Froggatt and Payne 2006; Kapo *et al.* 2007). Research had demonstrated that decisions to transfer a resident to hospital were usually taken by the physician, who, without consulting the resident, assesses the (in)ability of the home to address the dying resident's needs (Sidell *et al.* 1997). These decisions to transfer dying residents were ratified by care home staff acknowledging their limitations in providing adequate care.

In the UK, the primary care team is primarily responsible for the health care needs of care home residents. Unlike people residing in their own homes and also served by primary care teams, access to specialist teams for those dying in care homes in the UK is not necessarily automatic. To address this same problem, in the Netherlands, homes for the elderly as well as nursing homes are establishing separate units for residents requiring palliative care. These units are comprised of between five and ten single rooms to which dying people with complex problems are transferred from other settings. Residents in these rooms are looked after by a multidisciplinary palliative care team including nurses, care-givers, nursing home physicians, social workers, psychologists, physiotherapists, pastoral workers and volunteers (Francke and Kerkstra 2000; EAPC website 2002 accessed 26 August 2007).

The question of whether community palliative care teams could or should become involved in caring for residents dying in these settings in the UK has been debated primarily based on the argument that palliative care operates within a different paradigm from care home philosophy and that the latter may have its own 'successful' ways of accommodating dying residents' needs (Froggatt 2001a). It is essential to acknowledge that the dying trajectories of older people do not necessarily resemble those served by conventional palliative care. Older people have multiple pathologies, often including elements of dementia and do not necessarily die of cancer. Their needs may therefore differ from those in receipt of conventional palliative care services (Abbey *et al.* 2006). Therefore one crucial element, that of labelling someone as dying, can be difficult. This applies to many other aspects of 'conventional palliative care'. Abbey *et al.*'s (2006) thoughtful article explores these issues and calls for flexibility in the ways in which terminal care is delivered in these settings.

Both internal as well as external factors to the home influence the quality of terminal care. The role of the physician in deciding whether to admit a resident to hospital has already been mentioned. Only relatively recently palliative care has been introduced into medical education in a number of countries including the UK, Spain, Argentina and Canada (Bruera and

Sweeney 2002); consequently, older physicians are not very familiar with the principles and practices of palliative care, except insofar as they apply to younger people dying of cancer in their own homes (Katz 2003).

The quality of staff, their skill mix and their commitment to caring for dying residents is crucial (Sidell *et al.* 1997). Staff in care homes are traditionally very poorly paid. Yet, care workers were keen to retain residents till death in what they believed were their own homes (*ibid.*). However, the same care workers often felt ill-equipped to respond to residents' physical as well as their emotional needs. This related partly to their lack of training, but they perceived that the greatest difficulty related to staffing levels. Their demanding jobs meant that care workers were unable to provide what they perceived to be appropriate 'nursing care' such as included sitting with dying residents.

Staff in care homes, even including management, have limited understanding of the terms palliative care (Katz and Peace 2003) or end-of-life care (Froggatt and Payne 2006). Despite this, studies have demonstrated that home management can articulate what for them constitutes a good death, some components of which are embodied in the principles of palliative care. As in community hospitals, the level of staffing, availability of additional staff, whether bank (agency) or off-duty staff are used to ease the load is crucial when a resident becomes highly dependent. Many homes have minimal cover at night with staff members covering large numbers of residents, or assigned to particular areas of the home. As almost the same number of residents die at night as do in the daytime, this created tremendous pressure for care workers working at night, who in order to provide adequate care for a dying resident de facto needed to 'neglect' other residents (Sidell *et al.* 1997). This situation is exacerbated in the winter months when more residents die and there is increased staff sickness.

The location and design of the home influence the dying residents' care. Where homes are not close to public transport or primarily house 'out of town' residents, relatives are less likely to be involved in 'caring' activities or in decision-making. The layout of the home as well as the bedrooms also impact on the nature of terminal care. Many homes in the UK are converted from domestic dwellings which do not have spacious bedrooms permitting easy access to both sides of the bed for care workers.

Training for care staff in long-term settings is patchy and variable in the UK (Dalley and Denniss 2001) as it is elsewhere. However, since 2005 in the UK, 50 per cent of care workers in care homes are required by the National Minimum Standards for Care Homes (Department of Health 2002) to hold National Vocational Qualifications in Social Care at Level Two. Care Standard 11 of the Care Standards Act 2002 in the UK specifies that: 'Care and comfort are given to service users who are dying, their death is handled with dignity and propriety, and their spiritual needs, rites and functions observed.' The concept of dignity and privacy is also enshrined in the National Service Framework for Older People in the UK (Department of Health 2001). This acknowledges the importance of 'fitting services around people's needs'. Teaching care staff to respond to people's needs is complex and requires more than simply the availability of these programmes (Katz 2005). These include the ethos and culture of the home, and the value attached to staff development. Training designed for care homes has been developed in Australia (Maddocks *et al.* 2000) and in the UK (Macmillan 2004); however, concerted evaluation of these programmes needs to be undertaken to ascertain their effectiveness.

Payment for hospice services varies between countries. Palliative care services in the UK are 'free' for the end use, and in the USA through medical insurance schemes, 'hospice services' are bought in to an increasing, but still proportionately small, number of nursing homes, and where this occurs they take over a substantial proportion of the resident's total care. In the Netherlands there is a movement to move dying people into nursing homes or homes for the elderly and then apply the US model by bringing in specialist palliative care teams.

*My* Home Life: Quality of Life in Care Homes (Owen and NCHR&D Forum 2006) examined issues about the quality of living and dying in care homes and the following are some areas of good practice they highlight in relation to care at the end of life:

- Staff awareness of their own attitude to death and dying, and how that may influence decisions about care.

- Recognizing and valuing the principles of palliative care and a good death.

- An ability and willingness to involve outside support: What are the local support services? How does the care home get access?

- Ensuring that communication is open and sensitive; accepting that death is coming, yet recognizing that some residents and family may not want to talk openly about what is happening: family members may be reluctant to face the imminent death of their relative and can create problems for staff and resident alike.

- Ensuring that relatives who wish to be with a dying resident are enabled to and are given emotional and practical help.

- Recognizing the importance of not leaving a dying person alone; using volunteers if no staff member or relative available.

- Supporting other residents when someone is dying and offering bereavement support to residents and relatives.

- Supporting staff, some of whom may feel like 'family'.

- Offering the home before or after funeral, enabling other residents to participate.

- Holding annual service of thanksgiving for all those who died in previous year and inviting relatives.

(Adapted and summarized from *My* Home Life: Quality of Life
in Care Homes www.myhomelife.org.uk)

# Caring for dying prisoners – the US experience

Research into the care of prisoners dying from disease, as opposed to violent deaths, has been neglected by palliative care researchers in most countries. However, voluntary organizations in the USA have expressed interest in this field, and philosophers have considered the conflicts between the Hippocratic Oath and the custodial personnel's commitment to the penal harm movement which seeks to inflict pain on prisoners.

In the UK commentaries and reports have been published about the need for humane palliative care services to be available for dying prisoners (e.g. Yampolskaya and Winston 2003). As discussed by Koffman, the prison population in the UK includes older people likely to die of conventional diseases. In addition, the prison population is growing older, particularly with respect to male sex offenders who are unlikely to be released as they approach death. Personal communication with the UK prison health service suggests that prisoners are entitled to receive community palliative care services, including hospice admission, in the same way as the general population. Where feasible, prisoners who are believed to have less than three months to live are released on special licence on the grounds of deteriorating health (Bolger 2005). However, inevitably, considerations such as the safety of the public and staffing issues influence the extent to which the prison population receives these services.

Certain principles of palliative care, such as bereavement support, could help to reduce the use of drugs to cope with emotions (Finlay and Jones 2000). Prison authorities say (personal communication) that officers have training in communication skills and are supported by chaplaincy teams and voluntary groups. Individual prisoners have a personal officer who acts as their key worker, and distressed prisoners have constant access to 'listeners', fellow prisoners trained by the Samaritans. Dying prisoners are cared for by local specialist palliative care teams referred by the hospital consultant.

In the United States, over a number of years, much concern has been raised about the emphasis on living wills for prisoners as well as their access to palliative care. The living will issue is contested due to the perception that this may foster additional lack of trust between prisoners and prison services. The National Prison Hospice Association acknowledges some of the particularly thorny issues faced in caring for prisoners. For example, as in the UK, the volunteer is pivotal in delivering hospice care in the USA; however, when dealing with potentially dangerous prisoners, finding external volunteers is somewhat problematic. Price (2002) explores some of these issues:

> The basic concepts of a prison hospice are the same as those for a community hospice. The differences are only procedural. How will you train volunteers? How will you allow inmates' movement? To what degree do you allow special circumstances to supersede segregation time? To what extent do you change rules for visits by the family? How

do you give inmates control of their own care? And how do you define your team?

She cautions:

> if you forget the concepts of pain control, patient autonomy, multi-disciplinary team, patient and family as unit of care, volunteer – you can call your program comfort care, but don't call it hospice.

In the 1990s, the Grace (Guiding Responsive Action for Corrections in End of Life) Project was launched promoting compassionate end-of-life care in prisons and jails. Supported by the Robert Wood Johnson Foundation, the Grace Project has links with many prison, health and palliative care organizations in the USA and is administered by the Volunteers of America. It incorporates an online resource centre to distribute information about existing programmes and others being developed by other jails and prisons and to support embryonic projects. The Grace Project is connected to many correctional organizations in the USA, as well as hospice organizations.

Ratcliff (2001), in reviewing the Grace Project, notes that in the USA more than 2,500 inmates died of natural causes (including AIDS) but few died actually in prison for the following reason:

> Traditionally, there has been great discomfort and reluctance in allowing death to occur on-site for fear that the death would be equated with neglect. Often to avoid potential legal, ethical, and medical complications, facilities have found it easier to send all dying patients out of the facility. As one correctional professional explained, 'inmates are expected to go to the hospital "in shackles" to die, and not die behind bars'.
>
> (quoted in Ratcliff 2001: 13)

However, for many prisoners particularly after long periods of incarceration, the prison has become their home and their community, and other inmates, their family (personal communication UK prisons; Ratcliff 2001; Tillman 2001).

Ratcliff describes some of the challenges to providing good end-of-life care in prisons. These include a focus on conforming to administrative rule rather than enabling individual choice; crowded conditions which mitigate against treating dying people as individuals and involving their families in their care; concern about pain control and symptom relief medications being abused; problems in relation to liability and litigation with regard to heroic treatments; the need to involve prison staff whose primary responsibility is to ensure security and efficiency; and, lastly, problems posed by inmate classification. Through visiting prisons the Grace Project identified the most important issues to be addressed in prisons to enable prisoners to die there. These include:

- *Pain and symptom management.* The challenges include the attitude of health care and security personnel about the use and abuse of narcotics; prison formularies that severely limit available medications; possibility of theft and trafficking; and assurance of effective dosages.

- *Family visitation and involvement*. The challenges include the identification and reunification of families; the definition of other inmates as 'family' and arrangement for their visitation; visitor access to inmates who are unable to be transported to visitation areas (especially for children); and extended and off-hours visitation.

- *Training*. The challenges include orienting and training a diverse group that includes medical and nursing staff, security, and other administrative staff and volunteers; changing negative staff attitudes; adjusting staff assignments; and conflicting demands for staff time.

- *Inmate isolation*. The challenges include care for high security level inmates; transfer of inmates from one facility to another to access the programme; and lack of family or inmate family.

- *Volunteer involvement*. The challenges include securing administrative approval and security staff support for involvement of inmates as volunteers, as well as community volunteer engagement.

- *Attitude*. The challenges include creating what Tanya Tillman refers to as a neural zone where anger, fear and prejudice of inmates and staff can be set aside.

(Ratcliff 2001: 14)

The Grace Project produced End-of-Life Care Standards of Practice in Correctional Settings as well as a resource manual. The standards, which are subdivided into practices, are: care, safety, security, justice, programme and activity, administration and management. In summary, the most important standards include:

- involvement of inmates as volunteers
- increased visitation for families, including inmate family
- interdisciplinary team including physician, nurse, chaplain and social worker, at a minimum
- comprehensive plans of care
- advance care planning
- training in pain and symptom management
- bereavement services
- adaptation of the environment and diet for comfort.

(Ratcliff 2001: 15)

Hospice programmes are now operational in 20 federal or state jurisdictions in the United States and they work in a variety of ways. As noted by Koffman, the Louisiana State Penitentiary (LSP) Hospice Program provides palliative care to the state's men-only maximum security prison at Angola, Louisiana (Tillman 2001). This prison houses over 5,000 inmates, most of whom will die behind bars. The hospice programme established in 1998 is part of Angola's prison health system. A 40-bed ward in the prison infirmary is the setting where dying prisoners receive care from a multidisciplinary team, known as an interdisciplinary team in the USA. One innovative aspect of this team is the extensive use of inmate volunteers who undergo intensive training delivered by external as well as internal experts. Security personnel have also been taken on board in order to attempt to reduce the mutual distrust and suspicion between them and prisoners. Prisoners are admitted to the programme through personal choice but only if they meet stringent criteria, including knowledge of diagnosis and prognosis (not more than six months). The programme is very comprehensive and even includes a formal bereavement assessment early on, in order to anticipate future needs of family members and surviving inmates. Annual memorial services held to commemorate hospice patients are planned by inmate volunteers and future plans include attendance from patients' families in the newly completed chapel (Tillman 2001).

The goals of the hospice team at LSP, comprising the medical staff, security personnel and inmate volunteers, are as follows:

- to provide quality, compassionate end-of-life care to our patients and their families
- to redirect efforts at end of life to palliative of distressing symptoms rather than extension of life (at all costs) as indicated by vital signs
- to improve the institution's previous practice of withholding a patient's right to make health care choices for himself
- to recognize and acknowledge those relationships formed by the patient that he finds meaningful and life-affirming.

(Tillman 2001: 18)

The USA has led on hospice care in prisons and other correctional facilities, partly because of its large prison population. The voluntary sector has promoted palliative care in prison and although many of these programmes are still to be evaluated, their results should be of potential use to other countries with ageing prisoners with health problems.

## Conclusion and suggestions for further research

In exploring palliative care in institutions, this chapter has demonstrated that although there is some agreement about the goals of palliative care, the nature of the setting can determine the quality of palliative care delivered. Relationships between team members and the composition of 'teams' working in palliative care also vary from setting to setting – volunteers play a major role in hospices and prisons and less so in care homes and hospitals. There is need for further information to be gathered about the types of palliative care different organizations strive to deliver, as well as in-depth research to ascertain the appropriateness of adapting palliative care principles to a particular setting. It is also important to recognize that end-of-life care does not necessarily begin only at the very end of life, especially in view of the fact that most people who die, especially in Western societies, are old and have multiple health issues, including those that affect their mental competence.

# References

Abbey, J, Froggatt, K.A., Parker, D. and Abbey, B. (2006) Palliative care in long-term care: a system in change. *International Journal of Older People Nursing*, 1(1): 56–63.

Bolger, M. (2005) Dying in prison: providing palliative care in challenging environments. *International Journal of Palliative Nursing*; 11(12): 619–20.

Bruera, E. and Sweeney, C. (2002) Palliative Care Models: International Perspective. *Journal of Palliative Medicine*, 5(2): 319–27.

Carstairs, S. (2005) *Quality End-Of-Life Care: The right of every Canadian*. Sub-committee to update 'Of Life and Death' of the Standing Senate Committee on Social Affairs, Science and Technology.

Clark, D. and Seymour, J. (1999) *Reflections on palliative care*. Buckingham: Open University Press.

Clemens, K.E., Kumar, S., Bruera, E., Klaschik, E., Jaspers, B. and De Lima, L. (2007) Palliative care in developing countries: what are the important issues? *Palliative Medicine*, 21(3): 173–5.

Corner, J. and Dunlop, R. (1997) New approaches to care. In: D. Clark, S. Ahmedzai and J. Hockley (eds) *New Themes in Palliative Care*. Buckingham: Open University Press.

Cummings, I. (1999) Training of volunteers, in D. Doyle, G.W.C. Hanks and N. MacDonald (eds) *Oxford Textbook of Palliative Medicine*. Oxford: Oxford University Press.

Dalley, G. and Denniss, M. (2001) *Trained to Care? Investigating the skills and competencies of care assistants in homes for older people*. Centre for Policy on Ageing Report No.28. London: Centre for Policy on Ageing.

Department of Health (2001) *National Service Framework for Older People*. London: Department of Health.

Department of Health (2002) *Care Homes for Older People National Minimum Standards*. London: Stationery Office.

Doyle, D. (1999) The provision of palliative care. In: D. Doyle, G.W.C. Hanks and N. MacDonald (eds) *Oxford Textbook of Palliative Medicine*. Oxford: Oxford University Press.

Doyle, D. (2004) Palliative medicine in the home. In: D. Doyle, G. Hanks, N.I. Cherny and K. Calman (eds) *Oxford Textbook of Palliative Medicine*, 3rd edn. Oxford: Oxford University Press, pp. 1097–114.

Doyle, D., Hanks, G., Cherny, N.I. and Calman, K. (2005) (eds) *Oxford Textbook of Palliative Medicine*, 3rd edn. Oxford: Oxford University Press, pp. 1097–114.

Duffy. A. and Woodland, C. (2006) Introducing the Liverpool Care Pathway into Nursing Homes. *Nursing Older People*, 18(9): 33–6.

Edmonds, P., Stuttaford, J.M. and Penny, J. (1998) Do hospital palliative care teams improve symptom control? Use of a modified STAS as an evaluation tool. *Palliative Medicine*, 12: 345–51.

Edmonds, P., Karlsen, S. and Addington-Hall, J. (2000) Palliative care needs of hospital inpatients. *Palliative Medicine*, 14(3): 227–8.

Finlay, I.G. and Jones, N.K. (2000) Unresolved grief in young offenders in prison. *British Journal of General Practice*, 50(456): 569–70.

Francke, A.L. and Kerkstra, A. (2000) Palliative care services in The Netherlands: a descriptive study. *Patient Education and Counselling*, 41: 23–33.

Froggatt, K.A. (2000) *Palliative care education in nursing homes*. London: Macmillan Cancer Relief.

Froggatt, K.A. (2001a) Palliative care in nursing homes: where next? *Palliative Medicine*, 15: 42–8.

Froggatt, K.A. (2001b) Life and Death in English Nursing Homes: Sequestration or Transition? *Ageing and Society*, 21: 319–32.

Froggatt, K. and Payne, S. (2006) A survey of end-of-life care in care homes: issues of definition and practice. *Health and Social Care in the Community*, 14(4): 341–8.

Froggatt, K.A., Wilson, D., Justice, C., MacAdam, M., Leibovici, K., Kinch, J., Thomas, R. and Choi, J. (2006) End-of-life care in long-term care settings for older people: a literature review. *International Journal of Older People Nursing*, 1(1): 45–50.

Herxheimer, A., Begent, R., MacLean, D., Phillips, L., Southcott, B. and Walton, I. (1985) The short life of a terminal care support team: experience at Charing Cross Hospital. *British Medical Journal*, 290: 1877–9.

Higginson, I. (1993) Clinical audit: getting started and keeping going. In: I. Higginson (ed.) *Clinical Audit in Palliative Care*. Oxford: Radcliffe Medical Press.

Higginson, I.J., Finlay, I., Goodwin, D.M., Cook, A.M., Hood, K., Edwards, A.G.K., Douglas, H-R. and Norman, C.E. (2002) Do hospital-based palliative teams improve care for patients or families at the end of life? *Journal of Pain and Symptom Management*, 23(2): 96–106.

Hockley, J. (1997) The evolution of the hospice approach. In: D. Clark, J. Hockley and S. Ahmedzai (eds) *New Themes in Palliative Care*. Buckingham: Open University Press.

Hospice Information (2007a) *Minimum Data Sets – National Survey document*. www.hospiceinformation.info (accessed July 2007).

Hospice Information (2007b) www.hospiceinformation.info/factsandfigures/services.asp (accessed July 2007).

Jack, D., Oldham, J. and Williams, A. (2002) Do hospital-based palliative care clinical nurse specialists de-skill general staff? *International Journal of Palliative Nursing*, 8(7): 336–40.

James, N. and Field, D. (1992) The routinization of hospice: bureaucracy and charisma. *Social Science and Medicine*, 34(12): 1363–75.

Kapo, J., Morrison, L.J. and Liso, S. (2007) Palliative Care for the Older Adult, *Journal of Palliative Medicine*, 10(1): 185–209.

Katz, J.S. (2003) Training needs in the palliative approach of care home staff. *European Journal of Palliative Care*, 10(4): 154–6.

Katz, J.S. (2005) Palliative care in residential care facilities: a brief review. *International Journal of Palliative Nursing*, 11(3): 130–1.

Katz, J.T., Komaromy, C. and Sidell, M. (1999) Understanding palliative care in residential and nursing homes. In: *International Journal of Palliative Nursing*, 5(2): 58–64.

Katz, J.T., Sidell, M. and Komaromy, C. (2000a) *Investigating the Training Needs in Palliative Care*. Unpublished report for the Department of Health.

Katz, J.T., Komaromy, C. and Sidell, M. (2000b) Death in homes: bereavement needs of residents, relative and staff. *International Journal of Palliative Nursing*, 6(6): 274–9.

Katz, J.S. and Peace, S. (2003) *End of life in care homes: a palliative care approach* Oxford: Oxford University Press.

Lawton, J. (2000) *The dying process*. London: Routledge.

Macmillan Cancer Relief (2004) *Foundations in palliative care*. London: Macmillan Cancer Relief.

McNicholl, M.P., Dunne, K., Garvey, A., Sharkey, R. and Bradley, A. (2006) Using the Liverpool Care Pathway for a Dying Patient, *Nursing Standard*, 20(38): 46–50.

McQuillan, R., Finlay, I., Roberts, D. *et al.* (1996) The provision of a palliative care service in a teaching hospital and subsequent evaluation of that service, *Palliative Medicine*, 10: 231–9.

Maddocks, I., Abbey, J., Beck, K., De Bellis, A., Glaetzer, K., McLeod, A., Parker, D., and Pickhaver, A. (2000) *Palliative Care in Residential Care Facilities: Educational Resource Package*. Palliative Care Unit: The Flinders University of South Australia.

National Council for Palliative Care and NHS End of Life Care Programme (2007) *Building on Firm Foundations: Improving end of life care in care homes: examples of innovative practice*. www.endoflifecare.nhs.org.uk; www.ncpc.org.uk (accessed July 2007).

Office of National Statistics (2004) *Social Trends*. London: Stationery Office.

Owen, T. and National Care Home Research & Development Forum (2006) *My Home Life: A review of the literature*. London: Help the Aged.

Palliative Care Australia www.pallcare.org.au (accessed July 2007).

Pan, C.X., Morrison, R.S., Meier, D.E., Natale, D.K., Goldhirsch, S.L., Kralovec, P. and Cassel, C.K. (2001) How prevalent are Hospital-based Palliative Care Programs? Status Report and Future Directions, *Journal of Palliative Medicine*, 4(3): 315–24.

Partington, L. (2006) The challenges of adopting care pathways for the dying for use in care homes. *International Journal of Older People Nursing*, 1: 51–5.

Payne, S., Hawker, S., Kerr, C., Seamark, D., Roberts, H., Jarrett, N. and Smith, H. (2007a) Experiences of end-of-life care in community hospitals, *Health and Social Care in the Community*, 15(5): 494–501.

Payne, S., Hawker, S., Kerr, C., Seamark, D., Jarrett, N., Roberts, H. and Smith, H. (2007b) Health care workers' skills: perceived competence and experiences of end of life care in community hospitals. *Progress in Palliative Care*, 15(3): 118–25.

Price, C. (2002) To Adopt or Adapt? Principles of Hospice Care in the Correctional Setting. *National Prison Hospice Association News*, Issue 6, Boulder, CO.

Ratcliff, M. (2001) Dying inside the Walls. In: M.Z. Solomon, A.L. Romer, K.S. Heller and D.E. Weissman (eds) *Innovations in End-of-life Care*. New York: Mary Ann Liebert.

Salisbury, C., Bosanquet, N., Wilkinson, E.K. *et al.* (1999) The impact of different models of specialist palliative care on patients' quality of life: a systematic literature review, *Palliative Medicine*, 13(1): 3–17.

Seymour, J., Clark, D., Bath, P., Beech, N., Corner, J., Douglas, H-R., Halliday, D., Haviland, J., Marples, R., Normand, C., Skilbeck, J. and Webb, T. (2002) Clinical nurse specialists in palliative care. Part 3. Issues for the Macmillan Nurse role, *Palliative Medicine*, 16: 386–94.

Seymour, J., Witherspoon, R., Gott, M., Ross, H., Payne, S. with Owen, T. (2005)

*End-of-Life care: Promoting comfort, choice and well-being for older people.* Policy Press with Help the Aged.

Sidell, M., Katz, J.T. and Komaromy, C. (1997) *Dying in Nursing and Residential Nursing Homes for Older People: examining the case for palliative care.* Report for the Department of Health. Milton Keynes: Open University.

SCIE (2005) Research briefing 10: Terminal care in care homes. www.scie.org.uk/publications/briefings/briefing10/index.asp (accessed 21 May 2006 and 30 August 2007).

Tillman, T. (2001) Hospice in Prison: The Louisiana State Penitentiary Hospice Program. In: M.Z. Solomon, A.L. Romer, K.S. Heller and D.E. Weissman (eds) *Innovations in End-of-life Care.* New York: Mary Ann Liebert.

Thomas, K. and GSF central team (2007) Briefing Paper on the Gold Standards Framework in Care Homes (GSFCH) Programme. *GSFCH Briefing Paper 1.*

Yampolskaya, S. and Winston, N. (2003) Hospice care in prison: general principles and outcomes, *American Journal of Hospice and Palliative Care*, 20(4): 290–6.

Zerzan, J., Stearnes, S. and Hanson, L. (2000) Access to Palliative Care and Hospice in Nursing Homes, *JAMA*, 284(19): 2489–94.

Zinn, C. (2002) Australia: government subsidizes long term care by up to £22,000 a year, *British Medical Journal*, 324: 1543.

# 20

# Treatment decisions at the end of life

## A conceptual framework

*Bert Broeckaert*

---

**Key points**

- Ethical issues are important to the practice of palliative care.
- There is much debate about the term euthanasia.
- Key concepts in ethics are considered in the light of international research and legislation.

---

**Case Study 20.1**

Dorothy is 82 and suffering from advanced dementia. She stopped recognizing her husband and children more than three years ago. In the past few months, she has spent a large part of each day in bed and lost virtually all her capacities to interact with the world around her. Three days ago, swallowing became totally impossible for her. The physician who has been treating her during the many years she has already spent in the nursing home decided not to start artificial nutrition. Although she thought artificial nutrition would probably lengthen the patient's life, in this case she considered it to be futile treatment and thus decided not to start it. A nurse who has known the patient for many years felt very uncomfortable with this decision and talked to the local newspaper. In a front-page article, the physician is accused of performing euthanasia.

---

Rather than merely summing up the wide range of ethical questions that arise at the end of life, I would like to try to delve more deeply into the specific issue raised by cases like this one; that is, the confusion, discomfort and controversy associated with a number of difficult treatment decisions at the end of life. The most important reason why a treatment decision such as the one in our example is seen as problematic, is the fact that this decision has (or is thought to have) a life-shortening effect. Of course, we can accept that there exist situations where medical treatment no longer brings about a cure, but we still tend to expect that if treatment does not prolong life, it will at least sustain it. Yet, there are situations in which what health care workers consciously do has, or at least seems to have, an accepted or (in exceptional cases) intended life-shortening effect. Isn't euthanasia an appropriate term in all these cases? Or is there a clear boundary and an important difference between withholding artificial nutrition (as in our example) and euthanasia? Or between euthanasia and palliative sedation and other drastic forms of pain and symptom control?

What I will attempt to do in this short and modest chapter is offer nurses and other health care workers a conceptual framework that will permit them to develop further their own ideas about this complex and problematic field, and enter into dialogue about it. Without a shared set of words and concepts, any meaningful ethical discussion about this complicated matter is as good as impossible. Therefore, I offer in this chapter a typology about the different kinds of treatment decisions that can be taken in advanced stages of life-threatening illness.

## Euthanasia

'A case of euthanasia', the nurse felt and the newspaper wrote. But what is euthanasia? What do we mean when we use this word? Euthanasia is certainly a cause of major controversy, leading to very diverse and often very emotional reactions. For some, euthanasia is a right that ought to be recognized, as according to them it enables dying with dignity under undignified circumstances; for others, euthanasia is the very antithesis of palliative care, the opposite of a respectful and caring way to deal with dying patients and thus totally unacceptable. Nonetheless, in its original meaning 'euthanasia' gives little cause for such controversy. In ancient Greece, the word 'euthanasia' was used as a synonym for a gentle, fortunate and natural (certainly not medically induced) death without suffering, the sort of death that most people would hope for – *eu* (good) and *thanatos* (death): a good death. Though a shift of meaning can be observed already with Francis Bacon's use of the term in 1605 (the emphasis is more on what the physician does to reduce the dying person's suffering), it is only with people like Samuel C. Williams (1872) and Lionel A. Tollemache (1873) that the term 'euthanasia' acquires its contemporary meaning. Only at the end of the nineteenth century is euthanasia understood as 'suicide by proxy', or as 'suicide *in extremis*', where a physician intentionally administers lethal medication, at the patient's request, in order to relieve the patient of extreme and unbearable suffering (Emanuel 1994).

Around the beginning of the twentieth century, in reaction to the rise of this new pro-euthanasia movement, various forms of euthanasia came to be distinguished. For instance, an 1884 editorial in the *Boston Medical and Surgical Journal* already drew a distinction between active and passive euthanasia, rejecting the former (which was defended by people like Williams and Tollemache) and considering the latter – which amounted to withdrawing or withholding a possibly life-prolonging treatment – to be clearly acceptable. In 1899, *The Lancet* made another distinction, one which is also still well known, between direct and indirect euthanasia, where indirect refers to the fact that a medical treatment (such as pain relief) can have side effects which might shorten the patient's life, without this constituting the aim of the treatment: the actual (direct) aim is to bring the pain under control. Though the word 'euthanasia' in the Anglo-Saxon world is associated primarily with its voluntary character (the patient experiences life as unbearable and desires to escape from this suffering), the German discussion about the end of life was oriented differently from the outset. Long before the notorious work of Binding and Hoche (1922) and the euthanasia programmes of the Nazis, people such as Haeckel (1899) and Jost (1895) had already defended the killing of certain categories of incompetent incurably ill patients.

The discussion about euthanasia that has been ongoing since the end of the nineteenth century has made the word into a very complex term that covers a multiplicity of meanings. Various adjectives were and still are added to the term to make it clear what sort of life-shortening or life-terminating action one is speaking about. Thus, euthanasia is active or passive, direct or indirect, voluntary, involuntary or non-voluntary, and these adjectives can be used in all sorts of possible combinations. For instance, if one intentionally neglects to treat a lung infection with the aim of hastening the patient's death without the patient having requested this or given consent, then this could be seen as an example of direct passive non-voluntary euthanasia. In this way, the word 'euthanasia' as such becomes an umbrella term encompassing all possible forms of medical treatment (or non-treatment) that have a life-shortening effect.

Today there are still many authors and organizations that use this broad concept of euthanasia. On the other hand, in the Netherlands a very strict definition of euthanasia has been used since 1985 (and in Belgium since 1997) (Belgian Advisory Committee on Bioethics 1997; Adams and Nys 2005). In these countries, euthanasia is defined as 'intentionally terminating life by someone other than the person concerned, at the latter's request'. Thus, euthanasia becomes active, direct and voluntary by definition. A broad or general definition? A choice has to be made, as in delicate ethical decisions about the end of life employing a key term such as 'euthanasia' in both a narrow and a broad sense would only lead to confusion and misunderstandings.

One can present oneself as strongly for or against euthanasia and a legalization or regulation of this practice, or state that euthanasia is illegal everywhere except the Netherlands and Belgium. In such a case, one gives the word 'euthanasia' the specific and narrow meaning ascribed to it by

> **Box 20.1**
>
> *Euthanasia* (broad definition): a deliberate medical act or omission that has a life-shortening effect that is accepted or aimed at by the physician involved.
>
> *Direct euthanasia*: the intention and direct effect of the treatment is the death of the patient.
>
> *Indirect euthanasia*: the death of the patient is a foreseen but unintended side effect.
>
> *Active euthanasia*: the death of the patient is the result of the administration of lethal medication.
>
> *Passive euthanasia*: the death of the patient is the result of the withholding or withdrawing of a life-sustaining treatment.
>
> *Voluntary euthanasia*: the life of the patient is shortened conforming to his or her will.
>
> *Involuntary euthanasia*: the life of the patient is shortened contrary to his or her will.
>
> *Non-voluntary euthanasia*: the life of the patient is shortened while the will of the patient is not known.

people like Williams and Tollemache: the administration of lethal medication with the aim of ending the patient's life. Or one can use the word 'euthanasia' as an umbrella term, as I just described. But if one defends such a broad use of the term, then one must be consistent and thus recognize that in most countries certain forms of euthanasia (more precisely the passive and the indirect variants) can be accepted medical practice. Then it would be simply inconsequential to state that euthanasia is illegal everywhere except in the Netherlands and Belgium.

The counter-intuitive character of these conclusions shows that, in everyday speech, 'euthanasia' is usually used in a specific sense: when using the word euthanasia, people do not primarily think of *all* forms of possibly life-shortening medical actions or omissions, but of those specific cases where lethal medication is administered with the direct aim of ending the life of the patient. 'Euthanasia' in fact means active direct euthanasia. I would argue for using the narrow definition of euthanasia, not only because it is closer to everyday usage, to the idea immediately evoked by the term. More importantly, it is simply inopportune to use one and the same term for an entire series of actions that are judged quite differently, both ethically and legally. This would be tantamount to carrying out an unjustified conflation of the most controversial and often illegal practices with the most normal and perfectly legal (sometimes even legally required) acts. What is the benefit of talking about euthanasia in a case such as actively and intentionally ending the life of a quadriplegic patient (clearly controversial) and using the same terminology in the case of not reanimating a terminal cancer patient (it is precisely reanimation that would be controversial here)? Is it really wise to use the term 'euthanasia' (with all the connotations it invokes) when the intention to end life is clearly absent, as in the second case? Is it not precisely this intentional, active ending of life that is far removed from the healing and life-sustaining mission of the physician? Is it not this ending of life that creates all the controversy and thus deserves a term of its own?

When the words *indirect* euthanasia are used to refer to pain control with a life-shortening effect, we can say that, on the one hand, and completely erroneously, it is postulated or at least suggested that heavy pain treatment has an intrinsic life-shortening effect (Bercovitch *et al.* 1999) and, on the other hand, that the intention of pain control and direct euthanasia are so different that placing them both under the same heading (euthanasia) leads to more confusion than clarity. As far as the use of the words *passive* euthanasia is concerned, it is simply wrong to imply or suggest that as a rule withholding or withdrawing a life-sustaining treatment has a life-shortening effect and implies a life-shortening intention. More than enough reasons, it seems, to reject a broad interpretation of the concept of euthanasia and to opt for a more narrow use of the term (cf. Roy 2005). In the rest of this chapter, euthanasia refers only to the intentional and active ending of life.

## Medical end-of-life decisions

In opting for the strict sense of the term euthanasia, we will need to find a new umbrella term to cover the different treatment decisions taken at the end of life. In 1990, when he took on the task of carrying out a large-scale empirical study of Dutch euthanasia practice, Paul van der Maas and his team were confronted with the same problem. Restricting the use of the term euthanasia to the strict Dutch definition, they coined the new umbrella term 'medical decisions concerning the end of life' or 'medical end-of-life decisions'. Since then, the term has become standard usage in the Netherlands, and it regularly turns up in the international literature, especially as it informs a growing number of large-scale empirical studies (i.e. van der Maas *et al.* 1991, 1996; Kuhse *et al.* 1997; Deliens *et al.* 2000; van der Heide *et al.* 2003).

This new term comprises 'all decisions made by physicians about actions whose objective is to hasten the end of the patient's life, or where the physician can expect that the end of the patient's life will most probably be hastened as a result of such actions' (van der Maas *et al.* 1991). In other words, the term comprises all forms of life-shortening (or non-life-prolonging) medical action and thus basically covers the same area as the word euthanasia when used in its broad meaning.

---

**Box 20.2**

**Medical end-of-life decisions (van der Maas *et al.*)**
'all decisions made by physicians about actions whose objective is to hasten
the end of the patient's life, or where the physician can expect that the end of
the patient's life will most probably be hastened as a result of such actions'

- Non-treatment decisions: the withholding or withdrawal of potentially life-
  prolonging treatments

  - taking into account the possibility or certainty that this would hasten
    the patient's death
  - partly with the intention of hastening the patient's death.

- The alleviation of pain and symptoms with opioids in doses with a potential
  life-shortening effect

  - taking into account the possibility or certainty that this would hasten
    the patient's death
  - partly with the intention of hastening the patient's death.

- Physician-assisted death: the administration, prescription, or supply of
  drugs with the intention of shortening the patient's life

  - euthanasia (at patient's request)
  - physician-assisted suicide
  - ending of life without patient's explicit request.

---

How to evaluate the concept 'medical end-of-life decisions' and the typology behind it? Because of four reasons I feel compelled to reject this term and the framework involved. A first reason is the fact that this term unjustly gives the impression that we are dealing here essentially with medical-technical decisions, decisions that can only, or should only, be made by physicians, since only they possess the required expertise. This suggestion, which is inherent in the use of the term, is especially misleading and dangerous. To give an example: a decision is made to withdraw artificial administration of food and fluids in a patient in a persistent vegetative state (PVS) who has been in a deep coma for six months. This is a clear example of a medical decision concerning the end of life. It is also clear that such a decision will have a life-shortening effect. But is it really a decision that is essentially *medical*? I think the answer is clearly no. Admittedly, this decision does have an unmistakable and inevitable medical component. Without a correct assessment of the patient's medical condition, and without a proper idea of the available medical evidence in this area, it is impossible to make an appropriate decision. Nevertheless, my point is that the ultimate decision involves much more than just these medical facts, however indispensable they may be.

The more fundamental question being posed and answered here is whether the life of a PVS patient – a life which in principle can be prolonged, sometimes for several decades, until a natural death ensues – should be considered dignified and meaningful. Obviously, the decision to be made here is an *ethical* one, and in making essentially ethical decisions, I can think of no reason why the values and ideas of a single professional group (i.e. physicians) regarding what is dignified and meaningful should be the only ones that count. The ethical nature of many decisions and the fact that not everyone has the same ideas about what constitutes a meaningful human life are in themselves strong arguments in favour of involving other health care workers – and in the first place the patient and his or her family – in the decision-making process.

A second reason why I reject the term medical end-of-life decision is the fact that I find the term misleading. In their definition, van der Maas and colleagues refer to the various forms of life-shortening actions and omissions, so the meaning is actually the same as the term 'euthanasia' in the broad sense of the word (which I found problematic). The fact that what is at issue is the shortening or even ending of life is, however, not at all suggested by the rather euphemistic phrase 'medical end-of-life decisions'. Why would the decision to permit someone to spend his or her final days at home, the decision to prolong someone's life through a particular therapy and the decision to treat a specific symptom the dying person is confronted with not be included in this category? Use of a term such as 'medical decision concerning the end of life' only clouds the unique and troubling specificity – especially for physicians, who are assumed to seek a cure or at least to sustain life – of a number of acts one wishes to discuss; that is, the fact that the shortening of life is intended or at least accepted.

The third reason I have for rejecting the concept medical end-of-life decision is precisely its one-sided focus on life-shortening – one looks in fact at reality from a euthanasia-perspective. This of course doesn't come as a surprise: the term and the conceptual framework were specifically developed for the large-scale empirical study of Dutch euthanasia practice the authors were commissioned to do. It is, however, of the utmost importance that we, both in ethical discussion and in empirical research, do not just focus on life-shortening acts, but also keep life-*lengthening* treatment decisions in advanced disease in the picture. Otherwise, we lose sight of, for instance, the whole issue of futile treatment (cf. infra) and end up with a very one-sided picture that only problematizes and studies one aspect of the problem.

But the problem lies even deeper. The fourth and most important reason for resisting the medical end-of-life decision typology as coined by van der Maas, is the fact that many decisions at the end of life have nothing or little to do with either life-shortening or life-lengthening. The essential feature of pain control and palliative sedation is, for instance, *not* the fact that they are life-shortening (or life-lengthening) and the discontinuing of an ineffective curative treatment, for instance, does *not* have a life-shortening effect. Sometimes medical acts or omissions do have a life-shortening or life-lengthening effect, and this element should indeed be involved in ethical deliberation and in empirical study. However, this is only one element in a much broader discussion about dignified living and dying: palliative care is in fact, in accordance with the WHO's definition, neither focused on life-lengthening, nor life-shortening, but on the quality of life of the patient and his or her family. Therefore, it is out of the question that because of a most likely unintended but actual 'euthanatic prejudice' – the Dutch research framework was coined to answer questions regarding euthanasia practice in The Netherlands – treatment decisions in advanced disease should only or chiefly be seen and studied as life-shortening. An approach that is focused on life-shortening and takes a life-shortening effect as the common denominator – which is both the case in the classical broad euthanasia-typology and the Dutch medical end-of-life decisions typology – leads to a one-sided and skewed perception of the delicate ethical choices to be made at the end of life. With such a framework it is not possible to offer a fair empirical depiction of, for instance, pain control or a well-founded ethical assessment of palliative sedation.

## Treatment decisions in advanced disease

The rejection of both the broad classical euthanasia typology (direct/indirect, active/passive) and the Dutch medical end-of-life decisions typology brings us to an umbrella term and a typology that does not focus on life-shortening. Therefore, we simply talk about 'treatment decisions in advanced disease' (without implying that these necessarily shorten or lengthen life) and offer a typology about the different kinds of treatment decisions that can be taken in advanced stages of life-threatening illness. In other words, it is about the different ways medicine can help and support patients with advanced disease. We do not develop this typology because we are particularly keen on classifications but because each kind of treatment decision brings about specific ethical issues which can be misunderstood when no clear boundaries and differences have been set. In the absence of the kind of conceptual and terminological clarification I propose here, we are trapped in a conceptual mist that impairs our vision and judgement, a conceptual mist in which the lack of any shared understanding of the basic terms renders a meaningful ethical discussion impossible. We distinguish three major categories of treatment decisions in advanced disease:

* Choices with regard to *curative or life-sustaining treatment*: is such a treatment initiated or withheld, continued or withdrawn?
* Choices with regard to palliative treatment and *symptom control*: all treatments aimed at maximizing, in an active way, the incurably ill patient's quality of life and comfort.
* Choices with regard to *euthanasia and assisted suicide*, where lethal medication is purposefully administered.

In the remainder of this chapter we will look into each of these categories. Our aim with this is not to present an elaborate ethical evaluation, but just to clarify the different concepts. From the fact that we mention and describe a certain act it cannot, of course, be deduced that we approve of it or advocate it.

# (Forgoing) curative or life-sustaining treatment

When the treatment of a life-threatening disorder, despite all efforts, does not have the hoped-for effect, care-givers, patient and family face a number of difficult but unavoidable choices. A first series of decisions which has to be made relates to curative and life-sustaining treatment: are we going to continue or even radicalize our curative approach? Or are we, gradually or drastically, changing directions? Should we try to lengthen life? Or is that also not a realistic option anymore?

### *(Non)-treatment decisions*

Examples of difficult but necessary decisions regarding treatment – to start or not to start, to continue or not to continue – abound. Are we going to administer antibiotics when a patient in an irreversible coma develops pneumonia or will we refrain from doing this? Will we install or rather withhold tube feeding when a severely demented patient develops swallowing difficulties which make normal feeding impossible? Will we continue or discontinue a chemotherapy that might lengthen the patient's life a few months but that at the same time has a severe impact on the quality of life of the patient?

Decisions on curative or life-sustaining treatments are real choices: depending on the situation and the individuals concerned, they can turn out in two ways. One can choose to withdraw or withhold a certain treatment, since this treatment is no longer considered to be meaningful or effective in the given circumstances. Or one can choose to continue or initiate a treatment aimed at recovery or life sustainment. It is imperative to bear in mind both options, initiating and withholding, withdrawing and continuing, and not just to focus on one of them (e.g. non-treatment decisions) and then turn this option into a problem or put this option forward as the one and only choice.

The choices that need to be made here are indeed only rarely black-and-white choices where it would be perfectly clear what the real chances of success are and what is meaningful and what is futile. Consider once again the example of the PVS patient. It would be too simple to claim that continuing to artificially feed this patient is futile: from a physical standpoint it is not futile at all: the patient's life is clearly prolonged, the patient remains alive due to the treatment. Second, what is considered to be a meaningful and dignified human life? How should one weigh prolongation of life against quality of life? These are clearly matters where no objective standard exists, but where much depends on one individual's values and assessments. This is why it is of prime importance to get the patient, family and nurses and other health care workers involved as much as possible in the choices that are made. Using the phrase futile treatment too easily tends to ignore and underestimate this important ethical and personal dimension.

Typologies that only discuss *non*-treatment decisions and treat these as life-shortening acts or omissions, tend to neglect the fact that numerous non-treatment decisions have nothing to do with life-shortening (or rather the non-lengthening of life), as they involve the cessation of treatments which are no longer effective, which do *not* lead to the wished for recovery or lengthening of life. Treatments like this (for example, a chemo that isn't working) often have a serious and meaningless negative impact on the patient's comfort and quality of life, since they cause discomfort and suffering without offering any benefit to the patient. Stopping or not initiating such an ineffective treatment cannot be called life-shortening.

### Refusal of treatment

The motivation for withholding or withdrawing life-prolonging treatment can be two-fold: either it is done because in the given situation this treatment is deemed to be no longer meaningful or effective, or simply because the patient refuses treatment. Here, the textbook example is that of the Jehovah's Witness who refuses a needed blood transfusion and thus puts their life at stake. There is a growing international consensus that when a competent patient (such as a competent Jehovah's Witness) refuses a treatment, this refusal must be respected, even if such a refusal could lead to the patient's death. The relevant principle here is the principle of the right to physical integrity, a fundamental human right which can be found in the European Human Rights Treaty (Article 8) and which is just as clearly present in the Convention on Human Rights and Biomedicine (Council of Europe 1996). When applied to the field of health care, the right to physical integrity implies that medical intervention – which undeniably has an clear impact on a person's body – can take place only when the patient has given explicit consent to such action. When a patient refuses or withdraws this consent, this refusal must in principle be respected, even if in the view of the health care workers such a refusal will have deleterious consequences for the patient's chances of healing or quality of life. As health care workers, we may find it particularly regrettable and irresponsible if a patient who is diagnosed with breast cancer refuses surgery when it is clear to everyone that surgery would increase her chances considerably. In such cases, health care workers certainly have the right and the duty to express their concerns to the patient and to point out the great risk she is taking. However, if after all this the patient sticks to her decision to refuse surgery, then this decision must be respected.

# Pain and symptom control

When a life-threatening illness or disorder, despite all efforts, continues to evolve in an adverse way, the patient and their family are of course not left to their own devices, though an often gradual shift will take place from a curative and life-prolonging to a palliative approach. A second category of treatment decisions thus deals with the choices that have to be made with regard to palliative treatment and symptom control. These choices involve all treatments that are aimed at maximizing, in an active and interdisciplinary way, the incurably ill patient's quality of life and comfort. In what follows we will focus more specifically on the medicinal treatment of pain and on palliative sedation, as these specific forms of symptom control pose important ethical problems.

## *Pain control*

Unlike, for instance, euthanasia, nurses and physicians often regard pain relief as ethically unproblematic. The fact that the intention underlying pain control is said to be completely different from that of euthanasia ensures, it is often argued, an essential distinction between the two. Are we wasting our time then in looking more closely at pain control? I don't think so. The following is a telling example. A survey carried out by the Pallium group of the European and Israeli delegates to the sixth congress of the European Association of Palliative Care (Geneva 1999) revealed that only 5.3 per cent of the respondents thought that euthanasia should be permitted in palliative care under certain circumstances. On the other hand, 'the intentional shortening of life by raising opioid doses' commanded greater support: 15.4 per cent of the respondents stated that this action 'could be part of palliative care' (Janssens *et al.* 2002). It is strange that suddenly three times as many people should say yes, simply because the controversial word euthanasia is avoided and talking about opioid doses suggests pain relief and the ethical qualities linked with it. 'The intentional shortening of life', however, can hardly be regarded as the ultimate purpose of pain control or, more generally, symptom control. What is typical of pain and symptom control, I would argue, is not only the physician's underlying subjective intention (treating symptoms, not shortening life) but especially the adequacy and proportionality of what is occurring at the objective level. For this reason, I define pain and symptom control as follows: 'the intentional administration of analgesics and/or other drugs in dosages and combinations required to adequately relieve pain' (Broeckaert 2000a).

Striving for adequacy and proportionality – for a clear relation between the medication that is administered and the medication that is required – is absolutely essential for distinguishing pain control from euthanasia and assisted suicide. This is not simply hair-splitting, as can clearly be shown by the empirical 'end-of-life decisions' research. If we know that pain control is remarkably safe even when powerful medication is administered in extreme dosages (Bercovitch *et al.* 1999 are clear: 'high morphine dosage does not affect patient survival'), then we can conclude that when pain control is carried out according to the rules, it will hardly ever have a life-shortening effect, and as a result will hardly ever count as a form of euthanasia. In light of this, it is quite astonishing to read that in the Netherlands and Flanders, according to the physicians involved, pain control led to a marked shortening of life in no fewer than 19.1 per cent and 18.5 per cent of deaths, respectively (van der Maas *et al.* 1996; Deliens *et al.* 2000). If we look more closely at these numbers, it turns out that in 3 per cent (The Netherlands 1995) and even 5.3 per cent of all deaths (Flanders 1998), this pain control with life-shortening effect was administered 'in part with the aim of hastening the end of life'. One could reasonably conclude that in many of these cases the physicians were not very concerned about the aforementioned adequacy or proportionality of their dosages, and that they knowingly – precisely so as to shorten life – administered higher doses than were necessary to alleviate the pain. This very convincingly demonstrates the need for a good definition of pain control. A physician or nurse who deliberately and in full knowledge administers an overdose in order to shorten the patient's life, who is therefore unconcerned about adequacy and proportionality, is engaged in a form of euthanasia, and *not* pain control.

All this explains why we explicitly oppose phrases such as 'raising pain-killers' or 'intensifying pain control' as also used in a number of empirical studies. Indeed, the vagueness and ambiguity of these phrases perpetuate and strengthen the confusion and the abuse of the situation, for they include both those cases where with good reason – due to the insufficiency of a former, lighter treatment – the medication or the dosages are carefully increased, and those other cases where what is going on is actually (slow) euthanasia. Ambiguity in speech and action puts pain control in a poor light, as pain control and euthanasia all become one and the same, and causes fellow-care-givers, patients and their family to be afraid of the use of heavy pain medication, with undertreatment of serious pain as a tragic consequence.

### Palliative sedation

In a considerable number of terminal patients (15 to 36 per cent in Fainsinger *et al.* 2000) sedating the patient is necessary to control a number of refractory symptoms (dyspnoea, delirium, etc.). For many working in palliative care, sedation has nothing to do with euthanasia. Indeed, as ultimate therapy and most intense form of pain and symptom control, they believe sedation makes euthanasia superfluous. There are others, however, who think that sedation is nothing but 'slow euthanasia' (Billings and Bloch 1996): a disguised, hypocritical and barely humane form of euthanasia.

In dealing with a controversial practice like sedation, it is of supreme importance to determine what implicit and explicit messages and connotations are suggested by the terms used to indicate this practice (Broeckaert 2002). One of the major problems with 'terminal sedation' – one of the most well known but also the most disputed term – is that it is too general, so that cases which are quite different from an ethical viewpoint get included in the same category, with all the concomitant risks of confusion and levelling out. Whether a patient is sedated with the intention of shortening his or her life (the same intention as with euthanasia) or out of a desire to treat a refractory symptom (i.e. pure symptom control), there is nothing about the term 'terminal sedation' to suggest that it could not be applied in both cases, though they are completely different from an ethical point of view. On the other hand, the term is too narrow, suggesting very clearly that this sedation leads to the end, that it is a sedation 'unto death' or, in any event, a sedation that is maintained until death. I think such a narrow conception of sedation is extremely dangerous, precisely because it tends to blur the boundaries between euthanasia and sedation. In light of these difficulties with the term 'terminal sedation', I opted to introduce the term 'palliative sedation' (Broeckaert 2000a). This term makes clear what sedation is essentially about: palliation, symptom control, an attempt to relieve patients' suffering. The term is also sufficiently broad that it can include the various different forms of sedation employed in palliative care (deep sedation, mild sedation, continuous sedation, intermittent sedation, etc.).

Palliative sedation is not infrequently charged with being nothing more or less than a slow form of euthanasia. Although it is crucial to use a term that conveys the appropriate message, merely introducing a new term is of course not sufficient to refute this charge. Just like the term pain control, the term sedation is used (or abused) in some cases to indicate (or camouflage) practices that should be regarded more as forms of euthanasia. This is why a definition that clarifies what sedation in palliative care is and what it is not, one that explicates the meaning invoked by the term used, is a precondition for a meaningful debate on the relation between sedation and euthanasia. For several years, I have defined palliative sedation as follows: 'the intentional administration of sedative drugs in dosages and combinations required to reduce the consciousness of a terminal patient as much as necessary to adequately relieve one or more refractory symptoms' (Broeckaert 2000b).

The first thing to notice about this definition is that palliative sedation is clearly an intentional medical act. In palliative sedation, everything revolves around bringing symptoms under control, in this case refractory symptoms. *Refractory* symptoms are symptoms which cannot be relieved in a normal manner without resorting to consciousness reduction (sedation). Which symptoms this refers to is left intentionally vague by my proposed definition. This means of course that not only physical but also mental symptoms can be refractory. Note that I speak here explicitly about refractory, not difficult symptoms (Broeckaert and Nuñez-Olarte 2002). Now when a particular action is labelled 'symptom control' it not only means that the physician's underlying subjective intention is to control symptoms; it also means that what actually occurs on an objective level reflects this intention.

The upshot of all this can only be that, in a field where dosages and combinations are of crucial importance (if, for instance, too much is administered then the risk of shortening life is very real), the dosages and combinations that are actually administered are proportional to the specific suffering that one is attempting to alleviate. It is for this reason that this definition too places the emphasis on the adequacy and proportionality of what is done on the objective level. When a subjective intention to treat a refractory symptom does not get translated into an adequate and proportional action (i.e. administer as much as is needed), then either the intention in question was not the true intention or else it was genuine but got corrupted by other, competing intentions or by lack of experience or expertise. Any physician who deliberately and knowingly administers an overdose in order to shorten the patient's life must not try to delude himself or others. Whoever is not concerned with adequacy and proportionality is engaged in euthanasia, not sedation. Whoever administers more than required because they are not sure what they are doing is guilty of medical malpractice. It is clear that in neither case are we dealing with (adequate) palliative sedation. When, on the contrary, palliative sedation is performed properly, it has only in exceptional circumstances a life-shortening effect. The literature shows that within one and the same environment, there is no observable difference in survival periods between patients that have been sedated and those who have not (Ventafridda *et al.* 1990; Stone *et al.* 1997; Kohara *et al.* 2005). Because of obvious ethical objections no harder proof can be produced.

But what about artificial nutrition and hydration? The problem is obvious: those who are sedated can often no longer eat or drink normally. If such a patient is not being artificially administered food and fluids, death seems to be the inevitable result. This impression does, however, need to be adjusted immediately, as the vast majority of sedated patients are so close to death that the life-shortening effect of not artificially hydrating (let alone feeding) is practically zero. However, it should be clear that we did not include the withholding or withdrawing of artificial hydration in our definition (neither is it standard practice). When sedation is combined with the withholding of artificial nutrition and hydration, then it is not just sedation (inducing sleep) that is done, but it is sedation *and* the withholding or withdrawing of artificial nutrition and/or hydration. This needs to be communicated in this way.

# Euthanasia and assisted suicide

In our discussion of the concept of euthanasia, in the first part of this chapter, we clearly opted for a narrow understanding of this term. In our view the term euthanasia should only refer to those very unusual and controversial cases in which someone's life is actively and directly terminated, as painlessly as possible, in order to spare him or her from further suffering. In these cases death is the result not of withholding or withdrawing life-sustaining treatment, but of an active intervention. There is not only a life-terminating effect, but also a life-terminating intention. Euthanasia is thus, by definition, both active and direct.

As we think that there are more fundamental similarities than differences between voluntary and non-voluntary euthanasia (they share all characteristics mentioned in the previous paragraph), we feel it is appropriate not to restrict the use of the word euthanasia to only cases of voluntary euthanasia (as in the Dutch definition of euthanasia). Non-voluntary euthanasia does occur. Even though it is viewed in a very negative way and even though it is often equated with murder, such an assessment does not remove the need for a clear terminology. Again, the fact that we mention or describe an act, does not mean that we approve of it or advocate it.

With this third category of treatment decisions we leave normal medical practice. This last kind of treatment decision is obviously an exceptional and controversial category, clearly different from pain control and palliative sedation. There is indeed a big gap between the two and this is on three levels: the intention, the act and the result. As opposed to pain and symptom control (where relieving the symptom is the goal), euthanasia and assisted suicide by definition aim at shortening or terminating life: it is exactly the *intention* of the person involved to end or shorten the patient's life. Starting from this intention, one chooses the medication and determines the dosages (*act*): giving as much as needed to kill the patient (versus as much as needed to ease the symptom). The *result* of euthanasia and assisted suicide is by definition the patient's death (whereas symptom control only in exceptional cases has a life-shortening effect). We distinguish three kinds of acts that belong in this final third category in Box 20.3.

---

**Box 20.3**

|  | *Pain control* | *Palliative sedation* | *Euthanasia and physician assisted suicide* |
|---|---|---|---|
| Intention | Symptom control. | Symptom control. | Terminating life. |
| Act | Administering as much medication as needed to control the pain (proportionality). | Administering as much medication as needed to control the symptom (proportionality). | Administering as much medication as needed to terminate life. |
| Result | Shortens life only in very exceptional cases (a life-lengthening effect is observed quite regularly). | Shortens life only in exceptional cases. | Termination of life (by definition). |

### Voluntary euthanasia

In the case of euthanasia (both voluntary or non-voluntary) it is always an active intervention, in this case the administration of lethal medication, and not a withdrawing or withholding, which causes death. A second characteristic of euthanasia (again both voluntary and non-voluntary) is the fact that the lethal action is carried out by another person than the patient himself or herself. *Voluntary* euthanasia implies that the patient himself or herself requests that his or her life be ended. This does of course presupposes that the patient is capable of requesting this, in other words, that they are legally competent. Or that they have been competent, since sometimes euthanasia is not done on the basis of an actual request, but on the basis of a request written in a living will.

The Netherlands and Belgium are the only two countries in the world that have an Act on euthanasia (both voted in 2002) which allows voluntary euthanasia (in certain circumstances and provided that certain procedures are taken into account, exceptionally also on the basis of an advance directive). However, a legally enforceable right to voluntary euthanasia – which would jeopardize the physician's professional and moral autonomy – is out of the question, also in Belgium and the Netherlands. From the fact that the two euthanasia laws date from the same year and the fact that the Netherlands and Belgium are neighbouring countries that (partly) share the same language, it cannot simply be concluded that similar social processes are at the basis of both laws. This is clearly not the case. The Dutch euthanasia Act is little more than the codification of a case law which was the result of a broad euthanasia debate and a euthanasia practice that started more than three decades ago. Belgium, on the other hand, was a fairly 'regular' European country as far as euthanasia was concerned, until the political debate on euthanasia started in the summer of 1999, without any established euthanasia practice (Broeckaert 2001).

### Assisted suicide

The only and crucial difference between euthanasia and assisted suicide is the fact that with euthanasia, it is a person other than the person concerned who carries out the lethal act, while with assisted suicide, it is the patient who performs this act himself or herself. The Belgian Act on voluntary euthanasia does not mention a single word about assisted suicide; therefore, the legal status of assisted suicide in this country is obscure. Only the Netherlands allows both voluntary euthanasia and assisted suicide in the same way. In Switzerland assisted suicide is not punishable, when this assistance is not given from selfish motives. There is, however, not a Swiss law regulating this practice. Assisted suicide is only rarely physician-assisted suicide here: involvement of a physician is necessary nor implied (Hurst and Mauron 2003). Oregon's Death with Dignity Act came into effect in 1997 and allows physician-assisted suicide (but not voluntary euthanasia) in competent, terminally ill adult patients.[1]

### *Non-voluntary euthanasia*

Besides voluntary euthanasia and assisted suicide, we also have *non-voluntary* euthanasia: in these cases, lethal medication is purposefully administered *without*, and this is the difference with voluntary euthanasia, the patient's request. Disproportionally raising pain medication and/or sedatives (cf. supra) with the intention to speed up the end of life also belongs to this category and it does not matter whether this procedure takes a few minutes or a couple of days. Neither the Dutch nor the Belgian Act on euthanasia provides for this extremely delicate possibility.

---

**Box 20.4**   Treatment decisions in advanced disease – a conceptual framework (Broeckaert).

**(Forgoing) curative and/or life-sustaining treatment**

- Initiating or continuing a curative or life-sustaining treatment.
- Non-treatment decision: 'withdrawing or withholding a curative or life-sustaining treatment, because in the given situation this treatment is deemed to be no longer meaningful or effective.'
- Refusal of treatment: 'withdrawing or withholding a curative or life-sustaining treatment, because the patient refuses this treatment.'

**Pain and symptom control**

- Pain control: 'the intentional administration of analgesics and/or other drugs in dosages and combinations required to adequately relieve pain.'
- Palliative sedation: 'the intentional administration of sedative drugs in dosages and combinations required to reduce the consciousness of a terminal patient as much as necessary to adequately relieve one or more refractory symptoms.'

**Euthanasia and assisted suicide**

- Voluntary euthanasia: 'The intentional administration of lethal drugs in order to painlessly terminate the life of a patient suffering from an incurable condition deemed unbearable by the patient, at this patient's request.'
- Assisted suicide: 'intentionally assisting a person, at this person's request, to terminate his or her life.'
- Non-voluntary euthanasia: 'The intentional administration of lethal drugs in order to painlessly terminate the life of a patient suffering from an incurable condition deemed unbearable, not at this patient's request.'

---

# Conclusion

Palliative care aims to offer the best possible quality of life to terminally ill patients and their relatives. In order to do this, one often has to take delicate ethical decisions: with regard to curative or life-sustaining treatment, with regard to pain and symptom control, and maybe also with regard to euthanasia or assisted suicide. It is of utmost importance that in all these cases one tries to be as careful as possible. The patient's voice should play a central role; specialized advice and professional support is often required. Several choices can be made: some are widely accepted, others are a lot more controversial. Rather than expressing an ethical evaluation on this or that practice, this text intended to offer a conceptual framework, thus laying the necessary foundation of a meaningful ethical dialogue about a number of very delicate but at the same time very pressing issues.

# Note

1   www.oregon.gov/DHS/ph/pas (accessed 21 September 2007).

# Further reading

For an in-depth treatment of a number of ethical issues in palliative care, see ten Have, H. and Clark, D. (2002) (eds) *The Ethics of Palliative Care: European Perspectives*. Buckingham: Open University Press. For an introduction to the Belgian and Dutch euthanasia history and law, I refer to Schotsmans, P. and Meulenbergs, T. (2005) (eds) *Euthanasia and Palliative Care in the Low Countries*. Leuven – Paris – Dudley: Peeters. Lavi, S.J. (2005) *The Modern Art of Dying. A History of Euthanasia in the United States*. Princeton: Princeton University Press offers a convincing historical account of the changing attitudes towards death and dying in the USA.

# References

Adams, M. and Nys, H. (2005) Euthanasia in the low countries. Comparative reflections on the Belgian and Dutch euthanasia act. In: P. Schotsmans and T. Meulenbergs (eds) *Euthanasia and Palliative Care in the Low Countries*. Peeters, Leuven – Paris – Dudley, pp. 5–33.

Belgian Advisory Committee on Bioethics, Advice No 1 of 12 May 1997 concerning the desirability of a legal recognition of euthanasia www.health.fgov.be/bioeth (accessed 19 October 2007).

Bercovitch, M., Waller, A. and Adunsky, A. (1999) High dose morphine use in the hospice setting. A database survey of patient characteristics and effect on life expectancy. *Cancer*, 86(5): 871–7.

Billings, J.A. and Bloch, S.D. (1996) Slow Euthanasia. *Journal of Palliative Care*, 12(4): 21–30.

Binding, K. and Hoche, A. (1992) *Die Freigabe der Vernichtung lebensunwerten Lebens. Ihr Mass und ihre Form*. Leipzig: Felix Meiner Verlag.

Broeckaert, B. (2000a) Medically mediated death: From pain control to euthanasia. 13th World Congress on Medical Law, August 2000, Helsinki. *Book of Proceedings*, 1: 100.

Broeckaert, B. (2000b) Palliative sedation defined or why and when terminal sedation is not euthanasia. Abstract, 1st Congress RDPC, December 2000, Berlin (Germany). *Journal of Pain and Symptom Management*, 20(6): S58.

Broeckaert, B. (2001) Belgium: Towards a Legal Recognition of Euthanasia. *European Journal of Health Law*, 8: 95–107.

Broeckaert, B. and Nuñez-Olarte, J.M. (2002), Sedation in Palliative Care: Facts and Concepts. In: H. ten Have and D. Clark (eds) *The Ethics of Palliative Care. European Perspectives*. Buckingham: Open University Press, pp. 166–80.

Broeckaert, B. (2002) Palliative Sedation. Ethical Aspects. In: C. Gastmans (ed.) *Between Technology and Humanity. The Impact of Technology on Health Care Ethics*. Leuven: Leuven University Press, pp. 239–55.

Council of Europe (1996) Convention for the Protection of Human Rights and Dignity of the Human Being with regard to the Application of Biology and Medicine: Convention on Human Rights and Biomedicine (European Treaty Series, 164). 4 April 1997, Oviedo.

Deliens, L., Mortier, F., Bilsen, J., Cosyns, M., Vander Stichele, R., Vanoverloop, J. and Ingels, K. (2000) End-of-life decisions in medical practice in Flanders, Belgium: a nationwide survey. *The Lancet*, 356: 1806–11.

Emanuel, E.J. (1994) The history of euthanasia debates in the United States and Britain. *Annals of Internal Medicine*, 121: 793–802.

Fainsinger, R., Waller, A., Bercovici, M., Bengston, K., Landman, W., Hosking, M., Núñez-Olarte, J.M. and de Moissac, D. (2000) A multicentre international study of sedation for uncontrolled symptoms in terminally ill patients. *Palliative Medicine*, 14: 257–65.

Haeckel, E. (1899) *Die Welträthsel. Gemeinverständliche Studien über Monistische Philosophie*. E Strauss, Bonn.

Hurst, S.A. and Mauron, A. (2003) Assisted suicide and euthanasia in Switzerland: allowing a role for non-physicians. *British Medical Journal*, 326: 271–3.

Janssens, R., ten Have, H., Broeckaert, B., Clark, D., Gracia, D., Illhardt, F.-J., Lantz, G., Privitera, S. and Schotsmans, P. (2002) Moral values in palliative care: a European comparison: In: H. ten Have and D. Clark (eds) *The Ethics of Palliative Care. European Perspectives*. Buckingham: Open University Press, pp. 72–86.

Jost, A. (1895) *Das Recht auf den Tod*. Göttingen: Dietrich.

Kohara, H., Ueoka, H., Takeyama, H., Murakami, T. and Morita, T. (2005) Sedation for terminally ill patients with cancer with uncontrollable physical distress. *Journal of Palliative Medicine*, 8: 20–5.

Kuhse, H., Singer, P., Baume, P., Clark, M. and Rickard, M. (1997) End-of-life decisions in Australian medical practice. *Medical Journal of Australia*, 166: 191–6.

Roy, D.J. (2005) Euthanasia and withholding treatment. In: D. Doyle, G. Hanks, N. Cherny and K. Calman (eds) *Oxford Textbook of Palliative Medicine*, 3rd edn. Oxford: Oxford University Press, pp. 84–97.

Stone, P., Phillips, C., Spruyt, O. and Waight, C. (1997) A comparison of the use of sedatives in a hospital support team and in a hospice. *Palliative Medicine*, 11: 140–4.

Tollemache, L. (1873) The Cure for Incurables, *Fortnightly Review*, 13: 218–30.

van der Heide, A., Deliens, L., Faisst, K., Nilstun, T., Norup, M., Paci, E., van der

Wal, G. and van der Mass, P. (2003) End-of-life decision-making in six European countries: descriptive study. *The Lancet*, 361: 345–50.

van der Maas, P.J., van Delden, J.J.M., Pijnenborg, L. and Looman, C.W.N. (1991) Euthanasia and other medical practices concerning the end of life. *The Lancet*, 338: 669–74.

van der Maas, P.J., van der Wal, G., Haverkate, I., de Graff, C.L.M., Kester, J.G.C., Onwuteaka-Philipsen, B.D., van der Heide, A., Bosma, J.M. and Willems, D.L. (1996) Euthanasia, physician-assisted suicide, and other medical practices involving the end of life in the Netherlands 1990–1995. *New England Journal of Medicine*, 335: 1699–705.

Ventafridda, V., Ripamonti, C., deConno, F., Tamburini, M. and Cassileth, B.R. (1990) Symptom prevalence and control during cancer patients' last days of life. *Journal of Palliative Care*, 6(3): 7–11.

Williams, S.D. (1872) *Euthanasia*. London: Williams and Norgate.

# PART THREE

**Loss and bereavement**

# 21

## Overview

*Sheila Payne*

Most books present death as a clear junction between being alive and being dead. Similarly, being bereaved is regarded as a state that occurs following death. Therefore, the discussion of death and bereavement is usually relegated to the final chapter of a textbook. In this book, we have chosen to devote much more space than other nursing texts to loss and bereavement. We regard death not as a single event, but as a process in which nurses often have an important role to play (Quested and Rudge 2003). They manage and orchestrate the dying period, by controlling physical symptoms such as pain, noisy secretion (death rattle) or a dry mouth. Nurses work by containing and shaping the behaviours of the onlookers, for example by calling patients' relatives, medical staff or chaplains to the bedside at key times. Nurses also help to transform the newly dead body, making it presentable to family members, by washing and dressing the body, removing clinical equipment and any evidence of last resuscitation attempts. They are the professional workers most likely to be present during the final moments of life and at the time of death.

This section is concerned with nursing work and the social impact of this important transition – the end of life. It then moves on to discuss the impact of death on those who survive. Instead of explaining bereavement theories as entities to be proved or disproved, they are regarded as discourses – ways of talking about loss and conceptualizing the experience of bereavement. This chapter will introduce three major ways to understand bereavement: those which arise from psychological or psychiatric understanding of loss; those which arise from theories of stress and coping; and, lastly, those which are derived from sociological understandings of transitions in relationships and social networks. There are, of course, many other ways to understand bereavement which are located within major 'worldviews', such as the main religions or philosophies. Accounts are likely to be influenced by the culture, social class and life experience of those experiencing the loss. It will be emphasized that the experience of loss is important throughout the course of life-threatening illness, because the patient, families and friends will have encountered many losses throughout the person's illness, and for others who share the experience such as staff, fellow patients and co-residents in care homes. Bereavement should be thought of not as a single loss (the death), but as a culmination of losses and changes to previously taken-for-granted way of living and relationships.

The chapter goes on to explore the types of services and resources that are available to support bereaved people. However, it makes no assumption that all people need additional support. There is evidence that most people are very resilient and manage major life changes with their own resources and support from their families and communities. However, for some people bereavement presents such a challenge that they seek additional support from community-based organizations such as Cruse (a charity concerned with providing counselling and bereavement support), faith groups, hospice and specialist palliative care bereavement services, and other health and social care services (Joanna Briggs Institute 2006). There is a brief review of the evidence about the efficacy of interventions designed to support bereaved people. The chapter concludes by reviewing the content of the five chapters that make up Part Three, helping the reader to make links with the theories of loss and providing a framework for understanding the structure of this part of the book.

## Caring for the dead

In many cultures throughout history, women have cared for the dead. It is a common mark of respect that the newly dead are treated with dignity. As the place of death in some countries has moved more commonly into institutional environments, usually hospitals, it has generally been the role of nurses rather than family members to care for the newly dead. The nursing procedures and practices for performing the 'Last Offices' are thought to have changed little over the past 100 years (Wolf 1988). In an analysis of the procedure manuals of an Australian hospital, Quested and Rudge (2003) argue 'that to move from alive to dead involves a transition during which the individual is reconfigured conceptually, physically, socially and culturally through the care practices inflicted on the dead body' (p. 559). They highlight how nurses manage the newly dead person's body in ways that contain the physicality of the body as it changes colour, leaks urine or faeces, smells, stiffens and cools. It has been argued that nurses, especially those working in hospices and specialist palliative care services, collude in creating a certain image of the 'good death' (McNamara *et al.* 1994). Prior to death, the myth of peaceful dying is engineered by the use of sedation and, subsequently, nurses' actions help to create the impression that the person is asleep. This supports wider societal discourses that seek to pretend that the dead are merely asleep. This myth is exemplified in the use of metaphors like 'at peace' and 'the long sleep'.

While the dead person might be presented as though asleep, their body tends to be treated in very different ways from the bodies of living people. Quested and Rudge (2003) described how personal ornaments like jewellery are normally removed, the body is stripped of clothing, washed, dressed in a shroud, labelled and placed in a body bag or sheet. All these practices serve to remove the identity of the former living person from the now dead body. Even the way the person's body is spoken about positions them as different from the bodies of the living (see Box 21.1). Komaromy in the following chapter highlights how by regarding the body as unsightly and 'dangerous', it means that staff seek to shield the living from viewing the dead, such as drawing curtains to prevent fellow patients from seeing the removal of the body. Bryan (2007) in a review of the literature shows that there is little evidence for the widespread view that patients require protection from other dying patients. The reluctance by nursing staff to tell fellow patients when a person has died and their reasons for preventing them seeing the removal of the body is based on assumptions that it is distressing. Rather than directly addressing their concerns, patients become aware of social cues (like drawn curtains) which indicate a death has occurred and collude with staff in making death unspeakable and hidden.

Deaths enacted in intensive care units provide a good example of uncertainty as patients hover between living and death. In a detailed ethnographic study in the UK, Seymour (2001) provides accounts of how death is managed and contested between medical staff, nurses and family members in the intensive care unit. In patients with multiple organ failure, the treatment of each organ may become the work of different teams of medical experts – for example, renal failure may be treated by nephrologists, respiratory failure by chest physicians and heart failure by cardiologists. As previously discussed by Seymour and Ingleton in Chapter 10, the work of the medical team is directed at assembling a case to justify the withdrawal or continuation of life-prolonging medical treatment, while the nursing team attempts to provide integrated care that serves to maintain the integrity of the person as a whole individual (see Box 21.2).

---

**Box 21.1** Words used to describe the newly dead person's body

Mortal remains
The body
A 'stiff'
Corpse
The deceased
Cadaver

**Box 21.2**   'Nursing care only' (adapted from Seymour 2001)

The data from Seymour's study suggest that 'nursing' in intensive care is constituted dually. First, by the technical-medical work of medicine: this is the context within which 'nursing' operates and within which nurses must fashion their relationships with patients and their companions. And, second, by strategies which incorporate 'whole person work' into what is an essentially depersonalized context. Achieving and sustaining a balance between these constituents is a central, and inherently difficult, feature of nursing work in intensive care. The period during which nurses care for individuals who are approaching death is a time in which the contradictions associated with sustaining 'whole person' work become highly visible and highly problematic for nurses. A common feature of the case studies was the subtle change in emphasis, away from medicine and towards nursing, for both those individuals 'known' to be dying in a 'technical' sense *and* those 'felt' to be dying in a 'bodily' sense. 'Technical' dying is used here to represent a judgement informed by the collection of physiological data, while 'bodily' dying refers to 'intuitively' based clinical judgement. The common sense concept of 'nursing care only' was used to describe this time period.

An example from the case study concerns a young man, Richard, who had been fatally injured in a road traffic accident one week previously. In Richard's case, bodily dying started to outpace technical death. However, in spite of Richard's moribund appearance, there was a lengthy delay before active medical treatment was withdrawn. During this time, his nurse was largely left alone by the medical staff, who were conducting 'behind the scenes' negotiations about a withdrawal of drug therapies. The nurse described in her follow-up interview how:

> . . . we had to continue making up all his drips, washing him and cleaning, just doing the usual care that you give to other patients but I knew by looking at him . . . it was like 'Why am I doing this?' I knew I was doing it because they hadn't decided to withdraw but I just wanted to get someone in to look at him and say to them: 'How would you like your relative to look like this?' and: 'You're doing all this treatment but you're not doing anything.'

The dissonance between the requirement to care for the 'already dead' body and the ideology of the 'whole person' seemed to be solved by an attribution to the young man, 'Richard', of particular personal qualities by the nurse. Thus it became possible for her to describe him as 'fighting', as 'still living' and later:

> . . . he was strong and trying to say: 'I'm not giving up', although his body was saying: 'You can't survive with this', I felt his heart and his brain was fighting everything.

In this way, this particular nurse achieved a sense of meaning in her nursing work, albeit at considerable personal cost. She recalled how his image remained in her mind long after his death:

> Yes, Richard, really, I was – erm – I couldn't stop thinking about him. I can still see him.

# Pre-bereavement care and the care delivered near the time of death

Nurses, social workers and pastoral care staff have an important role in preparing families and friends for the death of the patient. Research evidence from the UK is contradictory, with some studies indicating that families found the care provided at this time by hospices as helpful in coping with loss (Field *et al.* 2007) and others indicating less impact (Grande *et al.* 2004). Box 21.3 offers suggestions about how nurses may support people immediately after a death.

# Definitions of terms in bereavement

It has been argued elsewhere that definitions of terms are closely related to the way loss is understood and the theories used to explain bereavement (Small 2001; Payne and Lloyd-Williams in press). However, for the purposes of this text, it might be useful to offer some broadly accepted definitions. Stroebe *et al.* (2002: 6) have provided brief definitions of the key concepts:

- *Bereavement* is understood to refer to the objective situation of having lost someone significant.

- *Grief* is the reaction to bereavement, defined as a primarily emotional (affective) reaction to the loss of a loved one through death.

- *Mourning* is the social expressions or acts expressive of grief that are shaped by the practices of a given society or cultural group.

Scholars have debated whether grief is universal. There is plenty of evidence that humans and other animals react to the loss of significant others in their environment but the nature of the expression and duration of grief are more likely to be contingent upon the meaning placed upon the loss (Lofland 1985) and cultural diversity (Morgan and Laungani 2003). So grief tends to refer to what is *felt*, while mourning refers to what is *done*. It is important for nurses and others working with bereaved people to realize that they should not infer the depth or intensity of grief from the overt behaviours displayed. Wailing at the bedside may be culturally sanctioned by some groups, while other social groups value stoicism and public emotional reserve, and both responses may be gender related (Walter 1999).

It is generally agreed that there are no single 'correct' or 'true' theories that explain the experience of loss or account for the emotions, experiences and cultural practices that characterize grief and mourning (Payne *et al.* 1999; Hockey *et al.* 2001; Joanna Briggs Institute 2006). A postmodern position suggests that individual diversity is paramount and that within broad cultural constraints each of us develops our own ways of *doing* bereavement (Walter 1999). The following is an example of the diversity of

**Box 21.3**    Suggestions for supporting people immediately after a death

- Tell the family member that the patient has died.
- Obtain medical confirmation and certification of death as soon as possible.
- Ask if the family member wishes to see the deceased person. Offer to accompany them to the room if the dead person is still on the ward or to view the body elsewhere.
- Warn them what their dead family member may look like, especially if they have visible injuries, bandages, etc. Many people have never seen a dead person and may be fearful.
- Offer to remain with them until they feel comfortable in the presence of the deceased person, and then offer to withdraw.
- Make it clear that they can touch the deceased person, kiss and caress them, and talk to them if they wish.
- Allow them as much time as they wish to remain with the body. Do not appear to be rushing them to leave.
- Enable family members to take mementoes of the deceased such as a lock of hair. For babies and young children, some parents wish to take photographs, hand or foot prints.
- Ask if family members wish to have a priest or faith advisor to pray with them or perform religious rituals.
- Enable family members to perform any cultural or religious practices that are meaningful for them.
- Help families to leave the hospital, care home or hospice when they are ready. Ensure that they are able to get home, assist with arranging transport and, if they wish, offer to contact friends or other family members who are able to offer support.
- Provide written information about procedures such as collection of the deceased's property, how to register the death and arrange a funeral.
- If there is to be a post-mortem examination and if body parts need to be removed for examination, request permission and obtain written consent. Make clear the reasons for any legal procedures such as an inquest.
- Provide family members with a contact telephone number in case they have questions they later wish to ask about the care of their loved one prior to or at the time of death.
- There are no 'right' words to say immediately after a death, but having the time and ability to listen to whatever the newly bereaved person may wish to talk about is generally valued.
- Help families to discuss organ or tissue donation if they wish. This may fulfill the wishes of the deceased.

expression of grief and memorialization practices within a family after the loss of a child: the grandparents may find comfort in religious rituals and prayer; the parents may react differently, the mother by retaining photographs, special items of clothing or toys, the father by 'burying' himself in work; and siblings may create a memory box, be disruptive at school or be 'super' good (see Riches and Dawson 2000). These examples of different responses to loss accord well with many nurses' experiences of relatives following a bereavement and their awareness of the variability of grieving. Some ways of talking and thinking about bereavement have become so popular that many people are unaware of their origins and they have become part of our taken-for-granted knowledge about bereavement – for example, the stage/phase models of loss. Although there may not appear to be strict social rules on how to behave when bereaved in mainstream White British society, Hockey (2001) has highlighted that there are more subtle injunctions: 'that the individual shall express their emotions, shall acknowledge the reality of their loss and shall share their thoughts and feelings with appropriate others' (p. 208). Many bereavement support services operate with these basic requirements of their clients.

# Understanding loss and bereavement

Much of the patients' and families' experience of advancing illness can be understood as coming to terms with a series of losses. These losses may be related to all aspects of a person's life, including their functional abilities to walk unaided, to talk and to be continent. In some conditions, such as Parkinson's disease, emotional expression may be blunted or emotional control may be lost such as in some dementias and following stroke. Advancing illness also impacts on social relationships and roles; for example, paid employment may be relinquished, leading to loss of self-esteem, financial hardship and loss of identity. Therefore, advancing illness provides a cascade of losses for both the ill person and their family members (Kitrungrote and Cohen 2006). Moreover, with open communication about the probable outcome of disease and greater awareness of prognosis, people in these circumstances may start to anticipate a series of losses that they have yet to experience. This has been described as anticipatory grief (Evans 1994). It has been argued that when life-threatening illness is very protracted as in dementia, family members may start to withdraw from the ill person before their death. Sudnow (1967) described social death as a loss of personhood and the dying person being treated as if they were already dead.

# Theories of loss and bereavement

In the following section, three types of theories used to understand loss and bereavement will be introduced briefly. This aims to provide the reader with sufficient information to critically evaluate the following chapters. Guidance on how to obtain more detailed information about each of these theories is available from 'Recommended reading' at the end of the chapter. The theories are grouped into three conceptual categories based on their major emphasis: psychological processes; stress and coping; and social and relational aspects of loss.

The ordering of the theories does not imply anything other than their historical emergence. Of course, the major religions and philosophies of the world also provide important accounts of loss and bereavement, which shape the way loss is understood and experienced for many people (Parkes *et al.* 1997). However, increasingly secularization of society, especially in parts of Europe, mean that religious explanations are arguably no longer the dominant way that loss is conceptualized. A review of the literature has highlighted common areas of disruption from the first year of bereavement including: cognitive disruption, dysphoria, health problems, and poor social and occupational functioning (Bonnano and Kaltman 2001). In a small minority (estimated to be 10–20 per cent), disruption to functioning becomes so severe as to warrant a label of 'complicated grief' (Bonnano and Kaltman 2001; Joanna Briggs Institute 2006). However, recent evidence suggests that most people demonstrate greater resilience than anticipated (Bonnano 2004).

# Theories that emphasize psychological processes

Over the past century, the most influential perspective on loss has been the focus on the experience of distressing emotions and the accompanying cognitions (thoughts) and behaviours. These ways to construe bereavement and grief have been derived from medical discourses, especially those that arise from psychiatric and psychological understandings. Attention has been directed predominantly to psychological processes. At one time bereavement has even been likened to an illness from which the person eventually recovers (Engel 1961). Thus, there has been an emphasis on describing the physical and psychological manifestations of grief as 'symptoms' and there has been an assumption that the typical trajectory of bereavement is from high distress to little or none. The time span of this trajectory has been variously estimated from weeks to years. However, the outcome of bereavement has been construed in terms of 'recovery' or 'resolution', rather like getting over a bad illness. The trajectory of bereavement has often been conceptualized as a series of stages or phases through which the person must progress (hence 'process'). The content and number of stages/phases vary but they tend to define the emotions and thoughts that are necessary to achieve 'resolution'. The tendency to map bereavement in terms of stages/phases has also given rise to notions of 'normal' and 'abnormal' grief (also described as complicated, complex and conflicted grief). This language of grief, therefore, suggests that there are 'right' and 'wrong' ways to grieve. Using this framework, most bereavement support workers have attempted to guide bereaved people along the 'right' path to resolution (Worden 1982, 1991, 2001; Parkes *et al.* 1996).

Freud (1917) is usually credited with the initial ideas that helped to shape the development of the phase/stage models of loss. Freud contributed much to twentieth-century thought and his psychoanalytic theory has been very influential in shaping our ways of understanding people. Writing during the turmoil and massive loss of life during the First World War in Europe, Freud was the first to point out the similarities and differences between grief and depression in his classic text *Mourning and Melancholia* (Freud 1917). His paper offered one of the first descriptions of normal and pathological grief. The thoughts discussed in it underpin psychoanalytic theory of depression and provide the basis for many current theories of grief and its resolution. In the light of the impact of Freud's theory of grief on subsequent theoretical developments, it is surprising to acknowledge that grief, as a psychological process, was never Freud's main focus of interest. Moreover, Freud's personal experiences of bereavement were not even compatible with his theoretical position. In *Mourning and Melancholia*, Freud argued that people became attached to others who are important for the satisfaction of their needs and to whom emotional expression is directed (cathexis). Love is conceptualized as the attachment of emotional energy to the psychological representation of the loved object (person). It is assumed that the more important the relationship, the greater the attachment. According to Freudian theory, grieving represents a dilemma because there is a simultaneous need to relinquish the relationship so that the person may regain the energy invested and a wish to maintain the bond with the love object. However, this is acknowledged to be painful work and so the bereaved person tends to hold on to an image of the dead person for as long as possible, until inevitably they have to face the reality of the loss and their new situation. According to Freud, the bereaved individual needs to accept the reality of the loss so that the emotional energy can be released and redirected. The process of withdrawing energy from the lost object is called 'grief work' (decathexis). He regarded this psychological processing as essential to the breaking of relationship bonds with the deceased, to allow the reinvestment of emotional energy and the formation of new relationships with others. Arguably, Freud's most important contributions to loss have been:

- introducing a developmental perspective (his personality theory emphasized early childhood development);
- introducing the 'grief work' hypothesis; and
- defining the difference between grief and depression.

His ideas were taken up and developed by many other people working within a psychodynamic tradition. An important follower was Bowbly (1969, 1973, 1980) who proposed a theory to account for the formation of close human relationships (attachments), especially between mothers and their babies, and to account for what happened when these relationships were interrupted, either temporarily or permanently (separation and loss). He suggested that through the process of human evolution, there had developed a need for mothers and infants to be in close proximity for survival and that this was achieved through an interactional process involving reciprocal behaviours and feelings between mothers and babies called attachment. Temporary separation was marked by characteristic behaviours and feelings such as distress, calling and searching, which usually resulted in people being reunited. He suggested that the nature of distress for infants and young children varied sequentially in the following ways (described as stages):

- *Protest* – marked by anger and loud crying, with constant searching for the lost mother and a hypervigilance anticipating her return.
- *Despair* – marked by withdrawal and less vigorous crying.
- *Detachment* – marked by an outward display of cheerful behaviour but the child remains emotionally distant.

Separation anxiety was thought to be an unpleasant state for infants. Therefore, infants quickly developed behaviours such as crying, which brought their mothers nearer to them, and other social behaviours that also served to maintain contact, such as smiling and later talking or physically clinging to their mother. Based on his knowledge about young children, Bowlby thought that permanent loss, such as bereavement, also triggered these feelings of intense distress and the same immediate behavioural responses of crying, searching, clinging, giving way to despondency, depression and later detachment. Bowlby proposed that the intensity of the grief was related to the closeness of the attachment relationship. For example, he predicted that we would be more distressed by the loss of a parent or sibling than a distant cousin because we had invested more emotional energy in that relationship. Recent research has demonstrated that patterns of attachment in childhood profoundly influence the way people grieve (Parkes 2006). However, this study is based on analysis of questionnaire responses from patients attending a psychiatric clinic and therefore they cannot be regarded as normal bereaved people.

In writing about the experience of loss, Bowlby was careful to emphasize that the phases were not discrete entities and that people may oscillate between them, although over the course of time it was anticipated that there would be linear progression. The four phases following loss were described by Bowlby (1980: 85) as:

1   Phase of numbing that usually lasts from a few hours to a week and may be interrupted by outbursts of extremely intense distress and/or anger.
2   Phase of yearning and searching for the lost figure lasting some months and sometimes for years.
3   Phase of disorganization and despair.
4   Phase of greater or lesser degree of reorganization.

As the experience of loss was related to the type of attachment, Bowbly suggested that 'abnormal' attachment patterns were likely to be associated with 'abnormal' grieving. For example, he noted that relationships that were very unequal, such as highly dependent or domineering relationships, were more likely to result in difficulties during bereavement. Like Freud, Bowlby emphasized the emotional aspects of loss and the need to 'work through' the loss to achieve an outcome where there was no longer any emotional investment in the dead person ('letting go'). Bowlby's ideas about attachment have been taken up by health and social care services; for example, in encouraging early contact between mothers and babies after birth. Bowlby's ideas were also influential in the development of Parkes's (1996) theories of loss. Both Bowlby and his colleague Parkes were psychiatrists and were in contact with patients struggling to understand the impact of their bereavements.

Parkes (1971, 1993, 1996) suggested that bereavement should be considered as a major psychosocial transition, which challenged the taken-for-granted world of the bereaved person. He argued that most people think of their world as relatively stable, in which they make assumptions of perceived control. Death, especially sudden death, challenges this, as people have to adapt to changes in relationships and social status (for example, from being a wife to a widow) and economic circumstances (living on a pension). He, like Bowlby, proposed that people progress through phases in coming to terms with their loss: numbness, pining, depression and recovery. Once again with a linear progression over time, although he acknowledges that there is great individual variability and that not everyone progresses at the same rate or that all phases are experienced. Parkes's ideas of 'normal' phases of grief have changed somewhat over time (Parkes 1972, 1986, 1996). The latest version of his theory emphasizes the emotional reactions experienced following the loss (Parkes 1996) rather than discrete phases. Parkes based his ideas on several research studies undertaken in the UK and the USA, as well as his clinical psychiatric work. Parkes was also influential in establishing one of the first hospice-based bereavement support services at St Christopher's Hospice, London, in which volunteers were trained to offer support to bereaved people.

Finally, there are two well-known models that are widely applied in specialist palliative care. Kubler-Ross (1969), a psychiatrist working in the USA who was heavily influenced by psychoanalytic ideas, proposed a stage model of loss in relation to dying that has been applied to bereavement. This model emphasizes changing emotional expression throughout the final period of life. Her model has become very popular with health professionals and aspects of it are now part of common lay taken-for-granted assumptions about how bereavement is experienced. It has been heavily critiqued over the years because it assumes that bereavement can be conceptualized as a series of sequential stages, and it focuses on emotional aspects of loss and largely ignores the social aspects (for a more detailed critique, see Payne *et al.* 1999). Despite the criticisms of her model, it continues to be dominant in the education of nurses, bereavement support workers and others.

Worden (1982, 1991, 2001) based his therapeutic model on phases of grief and what he called 'tasks of mourning'. According to Worden (1991), the goals of grief counselling, are to:

- increase the reality of the loss;
- help the counsellee deal with both expressed and latent affect;

- help the counsellee overcome various impediments to readjustment after the loss; and
- encourage the counsellee to say an appropriate goodbye and to feel comfortable reinvesting back into life.

Worden (2001) modified the final task to suggest a less final break with the dead person. He suggested that grief was a process not a state and that people needed to work through their reactions to loss to achieve a complete adjustment. Worden's books have been widely used as texts to guide counsellors and others working with bereaved people. It is therefore noteworthy that much of the language used presents bereavement as a medical condition and bereaved people as in need of therapy. He also describes pathological aspects of bereavement, highlighting how bereavement workers might identify different types of 'abnormal' grief.

Parkes, Kulber-Ross and Worden have modified and developed their ideas over time and the accounts presented here do not do justice to the complexity of their thinking. All these theories have been critiqued and challenged, especially in relation to notions of a linear progression through phases or stages and the need for 'grief work' (see Wortman and Silver 1989). However, many of these stage/phase theories are widely taught to student nurses and others working in health and social care. Moreover, they are frequently presented in a simplified form with little acknowledgement of the criticisms. In fact, the pervasiveness of psychological stage/phase models of grief means that they have largely been incorporated into everyday taken-for-granted assumptions about how people should feel and behave following a loss. In the following sections, two other ways of understanding loss will be introduced.

Stroebe (1992) challenged some aspects of the grief work hypothesis. While she recognized the cognitive processing element of the grief work hypothesis, she considered that it was limited because it focused attention on just the loss of the dead person and not on all the subsequent changes that are likely to arise for a bereaved person. She also challenged the notion that the lack of cognitive processing was potentially pathological by highlighting psychological research which showed that excessive rumination may also be harmful (Nolen-Hoeksema 2002). So just dwelling upon the loss may not be adaptive. She also argued that part of the experience of bereavement is coming to terms with psycho-social changes. In particular, she criticized the emphasis of the grief work hypothesis on psychological processing and its neglect of interpersonal relationships.

## Stress and coping models

Recent models of loss have concentrated on explaining grief as a transaction between the cognitive appraisal of the individual (how they understand their world) and what is happening in their environment. These models are based upon psychological theories of stress and coping, especially a transactional model developed by Lazarus and Folkman (1984), and subsequent modifications (Folkman 1997; Folkman and Greer 2000). This model proposed that while any event may be perceived as threatening by an individual, it is the meaning of the event and the resources available, which determines its stressfulness. Accordingly each event is thought about (called cognitive appraisal) to estimate its degree of threat (primary appraisal) and to determine and mobilize resources to cope with it (secondary appraisal). Coping may involve dealing directly with the threat (problem-focused coping) or may involve modifying the emotional response (emotion-focused coping). Stroebe and Schut (1999) developed these ideas to form a new model of loss, called 'the dual processing model'. They proposed that, following a death, people oscillate between 'restoration-focused' coping (e.g. dealing with everyday life) and 'loss-focused' coping (e.g. by expressing their distress). Examples of 'loss-focused' coping activities include thinking about the dead person, crying and talking about the loss. Examples of 'restoration-focused' activities include making new relationships, attending to everyday demands like parenting, 'forgetting' or being distracted from thinking about the loss, and returning to employment. They suggest that people move between these two forms of coping with grief depending upon their personality, age, gender and social roles, although many of the coping responses become progressively more 'restoration-focused'. From these ideas, they developed therapeutic interventions to help people address both types of coping to achieve a balance, especially for those people who have a tendency to retain loss- or restoration-focused modes of coping (Stroebe *et al.* 2002). For example, if a person is so overwhelmed by grief that they spend all their time crying, they may not be able to engage in everyday self-care activities such as cooking a meal or attending to the needs of their children. Similarly, some people may 'bury' themselves in activities such as paid employment, which functions well to distract their attention from their loss; however, in such cases, there is a danger that the emotional impact of the loss may not be fully acknowledged.

## Social and relational aspects of loss

In this section, I turn my attention to the writers who have emphasized the social aspects of bereavement and loss (e.g. Klass *et al.* 1996; Walter 1999). Most of these writers bring sociological or anthropological perspectives to the topic of bereavement. They emphasize the changes to social roles and relationships that bereavement precipitates. Social roles are very important in defining identity (as explained in Chapter 1). Moreover, in modern society, identity is usually not fixed but is constantly renegotiated throughout the life span. Therefore, social factors such as age, gender, social class and ethnicity all impact on the meaning of loss and the way bereavement is enacted (Field *et al.* 1997). From this perspective, grief is not merely a set of psychological responses that are largely biologically determined (as Bowlby has argued), as patterns of grief and possibilities for its expression are largely influenced by social and cultural factors (Reimers 2001; Field and Payne 2003). Historians and anthropologists have also noted the diversity of expressions of loss, in terms of the rituals associated with death, and the differing impact that different types of loss may have depending upon social status, age and gender. It is these social discourses about loss and bereavement that I explore next.

Lofland (1985) has drawn attention to the effects of the meaning of loss in different societies. She argues that the 'painful, debilitating and relatively long-lasting' (Lofland 1985: 172) grief typical of contemporary experience in North America and the UK arises from social conditions in which the majority of losses are experienced. Typically in the USA and the UK, deaths occur in older age and, therefore, spousal bereavement is common. In addition, the partner usually dies after a long joint relationship and, because of differences in male and female mortality, it is usually women who are left as widows with often little opportunity to form new partnerships. Some features of contemporary Western family structure and personal relationships – such as high investment in small numbers of children, high rates of divorce and marital separation, geographical mobility for education and employment, and increased numbers of people living in single-person households – may mean that, relative to other societies, older people are not very socially enmeshed in their local communities. Therefore, when bereavement occurs in older age, it may be experienced in relative isolation. The solitary widow living alone in the former family home may have plenty of opportunity to be constantly reminded of her lost partner.

Deaths that occur in younger people are almost always regarded as untimely and a tragedy. There are few agreed social responses to the loss of children in developed countries, so they tend to be regarded as highly abnormal and threatening (Riches and Dawson 2000). In addition, cultural expectations that bereavement should be an intensely personal and distressing experience are perpetuated through influential personal accounts (e.g. Lewis 1966) and by the self-help and popular literature, which tends to present a psychological and emotional account of grief (the types of information leaflets provided by hospices and specialist palliative care services are good examples). Lofland (1985: 181) argues that contemporary Western grief is expressed as it is because of four aspects of modern life:

- a relational pattern that links individuals to a small number of highly significant others;
- a definition of death as personal annihilation and as unusual and tragic except among the aged;
- selves which take very seriously their emotional states; and
- interactional settings that provide rich opportunities to contemplate loss.

Several writers have commented upon how the personal meaning of loss influences reactions to bereavement. Reimers (2001) highlights how Swedish society debated the 'proper' reaction to a major disaster, the sinking of a passenger ferry with the loss of 852 lives in 1994. Public debate centred on whether the bodies of the dead should be retrieved to permit burial or remain entombed in the sunken ship. Reimers argued that the public debates, which concluded that the bodies ought to be left in the ship, served to construct social discourses about 'normal' grieving. She concluded that this example demonstrated 'a societal ambition to discipline and control eruptions of strong sentiments, such as grief. One way to do this is to delineate the boundaries for what is to be considered as normal and permissive and to pathologise those who do not remain within those boundaries' (Reimers 2001: 244).

Other societies choose to memorialize certain deaths and not others. For example, memories of the many deaths that occurred during the First World War continue to haunt Britain and other countries (Hockey 2001). In the UK, the rituals associated with remembering the deaths of young soldiers in the First World War have increased rather than diminished in importance, although few people remain alive who witnessed these events almost a century ago. In comparison, no attempt is made to memorialize those killed in industrial accidents over the last century. While the British remembrance day is characteristically a sombre occasion, Mexicans celebrate the 'Day of the Dead' as a family festival (Salvador 2003).

Perhaps one of the most difficult types of bereavement for Western people at the present time is the death of a child (Riches and Dawson 2000). Low rates of infant mortality and the prevention and treatment of many acute medical conditions mean that the probability of babies, children and young people dying are generally very low in most developed countries. There are thus few socially accepted accounts to provide a meaning for these deaths. According to Riches and Dawson (2000), bereaved family members struggle to find a meaning for the death and differences between family members may give rise to different responses and ways of coping with grief. The devastating impact of child loss is not inevitable. Evidence from countries such as Brazil, where infant mortality rates are much higher, attest to different reactions, with some mothers describing their dead infants as angels returned to heaven and who are therefore safe and should not be mourned (Shepherd-Hughes 1972). Historically, the death of at least some children within large families was anticipated, but it is important not to attribute a lack of grief to parents in such circumstances. In modern society, childhood deaths are considered to be devastating to the parents because with smaller families relatively more emotional and material resources are invested in each child.

Riches and Dawson (2000) show that the death of a child challenges many of the taken-for-granted aspects of everyday life. Certain roles, such as being a parent, can only be enacted in the presence of a child; therefore, the death of an only child removes the possibility of this social role. Parenting is a highly valued social role from which the individual receives not only personal satisfaction but social esteem from others. Parents generally invest a great deal of themselves in the lives of their children and on the death of a child their role of protector and provider is taken away. The death of a child disrupts the sense of identity, not only because the person may feel guilt but because other people react to them in different ways. The loss of a sibling when family sizes are small leaves gaps that are hard or impossible to fill. Families are complex social structures in which there are reciprocal roles and shared identities, which are maintained over time by mutual support, collective memories and goals (Kissane and Bloch 2002). Families are also dynamic and may not be mutually supportive (as discussed in Chapter 1). Families are situated in cultural contexts that may frame the meaning of the loss, such as the major religions. They are also situated in social contexts that may constrain the possibilities and behaviours open to them. For example, stillbirth and neonatal deaths may not be openly recognized by some societies and the mourning rituals associated with them may not be similar to the rituals following the death of an adult. In the past in British hospitals it was unusual for miscarried foetuses and stillborn infants to be returned to their parents for burial. Hospitals tended to dispose of the infant in the way they would deal with unwanted biological material or even retain some body parts for research, without exploring the wishes of the parents or obtaining their consent. This was revealed to be deeply distressing (Sque *et al.* 2008). It is now common practice for parents to arrange burial or cremation themselves and that a more compassionate and careful approach is given to obtaining consent to post-mortem procedures.

Walter (1996) in the UK and Klass *et al.* (1996) in the USA have challenged the notion that successful resolution of grief involves 'moving on' and 'letting go' of the deceased person. Their views are based on the assumption that people wish to maintain feelings of continuity and that, even though physical relationships will end at the time of death, these relationships become transformed but remain important within the memory of the individual and community. Walter (1996, 1999) has proposed a biographical model of loss in which he suggests bereaved people seek to create a narrative that describes both the person who has died and the part they played in their lives. He argues that these narratives are socially constructed. Drawing upon his own personal experiences of grief, Walter argues that because postmodern societies are so fragmented and compartmentalized, people relate to others in different ways depending upon the social roles they occupy at any one time. For example, a person may be known to work colleagues as a hard driven boss, to his children as a kind but distant and largely absent father, to his wife as a generous but moody provider of finances, and to his Saturday morning golfing friends as a relaxed and easygoing man. The palliative care team may know this person as a difficult and demanding person. Each role and aspect of this person's identity may not be known to others because societies are no longer enmeshed. We may know little about the different aspects of the life of our loved ones because much of our lives are spent apart in paid employment, separate leisure pursuits and in travelling. Klass *et al.* (1996) also proposed a similar idea and illustrated this in relation to different types of loss. They argued that, for many people, adapting to loss involves incorporating some aspect of their previous relationship with the deceased person into their current lives but in a way that is tolerable and not distressing.

Walter (1996) proposed that the purpose of grief was to construct a durable biography in which the 'whole' person was revealed and this became integrated into the memory of survivors. Thus a grandchild would be told stories of what their dead grandfather did and what he was like as a person. In this model of grief, memories and relationships with the dead person are fostered and developed in ways that are helpful and supportive in the life of those still living. Walter (1999) has protested against counselling practices that urge people to 'let go' or 'break the bonds' of relationships with the deceased. From his perspective, it is thought that continuing to have a relationship with deceased friends and family members is helpful. These relationships are largely construed as taking place in shared memories or discussion about the dead person, but they may also be expressed in retained precious objects, photographs or mementoes from the dead person. He rejects the notion that 'holding on' to these aspects of the dead person represents a failure to resolve grief or is in anyway pathological. While Walter's analysis is helpful in challenging the dominance of psychological perspectives on loss, it is based on his autobiographical accounts rather than a body of empirical research. Walter is an articulate academic for whom words (in narrative accounts) come easily; it should not be assumed that others have a similar facility with language.

## How have these models influenced ways to help bereaved people?

Most bereaved people manage the experience of loss by drawing upon their personal resources, in terms of their personality and coping styles, and by mobilizing their social resources. These resources include family and friendship relationships in which grief can be acknowledged and shared, and faith groups and wider social structures that provide opportunities to express grief and perform mourning rituals. In the past, social concern for bereaved people largely focused on supplying financial help to widows and making arrangements for the care of orphans. Such endeavours continue to be vitally important in some areas of the world, following disasters such as the 2004 tsunami (Parkes 2005), or in parts of Africa for example, to help the bereaved following deaths from AIDS. In the latter half of the twentieth century in the UK, a number of self-help groups such as Cruse began to offer emotional support to bereaved people. By the end of the century, there had been a large increase in these types of groups, funded by charitable giving and catering for many different types of loss (e.g. by suicide) and different age groups (e.g. childhood bereavement services; see Chapter 26 by Rolls). Bereavement services associated with health care provision are unusual in many countries, the exceptions being specialist palliative care, a few accident and emergency departments and a few obstetric units. Statutory provision for bereavement support in the UK was largely confined to the activities of hospital chaplains and a few concerned individuals;

however, following public inquiries into the common practice of organ retention by pathology departments at British hospitals, acute general hospitals have started to provide bereavement services. Most bereavement support services in the UK remain outside the remit of statutory health and social care services.

From its early beginnings, hospice philosophy encompassed the care of patients and their families, which continued after death into bereavement. Most UK hospices and palliative care units regard the provision of bereavement support as integral to their services, although there remains great diversity in service provision (Field *et al.* 2007). For a number of reasons, bereavement support has been marginalized and, arguably, remains the least well-developed aspect of hospices and specialist palliative care services (Payne 2001a). Most services are based on an assumption that bereavement is a major stressful life event and that a minority of people experience substantial disruption to their physical, psychological and social functioning (Parkes 1996). Parkes (1993) has argued that offering support to people who have adequate internal and external resources can be disempowering and be detrimental to coping. This suggests that blanket provision of services to all bereaved family members may be at best wasteful of resources and, at worst, threatening to the coping responses of most people. A review of the literature about assumptions underpinning bereavement support in terms of facilitating emotional disclosure, grief work and counselling interventions reached ambiguous conclusions (Stroebe *et al.* 2005). There is some evidence that proactive and universal bereavement support is unnecessary and that only people who experience problems and seek help find bereavement interventions beneficial. This is in contrast to current practice in UK hospices, were adult bereavement support is generally offered to all rather than allocated following formal assessment of need (Field *et al.* 2007).

There is much that we do not know about what happens in hospice and specialist palliative care bereavement services and what constitutes good practice. There have been few methodologically rigorous evaluations of general bereavement support services and even fewer in relation to hospices (Payne *et al.* 1999). Two recent surveys suggest there are similar elements of hospice bereavement support in the UK (Field *et al.* 2004) and USA (Demmer 2003). Typically support may include a broad range of activities such as social evenings, social visits in the home by volunteers, counselling and support groups (Field *et al.* 2006; Reid *et al.* 2006). Such support may be provided by professionals and/or by trained volunteers. The use of bereavement support volunteers in hospices is common in some countries including the UK (Field *et al.* 2004) and in New Zealand (Payne 2001a). Two studies have demonstrated the effectiveness of volunteers in the provision of bereavement support (Parkes 1981; Relf 2001). Volunteers require careful recruitment, selection, training and supervision. Relf (2001) has pointed out that providing for the needs of volunteer workers in bereavement support is a demanding and skilled activity. Hospice bereavement support services also need to be able to identify when clients have such difficult and complex problems that they exceed their capacity to deal with them. Close and well-established links with other mental health services, such as liaison psychiatry or clinical psychology, are needed but may be difficult to access.

Providing bereavement services is difficult and demanding work. The emotional demand placed on those who witness grief and support bereaved people requires skill, knowledge and sensitivity (Payne 2001b). The paradoxical nature of bereavement support, which demands both professional standards of knowledge and skill and the warmth of human understanding and sensitivity, represents a challenge for all. There is a dilemma in training volunteers and professionals that the compassion and empathy, which lead them into this work, becomes constrained by a framework imposed by models of bereavement. Exposure to repeated distress needs to be acknowledged as potentially difficult to deal with. It is generally considered to be good practice to ensure that supervision is available to bereavement care workers, in which emotional off-loading and discussion of difficult circumstances can be dealt with on a regular basis (Payne 2002).

## Overview of chapters in Part Three

In the remainder of this chapter, I will briefly introduce the following five chapters. The themes of loss and the consequences of care at the time of death and during bereavement incorporate a number of perspectives. Authors of the following chapters draw on research, clinical practice and experience of bereavement support services from several domains.

In a revised Chapter 22, Komaromy focuses on nursing care during the process of dying. She draws on a large ethnographic study of older people dying in residential and nursing care homes in the UK. Komaromy and her colleagues have done much to reveal how difficult it is to achieve high-quality nursing care for dying people in these institutions. There are a cluster of factors that appear to conspire against optimal care. There is, of course, great diversity in the quality of care homes for older people in the UK and in other countries. In Australia, national guidelines have been developed to improve end-of-life in aged care (Commonwealth of Australia 2004). The protracted nature of dying for older people may also make it difficult for nurses to realize when they are dying and to predict when the death is likely to occur (Seymour *et al.* 2005). As Komaromy argues in her chapter, it is important for nurses to be able to predict when the person is dying to elicit additional resources and, if necessary, make a referral to a specialist palliative care team. Recognition of impending death also allows care to be modified; for example, regular pressure area care may involve disturbing the patient and contribute to pain and discomfort, and is not necessary if the person is in the final stages of dying. Changes to medication, food and fluid intake may all be appropriate as the person approaches death. The signs of dying may be harder to detect in very old people whose health declines slowly over many years. It may also be difficult for nurses in care homes to initiate discussions about dying with these people and their family members, if open discussion is not part of the culture of care. To achieve this they may need additional communication skills training and support from other staff members. Komaromy's chapter offers an illumination of these and other issues for nurses caring for those at the time of death.

The remaining chapters in Part Three focus on families and friends of the deceased person, who rapidly change their status in the minds of health and social care workers from 'carers' to become 'the bereaved'. In Chapter 23, Cobb writes about the role of nurses immediately after a death has occurred. He highlights the individuality of the experience of loss and the inadequacy of any one theoretical model to provide a template. Health care is increasingly being construed as the management of risk and public health messages are often conveyed in terms of reducing health risks associated with lifestyle choices such as smoking or eating high-fat foods. Relf applies the logic of risk management in Chapter 24 to a discussion of risk assessment in bereavement for poor outcome. She describes the use of standardized measures that predict the likelihood of poor bereavement outcome. This method has been used to allocate bereavement care to those most likely to benefit from it. It is argued that risk assessment not only targets costly and limited resources appropriately, but ensures that low-risk individuals are not disempowered by implying that they may not be able to cope with their loss and thus create dependency. Relf is critical of the notion of risk assessment and argues that it is embedded in a positivitist paradigm and is derived from the psychological/psychiatric models of bereavement. She explains how later models, introduced earlier in this overview, have challenged concepts such as 'recovery' and 'resolution' of grief. She concludes pragmatically by indicating the weaknesses and the strengths of using formalized risk assessment procedures. The debates about risk assessment in this chapter raise important issues for consideration in designing bereavement support services.

In a revised Chapter 25, Kissane provides an excellent summary of bereavement support activities provided by hospices and specialist palliative care services. Like Relf, he recommends the assessment of family members to identify needs, risks and dysfunctional relationships from first contact with hospice services. He proposes that support should be conceptualized at three levels:

- a general culture of support and understanding provided by all the members of the health and social care team in collaboration with the wider community;
- identification of those at risk and offers of support to prevent adverse outcomes; and
- recognition of those with existing problems and referral for psycho-therapeutic interventions.

Kissane describes the common activities and interventions that fit the different requirements of these categories of support. He considers the evidence base for the various activities and offers a summary of how nurses might engage in providing different types of support to bereaved people.

In a revised Chapter 26, Rolls focuses on families and childhood bereavement support. We have decided to include such a chapter in a book predominantly concerned with adult palliative care because adults relate to children in a number of important ways. For example, the terminal illness and death of an adult may impact upon children in their family system, including grandchildren, and following the death they will be bereaved. It is often difficult for adults, including nurses, to know how best to talk with children about approaching death and how best to deal with newly bereaved children. In the past the default position has been to not communicate with children in the mistaken believe that they can be shielded from family change and grief. Instead, this has tended to leave children alone with their fears unanswered. In this chapter, Rolls draws on a large study which mapped the characteristics of childhood bereavement services in the UK and how they work with children and families, and looked at their wider role in society (Rolls and Payne 2004). She argues that, in the past, loss and bereavement affecting children was contained within the family and was treated as a private matter but more recently services have developed specifically to support children and to help parents care for a bereaved child.

## Recommended reading

Firth, P., Luff, G. and Oliviere, D. (2005) *Loss, change and bereavement in palliative care*. Maidenhead: Open University Press.

Hockey, J., Katz, J. and Small, N. (eds) (2001) *Grief, Mourning and Death Ritual*. Buckingham: Open University Press.

Payne, S., Horn, S. and Relf, M. (1999) *Loss and Bereavement*. Buckingham: Open University Press.

Stroebe, M.S., Hansson, R.O., Stroebe, W. and Schut, H. (eds) (2002) *Handbook of Bereavement Research: Consequences, Coping and Care*. Washington, DC: American Psychological Association.

Walter, T. (1999) *On Bereavement*. Buckingham: Open University Press.

## References

Bonanno, G.A. (2004) Loss, trauma and human resilience: have we underestimated the human capacity to thrive after extremely aversive events? *American Psychologist*, 59(1): 20–8.

Bonanno, G.A. and Kaltman, S. (2001) The varieties of grief experience. *Clinical Psychology Review*, 21: 705.

Bowlby, J. (1969) *Attachment and Loss, Vol. 1: Attachment*. London: The Hogarth Press.

Bowlby, J. (1973) *Attachment and Loss, Vol. 2: Separation*. London: The Hogarth Press.

Bowlby, J. (1980) *Attachment and Loss, Vol. 3: Loss: Sadness and Depression*. London: The Hogarth Press.

Bryan, L. (2007) Should ward nurses hide death from other patients? *End of Life Care*, 1(1): 79–86.

Commonwealth of Australia (2004) *Guidelines for a Palliative Approach in Residential Aged Care*, www.palliativecare.gov.au (accessed June 2007).

Engel, G. (1961) Is grief a disease? *Psychological Medicine*, 23: 18–22.

Evans, A. (1994) Anticipatory grief: a theoretical challenge. *Palliative Medicine*, 8(2): 159–65.

Field, D., Hockey, J. and Small, N. (1997) *Death, Gender and Ethnicity*. London: Routledge.

Field, D. and Payne, S. (2003) Social aspects of bereavement. *Journal of Cancer Nursing*, 2(8): 21–5.

Field, D., Reid, D., Payne, S. and Relf, M. (2004) A national postal survey of adult bereavement support in hospice and specialist palliative care services in the UK. *International Journal of Palliative Nursing*, 10(12): 569–76.

Field, D., Payne, S., Relf, M. and Reid, D. (2007) An overview of adult bereavement support in the United Kingdom: Issues for policy and practice. *Social Science and Medicine*, 64(2): 428–38.

Field, D., Reid, D., Payne, S. and Relf, M. (2006) Adult bereavement in five English hospices: types of support. *International Journal of Palliative Nursing*, 12(9): 430–7.

Folkman, S. (1997) Positive psychological states and coping with severe stress. *Social Science and Medicine*, 45(8): 1207–21.

Folkman, S. and Greer, S. (2000) Promoting psychological well-being in the face of serious illness: when theory, research and practice inform each other. *Psycho-oncology*, 9: 11–19.

Freud, S. (1917) *Mourning and Melancholia*. London: The Hogarth Press.

Grande, G.E., Farquhar, M.C., Barclay, S.I.G. and Todd, C.J. (2004) Caregiver bereavement outcome: relationship with hospice at home, satisfaction with care, and home death. *Journal of Palliative Care*, 20: 69–77.

Hockey, J. (2001) Changing death rituals. In: J. Hockey, J. Katz and N. Small (eds) *Grief, Mourning and Death Ritual*. Buckingham: Open University Press.

Hockey, J., Katz, J. and Small, N. (eds) (2001) *Grief, Mourning and Death Ritual*. Buckingham: Open University Press.

Joanna Briggs Institute (2006) *Literature Review on Bereavement and Bereavement Care*. Aberdeen: The Robert Gordon University.

Kissane, D.W. and Bloch, S. (2002) *Family Focused Grief Therapy. A model of family-centred care during bereavement*. Buckingham: Open University Press.

Kitrungrote, L. and Cohen, M.Z. (2006) Quality of life of family caregivers of patients with cancer: A literature review. *Oncology Nursing Forum*, 33: 625–32.

Klass, D., Silverman, P.R. and Nickman, S.L. (1996) *Continuing Bonds*. Philadelphia, PA: Taylor & Francis.

Kübler-Ross, E. (1969) *On Death and Dying*. New York: Macmillan.

Lazarus, R.S. and Folkman, S. (1984) *Stress, Appraisal and Coping*. New York: Springer.

Lewis, C.S. (1966) *A Grief Observed*. London: Faber & Faber.

Lofland, L.H. (1985) The social shaping of emotion: a case of grief. *Symbolic Interaction*, 8(2): 171–90.

McNamara, B., Waddell, C. and Colvin, M. (1994) The institutionalization of the good death. *Social Science and Medicine*, 39: 1501–8.

Morgan, J.D. and Laungani, P. (2003) *Death and Bereavement around the World*. Amityville, NY: Baywood Publishing Company.

Nolen-Hoeksema, S. (2002) Ruminative coping and adjustment. In: M.S. Stroebe, R.O. Hansson, W. Stroebe and H. Schut (eds) *Handbook of Bereavement Research: Consequences, Coping and Care*. Washington, DC: American Psychological Association.

Parkes, C.M. (1971) Psychosocial transitions: a field for study. *Social Science and Medicine*, 5(2): 101–14.

Parkes, C.M. (1972) *Bereavement*. London: Routledge.

Parkes, C.M. (1981) Evaluation of a bereavement service. *Journal of Preventive Psychiatry*, 146: 11–17.

Parkes, C.M. (1986) *Bereavement*, 2nd edn. London: Routledge.

Parkes, C.M. (1993) Bereavement as a psychosocial transition: processes of adaptation to change. In: M.S. Stroebe, W. Stroebe and R.O. Hansson (eds) *Handbook of Bereavement*. Cambridge: Cambridge University Press.

Parkes, C.M. (1996) *Bereavement*, 3rd edn. London: Routledge.

Parkes, C.M. (2005) After the Tsunami. *Hospice Information Bulletin*, 4(2): 12.

Parkes, C.M. (2006) *Love and loss. The roots of grief and its complications*. London: Routledge.

Parkes, C.M., Relf, M. and Couldrick, A. (1996) *Counselling in Terminal Care and Bereavement*. Leicester: BPS Books.

Parkes, C.M., Laungani, P. and Young, B. (1997) *Death and Bereavement Across Cultures*. London: Routledge.

Payne, S. (2001a) Bereavement support: something for everyone? *International Journal of Palliative Nursing*, 7(3): 108.

Payne, S. (2001b) The role of volunteers in hospice bereavement support in New Zealand. *Palliative Medicine*, 15: 107–15.

Payne, S. (2002) Dilemmas in the use of volunteers to provide hospice bereavement support: Evidence from New Zealand. *Mortality*, 7(2): 139–54.

Payne, S. and Lloyd Williams, M. (in press) Bereavement care. In: M. Lloyd-Williams (2nd edn) *Psychosocial Issues in Palliative Care*. Oxford: Oxford University Press.

Payne, S., Horn, S. and Relf, M. (1999) *Loss and Bereavement*. Buckingham: Open University Press.

Quested, B. and Rudge, T. (2003) Nursing care of dead bodies: a discursive analysis of last offices. *Journal of Advanced Nursing*, 41(6): 553–60.

Reid, D., Field, D., Payne, S. and Relf, M. (2006) Adult bereavement in five English Hospices: participants, organisations and pre-bereavement support. *International Journal of Palliative Nursing*, 12(7): 320–7.

Reimers, E. (2001) Bereavement – a social phenomenon? *European Journal of Palliative Care*, 8(6): 242–5.

Relf, M. (2001) The effectiveness of volunteer bereavement care: an evaluation of a palliative care bereavement service. PhD thesis, University of London.

Riches, G. and Dawson, P. (2000) *An Intimate Loneliness: Supporting Bereaved Parents and Siblings*. Buckingham: Open University Press.

Rolls, L. and Payne, S. (2004) Childhood bereavement services: issues in UK service provision. *Mortality*, 9(4): 300–28.

Salvador, R.J. (2003) What do Mexicans celebrate on the 'Day of the Dead'? In: J.D. Morgan and P. Laungani (eds) *Death and Bereavement around the World Vol 2: Death and Bereavement in the Americans*. Amityville: Baywood Publishing Company.

Seymour, J. (2001) *Critical Moments – Death and Dying in Intensive Care*. Buckingham: Open University Press.

Seymour, J., Witherspoon, R., Gott, M., Ross, H. and Payne, S. (2005) *Dying in Older Age: End-of-Life Care*, Bristol: Policy Press.

Shepherd-Hughes, N. (1972) *Death Without Weeping. The Violence of Everyday Life in Brazil*. Berkeley, CA: University of California Press.

Small, N. (2001) Theories of grief: a critical review. In: J. Hockey, J. Katz and N. Small (eds) *Grief, Mourning and Death Ritual*. Buckingham: Open University Press.

Sque, M., Long, T., Payne, S., Roche, W. and Speck, P. (2008) The UK post-mortem organ retention crisis: a qualitative study of its impact on partners. *Journal of Advanced Nursing* 101: 71–77.

Stroebe, M. (1992) Coping with bereavement: A review of the grief work hypothesis. *Omega: Journal of Death and Dying*, 26: 19–42.

Stroebe, M. and Schut, H. (1999) The dual process model of coping with bereavement: rationale and description. *Death Studies*, 23: 197–224.

Stroebe, W., Schut, H. and Stroebe, M. (2005) Grief work, disclosure and counselling: Do they help the bereaved? *Clinical Psychology Review*, 25: 395–414.

Stroebe, M.S., Hansson, R.O., Stroebe, W. and Schut, H. (2002) *Handbook of Bereavement Research: Consequences, Coping and Care*. Washington, DC: American Psychological Association.

Stroebe, M., Stroebe, W., Schut, H., Zech, E. and Van, D. (2002) Does disclosure of emotion facilitate recovery from bereavement? Evidence from two prospective studies. *Journal of Consulting and Clinical Psychology*, 70: 169.

Sudnow, D. (1967) *Passing On*. Englewood Cliffs, NJ: Prentice-Hall.

Walter, T. (1996) A new model of grief: bereavement and biography. *Mortality*, 1(1): 1–29.

Walter, T. (1999) *On Bereavement*. Buckingham: Open University Press.

Wolf, Z. (1988) *Nurses' Work: The Sacred and the Profane*. Philadelphia, PA: University of Pennsylvania Press.

Worden, J.W. (1982) *Grief Counselling and Grief Therapy: A Handbook for the Mental Health Practitioner*. New York: Springer.

Worden, J.W. (1991) *Grief Counselling and Grief Therapy*, 2nd edn. New York: Springer.

Worden, J.W. (2001) *Grief Counselling and Grief Therapy*, 3rd edn. New York: Springer.

Wortman, C.B. and Silver, R.C. (1989) The myths of coping with loss. *Journal of Consulting and Clinical Psychology*, 57(3): 349–57.

# 22

# Nursing care at the time of death

*Carol Komaromy*

---

**Key points**

- Key professional groups such as nurses and care home staff are expected to be able to cope with death and dying as part of their routine care, while at the same time affording this type of care a special significance.
- The expectation on the provision of good quality end-of-life care that is enshrined in policy and practice still fails to take account of the needs of older people.
- Providing good quality care is dependent upon a diagnosis of dying which is not easy in chronic illness.
- The way in which death is managed can impact upon the experience of death and bereavement.

---

'We're expected to be able to cope with anything really. Sometimes you just have to pretend to be OK. 'Cos – you know – it's expected of you. You are it – the one who copes – while everyone else falls about' (Mary, staff nurse). This quote from Mary (whose name has been changed), a nurse in a care home for older people, is representative of the type of response that I commonly heard during the fieldwork on a project into the management of death and dying in these settings (Sidell *et al.* 1997). Indeed, nurses, as frontline workers, have to cope with death in all types of settings – hospitals, hospices and domestic homes as well as residential care homes. This chapter explores what happens at and around the time of death from a sociological point of view and how this impacts upon nursing care.

The chapter begins with a discussion of the importance of being able to predict when death will occur and goes on to ask what it is about death that makes it such a special event. An exploration of the different ways in which death is constructed and how that impacts upon the moment of death follow this discussion. The assumptions that underpin the notion of a 'good' death are challenged – both from the point of view of the possibility of being able

449

to define what this means as well as its achievement. The chapter concludes with a discussion of the body after death and its immediate impact upon any family and friends of the deceased.

## Where and when death occurs

The time, setting and place of death all have the potential to impact upon the way that professionals are able to provide care at the time of death. One of the key factors in being able to provide care is in knowing that someone is dying and when his or her death is likely to occur. The importance of being able to predict death and dying was something that Glaser and Strauss (1965) explored in a seminal ethnographic study based on the observations that they made in hospital wards in the USA. They found that, in order to plan terminal care, hospital staff needed to be able to predict when deaths might occur. However, these predictions were complex, needed to be updated and even 'renegotiated'. For example, they categorized predictions into three main types. First, they found that it was possible to be *virtually* certain about when the death would occur; second, for those patients for whom there was less certainty about the time of death, it might be possible *in the future* to establish a time when there could be certainty. The third and final category and the one that staff found most difficult to cope with, was that in which the time of death was *uncertain* and there was no clear time when any certainty could be established. In other words, there were patients for whom it was unlikely that staff would be able to predict the time of death. Studies into end-of-life care include explorations of the illness trajectories for people with chronic conditions, such as heart disease and renal impairment. In the slow decline towards death that is characterized by people dying over longer periods there are most likely to be slow and progressive periods of dying punctuated by acute exacerbations (Lynn *et al.* 2007). Perhaps in the 1960s, at the time of Glaser and Strauss's seminal work, the need for predictions about death could be viewed as part of the more instrumental treatment of dying people. But the need for accurate predictions of the time of death is even greater now as a result of changes in practice from general non-disclosure of diagnosis and prognosis to the current situation in which fuller disclosure is the norm. 'Hospice pioneers advanced a model of care in which patients were informed frankly and openly of their condition, and were actively encouraged to participate in all the decisions surrounding their treatment and care' (Abel 1986, cited in Lawton 2000: 42).

Underpinning this philosophy of disclosure is the assumption that pre-dicted deaths can be managed in the 'best' setting; that being the one that the dying person has chosen. The elite nature of palliative care has been well documented (Clark *et al.* 1997; Addington-Hall 1998; Lynn *et al.* 2007). There are people for whom a shared disclosure of death is not available or part of the philosophical approach to their care. Seymour (2001) for example, in her ethnographic account of end-of-life care, discussed the 'uncertain' deaths that occur in intensive care units. Likewise, death occurs in other settings in which it can be classified as being 'out of place', such as accident and emergency departments (Tinnermans 1998).

Changes in policy and practice in the UK have shifted the emphasis from providing good quality palliative care to those people with cancer and who meet the criteria for care, on to the needs of previously 'disadvantaged' dying people, of whom older people comprise the largest group. In the UK there are 450,000 older people resident in care homes for older people. The Department of Health for England and Wales and the Scottish Partnership for Palliative Care have been instrumental in policy development to extend palliative care to all dying people. This means that the right to provision of care is enshrined in policy documents which include: the End of Life Care initiative (DoH 2003), which supports the implementation of the Gold Standards Framework; the Liverpool Care Pathway for the Dying; and Preferred Priorities of Care tools. One key initiative that has arisen from the requirement that older people are entitled to end-of-life care, is the NHS end-of-life care programme working in partnership with the National Council for Palliative Care (see Froggatt 2004).

The key principle underpinning this shift is that care homes should implement strategies for care through a designated SHA link person. At the time of writing, the *NHS End of Life Care Programme Progress Report* (2006) had set up a steering group, written a series of reports and produced an introductory guide for staff working in care homes for older people. The guidance includes advice on being able to recognize a period of dying as the last few months of life, or less. This is an area that is problematic because care home staff are reluctant to categorize residents as dying until the last few weeks or days of life (Sidell *et al.* 1997).

This is not just confined to the needs of carers of dying people who wish to be able to plan end-of-life care and utilize the resources that are increasingly on offer. For everyone who is involved in death and dying, there is a premium upon being able to predict when a death is likely to occur. Not only is this due to the reality that being able to make an accurate prediction of death affects the ability of those involved to be able to choose the place of death and the manner of that death, including the form of supportive care. There are other reasons that explain why it is important to be able to predict death and it is some of these that I turn to next.

# The meaning of death

It has been argued that in a postmodern society death does not carry the same significance that it did in the past – particularly in the fifteenth century when people were more likely to believe that reward or punishment in the 'next' life was a result of their behaviour in this one. Bauman also suggests that the general decline in the belief in life after death in Western culture has reduced that power of creeds to dictate how we behave in this life. The result of this, he claims, is that in a postmodern society people are more likely to focus upon the intrinsic value of this life rather than postponing any investment in an 'afterlife'.

There are dangers in this type of generalized statement not least because it fails to acknowledge the detailed terrain of beliefs. It might be reasonable to claim that, in Western culture, there is no longer a unified belief neither in an 'afterlife' nor in the belief that admission to an afterlife is granted by some sort of moral or spiritual gatekeeper. But Davies (2002) argues that many people believe in a continuation of life after death and writes that, 'Death rites are as much concerned with the issues of identity and social continuity as with the very practical fact that human bodies decay and become offensive to the sight and smell of the living' (2002: 6).

With the focus for individuals on their social identity it seems to be very difficult to imagine a world in which we do not continue to exist in some way and even more difficult to remove ourselves from the influences in society that shape the way that death is treated. This makes what happens at the time of death still significant albeit to varying degrees. Furthermore, the practical fact of the decay of the material body that Davies refers to above does not mean that the body at the time of death is unimportant. For some who believe in a transition from one existence to another, the body plays a significant part. Davies (2002) argues that just as the living body is subjected to social rules on norms of behaviour, we also invest the corpse with meaning and feelings that reflect the values of society.

Yet, the body has different meanings associated with it and I would add that the body is also a container of death and as such is a 'taboo' object. When the bodies of residents in care homes are removed their exit is mostly concealed from other residents. 'Staff and funeral directors collude in conferring a dangerous status onto the body by covering the corpse with sheets or placing them into thick, black plastic bags. These covered up, enclosed bodies represent death in the form of a tightly wrapped corpse. . . . Having produced something unsightly it must be concealed' (Komaromy 2000: 311).

This diversity in beliefs about the meaning of death places a high premium on effective communication about what needs to happen at the time of death as well as the need to be able to predict the moment of death. Such diversity also suggests the potential for a lack of any clear understanding about what those needs might be. With so much invested in the significance of the moment of death, nurses, as key players at the time of death, face a potential minefield of incoherent, inconsistent, spiritual, emotional and physical needs all of which are in a relationship with each other and the dying person and any family and friends.

## The moment of death

The significance of the moment of death arises at several different levels: the medical, legal, spiritual, cultural and social. The impact of what happens at the moment of death is part of the understanding of the way that people are able to grieve. Institutional and social practices require action to be taken at the moment of death, in part arising from the professionalization of death. Perhaps it is unsurprising that there is a lot of anxiety about being present at the moment of death and doing the 'right' things at that moment. This places a burden upon those professionals who are involved at the time of death to get it 'right', because there is no second chance. Nurses present at the moment of death need to understand the significance of this moment on all of these levels.

### Medical and legal context

The need for information in order to be able to certify death is a legal requirement and one that places a great demand on being present at the moment of death. Paul Rossenbatt *et al.* (1976) argue that the medicalization of death is itself a form of ritual which involves medical people as the specialists who witness death. The medical construction of death defines it as a precise moment in time. The medicalization and legalization requires there to be a precise time given to the moment of death, even though there are ambiguities to this diagnosis (Turner 1987). Certainly, having the power to define a moment of death carries its own ritualistic power and this is particularly so when within the medical paradigm there are categories of death. For example, the status of the 'ventilated corpse' has been created to define the status of the body in the stage between the definition of brain death and the removal of organs for transplantation.

But what happens in the emergency resuscitations and the ambiguity of a cardiac arrest and the patient or person for whom the moment of death is one from which there is the possibility of recovery and who might be resuscitated? For people whose hearts are defined as having 'arrested', death is deemed to be 'out of place' and there are likely to be attempts made to resuscitate them. In her ethnographic study of a resuscitation team in a large teaching hospital, Page and Komaromy (2000) note the ritualistic aspects of cardio-pulmonary resuscitation (CPR): 'However, it is perhaps not difficult to see how a CPR event might be viewed in terms of a symbolic ritual, which, as van der Woning (1997) suggests, involves living out the myth of the superhuman, the heroic and "in control" and as such is illuminative of the culture in which it occurs.' They also claim that this ritual is an enactment of the power of medicine to be able to intervene and even possibly reverse death.

### Spiritual and cultural context

Any spiritual or religious belief system will invest meaning in the moment of death. If death is believed to be the time at which there is a transition from one existence to another, then there might be rituals that have to be carried out so that the passage is successful. The significance of taking cultural diversity into account rests on the need to recognize that a dying person's needs and beliefs will be shaped by beliefs and behaviours that are framed by his or her own cultural context, rather than that of the dominant culture within which care practices are often developed. For example, it is dangerous to assume that people who belong to particular ethnic or religious groups will all share the same needs and conform to the expectations of that group at the moment of death. The danger for care providers is that a rigid view of culture might result in a single representation of what someone's wishes might entail. In practice, care providers need to be sensitive to the needs associated within specific cultures but negotiated at the level of the individual. This would allow for a nuanced expression of individual diversity (Braun *et al.* 2000).

### Social context

Parkes (1971) argues that alongside death being conceived of as an event that is increasingly postponed in the Western world, there is an associated inability for people to face death. They also argue that the need for rituals associated with death have correspondingly declined. Rituals that surround death can be of different orders. But it could be argued that there are different forms of social ritual such as the professionalization and medicalization of death that serve the purpose of guiding people through the moment of death. The examples of medical rituals include the need for staff involved in deaths to be able to 'perform' (Goffman 1959). This means that everyone involved needs to be seen as concerned to get things right and must give a convincing performance of this, whatever their personal feelings. Goffman claims that 'impression management' is central to an understanding of what is taking place. In applying this idea to the moment of death it seems that the 'impression' is 'managed' according to routines and rituals that structure how staff members behave. To take the analogy of performance further, these 'scripts' are often written into organizational procedures and protocols as codes of behaviour. For example, it is as inappropriate for professionals to be too upset as it is for them to appear to be unaffected (Walter 1999).

   Family and friends often want to be present at the moment of death and might participate in a bedside vigil, or request to be notified when a death is imminent. The need to say 'good-bye' could be categorized as greater if there is not likely to be a meeting in another life. Whatever the level of need at a personal level, this is part of his or her social role when someone is dying.

### The role of nurses at the moment of death

It is not easy for nurses involved in end-of-life care and death to provide care that is appropriate at the time of death for individual dying people. As discussed above, there are dangers inherent in all of the interpretations of the purpose of death and the needs of dying people and their families. Likewise, there is a corresponding danger in not understanding the needs associated with someone's religious and cultural needs. These needs might conflict with the routines and rituals that are associated with the setting in which the death takes place. One of the care home managers told me of the resistance by her staff to leave a dead resident sitting in a chair for several hours while the family said their 'good-byes' (Sidell *et al.* 1997). She recounted how the staff tried to pressurize her into putting the resident to bed, straightening the body and getting the undertakers to remove the deceased resident. As head of home she had the power to resist, but it is difficult to imagine this being 'allowed' to happen in many institutional settings.

In an ideal situation the dying person would be able to articulate his or her needs in advance of death so that the care staff would understand their needs and try to meet them. This would allow for people who need to be present at the death to be invited to do so and for those things that need to be done to be performed. The difficulty arises when dying people are unable to make their wishes known and nursing staff have to make a judgement on their behalf. All of this discussion about the significance of the moment of death carries assumptions about the type of death that people could achieve and this is the subject of the next section.

# The 'good' death

Achieving a 'good' death clearly depends upon being aware of the imminence of death and the opportunity for the dying person to express their wishes as well as the capacity for care staff to be able to carry these out. The concept of a 'good' death is not new. Neither is it a straightforward concept. Its meaning has varied over time and between social and cultural groups. Bradbury (2001) has categorized the concept of a 'good' death into three types – the medicalized, the sacred and the natural, so that it is possible to analyse and evaluate deaths according to each of these types. For example, a 'good' medicalized death might be one that is anticipated and pain-free, but this conflicts with the criteria associated with the natural dimension of a 'good death'. What this ignores is the answer to the question good for whom? As early as 1972 Weismann had introduced the concept of 'appropriate deaths', which took much more account of the relational aspects of death and the fact that people do not die as isolated individuals but as members of a social group. However, this suggests that death can be well managed and controlled. More recently, Kellehear (2000) has argued that the understanding of the good death is twofold. First, there is a concern with the physical quality of life in the dying period and, second, a social concern with preparing for death. He argues further that these two concerns merge in the period of dying. Howarth (2007) offers a critique of the hospice movement and argues that the primary concern with the holistic view of the 'good death' adopted by the hospice movement has been overshadowed by a medical concern and signals a shift away from the social elements of the original palliative care philosophy.

In a study into physicians' emotional responses to the way that people in

456 Loss and bereavement

their care die, Good *et al.* (2004) take account of the technological changes that have impacted upon end-of-life care. Their findings suggest that: '. . . . dying is difficult, particularly in the modern hospital where there are so many treatment options and where relationships are short, discontinuous, without a perspective on the patient as a person, and with little time to acquire it. "Good deaths", if they exist, take place in the context of relationships in which the patient's personhood is known and valued' (2004: 23).

In homes for older people death is much more likely to be constructed as a 'natural and timely' event, coming as it does at the end of a long life. But there are still problems and concerns associated with death in old age. The care staff in homes for older people have to manage the difficult boundary between life and death. The staff in these settings to whom I talked described a 'good death' as one that was 'peaceful', 'pain-free' and 'accompanied'. 'Good death is neither protracted nor sudden, its shape constituting a straightforward trajectory from deterioration to death' (Komaromy and Hockey 2001: 75). Even when the 'ideal' death was achieved deathbed scenes were still constructed by staff as dramatic events, seemingly conferring significance on a life when the quality of that life had been lost (Komaromy 2000).

Concerns about the quality of the care of dying people in acute and community settings and the focus upon medical care and saving life regardless of its quality gave rise to a demand for a more holistic approach to death and dying. The hospice movement pioneered the approach that aimed to incorporate death and dying back into life through the high quality care of dying people. In order to do this the forms of distress of dying people had to be recognized and relieved. The hospice approach and palliative care have become synonymous with best quality care for dying people. Even so this type of death at a hospice is proscribed by moral ethics that means certain wishes such as euthanasia would not be granted. 'Palliative care professionals have, for a long time, been able to argue that the provision of palliative care relieves suffering to such an extent that euthanasia is no longer wanted by many people, even those who have previously been its advocates' (Oxenham and Boyd 1997: 284).

Dignity as part of a 'good death' is not easily defined. In a qualitative study into the way that dying people define dignity, Chochinov *et al.* (2002) discuss the way that the term dignity is used in clinical and philosophical discourse in an ambiguous manner. Responses from patients in the study that specifically relate to the time of death seemed to highlight what the authors call 'death anxiety' and which included concerns about what the terminal phase of the illness would be like. Several of the patients who are quoted in this study wanted a 'quick' ending.

### Sudden deaths as bad deaths

Most of the discussion of the achievement of a 'good death' so far implies that there is a possibility of preparation for death. As discussed above, not everyone wants to be able to prepare for death through a period of protracted dying. Some people would prefer to die quickly. However, there are deaths that cannot be anticipated and these create their own problems. The way that sudden death can complicate bereavement has been well documented (Walter 1999; Eyre 2001; Howarth 2001). The main focus has been upon the effect of sudden death upon bereaved people and comparatively little attention has been paid to the effect of sudden death upon the professionals involved, apart from the situation of violent death and disaster (Eyre 2001). Most significantly, for those settings where death is anticipated and considered to be 'natural' and 'timely' coming as it does at the end of a long life, such as care homes for older people, sudden death has an enormous impact on the care staff and sometimes other residents depending upon their awareness of what has taken place. Key concerns for care staff in homes for older people include coping with the shock of the unexpected death, informing the family and reporting such deaths to the coroner. Deaths that are not expected – often classified as 'sudden' deaths – cause equal distress to the professionals and any family and friends involved.

### The impact of the manner of death on bereavement

Michael Anderson (2000), writing about therapeutic response to grief, describes the event of death as something that is at the 'hub' of the stories of grief that are told during bereavement counselling and grief work. What he means by this is that all accounts lead to and from the event of the death. In grief counselling, people who are grieving are encouraged to talk about events that are categorized as being 'before' and 'after' the event. The death then is foregrounded as the most significant event in the grief process. This serves to place a greater focus upon the moment of death and how this is managed.

## Conclusion

In this chapter I have argued from a sociological point of view that the moment of death carries heavy responsibilities for nurses as the most likely professionals to be present. This is because the moment of death is affected by a number of key factors such as:

- the meaning of death which includes the medical and legal, the spiritual, religious and cultural significance
- the manner of death
- the quality of death and how that is translated
- the setting of death
- and the social significance of death and how the performance of death is carried out.

All of these factors are in a relationship with each other and provide the context in which death occurs. The premium on 'getting it right' is high given that the immediate aftermath of death affects the grief work of those who are bereaved.

## Further reading

Clark, D. and Wright, M. (2003) *Transitions in end of life care: hospice and related developments in Eastern Europe and Central Asia.* Buckingham: Open University Press.

Hockley, J. and Clark, D. (eds) (2002) *Palliative care for older people in care homes.* Buckingham: Open University Press.

Lynn, J., Chaudry, E., Noyes Simon, L., Wilkinson, A.M. and Lynch Schuster, J. (2007) *The Common Sense Guide to Improving Palliative Care.* Oxford: Oxford University Press.

## References

Abel, E. (1986) The hospice movement: institutionalising innovation, international Journal of Health Services. In: J. Lawton (2000) *The dying process.* London: Routledge, 16(1): 71–85.

Addington-Hall, J. (1998) Specialist palliative care in non-malignant disease. *Palliative Medicine,* 12(6): 417–27.

Anderson, M. (2000) 'You have to get inside the person' or making grief private: image and metaphor in the therapeutic reconstruction of bereavement. In: J. Hockey, J. Katz and N. Small (eds) (2000) *Grief, mourning and death ritual.* Buckingham: Open University Press, pp. 135–43.

Bradbury, M. (2001) The good death? In: D. Dickenson, M. Johnson and J. Samson Katz (2001) *Death, Dying and Bereavement.* London: Sage Publications, pp. 59–63.

Chochinov, H.M., Hack, T., McClement, S., Kristjanson, L. and Harlos, M. (2002) Dignity in the terminally ill: a developing empirical model. *Social Science and Medicine,* 54(3): 433–43.

Clark, D., Hockley, J. and Ahmedzai, S. (1997) *New themes in palliative care.* Buckingham: Open University Press.

Davies, D.J. (2002) *Death, ritual and belief.* London: Continuum.

Department of Health (DoH) (2003) *End of Life Care Initiative.* London: Department of Health.

Eyre, A. (2001) Post disaster rituals. In: J. Hockey, J. Katz. and N. Small (eds) *Grief, mourning and death ritual.* Buckingham: Open University Press, pp. 256–66.

Froggatt, K.A. (2004) *Palliative care in care homes for older people.* London: The National Council for Palliative Care.

Glaser, B.G. and Strauss, A. (1965) *Awareness of dying.* Chicago: Aldine Publishing Company.

Goffman, E. (1959) *The presentation of self in everyday life.* London: Penguin.

Good, M.J.D, Gadmer, N.M., Ruopp, P., Lakoma, M., Sullivan, A.M., Redinbaugh, E., Arnold, R.M. and Block, S.D. (2004) Narrative nuances on good and bad deaths internists' tales from high technology work places. *Social Science and Medicine*, 58(5): 939–53.

Howarth, G. (2001) Grieving in public. In: J. Hockey, J. Katz and N. Small (eds) (2001) *Grief, mourning and death ritual*. Buckingham: Open University Press, pp. 247–55.

Howarth, G. (2007) *Death and dying: a sociological introduction*. Cambridge: Polity.

Kellehear, A. (2000) Spirituality and palliative care: a model of needs. *Palliative Medicine*, 14: 149–55.

Komaromy, C. (2000) The sight and sound of death; the management of dead bodies in residential and nursing homes for older people. *Mortality*, 5(3): 299–315.

Komaromy, C. and Hockey, J. (2001) Naturalising death among older adults in residential care. In: J. Hockey, J. Katz and N. Small (eds) *Grief, mourning and death ritual*. Buckingham: Open University Press.

Lawton, J. (2000) *The dying process patients' experiences of palliative care*. London: Routledge.

*NHS End of Life Care Programme Progress Report* (2006) www.endoflifecare.nhs.uk (accessed 20 June 2007).

Lynn, J., Chaudry, E., Noyes Simon, L., Wilkinson, A.M. and Lynch Schuster, J. (2007) *The common sense guide to improving palliative care*. Oxford: Oxford University Press.

Oxenham, D. and Boyd, K. (1997) Voluntary euthanasia in terminal illness. In: D. Clark (ed.) (1996) *The future for palliative care*. Buckingham: Open University Press, pp. 275–87.

Page, S. and Komaromy, C. (2000) Lonely death: the case of expected and unexpected death. Paper presented to the *Fifth International Conference on Death, Dying and Disposal*, Goldsmiths College, London, September.

Parkes, C.M. (1971) The first year of bereavement: a longitudinal study of reaction of London widows to the death of their husbands. *Psychiatry*, 33: 444–67.

Rosenblatt, P., Walsh, R.P. and Jackson, D.A. (1976) Grief and mourning in cross cultural perspectives. Cited in D. Davies (2002) *Ritual and belief*. London: Continuum.

Seymour, J. (2001) *Critical moments in death and dying in intensive care*. Buckingham: Open University Press.

Sidell, M., Katz, J.T. and Komaromy, C. (1997) *Death and dying in residential and nursing homes for older people: examining the case for palliative care*. Department of Health Report.

Tinnermans, S. (1998) Resuscitation technology in the emergency department towards a dignified death. *Sociology of Health and Illness*, 20(2): 144–67.

Turner, B.S. (1987) *Medical power and social knowledge*. London: Sage Publications.

van der Woning, M. (1997) Should relatives be invited to witness a resuscitation attempt? A review of the literature. *Accident and Emergency Nursing*, 5: 215–18.

Walter, T. (1999) *On bereavement the culture of grief*. Buckingham: Open University Press.

# 23

# The care and support of bereaved people

*Mark Cobb*

---

**Key points**

- Nurses should be prepared for their encounters with people who are bereaved and are often in a good position to support them in the time immediately following death.
- Applying standard models of bereavement to people can devalue their experience and depersonalize care.
- People who are bereaved may involve nurses in establishing their narratives of loss.
- Simple follow-up contact may be all that many people who are bereaved require for support from nurses.
- Health professionals need to be aware of the wider resources of support and care available to bereaved people outside of the immediate health care context and be able to provide signposts to it.

---

## Introduction: In the company of the bereaved

Being present at the moment of someone's death is a familiar experience for many nurses and other health care professionals. Bearing witness to the consequence of fatal pathological events is an inevitable part of health care in which there are often procedures to guide the necessary practicalities of dealing with a dead body (Dougherty and Lister 2004), professional routines and cultural practices. This unexceptional biological reality, however, is an incomplete description because death is more than a clinical punctuation. In the presence of death we face the significance of human absence and loss, the deprivation of future possibilities, and the emptiness of an embodied space once filled with life. Most immediately nurses find themselves in the company of the bereaved wanting to care and console, concerned about the future, and aware that death imposes a loss that must be lived with.

Many people begin their bereavement in the company of health professionals and a common setting is the unfamiliar environment of a health care institution. An admission often follows a medical emergency resulting from a disease of the circulatory system or respiratory system or the impact of a neoplasm on a life system. In community settings it may be the health professional who is admitted into a domestic setting to control or palliate symptoms and provide support for informal carers. In such settings it is unlikely that consistent and well-resourced bereavement care is available beyond the practicalities and administration necessary for dealing with a deceased patient (Kissane 2000). In addition, professional boundaries, the discontinuities between care settings, and the relatively brief encounters that bereaved people can have with health professionals may contribute to both a neglect and paucity of bereavement care. This is particularly evident in acute hospital settings, where for example in the UK a common theme of complaints concerns the care provided to dying patients and the relationships between health care staff and family members following a patient's death (Healthcare Commission 2007).

It can be argued that bereavement has no part to play in health services and that nurses have no obligation to offer care to the bereaved beyond everyday compassion and the human desire to alleviate the suffering. There is also the criticism that as medicine provides a dominant framework to order death (Seale 1998), so bereavement may become subject to an equivalent regulation and expert clinical lore (Walter 1999). But bereavement has far-reaching consequences for people that can be detrimental to their well-being and health (Parkes 1998). While people may not choose to die in health care settings or the company of trained carers, many bereaved people have contact with and access to nurses both initially and following the death either through institutional or community based services. What this suggests is that nurses should be prepared for their encounters with people who are bereaved and should understand what role they may have in offering care and support within wider contexts of health promotion and care. This is a position familiar to those working in palliative and hospice care, but it is an area that has only recently received attention in mainstream and more acute health care (Department of Health 2005).

## Views of bereavement

Being bereaved is not a career, like teaching or acting. I can see that. But I wish it were. How much more comfortable if it were a recognised profession . . . I would like to be *engaged* in bereavement. An exacting job but a rewarding one, after the arduous period of preliminary training. Or even if it isn't a career there must be some ideal way of doing it.

(Bayley 2002 :213)

This chapter is premised on a palliative care philosophy that encompasses the bereaved within an overall remit of care that continues beyond a disease trajectory to encompass those who have to live with the consequences of death and the experience of bereavement (NCHSPCS 2002; NICE 2004). The exploration is based on an understanding of bereavement as a life event that requires people to revise and renegotiate the world (Parkes 2000). Many of the expectations, assumptions and meanings by which we navigate our lives and orientate ourselves can be invalidated as a result of bereavement. It therefore becomes necessary to relearn the world, not simply to take account of the absence of the person who has died, because the death of an individual can have a pervasive impact upon who we are and how we live. This requires attending to more than our internal world and may involve relearning the physical, temporal, spiritual and social aspects of our world (Attig 1996).

Relearning implies changing and this can be a creative, positive and fruitful journey. However, bereavement can also be a challenging or stressful transition in that it makes demands upon people beyond their resources as they attempt to deal with loss and renegotiate a meaningful life without the deceased. A recent empirically based model suggests that people may alternate between confronting the reality of loss and attending to the consequences of loss. This 'dual process' model proposes that bereaved people have to deal with two broad types of stressors – loss-orientated and restoration-orientated – and it recognizes that this dynamic process may include beneficial times in which people choose not to face or avoid aspects of loss (Stroebe and Schut 1999). This theoretical model integrates a range of existing ideas about bereavement and supports the differences and individuality that are evident in people's grieving. It is a model that informs the broad approach adopted in this chapter and it avoids some of the problematic assumptions, prescriptions and frameworks used by earlier models and theories (Wortman and Silver 2001).

In offering bereavement care and support we should be aware that we are guided and influenced not only by theories, but also by our own experiences, training, beliefs, attitudes and assumptions (Saunderson and Ridsdale 1999). In this sense, we have to acknowledge that while we stand in the company of the bereaved as professionals, we are also living with the losses characteristic of life some of which may be the result of death. Nurses need to develop and maintain a level of self-awareness and self-knowledge about areas of their own lives that are potential sources of difficulty or conflict in bereavement situations. People who are bereaved may become subject to the needs of the nurse who is living out, through either conscious or unconscious processes, their own bereavement. Equally nurses may develop strategies and practices that avoid or minimize the possibility or impact of caring for the bereaved when painful personal loss is evoked. There is a need therefore for nurses to be aware of the implicit boundaries in which care and support is offered. At one extreme, boundaries become effective barriers and at another, they become shaped by personal interests with a potential for a betrayal of trust, respect or intimacy that may be considered an abuse of the practitioner–client relationship (Nursing and Midwifery Council 2006). For these reasons nurses should ensure that their practice of bereavement care and support is the subject of clinical supervision, preceptorship or mentorship in which it can be safely and honestly explored.

# Respecting the diversity of individuals

All people have a finite future and death is an event that will apply to everyone. Bereavement, as the objective condition resulting from loss, can also be understood as a ubiquitous category. Standardized in this way, people who are bereaved can be expected to make conventional responses to loss and react to death in ways that can be reduced to explanatory theories and models. The logical consequence of this schema is that people who do not fit the accepted standard models present complications and abnormalities requiring interventions to resolve their deviant behaviour. However, the objectivity of death and bereavement required for their investigation and conceptualization is a limited and depersonalized perspective. The objective may appear to provide a vantage point in the care and support of the bereaved but it cannot provide an adequate position from which to appreciate the subjective value, meaning and impact of a particular death for the bereaved person.

In offering care and support to people who are bereaved we need to take the fullest possible account of the subjective view. However, if a theoretical view is necessarily insensitive to any individual, so a focus on the subjective view may not recognize any external references. People can also share much in common and their lives are inscribed through their social and cultural interactions and the contexts in which they live. Therefore, we may consider that a bereaved person is neither a predetermined abstract category nor a self-defining identity but an individual facing loss. A person in this situation will therefore draw upon his or her own unique understanding and experience which is embedded within a wider shared world in which people die. For these reasons becoming involved with bereaved people requires of us a broad understanding of the impact of loss upon personhood that is sensitive not only to psychological insights but also to other significant aspects of the person including history, gender, ethnicity (Field *et al.* 1997) and culture (Rees 2001).

# Dealing with the dead

The experience of a nurse in handling death and in understanding the necessary preparation and administration associated with a body for disposal can be a valuable and reassuring resource to those who are bereaved. In this situation the nurse can be a guide for those unfamiliar with what happens after death and an advocate for their wishes. In most countries the state has an interest in the cause of death and in the disposal of the dead body. Both of these can impose legal duties and limitations upon what happens to the dead body and health professionals may be required to act on behalf of the state to ensure these requirements are met.

A dead body is the location of a person who has died, the evidence of a fatal sequence and the site of decomposing material. The legal view of the body may trump the other perspectives but none should ignore the subjective impact of death upon the bereaved. In taking a more holistic and experiential perspective, a nurse may be well placed to support the bereaved in making choices about what happens to the body and in expressing their farewell. This requires sensitivity to personal needs and cultural/religious obligations, the dynamics of a mourning group, the limitations of certain contexts and the effect of bereavement upon the cognitive abilities of individuals.

It is helpful to establish if the people who are turned to for decisions about the dead body have any experience of this situation and if they have any particular expectations. Beliefs may come to play a key role at the time of death in relation to what is permissible and required. In addition the ethical framework by which people approach death may differ from the ethics of health care professionals or their institutions. Consequently, these should be carefully explored and understood by a nurse to avoid offence, to facilitate religious or cultural practices and to minimize the distress that may result from legal obligations, such as the requirement for a post-mortem examination or autopsy (Green and Green 2006).

People who are bereaved can easily be bewildered by the decisions they are required to make and the choices put before them about the person who has died. A nurse is often in an advantageous position in terms of information and access to key people in the post-mortem processes. This can be used with discernment to support and empower the bereaved in their responsibilities towards the person who has died in such things as involving them in last offices, providing access to chaplains or faith leaders, understanding their rights in relation to organ donation, and signposting sources of guidance and assistance in arranging a funeral.

# Sharing the story

Loss and change are unavoidable aspects of life and consequently people have to negotiate many types of disruptions and dislocations to their worlds over the years. In this sense bereavement is a normal situation that people find themselves in and which most will cope with and go on to reconstruct and revise their worlds. They do this without any particular professional intervention but they may often receive support and care from people they associate with and in whose circles they move. Family and friends, because of their proximity, can often be well placed to care for someone in their bereavement, providing accessible practical help as well as understanding companionship and a sympathetic ear. Such people can also be well placed to share in the storytelling about the loss and the person who has died. This narrative process may help people in transition to make some sort of sense and find meaning in their irreversibly changed world and lives. This human tendency to tell stories (in spoken and written form) can be both loss-orientated and restoration-orientated and Neimeyer and Anderson (2001) outline three types of narratives that seem to operate in accounts of loss:

- *External narratives*: these are accounts, descriptions and reports of what has happened. The objective form of these narratives provides ordered versions of external events from a personal perspective and therefore also relate to the storyteller. Descriptions of how the person died, reporting the actions of individuals and recounting what happened at the funeral are examples of external narratives.

- *Internal narratives*: these focus upon the affective responses to the death as experienced by the narrator or biographer. These self-expressions of what it feels like to experience the loss are emotion-based narratives and articulate the internal world of the bereaved person.

- *Reflexive narratives*: these build upon the primary narratives recalling what happened or expressing feeling and provide a secondary narrative of interpretation and reflection. Exploring the significance of the death, why it happened, and what the death means to the storyteller are examples of reflexive narratives.

Narratives of loss are ongoing projects and people who are bereaved may revise and revisit them individually and in association with others. Health professionals may also share in the stories of the bereaved because they may be part of the story. A person may need to establish a coherent account of how someone became ill and died with those who hold records of such events. A bereaved person may also feel confident in describing their feelings to someone who they expect might understand how people respond to loss. In this way a bereaved person may be checking out their own position and seeking validation for their feelings and thoughts. Finally, health professionals may also be turned to by a bereaved person in reflecting upon the meaning of the experience in terms of the past, present and future. A nurse involved in the care of the person who has died (directly or vicariously) may be considered by the bereaved person as someone who understands the context of loss and who therefore may be able to assist in conserving what has gone while negotiating what it means to live in the changed world.

The idea of storytelling can be considered a helpful approach to supporting bereaved people. Most people can tell stories and those who listen to stories do not require any particular expertise or specialist training, just the ability and time to listen. Stories can be told in the absence of other people through the written word and the internet provides a virtual world-wide space within which to share stories. But we must enter a caveat to this attractively simple proposition of support because some people will choose to remain solitary in their grief; a narrative may not be formed in spoken or written words; and silence may be just as important to someone as dialogue. If death imposes an absence, then for some people bereavement may not require anything to be said about it other than what is evident. Storytelling must not be an imperative to fill the silence. Equally we must resist the social convention of making people talk and we should question a professional convention that automatically refers the inarticulate to counsellors and therapists. Phillips suggests that the mourning process tends to make people more self-absorbed as well as in need of other people; however, he cautions that:

> If grief doesn't have a shareable story, if there is no convincing account of what happens to people when someone they know dies, grief will always be singular and secluding: as close as we can get to a private experience without it sounding nonsensical. When someone dies something is communicated to us that we cannot communicate. Hence the urgency that goes into making death a communal experience . . . The only taboo, where grief is concerned, is not experiencing it: not feeling it and performing it appropriately. There are no grief scandals in the way that there are sex scandals; there are only scandalous absences of grieving.
>
> (Phillips 2000: 257–8)

## Follow-up contact and aftercare

Most people do not die suddenly and from diagnosis to death both patients and carers may receive the support of professionals. Even death resulting from acute events and undiagnosed conditions can often be accompanied by a host of people paid to care. However, as we noted at the start of this chapter, many health services can come to a halt following a death. The exceptions to this are usually found in specialist services, of which palliative care is a particular example, and community services who are more likely to have to deal with long-term consequences of bereavement. What is evident is that some people who are bereaved experience the ending of what can be intensive levels of support and some may be offered support from new sources and for the first time.

Health services generally do not have the resources to offer more than a minimal amount of care and support to the bereaved. What care is offered is often targeted at those who are considered to be vulnerable to adverse bereavement outcomes and a risk assessment measure is used to identify susceptible people (Aranda and Milne 2000) (see the chapter by Relf). However, in the immediate period following a death there are many tasks that require the involvement of the bereaved, principally the funeral, which brings them to the attention of others and which can establish a transient cluster of support and people to turn to for help and advice. But within weeks this level of support has usually withdrawn and bereaved people may experience a further ending of care.

What may help bereaved people through these significant transitions of care and supportive company are relatively simple follow-up contacts. These can take the form of one-off meetings, domiciliary visits, telephone calls, letters and cards. The purpose of these contacts can include: the expression of concern into the well-being of the bereaved; an opportunity for the bereaved to say something of their current feelings and experiences; the opportunity to raise questions or concerns either about the death or the bereavement; the provision of information about sources of bereavement support in the community; the offer of further follow-up; and a means of ending the involvement of a service. Follow-up contacts should form part of a systematic approach to bereavement by services so that they are coordinated and adequately supported by staff. A bereavement aftercare programme introduced into one emergency department sends a letter to the named next of kin four to six weeks after the death. They are offered the opportunity to talk with a medical consultant about the death of their relative either in the department or over the telephone. Approximately one in seven of the next of kin accept the offer to talk with a consultant, the majority of which (81 per cent) happen in the department (Parris *et al.* 2007). In a study into the impact of a supportive telephone call, the bereaved people contacted mainly perceived the contact as positive in that it provided them with emotional support as well as the opportunity to ask questions about the illness and death (Kaunonen *et al.* 2000). The follow-up and aftercare services being reported are clearly supported by staff but to date there are insufficient systematic studies into their efficacy and benefit for people who are bereaved.

# Bereavement counselling and therapy

Bereavement results in diverse reactions of people with considerable variability in the manifestations of grief. Within this spectrum it is recognized that a minority of people (Bonano and Kaltman 2001) experience difficulties in their grieving to the extent that there may be a justification for psychological or pharmacological interventions. Persisting, troubling and excessive aspects of common grief which impair functioning may constitute a distinctive syndrome known as complicated grief, which can be understood as a state of chronic mourning such that, '[r]ecurrent, intrusive and distressing thoughts about the absence of the deceased make it difficult for persons with Complicated Grief Disorder to concentrate and to move beyond an acute state of mourning and live in the present' (Zhang *et al.* 2006). However, the natural response of health care professionals to want to help is offset by the lack of insufficient systematic evidence to date on which bereavement interventions are effective, with the exception of the pharmacological treatment of depression occurring in the context of bereavement (Forte *et al.* 2004).

People may be identified before a death has occurred as being in a high-risk category in terms of developing morbidities and disorders post-bereavement. This may be based upon assessing a range of factors or variables that may predict a poor bereavement outcome (Stroebe *et al.* 2006) (see the chapter by Relf). Screening for adverse outcomes may result in referrals to professionals who offer medical or psychological interventions. However, it may be much later after the death that a bereaved person feels that they are in difficulty or that they present to a health professional with symptoms of complicated grief. A common source of help for these people is counselling which is widely available through GP practices, voluntary agencies and private practices in the UK. A review of counselling in primary care in England concluded from the current evidence that it is more effective than usual care in the short-term but appears to provide no long-term benefits (Bower and Rowland 2006). In relation to people who have been referred to counselling because of their bereavement another review reported that while people with uncomplicated grief fail to derive benefits, '[n]evertheless, there are bereaved individuals who need help and who derive benefits from grief counseling and therapy. Most typically, these are individuals who have been unable to cope with their loss and for whom the grief reaction has in some way "gone wrong" ' (Stroebe *et al.* 2005).

## Support and care beyond health professionals

We have considered some of the general ways in which those who care for the dying may also care for the bereaved. There are some unique benefits that may be associated with professionals who become involved with people prior to death being able to offer some support to them in their bereavement. However, most people leave behind care settings or services and they face their bereavement not in the company of professionals but in the context of family, friends and the social networks provided in places of work, residence and the communities with which they associate. Health professionals need to be aware of the resources of support and care that may be available to bereaved people once they have returned to the places in which their lives continue.

Formal (paid) care of the bereaved may be provided through social care workers including professionally qualified social workers. Bereavement can be a significant aspect of social care services either because service users have experienced loss in this way or there is need for social care input as a result of a death (Currer 2001). However, much of the support available to bereaved people comes from voluntary and non-statutory organizations. One of the best-known voluntary community services in the UK is provided by the national charity Cruse Bereavement Care, who offer support through a network of over 178 branches and 6,300 trained volunteers. Cruse offers free information and advice to anyone who has been affected by a death; provides support and counselling one to one and in groups; offers education, support, information and publications to anyone supporting bereaved people; and increases public awareness of the needs of bereaved people through campaigning and information services (Cruse 2007).

Many national and local bereavement care resources have been established to meet the needs of specific groups. Winston's Wish is a charity offering support throughout the UK to bereaved children and young people through a national telephone helpline, practical resources and publications, and training and consultancy services for those working with bereaved families and those wishing to set up a grief support service in their own area (Winston's Wish 2007). More information about childhood bereavement services can be found in the chapter by Rolls. Another example is The Way Foundation which provides a self-help social and support network to people bereaved under the age of 50 and their children (Way Foundation 2007).

Bereaved people frequently come into contact with religious and cultural communities for the practical reason of arranging a funeral. These communities provide rituals, ceremonies and customs around death but many also offer some form of bereavement support. In Judaism, for example, the first seven days of intense mourning (*Shiva*) is a period in which the bereaved are exempt from the requirements of daily life and the Jewish community demonstrate practical care and condolence in the provision of meals (Rees 2001). In addition, there are Jewish support networks and counselling services. Christian churches, whose ministers conduct the majority of funerals, provide pastoral care to bereaved people and there are church-based bereavement visiting schemes offering community support through trained volunteers (Billings 2002).

Finally, the virtual community of the internet provides access for many people to a wealth of information and advice to help them in their bereavement, as well as a route to obtain personal support. The style, quality and up-to-date nature of the contents varies widely. There are sites provided by national organizations that provide practical information, such as www.bereavementadvice.org. In contrast, there are sites developed from personal experiences that many people will find helpful. www.ifishoulddie.co.uk was created following the death of the author's father. The site provides much practical information including details about the legal requirements following a death, organizing a funeral and a section on understanding and coping with grief (if i should die 2007). www.merrywidow.me.uk is a web-published guide for bereaved women needing clear practical advice based upon the author's experience following the death of her husband at the age of 37 (Merrywidow 2007).

# Conclusion

This chapter has brought together two major themes. The first derives from the fact that people die while known to health care services and that, therefore, these services have a responsibility for providing care and support to people who are bereaved. The second is derived from the changing views of scholars and clinicians who recognize that, in response to the death of someone significant to them, a bereaved person becomes involved in a dynamic process of relearning a changed world and reconstructing meaning in order to live with the experience of loss. Together these themes suggest a creative and challenging agenda for nursing and its important contribution to the care and support of bereaved people in terms of training, practice, service development and research. If most people begin their bereavement in the company of nurses, then nurses are uniquely placed in relation to the care of bereaved people and the contexts in which death occurs.

Storytelling can play an important role in the lives of bereaved people in their search to 'make sense' of what has happened and to assimilate their experience of loss into their life story. The challenge is that, '[l]ike a novel that loses a central character in the middle chapters, the life story disrupted by loss must be reorganized, rewritten, to find a new strand of continuity that bridges the past with the future in an intelligible fashion' (Neimeyer 2000: 263). The biographical nature of this narrative indicates each person's unique and varied response to bereavement. Storytelling reminds us that bereavement has a social context and involves other people. By implication, an important question for nurses concerns what narratives inform their understanding of bereavement and the care they offer bereaved people. Equally, we need to pay attention to whose language prevails: the person facing loss or the nurse who frames bereavement with professional and personal meanings?

Whatever the particular interests and skills of individual nurses, professional and service boundaries can impose their own disruption and discontinuity upon bereaved people. People who are bereaved can therefore find themselves estranged from both the context in which death has taken place and those professionals who they may expect to understand what it is that they are experiencing. Follow-up programmes, even of a basic form, that have been well thought through and, if properly organized, may offer an important element of continuity to bereaved people. However, it is also important that nurses should be actively aware of the resources available in the community to support bereaved people and be able to access relevant advice and information. None of this is to suggest that the care and support of bereaved people is a responsibility that nurses alone should be expected to hold, but neither is it one that they should neglect.

# References

Aranda, S. and Milne, D. (2000) *Guidelines for the assessment of complicated bereavement risk in family member of people receiving palliative care*. Melbourne: Centre for Palliative Care.

Attig, T. (1996) *How We Grieve: Relearning the World*. New York: Oxford University Press.

Bayley, J. (2002) *Widower's House*. London: Abacus.

Billings, A. (2002) *Dying and Grieving: A Guide to Pastoral Ministry*. London: SPCK.

Bonano, G. and Kaltman, S. (2001) Varieties of grief experience. *Clinical Psychology Review*, 21(5): 709.

Bower, P. and Rowland, N. (2006) Effectiveness and cost effectiveness of counselling in primary care. *Cochrane Database of Systematic Reviews*, 3: CD001025.

Cruse (2007) http://www.crusebereavementcare.org.uk.

Currer, C. (2001) *Responding to Grief: Dying, Bereavement and Social Care*. Basingstoke: Palgrave.

Department of Health (2005) *When a Patient Dies: Advice on Developing Bereavement Services*. London: Department of Health.

Dougherty, L. and Lister, S. (eds) (2004) *The Royal Marsden Hospital Manual of Clinical Nursing Procedures*. Oxford: Blackwell.

Field, D., Hockey, J. and Small, N. (eds) (1997) *Death, gender and ethnicity*. London: Routledge.

Forte, A.L., Hill, M., Pazder, R. and Feudtner, C. (2004) Bereavement care interventions: a systematic review. *BMC Palliative Care*, 3: 3.

Green, J. and Green, M. (2006) *Dealing with Death: A Handbook of Practices, Procedures and Law*. London: Jessica Kingsley.

Healthcare Commission (2007) *Spotlight on Complaints*. London: Commission for Healthcare Audit and Inspection.

if i should die (2007) http://www.ifishoulddie.co.uk (accessed July 2007).

Kaunonen, M., Tarkka, M-T., Laippala, P. and Paunonen-Ilmonen, M. (2000) The Impact of Supportive Telephone Call Intervention on Grief After the Death of a Family Member. *Cancer Nursing*, 23(6): 483–91.

Kissane, D.W. (2000) Neglect of bereavement care in general hospitals. *Medical Journal of Australia*, 173(9): 456.

Merrywidow (2007) http://www.merrywidow.me.uk/ (accessed July 2007).

NCHSPCS (National Council for Hospice and Specialist Palliative Care Services) (2002) *Definitions of Supportive and Palliative Care: Briefing Paper 11*. London: National Council for Hospice and Specialist Palliative Care Services.

NICE (National Institute for Clinical Excellence) (2004) *Improving Supportive and Palliative Care for Adults with Cancer*. London: National Institute for Clinical Excellence.

Neimeyer, R.A. (ed.) (2000) *Meaning Reconstruction and the Experience of Loss*. Washington: American Psychological Association.

Neimeyer, R.A. and Anderson, A. (2001) Meaning Reconstruction Theory. In: N. Thompson (ed.) *Loss and Grief: A Guide for Human Services Practitioners*. Basingstoke: Palgrave.

Nursing & Midwifery Council (NMC) (2006) *Registrant/client relationships and the prevention of abuse*. London: Nursing and Midwifery Council.

Parkes, C.M. (1998) Coping with loss: Bereavement in adult life. *British Medical Journal*, 216: 856–9.

Parris, R.J., Schlosenberg, J., Stanley, C., Maurice, S. and Clarke, S.F.J. (2007) Emergency department follow-up of bereaved relatives: an audit of one particular service. *Emergency Medicine Journal*, 24: 339–42.

Phillips, A. (2000) *Promises, Promises*. London: Faber and Faber.

Rees, D. (2001) *Death and Bereavement: The psychological, religious and cultural interfaces*. London: Whurr.

Saunderson, E.M. and Ridsdale, L. (1999) General practitioner's beliefs and attitudes about how to respond to death and bereavement: qualitative study. *British Medical Journal*, 319: 292–6.

Seale, C. (1998) *Constructing Death: The Sociology of Dying and Bereavement.* Cambridge: Cambridge University Press.

Stroebe, M. and Schut, H. (1999) The Dual Process Model of Coping with Bereavement: Rationale and Description. *Death Studies*, 23: 197–224.

Stroebe, W., Schut, H. and Stroebe, M.S. (2005) Grief work, disclosure and counseling: Do they help the bereaved? *Clinical Psychology Review*, 25: 395–414.

Stroebe, M.S., Folkman, S., Hansson, R.O. and Schut, H. (2006) The prediction of bereavement outcome: Development of an integrative risk factor framework. *Social Science & Medicine*, 63(9): 2440–51.

Walter, T. (1999) *On Bereavement: The Culture of Grief.* Buckingham: Open University Press.

Way Foundation (2007) http://www.wayfoundation.org.uk (accessed May 2007).

Winston's Wish (2007) http://www.winstonswish.org.uk/ (accessed June 2007).

Wortman, C.B. and Silver, R.C. (2001) The Myths of Coping with Loss Revisited. In: M.S. Stroebe, R.O. Hansson, W. Stroebe and H. Schut (eds) *Handbook of Bereavement Research: Consequences Coping and Care.* Washington: American Psychological Association.

Zhang, B., El-Jawahri, A. and Prigerson, H.G. (2006) Update on Bereavement Research: Evidence-Based Guidelines for the Diagnosis and Treatment of Complicated Bereavement. *Journal of Palliative Medicine*, 9(5): 1188–203.

# 24

# Risk assessment and adult bereavement services

*Marilyn Relf*

---

**Key points**

- Factors that account for diversity in grief experiences.
- Assessment of risk, vulnerability and resilience.
- Problems associated with current assessment methods.
- Implications for palliative care bereavement services.

---

There is substantial evidence that bereavement is associated with risks to health and well-being. However, experiences vary; while most people suffer intense grief after a significant bereavement, many adapt well and only a minority suffer long-term problems. One line of enquiry has focused on identifying the factors that influence the course of grief. If we can predict those who may be more vulnerable, or 'at risk', then it may be possible to intervene to prevent 'pathological' or 'complicated' grief by offering appropriate help. This chapter explores 'risk' in relation to bereavement, risk factors and their use in palliative care. Can we predict those who may need help? If so, what are the implications for bereavement services and are methods pioneered in palliative care transferable to other health care settings?

---

## Bereavement and health

The relationship between health and illness is increasingly explained in terms of risk (Petersen and Lupton 1996). A major focus has been to identify personal characteristics, behaviours and environments that predispose individuals to ill health. The health consequences of bereavement have been widely investigated. Bereaved people frequently experience short-term health problems often arising from behavioural change such as poor diet, altered sleep patterns and increased use of alcohol. Bereavement may negatively affect the endocrine (Kim and Jacobs 1993) and immune systems particularly among those who are depressed (Irwin and Pike 1993). A substantial minority of bereaved people are at elevated risk of experiencing persisting physical and mental health problems (Stroebe and Schut 2001) including depression, anxiety and poor general health. It is not surprising that bereaved people visit doctors more frequently and increase their use of psychotropic drugs.

Lasting poor health is viewed as an indicator that grief has become 'pathological' (Parkes 1990) or 'complicated' and identifying the factors that influence the course of grief is a major theme of bereavement research. A number of early prospective studies found that those who had enduring problems shared common characteristics that were apparent soon after bereavement. Parkes (1981) and Raphael (1977) used these 'risk factors' to assess vulnerability and provided evidence that counselling could reduce health risks from 'high' to 'low'. While 'bereavement counselling' is often used indiscriminately to refer to a range of interventions from befriending through to therapy, there is little evidence that untargeted bereavement services are effective (Schut and Stroebe 2005).

NICE (2004) views assessment as integral to palliative care bereavement services and recommends a three-component model of service provision. All bereaved people should receive information about grief and how to access services. A small group may need the level of support that can be provided by volunteers and a minority may need specialist counselling or therapy. In practice, the distinction between specialist bereavement services provided by volunteers and professional counselling services is not always clear. However, the principle that different levels of need should be identified is now widely endorsed (Davies and Higginson 2004). Estimates of need vary but the consensus is that up to 20 per cent of bereaved widows and widowers experience complicated grief (Jacobs 1993).

Relf *et al.* (in press) summarize the rationale for assessing need in palliative care as follows:

- Palliative care encompasses family needs and is well placed to provide continuity of care after bereavement.
- Offering support proactively may minimize the health risks associated with bereavement.
- Support should be channelled towards those who are more vulnerable.
- Assessment can clarify concerns and support decision-making about the type and level of help that may be needed.

Bereavement assessment developed within a philosophical framework that is often referred to as a 'medical model'. In this view, vulnerability is predictable and measurable and intervention is a form of treatment to prevent, or cure, 'pathological' grief. Silverman and Klass (1996) argue that traditional models of grief are also framed within this paradigm. Such models view 'healthy' adjustment as dependent on the capacity of the individual to 'work through' a 'normal' grief process, encompassing experiencing emotional pain and detaching from the deceased. Both failure to engage (absent or delayed grief), and failure to disengage (chronic grief), with this process is conceptualized as dysfunctional and predictive of poor health (Parkes and Weiss 1983). According to this view, intervention should encourage people to work through their grief (Worden 2003). Before exploring criticisms of this 'grief work' model (Wortman and Silver 1989; Stroebe 1992; Klass *et al.* 1996) and the implications for assessment, I will first provide an overview of risk factors.

# Risk factors

There are a number of detailed reviews of the extensive literature on risk factors (Aranda and Milne 2000; Stroebe and Schut 2001). These reviews conclude that differences in outcome are influenced by the:

- events and circumstances surrounding the death
- meaning of the relationship with the deceased
- internal resources of the individual
- quality of social support and external resources.

In summary, risk factors are the characteristics of bereaved people and the features of their situation that increase the probability of vulnerability (Parkes 1990). There are three groups of risk factors: situational, personal and environmental, and in the following section I will highlight key findings. I will use 'family' broadly to include those who have strong emotional and social ties with the deceased. It should be noted that the literature is limited; most studies focus on widowhood and have been carried out in the USA with a smaller number undertaken in the UK, Australia, Germany and the Netherlands.

## Situational factors

These factors reflect the circumstances surrounding the death and the impact of concurrent life events.

### Circumstances of the death

There is conflicting evidence about the influence of the mode of the death. Some studies have found that sudden, untimely or violent bereavements may be more difficult than those that are anticipated. Sudden death is associated with persisting feelings of shock, disbelief and anxiety (Stroebe *et al.* 1988). Violent or accidental deaths may cause post-traumatic stress disorder with high levels of anxiety, flashbacks and nightmares. Suicide is associated with high levels of anger and guilt and the associated stigma may decrease social support.

It is often argued that anticipated losses are less problematic because a period of forewarning provides a context for understanding that loss is inevitable and offers an opportunity to make amends, to take a gradual leave taking and to begin to grieve and adjust. Caring for the patient may also be a positive experience and the death may bring feelings of relief. However, forewarning is not always related to outcome (Cleiren *et al.* 1988) and a protracted terminal illness, such as cancer, is also associated with increased health risks (Sanders 1983). Cleiren (1991), comparing the impact of road traffic accidents, suicide and long-term illness, concluded that mode of death was too general a risk factor and not as important as coping strategies and social support.

### Concurrent life events

People facing multiple crises, such as other losses or financial difficulties, may experience more stress-related health problems (Sanders 1993). It is difficult, however, to disentangle the relationship between bereavement, socio-economic factors and health because of the main effect of deprivation, poor housing and low socio-economic status on health in the general population.

### **Personal factors**

These factors are concerned with what the individual brings to the experience; their life experience, history and personality.

### Age

As people get older they experience more ill health. However, bereavement studies indicate that younger widows and widowers have higher mortality and increased morbidity. These differences may be explained by the concept of 'timeliness' (Parkes 1996); bereavement later in life may be less distressing because it fits societal expectations about longevity. Older people may receive more support because their friends are also more likely to have experienced bereavement. However, there is evidence that older people also experience psychological problems (Gallagher-Thompson *et al.* 1993). For example, Sanders (1981) found that while younger people react to bereavement with greater shock and emotional intensity, older people experience problems arising from isolation and loneliness.

### Gender

Studies that compare widows and widowers with non-bereaved married people consistently show significant differences between the health of widowers and married men but not between widows and married women. These findings are usually explained by gender differences in use of social support. Widowers may have relied on their partners to maintain social contacts (Stroebe and Stroebe 1983) and may find it difficult to seek support (Wortman *et al.* 1993). Moreover, in some cultures (such as the UK) men may be socialized to hide distress in order to conform to masculine ideals (Riches and Dawson 1997).

### Relationship to the deceased

The loss of a close relationship, such as a spouse, parent or child, is related to greater vulnerability. However, the subjective meaning of the lost relationship is more important than the degree of kinship (Neimayer 2000).

### Pre-existing health

Poor health may be exacerbated by the stress of bereavement.

### Personality

Relatively few studies have focused directly on the relationship between personality and grief. There is evidence that people who are insecure, anxious, have low self-esteem (Parkes and Weiss 1983), low self-trust (Parkes 1990) or who cope by denial (Sanders 1981), or extreme self-reliance (Parkes 1990) are likely to find bereavement more problematic. Personality factors indicative of resilience include the ability to communicate feelings and thoughts to others, high self-esteem and personal competency (Lund *et al.* 1993).

Personality traits influence the quality of relationships. Both dependent and ambivalent relationships are associated with vulnerability. Parkes and Weiss (1983) found that intense clinging is associated with a 'grief prone personality' and protracted high levels of distress or 'chronic' grief. People in dependent relationships may have little support outside the primary relationship (Cleiren 1991). Grief may be 'conflicted' following the loss of an ambivalent relationship. Feelings of relief may be accompanied by guilt at not having been able to resolve difficulties. According to attachment theory (Bowlby 1980), the security of childhood attachment bonds has a powerful influence on personality, the nature of adult relationships and vulnerability to loss. Parkes (2006) provides evidence to support these claims in a retrospective study of people referred to psychiatric care for bereavement therapy.

### Spiritual and religious beliefs

Spiritual and religious beliefs are associated with resilience following bereavement. However, the evidence is weak because of methodological flaws in many studies. Moreover, the majority of studies have been undertaken in the USA where religious beliefs are more widespread than in the UK and many other European countries (Becker *et al.* 2007).

### Environmental factors

Environmental factors reflect the social and cultural context of individual loss. This includes the family and wider social network and the influence of culture on attitudes and beliefs about grief.

#### Social support

Social integration and support is a significant factor in resilience (Greene 2002) and there is general agreement that the perception that social support is inadequate is a robust indicator of vulnerability. A number of factors influence the availability of social support following bereavement:

- Bereavement may deprive individuals of their main source of emotional support and geographical mobility may mean that family and close friends are not easily accessible (Stroebe *et al.* 1988).

- Members of social networks do not necessarily grieve in similar ways, they may lack the emotional energy to help each other and bereavement may precipitate a network crisis (Stylianos and Vachon 1993). Family members may avoid talking about problems because they do not want to burden each other (Cleiren 1991) and family discord is a common source of additional stress. Family therapy provided pre-bereavement to families with high levels of conflict can promote resilience (Kissane and Bloch 2002).

- Although grief is universal, the way it is expressed varies across cultures (Parkes *et al.* 1997). In postmodern societies a decline in ritual is believed to contribute to a lack of shared understanding and is associated with anxiety and adjustment problems. For example, in the UK, despite professional beliefs that expressing feelings is helpful, the prevailing norm is to keep grief private and great value is placed on self-reliance, independence and autonomy (Walter 1999). Revealing feelings may be equated to weakness and bereaved people may feel that they should suppress emotions and hide distress. These social norms influence the behaviour of both men and women (Riches and Dawson 1997; Martin and Doka 2000).

- Anxiety about responding inappropriately may inhibit helping behaviour and block expressions of concern (Lehman *et al.* 1986).

- Grief may be 'disenfranchised' (Doka 1989) if the lost relationship is not acknowledged or socially sanctioned, e.g. the loss of a lover or same-sex partner.

- The ability to mobilize or use social support may be influenced by pre-existing personality traits. Bereaved people who are angry, inconsolable or depressed may be less likely to seek support and may alienate or exhaust supporters (Stroebe and Stroebe 1987). Some people attract warmth and compassion while others perceive hostility when none is intended and feel that their needs are not being met despite the good intentions of others. Helpers are likely to withdraw if they feel their support attempts are not helpful (Schilling 1987).

### *Summary*

Risk factors may be divided into three groups: situational, personal and environmental (Figure 24.1). The key areas for assessment for each group are given in Table 24.1. The relative impact of individual risk factors and the interaction between them is unclear. For example, age and kinship may be less important than the quality and meaning of the lost relationship. The

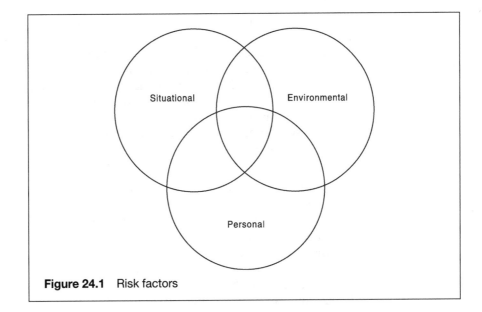

**Figure 24.1**   Risk factors

**Table 24.1**   Key areas for assessment

| *Risk factors* | *Key areas for assessment* |
| --- | --- |
| **Situational** | • How did the individual experience and react to the illness and death? <br> • Are there any concurrent life events that may cause additional stress? |
| **Personal** | • Who has been lost? What is the meaning of the lost relationship? <br> • How is the individual's life experience and personality affecting their reactions and way of coping? <br> • Are there any pre-existing psychological or physical health problems? |
| **Environmental** | • How much support is available and to what extent is it perceived as helpful? |

importance of beliefs, attitudes and cultural factors such as the norms that influence the expression of grief are important but have received little attention.

# Assessing vulnerability

Traditionally it has been assumed that an accumulation of risk factors increases vulnerability. Parkes emphasizes the interrelationship of risk factors as follows:

> Statistical studies confirm what common sense leads one to suspect – that secure people whose experience of life has led to a reasonable trust in themselves, and others, will cope well with anticipated bereavements, provided they are well supported by a family who respects their need to grieve. However, multiple or unexpected and untimely losses of people on whom one depends or who depended on the survivor can overwhelm the most secure person and lack of security and support can undermine a person's capacity to cope with all types of bereavement.
>
> (Parkes 1990: 309)

Figure 24.1 provides a simple diagram to illustrate this interrelationship and how the cumulative presence of risk factors may be used to decide the level of support needed. Thus, those in the centre may need therapeutic counselling, those in the overlapping areas may benefit from supportive counselling and those with few factors present are unlikely to need external help.

Checklists of risk factors have been used to assess need in relation to bereavement since the 1980s. The Bereavement Risk Index (Parkes 1981; Parkes and Weiss 1983), and variations of it, are widely used in palliative care in the UK (Payne and Relf 1994), in Australia (Gibson and Graham 1991) and in the USA (Beckwith *et al.* 1990; Levy *et al.* 1992). In the UK and USA nurses usually have responsibility for making assessments and volunteers are widely involved in providing support (Demmer 2003; Field *et al.* 2004). Risk factors may be used to assess the needs of people seeking help after bereavement and measures have been developed to assess complicated grief (Prigerson *et al.* 1995; Jordan *et al.* 2005).

Although routine assessment using formal methods is highly recommended in the literature, a recent study in the UK found that this is not always adopted in practice (Field *et al.* 2004). Half of UK palliative care bereavement services do not use formal methods to assess need but adopt a universalistic approach and offer support to all. However, the study also found evidence that these services were more proactive in contacting those who caused staff to feel particularly concerned. Such decision-making relied on clinical experience and 'gut feelings'. It would seem that for a large number of services in the UK the assessment of need is rather ad hoc and the evidence suggests that there may be problems in routinely applying research findings about risk in practice. I will refer to the UK to illustrate what these problems may be.

## Problems with current methods of assessment in the UK

1   The diversity of grief is increasingly recognized. In order to be responsive to individual needs, UK bereavement services are urged to offer a multiplicity of supportive strategies (Bereavement Care Standards 2001). There may be a tension between providing choice and accessible services and assessing need. Formal methods of assessment may be viewed as limiting access. For example, Payne and Relf (1994) found that nurses had concerns about withholding services from people who may need them.

2   Assessment relies on nurses' knowledge and understanding of families and care-givers as well as patients. However, there is evidence that pre-bereavement work with family members may be limited by constraints on time, skills and resources. Attending to psychosocial needs may be given low priority (Field *et al.* 1992) and information may be inadequate or inaccurate (Agnew *et al.* 2007). Pottinger (1991), for example, found that those who wanted support, but did not receive it, showed marked feelings of anxiety and intense grief. The time available to work with relatives as well as patients may be limited and lack of time may mean that the focus of care is inevitably on the patient rather than on the family, making it difficult to carry out assessments. Education to support assessment may be lacking or inconsistent (Agnew *et al.* 2007).

3   Assessment relies on care-givers being prepared to talk about themselves at a time when their energies are often focused on the patient. In addition, nurses may fear that asking questions pertaining to assessment will be intrusive (Payne and Relf 1994).

4   Studies of the Bereavement Risk Index (BRI) suggest that it has limited reliability. In the USA, Beckwith *et al.* (1990) found that the index was predictive of outcome only at three months after bereavement. Levy *et al.* (1992) found that the BRI has low internal consistency and concluded that it is flawed.
    The lack of reliability may reflect a number of factors. Following the BRI, assessment checklists include difficult to rate concepts such as 'unusual' levels of anger or guilt. This means that objectivity may be undermined; what one nurse considers 'unusual' may be 'normal' to another. The BRI was derived from the Harvard Bereavement Study in the USA (Parkes and Weiss 1983). This study focused on an atypical group of young widows and widowers (mean age 45) and the BRI may lack sensitivity across cultures, with older people or with non-spouses. Similarly, many studies of the relationship between bereavement and

health have focused on the experiences of younger widows, often obtaining low response rates and relying on self-report. These problems with the reliability of research findings have been described elsewhere (Payne *et al.* 1999).

5   The scope of checklists is limited to factors associated with vulnerability. Factors that may increase resilience, such as secure attachment or positive reappraisal, have only recently received attention (Bonanno *et al.* 2004). The coping processes and pathways between the experience of bereavement and outcome have also been neglected (Stroebe *et al.* 2006).

6   Informal methods are more likely to be associated with an inconsistent approach to needs assessment and offers of bereavement support may be ad hoc and influenced by personal assumptions.

Despite these problems, assessment can be remarkably consistent. Relf and Lines (2005) examined records of assessment decisions over a 13-year period in one UK hospice. The proportion of main carers assessed as 'at risk' was approximately 40 per cent per annum.

To summarize, making decisions about who may be vulnerable after bereavement is a complex process that relies on nurses' knowledge of risk factors and having sufficient time and skills to work with family members. While the need to target ongoing support is widely accepted, current methods are problematic and widely used formal tools lack reliability and are limited in scope. It is not surprising that there is discontent with existing methods (Agnew *et al.* 2007). Suggestions for improving assessment tools include incorporating measures of resilience (Payne and Relf 1994).

## Implications for practice

Given these problems, is assessment feasible? One solution would be to abandon assessment and either to offer support to all or to wait for people to seek help. Offering support to all would be resource consuming and ignores the evidence that the majority of people will not need ongoing help. Systematically contacting all bereaved people involves assessment decisions (such as deciding who to contact in a family). Rather than abandoning the practice, there are good reasons to seek to improve it.

First, it is important to clarify the place of assessment within practice. As described earlier, both assessment and intervention have been framed within a paradigm that considers behaviour to be measurable and predictable. However, this view is simplistic. Many factors influence the way individuals express grief and pathological grief can no longer be thought of as a unitary concept. Models that conceptualize grief as primarily an emotional, linear process of stages or phases are too narrow. It is now accepted that 'normal' grief is multidimensional (Shuchter and Zisook 1993). Bereavement affects cognitive processes as well as emotions, is experienced within a social context and may influence behaviour, social interaction, role

performance, self-esteem and spiritual beliefs. These theoretical developments change our understanding of normal and complicated grief and
'risk'.

Studies of childhood and parental grief have demonstrated that adjustment does not depend on severing attachment bonds (Klass *et al.* 1996). This
means that there may not be a definite point that marks 'recovery' or
'closure'. Successful mourning does not involve relinquishing attachment.
Important relationships continue to influence us whether or not the person is
physically present. Mourning involves understanding the meaning of the
loss and all that has happened (Walter 1996). This is not merely a cognitive
process but also a 'tacit, passionate process that unfolds in a social field'
(Neimeyer 2000: 552). In palliative care, an important aspect of support may
be to help mourners to mobilize their own resources and to make sense of
all that has happened to them on the roller coaster journey from diagnosis to
the reality of living without the deceased. Neimeyer and Anderson (2002)
describe personal 'stories' as having three elements:

- what happened and when (external narrative)
- the personal impact of events (internal events)
- the way that the person makes sense of the experience (reflexive
  narrative).

Asking questions about these different aspects of narrative helps to identify
resilience and vulnerability (Relf *et al.* in press).

Stroebe and Schut (1999) conceptualize grief as a dual process. Bereaved
people cope by oscillating between behaviour that is focused on their loss
(e.g. thinking about the deceased, pining, holding onto memories, expressing
feelings) and behaviour that is focused on managing everyday life (e.g. sup-
pressing memories and taking 'time off' from grief, keeping busy, regulating
emotions). Neither mode is inferior and the degree of oscillation is influenced
by such factors as personality, gender and cultural background. This model
suggests that avoidance of emotion may be functional rather than problematic. However, as in traditional models, coping behaviour that focuses
exclusively on emotional expression (chronic grief) or on distraction (absent
grief) is seen as problematic.

Martin and Doka (2000) argue that personality has a major influence on
ways of experiencing and expressing grief. People who are primarily in touch
with their feelings experience 'intuitive' grief as described in the traditional
models. However, people who are primarily thinkers experience grief as a
cognitive process or 'instrumental' grief. They prefer to cope by seeking information, thinking through problems, taking action and seeking diversion.
Most people will have one mode as dominant and the other as subordinate.
However, 'instrumental' grief may be viewed as problematic rather than
functional. For example, controlling emotions may be seen as indicative of
successful coping by some people but be judged as risky by professionals
who rely on traditional models to inform their work. Martin and Doka
(2000) suggest that helpers should seek to understand and validate individual

ways of coping to enable people to build on their strengths while developing their range of coping strategies.

These developments point to the importance of individual coping resources as a major factor in determining resilience and vulnerability. Adults have preferred ways of coping with life events and one way to improve assessment is to consider how individuals are responding to the demands of their situation. Individual coping resources mediate between the presence of risk factors and health outcomes, and assessment will be improved if coping processes are taken into account (Stroebe *et al.* 2006). This approach has not been tested. However, a recent UK guidance for specialist palliative care bereavement services suggests a framework to assess need by focusing on coping (Relf *et al.* in press). This framework draws on Machin's 'Range of Responses to Loss' (Machin 2006). The guidance includes a pathway for assessing need and stresses that family assessment will be improved if it:

- is based on conversations with family members as well as observations
- is supported by education and training
- is ongoing from first point of contact with palliative care rather than 'one-off' after bereavement.

In palliative care, the regular review of the psychosocial needs of both care-givers and patients will contribute to improved decision-making in relation to bereavement support. Those who are likely to be more vulnerable should be offered support by skilled people whose understanding of grief goes beyond a simplistic notion of stage models of grief. It is important that individuals who do not want support should not feel pressured into accepting help. While great care should to be taken to avoid pathologizing grief by offering counselling services to those who do not need them, it should also be recognized that many people will want to check out that their reactions are 'normal'. They are unlikely to need professional support and volunteer services aimed at listening, understanding and helping people to mobilize their own resources are likely to support resilience.

How transferable are methods of bereavement needs assessment pioneered in palliative care to acute health care? Clearly it will be more difficult to assess vulnerability in settings where psychosocial needs are a low priority and the patient is the focus of care rather than the family. However, understanding the factors that influence the course of grief, particularly the importance of the circumstances surrounding the death, can help to ensure care-giver's needs are recognized. What happens at times of crisis is very important and poor communication, failures, frustration and suffering will be remembered and dwelt on after bereavement. Written information about grief and signposting of support services should always be provided.

# Conclusion

The health consequences of bereavement are well documented. Both assessment and intervention have been conceptualized within a framework that views the course of grief as predictable. Risk factors relating to lasting health problems after bereavement may be divided into three groups: situational, personal and environmental. Strong arguments have been made that these should be used to assess need in order to channel resources to those who may be more vulnerable. Assessment is recommended as integral to specialist palliative care. Currently, decisions are made either by relying on clinical judgement or by using more formal methods involving assessment checklists. A number of factors have been considered that limit the reliability of these methods. Needs assessment may be improved by incorporating it into an ongoing process of assessment of individual and family coping that begins pre-bereavement and considers resilience alongside vulnerability.

# References

Agnew, A., Manktelow, R. and Jones, L. (2007) *A systematic literature review and a national audit of bereavement risk assessment practice in Marie Curie hospices.* Report. London: Marie Curie Cancer Care.

Aranda, S. and Milne, D. (2000) *Guidelines for the assessment of complicated bereavement risk in family members of people receiving palliative care.* Melbourne Centre for Palliative Care.

Becker, G., Xander, C.J., Blum, H.E., Lutterbach, J., Momm, F., Gysels, M. and Higginson, I.J. (2007) Do religious or spiritual beliefs influence bereavement? A systematic review. *Palliative Medicine,* 21: 207–17.

Beckwith, B.E., Beckwith, S.K., Gray, T.L., Micsko, M.M., Holm, J.E., Plummer, V.H. and Flaa, S.L. (1990) Identification of spouses at high risk during bereavement: a preliminary assessment of Parkes and Weiss' risk index. *The Hospice Journal,* 6: 35–45.

Bereavement Care Standards (2001) *Standards for Bereavement Care in the UK.* London: London Bereavement Network.

Bonanno, G., Wortman, C. and Nesse, R. (2004) Prospective patterns of resilience and maladjustment during widowhood. *Psychology and Aging,* 19: 260–71.

Bowlby, J. (1980) *Attachment and Loss (Volume 3) Loss, Sadness and Depression.* London: The Hogarth Press.

Cleiren, M.P.H.D. (1991) *Bereavement and Adaptation: A Comparative Study of the Aftermath of a Death.* Washington: Hemisphere Publishing.

Cleiren, M.P.H.D., van der Wal, J. and Diekstra, R.F.W. (1988) Death after a long term disease: anticipation and outcome in the bereaved – part II. *Pharos International,* 54: 136–9.

Davies, E. and Higginson, I.J. (eds) (2004) *Better Palliative Care for Older People.* Copenhagen: World Health Organization.

Demmer, C. (2003) A national survey of hospice bereavement services. *Omega*, 47: 327–41.

Doka, K.J. (1989) *Disenfranchised Grief*. Lexington, MA: Lexington Books.

Field, D., Dand, P., Ahmedzai, S. and Biswas, B. (1992) Care and information received by lay carers of terminally ill patients at the Leicestershire Hospice. *Palliative Medicine*, 6(3): 237–45.

Field, D., Reid, D., Payne, S.A. and Relf, M. (2004) Survey of UK hospice and specialist palliative care adult bereavement services. *International Journal of Palliative Nursing*, 10(12): 569–76.

Gallagher-Thompson, D.E., Futterman, A., Farbarrow, N. and Peterson, J.A. (1993) The impact of spousal bereavement on older widows and widowers. In: M.S. Stroebe, W. Stroebe and R.O. Hansson (eds) *Handbook of Bereavement*. Cambridge: Cambridge University Press.

Gibson, D.W. and Graham, D. (1991) *Bereavement risk assessment in Australian hospice care centres: a survey*. Victoria, Australia: Ballarat University College.

Greene, R. (2002) Holocaust survivors: a study in resilience. *Journal of Gerontological Social Work*, 37(1): 3–18.

Irwin, M. and Pike, J. (1993) Bereavement, depressive symptoms and immune function. In: M.S Stroebe, W. Stroebe and R.O. Hansson (eds) *Handbook of Bereavement*. Cambridge: Cambridge University Press.

Jacobs, S. (1993) *Pathologic Grief: Maladaptions to Loss*. Washington, DC: American Psychiatric Press.

Jordan, J.R., Baker, J., Matteis, M., Rosenthal, S. and Ware, E.S. (2005) The grief evaluation measure (GEM): an initial validation study. *Death Studies*, 29: 301–32.

Kim, K. and Jacobs, S. (1993) Bereavement and neuroendocrine change. In: M.S. Stroebe, W. Stroebe and R.O. Hansson (eds) *Handbook of Bereavement*. Cambridge: Cambridge University Press.

Kissane, D.W. and Bloch, S. (2002) *Family Focused Grief Therapy*. Buckingham: Open University Press.

Klass, D., Silverman, P.R. and Nickman, S.L. (1996) *Continuing Bonds*. Washington, DC: Taylor and Francis.

Lehman, D.R., Ellard, J.H. and Wortman, C.B. (1986) Social support for the bereaved: recipients' and providers' perspectives on what is helpful. *Journal of Consulting and Clinical Psychology*, 54: 438–46.

Levy, L.H., Derby, J.F. and Martinowski, K.S. (1992) The question of who participates in bereavement research and the bereavement risk index. *Omega – Journal of Death and Dying*, 25: 225–38.

Lund, D., Caserta, M.S. and Dimond, M.F. (1993) The course of spousal bereavement in later life. In: M.S Stroebe, W. Stroebe and R.O. Hansson (eds) *Handbook of Bereavement*. Cambridge: Cambridge University Press.

Machin, L. (2006) The landscape of loss. *Bereavement Care*, 25(1): 7–11.

Martin, T.L. and Doka, K.J. (2000) *Men Don't Cry . . . Women Do*. Philadelphia: Taylor and Francis.

National Institute for Clinical Excellence (2004) *Improving Supportive and Palliative Care for Adults with Cancer*. London: National Institute for Clinical Excellence, 12: 155–67.

Neimeyer, R.A. (2000) Searching for the meaning of meaning: grief therapy and the process of reconstruction. *Death Studies*, 24: 541–58.

Neimeyer, R. and Anderson, A. (2002) Meaning reconstruction theory. In: N. Thompson (ed.) *Loss and Grief*. Basingstoke: Palgrave, pp. 45–64.

Parkes, C.M. (1981) Evaluation of a bereavement service. *Journal of Preventive Psychiatry*, 1: 179–88.

Parkes, C.M. (1990) Risk factors in bereavement: implications for the prevention and treatment of pathologic grief. *Psychiatric Annals*, 20: 308–13.

Parkes, C.M. (1996) *Bereavement. Studies of Grief in Adult Life*, 3rd edn. London: Penguin.

Parkes, C.M. (2006) *Love and Loss*. London: Routledge.

Parkes, C.M., Laungani, P. and Young, B. (1997) *Death and Bereavement Across Cultures*. London: Routledge.

Parkes, C.M. and Weiss, R.S. (1983) *Recovery From Bereavement*. New York: Basic Books.

Payne, S., Horn, S. and Relf, M. (1999) *Loss and Bereavement*. Buckingham: Open University Press.

Payne, S. and Relf, M. (1994) A survey of bereavement needs assessment and support services. *Palliative Medicine*, 8: 291–7.

Petersen, A. and Lupton, D. (1996) *The New Public Health: Health and Self in the Age of Risk*. London: Sage Publications.

Pottinger, A.M. (1991) Grieving relatives' perception of their needs and adjustment in a continuing care unit. *Palliative Medicine*, 5: 117–21.

Prigerson, H.G., Maciejewski, P.K., Reynolds, C.F., Bierhals, A.J., Newsom, J.T., Fasiczka, A., Frank, E., Doman, J. and Miller, M. (1995) Inventory of complicated grief: a scale to measure maladaptive symptoms of loss. *Psychiatry Research*, 59: 65–79.

Raphael, B. (1977) Preventive intervention with the recently bereaved. *Archives of General Psychiatry*, 34: 1450–4.

Relf, M. and Lines, C. (2005) *Who uses bereavement care?* Paper presented at the 7th International Conference on Grief and Bereavement, London. View at www.crusebereavementcare.org.uk.

Relf, M., Machin, L. and Archer, N. (in press) *Guidance for Bereavement Needs Assessment in Palliative Care*. London: Help the Hospices.

Riches, G. and Dawson, P. (1997) Shoring up the walls of heartache: parental responses to the death of a child. In: N. Small and D. Field (eds) *Race, Gender and Death*. London: Routledge.

Sanders, C.M. (1981) Comparison of younger and older spouses in bereavement outcome. *Omega – Journal of Death and Dying*, 11: 217–32.

Sanders, C.M. (1983) Effects of sudden versus chronic illness death on bereavement outcome. *Omega – Journal of Death and Dying*, 11: 227–41.

Sanders, C.M. (1993) Risk factors in bereavement outcome. In: M.S Stroebe, W. Stroebe and R.O. Hansson (eds) *Handbook of Bereavement*. Cambridge: Cambridge University Press.

Schilling, R.F. (1987) Limitations of social support. *Social Services Review*, 61: 19–31.

Schut, H. and Stroebe, M.S. (2005) Interventions to enhance adaptation to bereavement. *Journal of Palliative Medicine*, 8: S140–S146.

Shuchter, S.R. and Zisook, S. (1993) The course of normal grief. In: M.S. Stroebe, W. Stroebe and R.O. Hansson (eds) *Handbook of Bereavement*. Cambridge: Cambridge University Press.

Silverman, P.R. and Klass, D. (1996) Introduction: What's the problem? In: D. Klass, P.R. Silverman and S.L. Nickman (eds) *Continuing Bonds*. Washington: Taylor & Francis.

Stroebe, M.S. (1992) Coping with bereavement: a review of the grief work hypothesis. *Omega – Journal of Death and Dying*, 26: 19–42.

Stroebe, M.S., Folkman, S., Hansson, R.O. and Schut, H. (2006) The prediction of bereavement outcome: development of an integrative risk factor framework. *Social Science and Medicine*, 63: 2440–51.

Stroebe, M.S. and Schut, H. (1999) The Dual Process Model of coping with bereavement: rationale and description. *Death Studies*, 23: 197–224.

Stroebe, W. and Schut, H. (2001) Risk factors in bereavement outcome: a methodological and empirical review. In: M.S. Stroebe, R.O. Hansson, W. Stroebe and H. Schut (eds) *Handbook of Bereavement Research: Consequences, Coping and Care*. Washington, DC: American Psychological Association, pp. 349–71.

Stroebe, M.S. and Stroebe, W. (1983) Who suffers more? Sex differences in health risks of the widowed. *Psychological Bulletin*, 93: 279–301.

Stroebe, W. and Stroebe, M.S. (1987) *Bereavement and Health*. Cambridge: Cambridge University Press.

Stroebe, W., Stroebe, M.S. and Domittner, G. (1988) Individual and situational differences in recovery from bereavement: a risk group identified. *Journal of Social Issues*, 44: 143–58.

Stylianos, S.K. and Vachon, M.L.S. (1993) The role of social support in bereavement. In: M.S. Stroebe, W. Stroebe and R.O. Hansson (eds) *Handbook of Bereavement*. Cambridge: Cambridge University Press.

Walter, T. (1996) A new model of grief: bereavement and biography. *Mortality*, 1: 7–25.

Walter, T. (1999) *On Bereavement: The Culture of Grief*. Milton Keynes: Open University Press.

Worden, J.W. (2003) *Grief Counselling and Grief Therapy*, 3rd edn. London: Brunner Routledge.

Wortman, C.B. and Silver, R.C. (1989) The myths of coping with loss. *Journal of Consulting and Clinical Psychology*, 57: 349–57.

Wortman, C.B., Silver, R.C. and Kessler, R.C. (1993) The meaning of loss and adjustment to bereavement. In: M.S. Stroebe, W. Stroebe and R.O. Hansson (eds) *Handbook of Bereavement*. Cambridge: Cambridge University Press.

# 25

# Bereavement support services

*David Kissane*

---

**Key points**

- Bereavement care starts at entry to palliative care services with screening for risk factors, including family dysfunction, and the service sustaining continuity of care for those deemed 'at risk'.
- Risk factors for complicated grief include personal vulnerability, a pathological relationship with the patient, poor family and social support and eventually witnessing a difficult death.
- Documentation of bereavement care plans, based on risk factors and recording 'which staff member does what' is crucial to avoid missing follow-up of 'at risk' relatives.
- Specialist bereavement services should target those 'at risk' or with morbid complications; resilient individuals and families are the responsibility of the general community.

---

A natural continuity ought to exist between support for the grieving process in patients and their carers during palliative care and its maintenance for the bereaved after the death. Health care organizations caring for the dying have an invaluable opportunity to deliver such seamless care and thus minimize the rates of pathological consequence arising in the bereaved (Field *et al.* 2007). The configuration of bereavement support services is the practical manner in which this ideal is achieved (Reid *et al.* 2006).

Nurses at the coalface of clinical care are intimately involved not only with the dying but also their loved ones and carers – those family members and friends who subsequently become the bereaved. Moreover, knowledge of and familiarity with these people enables nurses to sustain a supportive role during that peak time of emotional distress, the early phase of bereavement. Their contribution to any programme of bereavement support is crucial to its success (Foliart *et al.* 2001).

In this chapter, the nature of grief and the mourning process is assumed, as is the care of the newly bereaved present at the moment of death. Here the focus is on the formal and informal support services provided by hospices and specialist palliative care services, with particular attention to the nurse's role, given the principles, stated above, of continuity of care and the nurse's intimate, prior connection with those who become bereaved.

## Aims of bereavement support programmes

The goal of these programmes is to deliver relevant and effective support to the bereaved in a manner that is both clinically appropriate and cost-effective. A targeted response is necessary to reach certain groups whose needs might otherwise be neglected (Schut and Stroebe 2005), while a preventive approach is worthwhile for its capacity to reduce costs significantly by assisting those at high risk of a pathological outcome before more serious difficulties arise.

Three broad levels of care of the bereaved therefore emerge:

- generic support for all the bereaved provided by the whole treatment team and broad community;
- targeted support for those at high risk to prevent morbid grief;
- specific interventions for those experiencing complicated grief.

Such a multi-level approach helps to separate generic support from specialist bereavement services as well as ensure that programmes are indeed focused in a cost-effective manner. Studies suggest that approximately 30 per cent of family care-givers use bereavement services, especially in the first six months post loss (Yi *et al.* 2006; Cherlin *et al.* 2007).

Appropriate credentialing of staff holding special skills is required to competently deliver the highest or third level of bereavement care provision, in which specific interventions are applied when complicated grief has intervened (Field *et al.* 2004; Yi *et al.* 2006). In contrast, team education and in-service up-skilling about bereavement care underpins the generic delivery of support to all involved with a hospice or palliative care programme. The middle level of bereavement service provision is addressed by a mixed contribution from general and specialist staff.

Potential staff involved with bereavement support programmes therefore include both generalist and specialist palliative care nurses, the general practitioner, the allied health team incorporating social worker, psychologist, psychiatrist, occupational therapist, pastoral care worker or chaplain, and finally the team of trained community volunteers. The palliative care medical consultant, and for that matter others such as the medical oncologist, surgeon or consultant physician, are generally the least involved beyond ensuring that the members of the team are appropriately engaged in such relevant supportive work. An understanding of the operation of bereavement support services is highly pertinent to nurses working in hospice and palliative care (Field *et al.* 2004).

# Generic bereavement support programmes

These services are intended for all of the bereaved in a non-discriminatory manner. They form the bedrock of any bereavement support programme, and are the common starting point when a new palliative care service is established. Key components of such a generic programme include: attendance at the funeral; expression of sympathy via cards or telephone calls; brochures about grief; follow-up visits to the home; and commemorative services as the year unfolds (Foliart *et al.* 2001; Field *et al.* 2004; Yi *et al.* 2006).

## *Attendance at the funeral*

Not only is the funeral a key social ritual in which the life of the deceased is celebrated, it also symbolizes continuity for the living, albeit without the family member that has died. Such rituals have great cultural relevance and personal meaning to the bereaved, who are usually therefore touched by the presence of representatives of the health care team.

Of their nature, funerals are time-consuming, and necessarily costly in terms of the staff time involved in attendance. Does a single person represent the team, or do they feel the need for companionship as well? It quickly becomes burdensome to the palliative care service if two or more staff attend every funeral. Routine consideration of whether the service needs to be represented and who should be involved is therefore desirable.

First, where a series of health care teams have been involved in the patient's and family's care, identification of who was primarily involved seems sensible. For instance, sometimes an oncology service has had several years of intense involvement in contrast with the palliative care services where, in the USA, there may only be contact in the final week. Knowing that the oncology nursing staff intends to attend the funeral can free the palliative care team from unnecessary duplication. Similarly, a long period of time with the home care team might contrast with a short time as an inpatient. In different circumstances, a patient dying from stroke or respiratory disorder may have had negligible contact with any service, in which case, attendance may signify willingness to help in a manner that both inspires the family and connects staff with needy relatives.

What are the reasons for involvement in a funeral service? While the health care team hopes to benefit the bereaved through attendance, no harm should ever be caused by intrusiveness (Kissane and Bloch 2002). The latter might arise when the palliative care service has been viewed ambivalently by the relatives, sometimes associated with treatment complications or poor health outcome. From time to time, particular staff 'get offside' with relatives due to some attitudinal or personality clash. In any setting of conflict, the bereaved will want respect and privacy, which may lead to an active decision that the palliative care service will not be represented at the funeral.

How might attendance prove beneficial to the bereaved? Generally it symbolizes connectedness with and concern for the bereaved, conveying considerable respect while also providing an opportunity for the attendee to invite continued contact. 'Please let me know if I can be of assistance.' Where the attendee has both known and cared for the deceased, their presence communicates a strong commitment to support. They may become the logical choice for contact should the bereaved later perceive difficulties to be developing.

The literature on clinician burnout also identifies attendance at funerals as a means of the health professional attending to their own grief (Rickerson *et al.* 2005). They may have lost a person they felt especially attached to. An ethical caution is however needed here. When the actions of any professional are directed to their own rather than the patient's or family's needs, there is a potential danger of abuse through boundary transgression. Careful reflection about the motivations of the professional serves to guide this decision-making. If personal gain was the primary reason for attendance at the funeral, some alternative approach to grieving with their professional colleagues is warranted, exemplified by a debriefing group for staff (Demmer 1999). The ethical rationale for nurses' attendance at funerals ought to be its potential benefit to the bereaved.

A common quandary is the level of involvement that follows during the funeral service. Attendance at the church or funeral parlour for a commemorative service has different connotations to presence at the graveside, which, in turn, is different from returning home with the bereaved for a wake following the burial. What meaning does each level of involvement convey and what message does it give to the family? Differences exist here in the involvement of the doctor or nurse involved in physical health care, with the chaplain or pastoral care worker involved in the spiritual and religious aspects of the ritual. In general, it is sufficient for clinical staff to pay their respects in association with the commemorative service and then discreetly withdraw to allow the family to grieve with their own community and friends.

From time to time, conflict arises within palliative care teams about who should attend. On what basis does one select between a nurse who has had daily contact for several weeks and a social worker who has had a single, extended session? Generally, the greater the sense of connectedness, the more supportive that person's attendance will be perceived. However, consideration might be given to future support needs, and where greater risk prevails of morbid outcome, one professional could be of greater potential benefit than another. In such decisions, the focus is clearly on the needs of the bereaved rather than the staff members involved. Occasionally joint attendance evolves, worthwhile when one is relatively inexperienced and likely to benefit from a colleague's support until greater experience is established.

In summary, then, palliative care teams do well to discuss the who and why of funeral attendance in every case of death, so that cogent reasons underpin any staff attendance, rather than having random, or worse, routinized patterns prevail.

### The sympathy card or telephone call

Not uncommonly, nurses can be off duty at a time when a patient with whom they have been considerably involved dies. In these circumstances, a telephone call to the bereaved from a key individual will be greatly appreciated over subsequent days (Reid *et al.* 2006). For a team, however, a sympathy card enables several to sign where multiple phone calls would be inappropriate. Furthermore, a message of continued availability for advice and support can helpfully be added. This not only serves as a source of reassurance but, not surprisingly, key nurses become the first point of contact when relatives are distressed because these nurses have been prime sources of support during the final illness of the deceased. In this sense, the card or telephone call symbolizes an important link (Wilkes 1993).

Sometimes the final admission of a dying patient breaks continuity for nurses who may have been involved for months. They are not present at the time of death but learn about it over the next few days. Calls or correspondence are then a sensitive means of expressing sympathy to the bereaved once death has occurred. Hospices or home care services around the world employ a number of variations on this theme, dependent on local conditions (deCinque *et al.* 2004; Field *et al.* 2004; Yi *et al.* 2006; Cherlin *et al.* 2007). When several deaths occur each week, staff may have a fortnightly or monthly card writing session. Attention to some systematic process ensures that families are not overlooked through temporary circumstance (Street *et al.* 2004). Some teams select the primary author of the correspondence from within their core group, based on who knew the relatives best or felt some affinity to the carer. Others see this as a duty of the nurse in charge.

Whatever the local method, documentation of this activity fosters compliance and ensures that the process is not postponed. All services discover that care of the current workload of patients takes precedence over those lost, and the bereaved are readily neglected by well-intentioned people (Lattanzi-Licht 1989). Implementation of a structured process with its own documentation protects against avoidance, delay or neglect, and later facilitates follow-up when periodic memorial services are being planned for these relatives and friends of the deceased.

The anniversary of the death is another occasion when a card offers support and may provide an opportunity for someone who is struggling to receive appropriate care (Gibson and Graham 1991). A systematic yet personalized method of generating such cards is essential.

### Brochures and educational material

Information about what to expect emotionally and the normal course of mourning is greatly appreciated by the bereaved. A survey of Californian hospices identified that over 90 per cent offer educational material routinely (Foliart *et al.* 2001); Spanish programmes similarly reach 89 per cent (Yi *et al.* 2006). Many hospices also permit library books to be borrowed by the bereaved.

### Follow-up visits

Where community teams have supported a dying person and their family in the home, follow-up visits to the bereaved are greatly appreciated (Matsushima *et al.* 2002). From the point of view of the team, dialogue about such practice is worthwhile when allied health members have also been involved. Is there confidence about the resilience of the bereaved (Bonanno *et al.* 2005), or some concern about risk, which warrants consistent follow-up? Is there a general practitioner involved? Does the team know the GP's usual practice regarding follow-up of the bereaved? Has this been discussed or is it worth a call to clarify? Especially when a nurse has concern about the welfare of a recently bereaved carer, discussion with the general practitioner usefully engages that person in a plan of continued preventive care.

What is the ideal timing of follow-up visits to the home of a widow or widower? No single guideline will suffice as circumstances can be so varied. A visit one to two weeks post-death proves the commonest pattern, but some of the bereaved will stay with other relatives for a time, making a visit one to two months later the practical option. Insight into family plans is clearly helpful here.

The content of conversation with the bereaved is worth special comment. Not only should the nurse ask about their welfare and coping, but questions that review the dying process are also valuable. Thus,

- How do you think X's death evolved?
- Were there difficult moments for you?
- Were you left with questions about what happened?
- Did you talk to the doctor about what would go on the death certificate?
- How did the funeral go?
- Are there family members you are concerned about?
- How are you coping now?

This conversation, typically occurring over a cup of tea or coffee, will precipitate active grieving, and the nurse should feel quite comfortable about the normality and appropriateness of this. Within appropriate cultural norms, tearfulness should be understood as natural, even desirable, and with time and patient listening, the nurse will generate a sense of valuable support. Beyond affirmation of the appropriateness of grief, accompaniment is the key therapeutic activity; solutions are generally not needed, as the context now exists that grief will unfold over many subsequent months. A new phase of life has been entered in which the bereaved will be required to effect considerable change and adaptation, but there is plenty of time in which to accomplish this (Parkes 1998). The nurse might conclude the visit by offering congratulations about the care and dedication given to the dying relative. An offer of availability in the future – 'simply call me if needed' – sustains the continuity of the preceding care. The nurse can thus be a genuine reference point of enquiry should problems develop.

### Memorial services

As many societies have become less religious, a tradition of palliative care teams running memorial services has been established (Reid *et al.* 2006). The rationale is to both provide a multidenominational ritual to facilitate normal grieving and to provide a contact point as time passes at which staff have the opportunity to meet the bereaved and check on their overall coping. Nurses are a pivotal part of this process because of their personal knowledge of the relatives involved. If the local culture has a very high level of involvement with religious ceremonies, exemplified by Buddhist ceremonies in Japan, the spirit of bereavement care may be embodied in the existing ceremonies (Matsushima *et al.* 2002). Nonetheless, palliative care staff can be actively involved.

Dependent of the size of any palliative care programme, these commemorative services are usually conducted six monthly or yearly. Practical considerations such as the size of a chapel and what is manageable for the staff usually prevail. Planning may be designated to key staff members but a team is generally needed to cope with the multiplicity of arrangements. Planning becomes systematized once a few have been conducted.

When the team meets, the list of potential invitees is reviewed for the relevant period, and invitations are issued on behalf of the programme. Some services select team members who will be remembered by the bereaved to sign the invitations, using linkages that will foster attendance.

Chaplains usually assist with the content of the ceremonies, which can combine prayers, song or hymns and readings from a variety of religious traditions. Families are often invited to write the name of their deceased relative in a commemorative book, these names being read out at an appropriate moment during the ritual. Family members can be invited to come forward and light a candle in memory of their loved one. Having medical, nursing or allied health staff read Scripture or other spiritual prayers and poetry during the ceremony is appreciated by the families and proves to be one way of ensuring that such staff attend. Once medical practitioners appreciate the benefits of the memorial to families and enjoy hearing how they are coping several months after their relative's death, they tend to return for subsequent memorials. The serving of refreshments following the ceremony is a *sine qua non* of the format as it facilitates reunion.

Attendance by the bereaved at such memorial services tends to signify a reasonable adaptation to the loss. Non-attendance, when based on avoidance mechanisms, may be associated with the development of complicated grief. Hence a review of those who apologized or did not attend is as important a feature of the bereavement support programme as the memorial itself. What is known about the mourning of the non-attendees? Did any of them carry high risk factors for the development of complicated grief (Zhang *et al.* 2006)? A team member could make contact to review the coping of any who appear to be a concern.

The memorial programme has many covert benefits for the contributing staff through building cohesion, a spirit of generosity and a spiritual dimension to the team as a whole (Rickerson *et al.* 2005). It is generally perceived to be a worthwhile extracurricular activity for the multidisciplinary team.

# Targeted support for those at high risk

Factors that increase the risk of complicated grief developing in the bereaved were described in Chapter 24 and are summarized here in Table 25.1. The goal of this aspect of a bereavement support programme is to select and

**Table 25.1**  Classification of evidence-based risk factors for the development of complicated grief in the bereaved

## 1. Antedecedent factors

*Nature of the carer's personality and individual vulnerabilities*

- Their coping style and prior history in dealing with loss (e.g. anxious worrier or low self-esteem).
- Any past history of psychiatric disorder (e.g. depression).
- The build-up of cumulative experiences of loss.

*Nature of their relationship with the dying patient*

- An ambivalent relationship (e.g. anger and hostility at alcoholism, gambling, infidelity, financial ruin).
- An overly dependent relationship (e.g. clinging and possessive from basic insecurities).
- An avoidant relationship (e.g. distant and awkard in an insecure manner).
- An unrecognized relationship (e.g. secret).

## 2. Decedent factors

*Nature of the death*

- One that is untimely in the life cycle (e.g. death of a child).
- Sudden or unexpected at that time (e.g. event related, for instance sepsis or pulmonary embolism).
- Traumatic (e.g. large bedsores with debility).
- Stigmatized or disenfranchising (e.g. AIDS or suicide).

## 3. Post-death factors

*Nature of their family*

- Dysfunctional (e.g. poor communicators, high conflict, poor cohesion).
- Reconstituted in a problematic manner (e.g. remarriage creating ambivalent step relationships; estate and legal conflicts).

*Nature of their support network*

- Isolated from extended family and friends (e.g. new migrant).
- Alienated from neighbours (e.g. perception of poor community support carried by the individual).

apply a preventive model of care to counter and minimize the likelihood of morbidity in a proactive and cost-effective manner. To optimize compliance with such a programme, standardization of the risk assessment procedure is strongly recommended. In the early 1990s, surveys of palliative care teams in Australia revealed that only between one-quarter and one-third utilized a standardized risk assessment procedure, and for 85 per cent of these, it was done by a nurse (Gibson and Graham 1991). These rates are improving globally in the twenty-first century, but are still limited by inadequate staffing (Yi *et al.* 2006; Field *et al.* 2007).

Such targeted support can be delivered individually, or via a group or family approach. Usually time-limited in their design, the therapeutic approach is commonly supportive-expressive or psycho-educational in its application. The former utilizes the notion of encouraging active grieving through the sharing of thoughts and feelings with the counsellor; the latter offers information about the nature and course of the grief journey, a group environment being selected as a means of the bereaved sharing their experiences with others in a comparable predicament (Lieberman and Yalom 1992).

Credentialing processes require the choice of a therapist who has been formally trained in bereavement counselling for these models to be competently applied. Nurses, however, make a valuable contribution as co-facilitators of a bereavement group, particularly when they bring a sense of continuity through having known the deceased relative.

### Preventive individual therapy with the bereaved

Where factors indicative of high risk for morbid outcome are present in the bereaved, a preventive approach in which a counsellor provides a limited number of sessions (for instance six) over the next 6–12 months has been shown to reduce morbidity (Raphael 1977). There are certain risk factors that point to the appropriateness of an individual model of preventive support: personal vulnerabilities, for instance a past history of depression, or an anxious worrying style with limited coping reserves; ambivalent relationships, including a lot of anger; the disenfranchised, where the loss cannot be openly acknowledged and publicly mourned (Doka 1989); and a degree of avoidance or shyness suggesting they will be less willing to join a group environment.

The danger of an individual model is the development of dependence on the counsellor, for which reason this approach is often combined with a group or family approach for the added socialization the latter can provide. Sometimes two or three individual sessions will build up sufficient trust in the counsellor to allow movement into a group that this counsellor also facilitates.

The therapy model in individual preventive interventions is generally supportive-expressive. Attention is given both to nurturing the expression of grief through remembering and sharing stories, and, in parallel, adjustment to life without the deceased through active coping. Stroebe and Schut (1999) have termed this the dual process model of coping with loss.

### *Preventive group therapy with the bereaved*

Group therapy is very cost-effective and serves to connect the bereaved with others caught up in the loneliness and isolation that often follows loss of a significant companion. Risk factors that point to the value of a group approach include: a poorly supportive social network, where the individual is isolated or alienated from others; an overly dependent relationship with the deceased, leaving the bereaved isolated and vulnerable as a result; and an identifiable subgroup within society, who will profit from linking with others that share a comparable experience of loss. Examples of the latter include the spousally bereaved (Lieberman and Yalom 1992), adolescent or sibling groups (Stokes *et al.* 1997), and relatives of people who have committed suicide or died in a traumatic natural disaster (Schwab 1995–96; Goodkin *et al.* 1996–97). Strong satisfaction is generally reported with any group experience but it varies with both the group's objectives and its setting (Hopmeyer and Werk 1994).

Group approaches can be facilitated by a trained counsellor or operate at a self-help level, incorporating the assistance of volunteers (Field *et al.* 2007). The greater the risk of morbid complications for the bereaved, the more important that the former criterion operates; the latter approach can complement an individual supportive programme run by a trained counsellor (Thuen 1995; Foliart *et al.* 2001). High participant satisfaction with bereavement support groups is relatively strongly related to the quality of group leadership (Thuen 1995). Self-help groups need the wisdom of experience to draw the wary into a safe environment, avoid cliques, provide variety and foster socialization. Organizations such as Cruse Bereavement, Solace or Compassionate Friends are very helpful to bereavement counsellors in running such group programmes (Kirschling and Osmont 1992–93; Wheeler 1993–94).

The models of therapy used when a trained counsellor leads groups include psycho-educational, supportive-expressive and psychodynamic (Yalom and Vinogradov 1988). Hospice programmes will typically adopt the psycho-educational approach because of its time-limited nature (six to eight sessions) and its ability to reassure the bereaved about normal grieving through some informational content. All groups deliver support and the opportunity for expression of feelings about the loss. Facilitators foster cohesion through the use of refreshments and active invitation to the members to exchange their contact details. A successful short-term bereavement group will have its members continue to support one another long beyond the formal life of the group.

Short-term groups are usually closed in that new members are not added once the group process has begun. Longer-term groups may be open, with new members (who are generally more recently bereaved) being added as some more senior members withdraw. In the latter setting, the relative improvement of older group members is used therapeutically to support the fragility of more recent members, while a psychodynamic approach may make use of patterns of relationship evident across a life-span to provide insight into problems that repeatedly interfere with relationships in the present. Longer-term groups are generally conducted by regionally based bereavement counselling services rather than smaller hospice programmes and they seek to meet the needs of the especially high-risk bereaved (Foliart *et al.* 2001).

Group processes address unmet dependency needs in the lonely bereaved through connecting them to a network of people rather than a single therapist. The greater the homogeneity of membership in age and other social circumstances, the easier will connectedness develop. Care needs to be taken whenever a group becomes unbalanced through a member being noticeably different in some characteristic and potentially challenging to integrate with others. Formal training in group therapy is invaluable to ensure that facilitators develop a healthy and nurturing environment.

### Preventive family therapy with the bereaved

As the family is often the primary social network of the bereaved, identification of families at high risk of morbid bereavement outcome enables adoption of a family-centred model of care in keeping with the goals and rhetoric of the hospice movement. Risk factors that identify families suitable for a preventive family approach include: a dysfunctional method of relating as a family unit through poor communication, cohesiveness or conflict resolution (Kissane *et al.* 1996); a stage in the life cycle when the family especially matters to the health and development of its membership – for instance, death of a child or adolescent (Davies *et al.* 1986); and the cumulative experience of losses through multiple illnesses, disabilities or deaths in a family that is stretched to its limits, including a stigmatized or traumatic death – for instance, death from AIDS, suicide or homicide (Walsh and McGoldrick 1991).

The model of therapy is typically brief (six to ten sessions) and its focus can be supportive-expressive or directed to the family's functioning (Kissane *et al.* 1998). The latter approach, termed Family Focused Grief Therapy (FFGT), makes use of a screening strategy that identifies families at greater risk of morbid outcome through the routine administration of the Family Relationships Index (FRI) (Moos and Moos 1981), a 12-item pencil and paper questionnaire that informs about family functioning. The FRI is completed when the patient is first admitted to the palliative care or hospice unit. Continuity of family work is then established before the death of the ill family member, and the therapist's intimate knowledge and memory of this deceased person is hugely advantageous to later work during bereavement. Optimizing family functioning while promoting sharing of grief facilitates the development of a supportive environment with those most touched by the death – the immediate family (Kissane and Bloch 2002; Kissane *et al.* 2006).

Therapists leading such family interventions need formal training in family therapy and typically come out of disciplines such as social work or psychology. However the co-therapy approach strengthens the overall application of FFGT when it combines input from clinical staff with a detailed understanding of the care needs of the dying family member. The nurse plays a useful role here. Moreover co-therapy deepens the involvement of the multidisciplinary team with the family in a therapeutically powerful manner.

Grieving families who have lost a child clearly benefit from a family-centred approach to support (deCinque *et al.* 2004; Auman 2007). Dora Black's group (1985) in the UK and Betty Davies (1986) in the USA provide outstanding examples of such family-oriented approaches. A family approach to bereavement support is also remarkably suitable for many adult families who have lost a parent and seek to more effectively support their remaining parent.

## Specific interventions for those experiencing complicated grief

The kernel of specialist bereavement counselling is with the 20 per cent of the bereaved who develop some form of complicated grief (Middleton *et al.* 1993). No longer is the intervention preventive as the morbidity associated with such distortion of normal grieving calls for specific interventions to alleviate the distress. Over the past decade, considerable research has sought to define diagnostic criteria to empower better recognition of those who develop forms of pathological grief but do not meet DSM criteria for psychiatric disorders such as Major Depressive Disorder or Post Traumatic Stress Disorder (Horowitz *et al.* 1997; Prigerson *et al.* 1999).

Accumulating evidence is that the symptoms, course and response to treatment of a disorder, proposed to be called Prolonged Grief Disorder (PGD), are distinct from normal grief. Diagnostic criteria for PGD are shown in Table 25.2 (Prigerson *et al.* 2007). Risk factors for PGD include insecure attachment styles and childhood separation anxiety; controlling parents, parental abuse or early death of a parent; a close relationship to the deceased including excessive dependency; and a lack of preparation for the death (Prigerson *et al.* 2007).

In controlled studies, complicated grief (such as PGD) has responded better to a cognitive-behavioural than interpersonal model of therapy, where, in the former, greater socialization is accomplished by activity scheduling and the bereaved person is drawn out of an entrenched pattern of retreat and avoidance (Shear *et al.* 2005). Similar greater improvement resulted from cognitive restructuring and exposure therapy than from supportive counselling (Boelen *et al.* 2007). In group therapy for complicated grief, improved outcomes were seen in groups whose members had a history of relatively mature relationships compared to those with immature object relations (Piper *et al.* 2007).

Depression as a complication of grief is appropriately treated with anti-depressant medication alongside psychotherapies (Hensley 2006). Traumatic

**Table 25.2** Criteria for Prolonged Grief Disorder proposed for *DSM-V* (after Prigerson *et al.* 2007)

1. **Event criterion**: Bereavement (loss of a loved person)

2. **Separation distress**: The bereaved person experiences at least one of the three following symptoms, which must be experienced daily, and to a distressing or disruptive degree:

   - intrusive thoughts related to the lost relationship
   - intense feelings of emotional pain, sorrow or pangs of grief
   - yearning for the lost person.

3. **Cognitive, emotional, and behavioural symptoms**: The bereaved person must have five (or more) of the following symptoms, experienced daily, and to a distressing or disruptive degree:

   - confusion about one's role in life or diminished sense of self (i.e. feeling that a part of oneself has died)
   - difficulty accepting the loss
   - avoidance of reminders of the reality of the loss
   - inability to trust others since the loss
   - bitterness or anger related to the loss
   - difficulty moving on with life (e.g. making new friends, pursuing interests)
   - numbness (absence of emotion) since the loss
   - feeling that life is unfulfilling, empty and meaningless since the loss
   - feeling stunned, dazed or shocked by the loss.

4. **Duration**: Duration at least six months from the onset of separation distress.

5. **Impairment**: The above symptomatic disturbance causes clinically significant distress or impairment in social, occupational or other important areas of functioning (e.g. domestic responsibilities).

6. **Medical exclusion**: The disturbance is not due to the physiological effects of a substance or a general medical condition.

7. **Relation to other mental disorders**: Not better accounted for by Major Depressive Disorder, Generalized Anxiety Disorder or Post-traumatic Stress Disorder.

grief warrants desensitization to the cues that trigger recurrent distress. Special skills are needed in responding to these forms of complicated grief that warrant appropriate professional training and credentialing of therapists (Raphael *et al.* 2001; Jordan and Neimeyer 2003).

An important nursing role is the recognition of poor coping and the sensitive referral of people with complicated grief to specialist bereavement counsellors – psychologists and psychiatrists – for appropriate interventions. Resistance to referral may be based on avoidance, fear, ignorance of the possible help available or a sense of stigma about needing help. Here the trust that the nurse has established as a sensible and caring advocate will help the bereaved accept guidance about appropriate referral.

# Efficacy of bereavement support services

Evaluations of bereavement support services tend to report high levels of satisfaction with the care provided (Hopmeyer and Werk 1994; Thuen 1995), but there are several methodological difficulties with such endeavours, particularly the social desirability of such a response, and the effect size has generally been small (Harding and Higginson 2003; Stroebe *et al.* 2005).

The majority of palliative care or hospice programmes in the United Kingdom, United States, Canada, Australia and New Zealand now accept bereavement support as integral to their services. The current challenge is to integrate this support to deliver continuity of care rather than have bereavement support added on as 'an extra' after death.

A survey by the Californian Hospice and Palliative Care Association identified that volunteers accounted for almost one-quarter of bereavement staff (Foliart *et al.* 2001). Payne (2001) explored this contribution of volunteers to bereavement support in New Zealand. While two-thirds had generic volunteer training, only one-third had specific training in bereavement and most (71 per cent) recognized previous personal bereavements. That half found their work emotionally distressing and one-quarter had problems with 'boundaries' points to the imperative for both training and supervision. Volunteers are a valuable asset but should not be the main form of service for those at high risk or who have developed complicated grief (Raphael *et al.* 2001; Jordan and Neimeyer 2003).

In the USA, 55 per cent of a random sample of teaching hospitals reported some form of bereavement support, generally provided by a social worker or chaplain (Billings and Pantilat 2001). A comprehensive survey of hospice settings across Japan found that three-quarters provided some form of bereavement follow-up, most frequently using cards (84 per cent) and memorial services (59 per cent) (Matsushima *et al.* 2002). Nurses were actively involved. The prevalence of social groups was 35 per cent, telephone calls 32 per cent, home visits 22 per cent, individual counselling 22 per cent, self-help groups 11 per cent and family counselling 8 per cent.

# Guidelines for setting up bereavement services

Where services are establishing bereavement support programmes, attention to published guidelines about their development can prove helpful (Sandler *et al.* 2005). The National Association of Bereavement Services in the United Kingdom published guidelines in 1994 (see Stewart 1994), the National Hospice Organization in the USA in 1997 and the Centre for Palliative Care in Australia in 1999.

# References

Auman, M.J. (2007) Bereavement support for children, *Journal of School Nursing*, 23(1): 34–9.

Billings, J.A. and Pantilat, S. (2001) Survey of palliative care programs in United States teaching hospitals, *Journal of Palliative Medicine*, 4: 309–14.

Black, D. and Urbanowicz, M. (1985) Bereaved children – family intervention. In: J. Stevenson (ed.) *Recent Research in Developmental Psychopathology*. Oxford: Pergamon, pp. 179–87.

Boelen, P.A., de Keijser, J., van den Hout, M.A. and van den Bout, J. (2007) Treatment of complicated grief: A comparison between cognitive-behavioral therapy and supportive counseling, *Journal of Consult Clinical Psychology*, 75(2): 277–84.

Bonanno, G., Moskowitz, J. and Tedlie, J. (2005) Resilience to loss in bereaved spouses, bereaved parents, and bereaved gay men. *Journal of Personality & Social Psychology*, 88: 827–43.

Centre for Palliative Care (1999) *Bereavement Risk Assessment Guidelines*. Melbourne: Centre for Palliative Care.

Cherlin, E.J., Barry, C.L., Prigerson, H.G., Green, D.S., Johson-Hurzler, R., Kasl, S.V. and Bradley, E.H. (2007) Bereavement services for family caregivers: how often used, why, and why not, *Journal of Palliative Medicine*, 10(1): 148–58.

Davies, B., Spinetta, J., Martinson, I., McClowry, S. and Kulenkamp, E. (1986) Manifestations of levels of functioning in grieving families, *Journal of Family Issues*, 7: 297–313.

deCinque, N., Monterosso, L., Dadd, G., Sidhu, R. and Lucas, R. (2004) Bereavement support for families following the death of a child from cancer: Practice characteristics of Australian and New Zealand paediatric oncology units, *Journal of Paediatric Child Health*, 40(3): 131–5.

Demmer, C. (1999) Death-related experience and professional support among nursing staff in AIDS care facilities, *Omega*, 39: 123–32.

Doka, K.J. (1989) *Disenfranchised Grief: Recognizing Hidden Sorrow*. Lexington, MA: Lexington Books.

Field, D., Payne, S., Relf, M. and Reid, D. (2007) Some issues in the provision of adult bereavement support by UK hospices, *Social Science Medicine*, 64(2): 428–38.

Field, D., Reid, D., Payne, S. and Relf, M. (2004) Survey of UK hospice and specialist palliative care adult bereavement services, *International Journal of Palliative Nursing*, 10(12): 569–76.

Foliart, D.E., Clausen, M. and Siljestrom, C. (2001) Bereavement practices among California hospices: results of a state-wide survey, *Death Studies*, 25: 461–7.

Gibson, D.W. and Graham, D. (1991) *Bereavement risk assessment in Australian hospice care centres: a survey*. Unpublished dissertation, Ballarat University College, Australia.

Goodkin, K., Burkhalter, J.E., Tuttle, R.S., Blaney, N.T., Feaster, D.J. and Leeds, B. (1996–97) A research derived bereavement support group technique for the HIV-1 infected, *Omega*, 34: 279–300.

Harding, R. and Higginson, I.J. (2003) What is the best way to help caregivers in cancer and palliative care? A systematic literature review of interventions and their effectiveness. *Palliative Medicine*, 17: 63–74.

Hensley, P.L. (2006) Treatment of bereavement-related depression and traumatic grief, *Journal of Affective Disorder*, 92(1): 117–24.

Hopmeyer, E. and Werk, A. (1994) A comparative study of family bereavement groups, *Death Studies*, 18: 243–56.

Horowitz, M.J., Siegel, B., Holen, A., Bonanno, G.A., Milbrath, C. and Stinson, C.H. (1997) Diagnostic criteria for complicated grief disorder. *American Journal Psychiatry*, 154: 904–10.

Jordan, J.R. and Neimeyer, R.A. (2003) Does grief counselling work? *Death Studies*, 27: 765–86.

Kirschling, J.M. and Osmont, K. (1992–93) Bereavement network: a community based group. *Journal of Death and Dying*, 26(2): 119–27.

Kissane, D.W., Bloch, S., Dowe, D.L., Snyder, R.D., Onghena, P., McKenzie, D.P. and Wallace, C.S. (1996) The Melbourne family grief study, I: perceptions of family functioning in bereavement, *American Journal of Psychiatry*, 153: 650–8.

Kissane, D.W., Bloch, S., McKenzie, M., McDowall, A.C. and Nitzan, R. (1998) Family grief therapy: a preliminary account of a new model to promote healthy family functioning during palliative care and bereavement, *Psycho-Oncology*, 7(1): 14–25.

Kissane, D.W. and Bloch, S. (2002) *Family Focused Grief Therapy. A model of family-centred care during palliative care and bereavement*. Buckingham: Open University Press.

Kissane, D.W., McKenzie, M., Bloch, S., Moskowitz, C., McKenzie, D.P. and O'Neill, I. (2006) Family focused grief therapy: a randomized controlled trial in palliative care and bereavement. *American Journal of Psychiatry*, 163: 1208–18.

Lattanzi-Licht, M.E. (1989) Bereavement services: practice and problems. *Hospice Journal*, 5: 1–28.

Lieberman, M.A. and Yalom, I. (1992) Brief group therapy for the spousally bereaved: a controlled study, *International Journal of Group Psychotherapy*, 42: 117–32.

Matsushima, T., Akabayashi, A. and Nishitateno, K. (2002) The current status of bereavement follow-up in hospice and palliative care in Japan, *Palliative Medicine*, 16(2): 151–8.

Middleton, W., Raphael, B., Martinek, N. and Misso, V. (1993) Pathological grief reactions. In: M.S. Stroebe, W. Stroebe and R.O. Hansson (eds) *Handbook of Bereavement*. Cambridge: Cambridge University Press.

Moos, R.H. and Moos, B.S. (1981) *Family Environment Scale Manual*. Palo Alto, CA: Consulting Psychologists Press.

National Hospice Organization (1997) *A pathway for patients and families facing terminal illness: self-determined life closure, safe comfortable dying and effective grieving*. Alexandria, Virginia: National Hospice Organization.

Parkes, C.M. (1998) *Bereavement: Studies of Grief in Adult Life*, 3rd edn. Madison, CT: International Universities Press.

Payne, S. (2001) The role of volunteers in hospice bereavement support in New Zealand, *Palliative Medicine*, 15(2): 107–15.

Piper, W.E., Ogrodniczuk, J.S., Joyce, A.S., Weidman, R. and Rosie, J.S. (2007) Group composition and group therapy for complicated grief, *Journal of Consult Clinical Psychology*, 75(1): 116–25.

Prigerson, H.G, Shear, M.K., Jacobs, S.C., Reynolds, C.F., Maciejewski, P.K., Davidson, J.R., Rosenheck, R.A., Pilkonis, P.A., Wortman, C.B., Williams, J.B., Widiger, T.A., Frank, E., Kupfer, D.J. and Zisook, S. (1999) Consensus criteria for traumatic grief. A preliminary empirical test. *British Journal Psychiatry*, 174: 67–73.

Prigerson, H.G., Horowitz, M.J., Jacobs, S.C., Parkes, C.M., Aslan, M., Raphael, B., Marwit, S.J., Wortman, C., Goodkin, K., Neimeyer, R.A., Bonanno, G., Block, S.D., Kissane, D.W., Boelen, P., Maercker, A., Litz, B., Johnson, J.G., First, M.B. and Maciejewski, P.K. (2007) Field trial of consensus criteria for prolonged grief disorder proposed for DSM-V. *American Journal of Psychiatry*, in press.

Raphael, B. (1977) Preventive intervention with the recently bereaved, *Archives of General Psychiatry*, 34: 1450–4.

Raphael, B., Minkov, C. and Dobson, M. (2001) Psychotherapeutic and pharmacological interventions for bereaved persons. In: M.S. Stroebe, R.O. Hansson, W. Stroebe and H. Schut (eds) *Handbook of Bereavement Research*. Washington, DC: American Psychological Association.

Reid, D., Field, D., Payne, S. and. Relf, M. (2006) Adult bereavement in five English hospices: types of support, *International Journal of Palliative Nursing*, 12(9): 430–7.

Rickerson, E.M., Somers, C., Allen, C.M., Lewis, B., Strumpf, N. and Casarett, D.J. (2005) How well are we caring for caregivers? Prevalence of grief-related symptoms and need for bereavement support among long-term care staff, *Journal of Pain and Symptom Management*, 30(3): 227–33.

Sandler, I., Balk, D., Jordan, J., Kennedy, C., Nadeau, J. and Shapiro, E. (2005) Bridging the gap between research and practice in bereavement: Report from the Center for the Advancement of Health. *Death Studies*, 29: 93–122.

Schut, H. and Stroebe, M.S. (2005) Interventions to enhance adaptation to bereavement, *Journal of Palliative Medicine*, 8(Suppl 1): S140–S147.

Schwab, R. (1995–96) Bereaved parents and support group participation, *Omega*, 32: 49–61.

Shear, K., Frank, E., Houck, P.R. and Reynolds, C.F. (2005) Treatment of complicated grief: A randomized controlled trial. *Journal of the American Medical Association*, 293: 2601–8.

Stewart, J. (1994) *Guidelines for setting up a bereavement service*. London: National Association of Bereavement Services.

Stokes, J., Wyer, S. and Crossley, D. (1997) The challenge of evaluating a child bereavement programme, *Palliative Medicine*, 11: 179–90.

Street, A.F., Love, A.W. and Blackford, J. (2004) Exploring bereavement care in inpatient settings, *Contemporary Nurse*, 17(3): 240–50.

Stroebe, M. and Schut, H. (1999) The dual process model of coping with bereavement: rationale and description, *Death Studies*, 23: 197–224.

Stroebe, W., Schut, H. and Stroebe, M. (2005) Grief work, disclosure, and counselling: Do they help the bereaved? *Clinical Psychology Reviews*, 25: 395–414.

Thuen, F. (1995) Satisfaction with bereavement support groups. Evaluation of the Norwegian Bereavement Care Project, *Journal of Mental Health*, 4: 499–510.

Walsh, F. and McGoldrick, M. (eds) (1991) *Living beyond Loss: Death in the Family*. New York, NY: Norton.

Wheeler, I. (1993–94) The role of meaning and purpose in life in bereaved parents associated with a self-help group: compassionate friends, *Omega*, 28: 261–71.

Wilkes, E. (1993) Characteristics of hospice bereavement services, *Journal of Cancer Care*, 2: 183–9.

Yalom, I.D. and Vinogradov, S. (1988) Bereavement groups: techniques and themes, *International Journal of Group Psychotherapy*, 38: 419–46.

Yi, P., Barreto, P., Soler, C., Fombuena, M., Espinar, V., Pascual, L., Navarro, R., Gonzalez, R., Bernabeu, J. and Suarez, J. (2006) Grief support provided to caregivers of palliative care patients in Spain, *Palliative Medicine*, 20(5): 521–31.

Zhang, B., El-Jawahri, A. and Prigerson, H. (2006) Update on bereavement research: evidence-based guidelines for the diagnosis and treatment of complicated bereavement. *Journal of Palliative Medicine*, 9(5): 1188–203.

# 26

# Helping children and families facing bereavement in palliative care settings

*Liz Rolls*

---

**Key points**

- Bereavement occurs within the particular social context of a child and their family.
- The death of a parent or sibling has an immediate and lasting effect on this environment, although the long-term effects on the child are uncertain.
- This context needs to be taken into account when providing support.
- Staff working in palliative care settings are in a unique position to both formally and informally provide an 'ecological niche' for children and families facing bereavement.

---

# Introduction

This chapter describes how children and families facing bereavement can be supported in palliative care and other settings. Drawing on international, contemporary literature, it contextualizes children's bereavement within the broader context of theories of human development and bereavement. It situates the experience of children and family bereavement within an ecological framework, and uses this to identify how a bereaved child's experience is mediated by their social context. It then draws on a UK-based research study of childhood bereavement services to illustrate some of the ways in which services act as an 'ecological niche' through which the needs of bereaved children and their families can be met. Finally, it focuses on how practitioners in palliative care settings can become an ecological niche, and support children and families both pre- and post-bereavement. For clarity, the way in which the terms 'children' and 'families' are being defined is described in Box 26.1.

---

**Box 26.1**   Definitions

**'Child', 'children' and 'childhood':**
Unless otherwise stated, these terms refer to children, young people and young adults between 0 and 18 years.

**'Parents' and 'family':**
The term 'parent' is used to mean biological and adoptive parents. The term 'family' is used to mean the 'network of people in the child's immediate psychosocial field' (Carr 1999: 3) including those who play a significant role.

**The use of these terms:**
The broad use of these terms does not intend to ignore the variety of family compositions within the UK, nor foreclose on later consideration of the impact of the individual family constellation on a child who has been bereaved.

---

# Children and families facing bereavement: a theoretical context

There are two theoretical contexts in which it is helpful to situate the challenges for children and families facing bereavement. First, as bereavement occurs at a particular time in a child's life, theories of human development help identify the potential impact of bereavement on the child's maturation, as well as indicate appropriate ways to support them. Second, theories of bereavement contribute to deepening our understanding of a child's responses to a death in the family, and each of these will be explored in turn.

# Competing models of human development

There are competing theories of how humans develop. In biologically deterministic models, development from infancy is seen as a 'forward-looking' linear process, the outcome of which is adulthood. Working in the UK, Corsaro (1997) argues that, as the model involves socializing children through training, sometimes viewed as 'taming' them to become a competent adult member of society, this perspective focuses on children's *futures* not their *present*. In contrast, the constructivist model sees the child as an active, creative agent in their development. Theorists such as the French educationalist Piaget (1937/1954) believed that, from infancy, we interpret, organize and use information from the environment, and construct conceptions of the physical and social worlds to which we then respond. This sociocultural perspective is shared by the Russian educationalist Vygotsky (1978), who argues that rather than being appropriated by, and consumers of, adult society, children are themselves appropriators of society through their active, creative, social agency (Corsaro 1997).

However, these competing perspectives ignore the *relationship* between the biological, genetic inheritance of an individual and the particularity of its environment. A more inclusive model of human development has been developed by Bronfenbrenner (1992) in the United States. His bioecological model of development not only emphasizes the importance of the interpersonal, social relationships on the development of the child and their capacity to act on their social world, but the set of *processes* thorough which these interact *over the life course* (Bronfenbrenner 1992). These processes take place through progressively more complex reciprocal interactions between individuals and their environment. This notion of 'social ecology' occurs in the context of the four systems or environments outlined in Figure 26.1.

Importantly, it is within this *dynamic* of relationships that the death of a parent or sibling – the bereavement of a child – occurs.

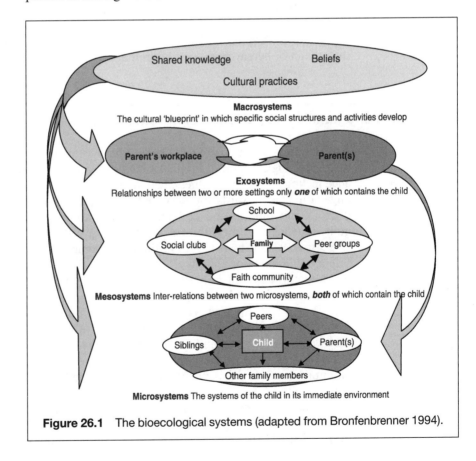

**Figure 26.1**   The bioecological systems (adapted from Bronfenbrenner 1994).

# Theories of bereavement

During the past 50 years, there has been increasing international literature on bereavement, including the varied definitions of mourning, grief and bereavement, and the development of the broad range of bereavement discourses. However, what is of note is that there are very few models in the literature of bereavement that reflects the contemporaneous experience of children and young people, derived from their own voice. Rather, ideas about their bereavement experience are borrowed and adapted from theories and models that apply, in the first instance, to adults. Exceptions to this include Holland's (2001) retrospective UK study of *adults* who experienced loss in childhood, and Christ's (2000) US study on the responses children, at 6 and 14 months following the death of a parent. However, the outcome – following a Parent Guidance Intervention or a supportive reflective intervention – was based on *adult determined* levels of functioning. Chowns *et al.*'s (2005) UK-based collaborative study of children living with the uncertainty of life-threatening parental illness is one of the few that privileges children's own voice (Rolls and Payne 2007). Despite this lack, there are a number of theoretical accounts of the impact of bereavement on children and it is to these we now turn.

# Children's and families' experience of bereavement

Unlike adults, children are less likely to have strategies to minimize or avoid the psychological pain of grief (Archer 1999), and they are likely to experience feelings of denial, sadness, fear, anxiety expressed in bodily symptoms; anger directed towards the deceased parent, the remaining parent and/or doctors and nurses; and feelings of panic about abandonment, despair, guilt, loneliness, responsibility, isolation and self-reproach (Bowlby 1961; Dyregrov 1991). Christ (2000) in the USA argues that children may constitute a vulnerable population at increased risk for social impairment and/or psychopathology, not only during the immediate post-bereavement period but extending into adulthood; although Harrington and Harrison (1999) in the UK contest this view. However, there are unresolved questions arising from studies which argue that, one year after parental bereavement, bereaved children are comparable to their peers, and Worden and Silverman (1996) in the USA suggest that the findings on the emotional impact of parental death for dependent children have not been consistent due to serious methodological limitations.

What is more certain is that how a child experiences and responds to the death of a significant person, and the accommodation, or 'timely reconstitution' (Christ 2000) that a child is able to make, is the result of a complex set of processes or interactions between the significant relationships in the ecological systems of which they are a part. Drawing on international literature, a number of mediators have been identified.

### The child's characteristics, including their age and stage of cognitive and emotional development

The child's characteristics differentiate and affect the experience of bereavement. The significance of gender is unclear. Worden *et al.* (1999) suggest that boys are more affected than girls by the loss of a parent, and girls more than boys by the loss of a sibling, while Raveis *et al.* (1999) found that boys reported lower levels of depressive symptoms than girls. There is also uncertainty about the age at which a child develops a capacity to mourn, which itself may be related to their capacity to understand the concept of death as permanent, irreversible, inevitable and universal. This capacity is influenced by a number of factors including the child's experience of death, religious beliefs and what children are told (Stambrook and Parker 1987; Anthony and Bhana 1988–9). Thus, more recent writers locate a child's understanding of death in their social experience, rather than in their developmental age. However, a number of commentators argue that even very young children have a concept of death (Black 1996) although, as Corr (1991) notes, the capacity to *conceptualize* is different from *understanding the significance* of it. Furthermore, the expression of sadness does not require the child to have a concept of death (Furman 1974); an argument supported by Bowlby (1960, 1980/1998) who suggests that children can show grief reactions as soon as they have developed attached relationships, and that these can be seen in children as young as six months old.

Adolescents are less physically dependent on adults for their care. Nevertheless, the death of a parent or sibling has significance. Young people may have a desperate struggle in trying to understand and cope with overwhelming and unexpected feelings following a deeply felt bereavement (Ribbens McCarthy 2006). The conflicts they experience are between separation versus reunion, abandonment versus safety, independence versus dependence, and closeness versus distance, and these echo the processes in adolescent mourning: experiencing the need to separate, protest at this experience, a search for ways to overcome, being challenged by a situation not of their making, feeling disorientated/disorganized, and being called upon to reorganize their lives (Corr 1991).

### Who has died and who remains

The death of a parent or a sibling occurs in the child's close family system and has an immediate and lasting effect on this environment. The death of a parent is one of the greatest crises in the life of a child and one of the most fundamental losses they can face (Dyregrov 1991; Worden 1996). As a consequence of parental death, the familiar design of family life is completely disrupted, creating changes in the relationships that surround the child (Schuchter and Zisook 1993). When the death of a sibling occurs, there will have been a history of a complex set of sibling relationships, and their death presents a different set of challenges for the bereaved child, who has been described as the 'forgotten mourner' (Hindmarch 1995).

These include negotiating the ambivalent feelings often found in sibling relationships (Dyregrov 1991). Furthermore, when a child has died of a life-limiting illness, the well siblings will have already been living in 'houses of chronic sorrow' (Bertman 1991: 320, citing Bluebond-Langner 1989).

Following a parental or sibling death, the child continues in a relationship with those who remain. Where a parent has died, the presence of young children in the home represents a considerable burden for the surviving bereaved parent (Parkes 1986). In addition, the child suffers not only the loss of the parent, but is often deprived of the attention they need at a time when extra reassurance is needed (Grollman 1967), creating 'a new terror for a bereft child: the loss of one parent, and the symbolic or temporary loss – the unavailability – of the other' (Bertman 1991: 321). Riches and Dawson (2000) term this experience a 'double jeopardy'.

Following the death of a sibling, as well as experiencing the loss of that relationship, the bereaved child will now be in the environment of parents who have lost a child, and on whom there is now a 'need to mourn their *separate* relationships with the child [and] conflicting demands both to let go of the parent role (in the case of the child who died) and, at the same time, to continue to be a parent to the remaining sibling' (Bertman 1991: 322, emphasis in the original). In grieving for their deceased child, the ability of parents to maintain balanced interaction with the surviving children is difficult (Rubin 1993). Furthermore, they may put an intolerable emotional burden on their remaining children (Pettle and Britten 1995) because of increased parental anxiety and over-protection (Dyregrov 1991).

The active coping style of the surviving parent appears to affect the outcome for the child (Christ 2000). Hurd's (1999) US-based study suggests that Bowlby's prediction – that healthy mourning during childhood can be influenced by certain positive family factors – is corroborated by adults' retrospective view of their childhood bereavement experience. Key factors contributing to healthy childhood mourning included positive relationships between the child and both parents, ample emotional and psychological support from the surviving parent, and open and honest communication with the child about the death and its impact on the family (Hurd 1999; Raveis *et al.* 1999).

These are important factors to take into account when providing support to a bereaved child and their family, and will be discussed more fully later.

### The circumstances around the death

The circumstances surrounding the death involve a number of aspects, including how the person died, how and what children are told and how involved they are in the funeral, and what life is like afterwards.

### How the person died

An anticipated death in which there is some warning helps lower anxieties (Black 1998) and provides an opportunity for families to redefine their expectations of themselves and their relationships (Altschuler 2005). By contrast, a sudden death is a shock to the family system (Handsley 2001) placing it under great strain. These deaths often have a traumatic aspect resulting in a stronger impact on adults and the desire to protect children from too much detail (Dyregrov 1991). Indeed, children who have witnessed a violent death may develop post-traumatic stress disorder (Pynoos *et al.* 1987) and the children of murdered parents may well need specialized help (Black *et al.* 1992). The death of a parent or sibling by suicide presents particular difficulties for a child, not only because these are invariably violent deaths but also because they challenge the child's notions of the world and what people can do (Dyregrov 1991). In addition, murder and suicide are often accompanied by stigma and notoriety, which have consequences for the bereaved person's future life, including fears for their own safety (Riches and Dawson 2000).

### How and what children are told and how involved they are in the funeral

As well as learning about the illness, hearing about the death is a significant moment (Worden 1996), and parents are confronted with decisions about what, when and how to tell their children about the events surrounding the illness and death. Although children vary in their emotional and behavioural reactions, their responses are strongly influenced by those of the surviving parent and other adults (Worden 1996). Forewarning can help the child prepare (Black 1998), but for many reasons parents will deny their children information (Black 1996; Silverman 2000), or provide information at the time of diagnosis, but not keep the child updated (Dyregrov 1991). Children benefit from attending funerals and other rituals (Black 1998), as these help children to acknowledge the death, honour the life of the deceased, and provide support and comfort for the bereaved children (Worden 1996).

### What life is like afterwards

As well as creating dramatic changes in the relationships that surround the child (Schuchter and Zisook 1993), bereavement also has an impact on the practical aspects of everyday life (Melvin and Lukeman 2000), and on the 'internal working models' of the family (Riches and Dawson 2000: 5). According to Worden (1996), positive adjustment is associated with fewer daily life changes, but change is inevitable. The most frequent changes are experienced in the first four months, and there may be increased resentment at added responsibilities, especially following the death of a mother (Worden 1996). However, with changing roles between partners and the increasing inclusion of children within the social economy of the household, this may not always be the case. Death may also involve significant changes in the family's financial status, creating difficulties for the surviving members to manage (Corden *et al.* 2002). When the parent(s) are unavailable, the child needs support from outside, and access to a replacement person can have positive effects on the child (Dyregrov 1991; Melvin and Lukeman 2000), although the surviving parent's new relationships may present the child with difficulty. Significant changes in communication patterns also occur, including difficulty talking about the dead person or particular topics that may cause distress, the censoring of information, and in who talks to whom (Moos 1995). Balk (1990) argues that siblings, in trying to appear to cope, may not be given opportunities to talk, but children may also understand the burden under which the parent(s) struggle and adjust their behaviour accordingly (Silverman 2000). In addition, parents may be unwilling to discuss details of the death and their own feelings about it (Riches and Dawson 2000).

## Child's relationship to peer and school

The school is an important setting for a bereaved child; it is a social environment that influences the meaning of loss (Rowling and Holland 2000; Rowling, 2003), either providing a potential haven of peace and normality (Pennells and Smith 1995) and peer support (Ribbens McCarthy 2006), or being a source of increased distress and isolation (Hindmarch 1995; Rowling 2003). Peers are both sources of comfort, especially having a friend who has had a similar experience, having older friends, or friends who knew the person who has died. However, children may not talk to friends for a number of reasons including their fear of crying, awkwardness on the part of friends, their friends not knowing or caring about the death, and it feeling too personal (Worden 1996). The maintenance of contact with other children at school is important, especially if there is also parental grief (Walsh and McGoldrick 1991). However, many siblings feel peers and teachers do not understand their feelings (Hindmarch 1995), and school problems arise because of increased teasing (Rowling 2003); not being understood by peers and teachers; and through poor concentration (Pettle and Britten 1995). In some cases, the school community itself may be experiencing the loss of one of its students or staff. Schools that provide both open discussions about life and death for its pupils, as well as individual support if a death occurs, offer a protective moderating factor to the bereaved child (Dyregrov 1991).

## Providing an ecological 'niche' for bereaved children and their families

Bronfenbrenner's (1992) model identifies that the capacity to develop psychological health rests on successful adaptation to events that have occurred.

This adaptation – or its opposite, a failure to adapt – occurs in 'ecological niches'; events that are 'favourable or unfavourable for the development of individuals' (Bronfenbrenner 1992: 194). This section uses the work of UK childhood bereavement services as an example of the way in which services can provide an 'ecological niche' through which to help and support bereaved children and families. It draws on a UK study of childhood bereavement services that examined their nature and purpose. For full details of the research design and methods, and the broad findings on UK service provision, and children's experience of their use, see Rolls and Payne (2003, 2004, 2007).

# The work of UK childhood bereavement services

UK childhood bereavement services offer a range of interventions which impact on the environments of the child. In Bronfenbrenner's ecological model, childhood bereavement services exist as part of the exosystem, whether or not a child has been bereaved. Once a bereaved child uses a childhood bereavement service, it becomes a setting in the mesosystem in which the restorative 'proximal processes' between the child and childhood bereavement service providers can occur.

### Childhood bereavement services: A mesosystem of the child

Services offer support to children in different ways – either directly, or indirectly through websites and newsletters. Direct support is also offered in two modes: either individually or in groups, with the child only or with their family, and Figure 26.2 identifies the types of activity that each dimension might include.

The service's focus is always on the child but parents also need to have their feelings recognized (Monroe 1995), and the extent to which a service focuses on the bereavement needs of parents varies. This may be undertaken in a parents' group, as part of family work, or parents may be referred to an adult service such as Cruse.

Service providers engage in a purposeful relationship with the child, and it is through these relationships – the proximal processes – that the child's bereavement experience is transformed. The relationships and activities are not random, and while the specific activities may differ, *between* services and *within* services, they are purposeful. Underlying the activities are a set of objectives that would enable the child to:

*Remember the person who has died and create a 'story' that the child can integrate into their life narrative*

Services help children remember the person who has died through a number of activities, including making a 'memory jar', collecting important items in

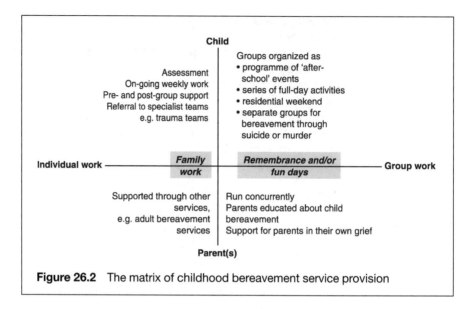

**Figure 26.2** The matrix of childhood bereavement service provision

a special 'memory' box, or making and decorating a photograph frame. What is crucial to these activities is not just the making or collection of the artefact(s), but helping the child talk about the meaning these have for them (Riches and Dawson 2000). This process supports 'continuing bonds' (Potts *et al.* 1999); helps create a narrative; and forms part of helping a child understand, name and enable them to express their feelings.

### Understand and express their feelings

Opportunities for mentally processing the traumatic changes and unfamiliar feelings of bereavement are crucial (Riches and Dawson 2000). This includes an opportunity for 'cognitive mastery' of the event, as well as stimulating emotional coping (Dyregrov 1991). There are many creative ways in which services help children understand and express their feelings, such as through the use of story telling, puppets, 'anger walls' or other games, watching and talking about videos, and through other symbolic activities.

### Understand the 'normality' of bereavement and reduce isolation

There is a need to appreciate the normality of parental and sibling grieving, and both parents and children often feel isolated in such an extremely important event (Riches and Dawson 2000). Sibling groups can help over-come these feelings (Wright *et al.* 1996). Within the wider group, services usually run age-specific activities, and children can become supportive of each other both during and after these.

### *Childhood bereavement services: An exosystem of the child*

UK childhood bereavement services also work with those who have an impact on the environments of a child, for example, the emergency services and schools. Their work includes:

*Providing advice and information to the families of children who have been bereaved (influencing the microsystem)*

As we have seen, what and how children are told about events surrounding the death is important, and parents may need help in thinking about what to say to their child (Monroe 1995). Parents may also be confused about their child's response to the death, and uncertain how to help them understand both the events surrounding the death and the confusing set of feelings they are experiencing. Giving appropriate advice and information is, therefore, crucial in supporting parents to respond appropriately to their children's needs, and in helping them anticipate difficulties. Services clearly feel this is an important aspect of their work, as 95 per cent of childhood bereavement services in the study offered information and advice to bereaved families, while 88 per cent of services provided resources, such as books and leaflets (Rolls and Payne 2003).

*Supporting schools where either a member of staff or a child has died, or where a child has been bereaved (influencing other mesosystems)*

As an important setting for a bereaved child, the school can be enhanced in a number of ways. Those that provide both open discussions about life and death for its pupils, as well as individual support if a death occurs, offer a protective moderating factor to the bereaved child (Dyregrov 1991). In the study, 66 per cent of childhood bereavement services provided support to schools where there has been a death in the school community itself, or where a child in the school has been bereaved. The level and type of support ranged from advising teachers on how to support the bereaved child, to supporting and assisting them in their own bereavement.

The Childhood Bereavement Network (a network of UK service providers, organizations and individuals working to improve access and service provision) is campaigning for every school to promote the well-being of bereaved children and young people through a whole-school approach, including flexible pastoral support, developing systems for communicating important information about children's bereavements, and school policy development.

*Educating and training health, social care and other professionals (influencing other exosystems)*

While children may not have access to, or want to use, a specialized bereavement service, they are often in contact – during the course of their everyday life – with a range of professionals such as teachers, doctors and school nurses. Furthermore, groups of people, such as staff of the emergency services and specialist palliative care settings, may be present in the environment where death occurred. These groups are therefore important mediators of help and information about bereavement. In the study, 32 per cent of services offered education and training to these groups (Rolls and Payne 2003).

*Influencing the social constructions, cultural assumptions and beliefs about childhood bereavement (influencing the macrosystems)*

There is now an ambivalent and contradictory attitude to death in modern society; death is both present, for example, through the mass media and, at the same time, serious discussion about our own deaths is still considered morbid (Riches and Dawson 2000).

Death has been removed from public space and communal religious practices into hospital and has become a technical matter. Funerals are now organized by specialists and rituals have been deconstructed so people do not know how to act (Mellor 1993). This privatization and subjectivization of the experience has consequences for individuals, as 'the absence of death from the public space makes its presence in the private space an intense and potentially threatening one' (Mellor 1993: 21). Furthermore, it is not only death and bereavement that is sequestered into the private domain. Children themselves are subsumed within the privatized nuclear family and hidden statistically from significant events that affect them (for example, from how many children are bereaved annually). This may be because 'they are not expected to have a stake in the present, social, economic or political arrangements' (Qvortrup 1997: 25). In their response to children's bereavement, childhood bereavement services are influencing cultural attitudes and beliefs. These influences are outlined diagrammatically in Figure 26.3.

## Providing an ecological 'niche' for children and their families facing bereavement in palliative care settings

Staff working in palliative care settings are in a unique position to provide an 'ecological niche' for children and families facing bereavement. The pre-bereavement phase offers particular opportunities for staff to influence their experience of both the death and the immediate aftermath. Being in close contact during this time means that staff – while not being able to change the reality of the fact of dying and death – are able to contribute to making order out of chaos and help give a language for, and meaning to, children and families experience of grief. This contribution can be both informal through the 'everyday' interaction with children and their families, or through more formally arranged (individual or group) sessions. It is not possible – nor desirable – to provide a 'formula' of appropriate responses or

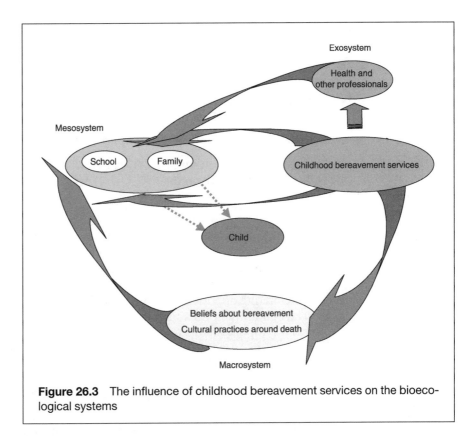

**Figure 26.3** The influence of childhood bereavement services on the bioecological systems

actions, but Bronfenbrenner's framework can be a useful tool to enable staff to think about the needs of children and families, and how best to respond and support them.

## Using Bronfenbrenner's framework

Although this list is not exhaustive, there are four ways in which Bronfenbrenner's framework can be used by staff to frame their responses and support to children and their families.

### Understanding the specific context of the child and their family

Understanding the 'ecological' context helps inform staff about factors they need to take into account in their responses to a child's needs. Useful information that helps shape an appropriate response or course of action includes:

- the meaning of the child's relationship to the person who is dying or has died (in the child's terms);

- the child's capacity to understand the nature of the illness, its life-limiting potential, and the permanency of death;
- the family's cultural beliefs and practices in relation to death, the disposal of bodies, and mourning;
- what the child has been told about the illness, dying and death.

### *Being an ecological niche for the child in the palliative care setting*

Staff in palliative care settings are well-placed to provide an ecological niche for children by helping them to:

- Create memories of their relative, by:
  - encouraging the child to talk, for example about: what has been happening during the illness; what memories they have of the person before they became ill; things the child enjoys about them and loves them for, incidents that are important;
  - encouraging the child to write or draw this story;
  - facilitating opportunities where the child and their dying relative can talk about their life together;
  - clarifying the child's understanding about the illness, and telling the 'truth' in answers to questions about the disease in ways the child can understand.
- Understand and express their feelings, by:
  - taking them seriously – even when being 'light-hearted' and having fun;
  - wondering what the child is asking and saying (that is, is the child asking a concrete question for which they need a concrete answer, or are they giving a clue to an aspect of their underlying mental/emotional state that needs addressing);
  - reflecting back the feeling that is being expressed rather than responding to the concrete question/expressed emotion. This allows the child to: reflect more; feel safe in the knowledge that their feelings have being taken seriously; and clarifies whether what they have said is really the problem;
  - inviting the child to say more;
  - asking them what they think would help them, rather than assuming anything.
- Understand the 'normality' of bereavement and reduce isolation, by:
  - responding honestly in age-appropriate language. This signals the 'normality' of dying and death as something that can be spoken about, even if it feels sad or difficult to do so;
  - encouraging groups of children to come together and providing opportunities for them to share their experiences and support each other;
  - encouraging children to talk to their parents, reassuring them that while parents may be sad, they will still want to know how the child is doing;

  ○   encouraging children to talk to a trusted person, such as a friend or their teacher.

### *Being an ecological niche for the parents in palliative care settings*

Staff in palliative care settings are well-placed to provide an ecological niche for parents by:

- enhancing their capacity to parent, through advice and support;
- relieving them, at times, of the responsibility for the care of their child;
- encouraging and helping them think about how, what and when they tell their child about the illness, and about death;
- inviting them to think about whether the child sees the dead body and, if so, to mediate this experience;
- inviting them to think about how to include the child in the funeral arrangements;
- giving parents a language for some of the medical aspects that children may ask about;
- encouraging them to talk as a family about what is happening, and to their child about how the child is feeling;
- putting them in touch with other parents or support services.

### *Influencing others*

In addition, staff in palliative care settings have the capacity to influence others and their responses to bereaved children and their families, through educating and training others, and by influencing the social constructions, cultural assumptions and beliefs about dying, death and childhood bereavement.

Useful resources and information for practitioners and families can be found on a number of worldwide websites. A few examples are listed in Box 26.2.

---

**Box 26.2**   Useful websites for families and practitioners

http://www.childbereavement.org.uk/
http://www.dougy.org/
http://www.grief.org.au/
http://www.paradisekids.org.au/services.htm
http://www.skylight.org.nz/
http://www.winstonswish.org.uk/

---

# Conclusion

Locating this brief review of the impact on bereavement on a child in Bronfenbrenner's (1992) ecological systems model shows that the event occurs in, and is mediated by, a complex set of inter-relationships within the micro- and mesosystems of the child. Thus, each child in a family will experience the bereavement differently, not only because of the different qualitative relationship that they had to the deceased, but also because of the proximal processes of the micro- and mesosystems of which each of them is a part. Through their knowledge and place within a mesosystem of the child, staff in palliative care settings, *in any cultural context*, are uniquely placed to provide an 'ecological niche' of support to children and their families both pre- and post-bereavement in each of these systems.

# References

Altschuler, J. (2005) Illness and loss within the family. In: P. Firth, G. Luff, and D. Oliviere, *Loss, change and bereavement in palliative care*. Maidenhead: Open University Press, pp. 53–65.

Anthony, Z. and Bhana, K. (1988–9) An exploratory study of Muslim girls' understanding of death. *Omega*, 19: 215–27.

Archer, J. (1999) *The nature of grief: the evolution and psychology of the actions to loss*. London: Routledge.

Balk, D. (1990) The self-concepts of bereaved adolescents: Sibling death and its aftermath. *Journal of Adolescent Research*, 5(1): 112–32.

Bertman, S. (1991) Children and death: Insights, hindsights and illuminations. In: D. Papadatos and C. Papadatou (eds) *Children and death*. New York: Hemisphere, pp. 311–29.

Black, D. (1996) Childhood bereavement. *British Medical Journal*, 312(7045): 1496.

Black, D. (1998) Bereavement in childhood. *British Medical Journal*, 316(7135): 931–33.

Black, D., Harris-Hendricks, J. and Kaplan, C. (1992) When father kills mother: Post traumatic stress disorder in the children. *Psychotherapy and Psychosomatics*, 57(4): 152–7.

Bluebond-Langner, M. (1989) Worlds of dying children and their well siblings. *Death Studies*, 13: 1–16.

Bowlby, J. (1960) Grief and mourning in infancy and early childhood. *Psychoanalytic Study of the Child*, 15: 9–52.

Bowlby, J. (1961) Process of mourning. *International Journal of Psychoanalysis*, 42: 317–40.

Bowlby, J. (1998) *Attachment and loss: Vol. 3: Loss, sadness and depression*. London: Pimlico (first published in 1980 by London: Hogarth Press).

Bronfenbrenner, U. (1992) Ecological systems theory. In: R. Vasta (ed.) *Six theories of child development: Revised formulations and current issues*. London: Jessica Kingsley, pp. 187–249.

Bronfenbrenner, U. (1994) Ecological models of human development. In: T. Husen and T.N. Postlethwaite (eds) *International Encyclopaedia of Education*, 2nd edn. Oxford: Pergamon, 3: 1643–7.

Chowns, G., Bussey, S. and Jones, A. (2005) 'No – You don't know how we feel'. Lessons learnt from a collaborative inquiry with children facing the life threatening illness of a parent. Paper presented at the 7th International Conference of the Social Context of Death, Dying and Disposal. University of Bath, UK.

Christ, G.H. (2000) *Healing children's grief: Surviving a parent's death from cancer*. Oxford: Oxford University Press.

Corden, A., Sloper, P. and Sainsbury, R. (2002) Financial effects for families after the death of a disabled or chronically ill child: A neglected dimension of bereavement. *Child: Care, Health and Development*, 28(3): 199–204.

Corr, C.A. (1991) Understanding adolescents and death. In: D. Papadatou and C. Papadatos (eds) *Children and Death*. New York: Hemisphere, pp. 33–51.

Corsaro, W.A. (1997) *The sociology of childhood*. London: Pine Forge Press.

Dyregrov, A. (1991) *Grief in children: A handbook for adults*. London: Jessica Kingsley.

Furman, E. (1974) *A child's parent dies: Studies in childhood bereavement*. London: Yale University Press.

Grollman, E. (1967) Prologue. In: E. Grollman (ed.) *Explaining death to children*. Boston: Beacon Press, pp. 3–27.

Handsley, S. (2001) 'But what about us?' The residual effects of sudden death on self-identity and family relationships. *Mortality*, 6(1): 9–29.

Harrington, R. and Harrison, L. (1999) Unproven assumptions about the impact of bereavement on children. *Journal of the Royal Society of Medicine*, 92(5): 230–3.

Hindmarch, C. (1995) Secondary losses for siblings. *Child: Care, Health, and Development*, 21(6): 425–31.

Holland, J. (2001) *Understanding children's experiences of parental bereavement*. London: Jessica Kingsley.

Hurd, R.C. (1999) Adults view their childhood bereavement experiences. *Death Studies*, 23(1): 17–41.

Mellor, P.A. (1993) Death in high modernity: The contemporary presence and absence of death. In: D. Clark (ed.) *The sociology of death*. Oxford: Blackwell, pp. 11–30.

Melvin, D. and Lukeman, D. (2000) Bereavement: A framework for those working with children. *Clinical Child Psychology and Psychiatry*, 5(4): 521–39.

Monroe, B. (1995) Helping the grieving family. In: S.C. Smith and M. Pennells *Interventions with bereaved children*. London: Jessica Kingsley.

Moos, N.L. (1995) An integrative model of grief. *Death Studies*, 19(4): 337–64.

Pennells, M. and Smith, S.C. (1995) *The forgotten mourners: Guidelines for working with bereaved children*. London: Jessica Kingsley.

Parkes, C.M. (1986) *Bereavement: Studies of grief in adult life*, 2nd edn. London: Routledge.

Pettle, S.A. and Britten, C.M. (1995) Talking with children about death and dying. *Child: Care, Health and Development*, 21(6): 395–404.

Piaget, J. (1937/1954) *The construction of reality in the child*. New York: Basic Books.

Potts, S., Farrell, M. and O'Toole, J. (1999) Treasure Weekend: Supporting bereaved siblings. *Palliative Medicine*, 13: 51–6.

Pynoos, R.S., Frederick, C., Nader, K., Arroyo, W., Steinberg, A., Eth, S., Nunez, F. and Fairbank, L. (1987) Life threat and post-traumatic stress in school age children. *Archives of General Psychiatry*, 44: 1057–63.

Qvortrup, J. (1997) A voice for children in statistical and social accounting: A plea for children's right to be heard. In: A. James and A. Prout (eds) *Constructing and reconstructing childhood*, 2nd edn. London: Falmer Press, pp. 78–98.

Raveis, V.H., Siegel, K. and Karus, D. (1999) Children's psychological distress following the death of a parent. *Journal of Youth and Adolescence*, 28(2): 165–80.

Ribbens McCarthy, J. (2006) *Young people's experience of loss and bereavement: Towards an interdisciplinary approach*. Maidenhead: Open University Press.

Riches, G. and Dawson, P. (2000) *An intimate loneliness: Supporting bereaved parents and siblings*. Buckingham: Open University Press.

Rolls, L. and Payne, S. (2003) Childhood bereavement services: A survey of UK provision. *Palliative Medicine*, 17: 423–32.

Rolls, L. and Payne, S. (2004) Childhood bereavement services: Issues in UK provision. Mortality, 9(4): 300–28.

Rolls, L. and Payne, S. (2007) Children and young people's experience of UK childhood bereavement services. *Mortality*, 12(3): 281–303.

Rowling, L. (2003) *Grief in school communities: Effective support strategies*. Buckingham: Open University Press.

Rowling, L. and Holland, J. (2000) Grief and School communities: The impact of social context, a comparison between Australia and England. *Death Studies*, 24: 35–50.

Rubin, S. (1993) The death of a child is forever: The life course impact of child loss. In: M. Stroebe, W. Stroebe and R.O. Hansson (eds) *Handbook of bereavement: Theory, research and intervention*. Cambridge: Cambridge University Press, pp. 285–99.

Schuchter, S. and Zisook, S. (1993) A course of normal grief. In: M. Stroebe, W. Stroebe and R. Hannson (eds) *Handbook of bereavement: Theory, research and intervention*. Cambridge: Cambridge University Press, pp. 23–43.

Silverman, P.R. (2000) *Never too young to know: Death in children's lives*. Oxford: Oxford University Press.

Stambrook, M. and Parker, K.C.H. (1987) The development of the concept of death in childhood: A review of the literature. *Merrill Palmer Quarterly*, 33: 133–57.

Vygotsky, L.S. (1978). *Mind in society*. Cambridge, MA: Harvard University Press.

Walsh, F. and McGoldrick, M. (1991) Loss and the family: A systemic perspective. In: F. Walsh and M. McGoldrick (eds) *Living beyond loss: Death in the family*. New York: Norton, pp. 1–29.

Worden, J.W. (1996) *Children and grief: When a parent dies*. New York: Guilford Press.

Worden, J.W., Davies, B. and McCown, D. (1999) Comparing parent loss with sibling loss. *Death Studies*, 23(1): 1–15.

Worden, J.W. and Silverman, P.R. (1996) Parental death and the adjustment of school-age children. *Omega*, 33(2): 91–102.

Wright, J.B., Aldridge, J., Gillance, H. and Tucker, A. (1996) Hospice-based groups for bereaved siblings. *European Journal of Palliative Care*, 3(1): 10–15.

# PART FOUR

## Contemporary issues

# 27

# Overview

*Christine Ingleton and Jane Seymour*

Changes in population demographics, health needs and reforms in health care delivery and work practices have had a major impact on the nursing profession in many developed countries. The need for reform in nursing emerges from challenges in four main areas: education, service, recruitment and retention, and changes both in health needs and models of care delivery. The widespread shortage of nurses and their high turnover are global issues that are of increasing importance to all health care systems as they strive to find solutions to satisfy demands for nurses in all areas of health care (While 2005). Nurses prefer to work with healthy people and those who will regain health, or with children, or in highly technical areas such as the operating theatre (Kluster *et al.* 2007), and this situation could present problems for the recruitment and retention of nurses working in palliative care.

At the same time, increases in the age profile of populations, the rising incidence of cancer and the worldwide spread of HIV/AIDS, point to an increase in the need for palliative care in the coming years. As the need for palliative care increases, so the need for general and specialist palliative care education both pre- and post-registration continues to grow. However, meeting those needs is particularly challenging because the nature of palliative care means that teaching and learning about it can be complex and problematic (Wee 2007). Box 27.1 shows the particular challenges facing nursing and other disciplines in palliative care education. These will be discussed in turn.

## Changes in the initial preparation of nurses

Palliative care education worldwide has undergone massive reforms in terms of where and how nurses are prepared in both pre-registration training and in subsequent continuing professional development. To date, most studies have been concerned predominantly with the post-registration preparation

**Box 27.1** Challenges in palliative care education

- Changes in the initial preparation of nurses
- Changes in the continuing education of nurses
- The scarcity of resources and teaching staff with skills in general palliative care
- Delivering education in resource poor countries
- The paucity of evidence to indicate the effect of education on practice
- Distance, cost and access to effective programmes of education

of nurses to work in cancer and palliative care, such as the identification of deficiencies in education and factors that may enhance nursing competence in palliative and end-of-life care. Those studies that exist show that nurses in the UK are inadequately prepared to undertake this type of care and experience considerable stress (Lloyd-Williams and Field 2002).

Brajtman *et al.* (2007) suggest that Canadian nurse educators have embraced palliative care only to a limited extent, and there is wide variation in the degree to which end-of-life care is addressed within the undergraduate nursing curriculum. Reporting results from a purposive sample of 58 undergraduate students who completed a questionnaire survey, findings indicated that student nurses held positive attitudes towards caring for dying patients; however, they had modest knowledge levels, and only one-third did not feel adequately prepared to care for dying people. Although end-of-life care education tended to be threaded throughout the programme, the emphasis was dependent upon the commitment of individual staff members of faculty staff with experience and/or expertise.

In the USA, Dickinson (2006) conducted a study to compare the status of current death education and end-of-life issues in undergraduate nursing programmes with those in 1984. In common with the Canadian study, Dickinson reported that the prominence of end-of-life care within the curriculum was contingent upon the skills and interests of faculty staff. In the intervening 22-year period, he noted that slight changes in the programme of the US nursing schools regarding end-of-life/death issues were discernable: 'the number of offerings has increased, though nursing schools were well into an emphasis on death and dying in 1984' (p. 166).

In the UK, there are relatively few cancer and palliative care specific modules within pre-registration education programmes (RCN 2003). This has raised concerns about the ability of newly qualified nurses to care effectively for palliative care patients in non-specialist settings (RCN 2003).

From the information that is currently available, it would appear that palliative care education has not been incorporated adequately within undergraduate training with any degree of uniformity. Given the growing volume of work in both the acute and community sectors in providing care for those patients with chronic, life-limiting diseases, palliative care education should take greater prominence than at present.

# Changes in the continuing education of nurses

In the past, nursing has been viewed as a practice-based profession, with little expectation of education beyond that needed to inform and perform practical tasks. As the academic profile of nursing has developed, the number of post-registration practitioners seeking higher education courses to update their academic qualifications to first or higher degree level has increased markedly. Currently, a major issue facing registered nurses is the ongoing challenge of maintaining professional competence in the context of rapidly changing health care systems.

Research has demonstrated worldwide that there are major deficiencies in post-registration nursing education for end-of-life care (Mallory 2003; Easom *et al.* 2006). For example, Barclay *et al.* (2003) report that health care practitioners in Wales are inadequately trained in the areas of symptom management; health care providers in China and Japan both report a small increase in training focused on end-of-life care but highlight the need for more educational preparation (Takeda 2002; Wang *et al.* 2002). In the context of other care environments such as nursing homes, there is a lack of sufficient education and training (Froggatt 2004). Similarly in the USA, there is lack of training in overall end-of-life care management in assisted living facilities (Robinson 2004). Despite this, the number of nurses undertaking post-registration education remains worryingly low (O'Connor and Fitzsimmons 2005).

Delivering continuing professional education in palliative care is complex and involves increasing knowledge, developing approaches to care, the ability to work with emotionally difficult situations and the skills of networking with colleagues (Hughes *et al.* 2006). One of the most difficult dilemmas for the palliative care educator is to achieve some kind of standardization across programmes. In 1997 the European Association for Palliative Care (EAPC) proposed that the collective member association in each country should create a national education network to establish minimum recommendations for training for both nurses and doctors, and also identify those training skills most appropriate for palliative care educators (Vlieger *et al.* 2004). The report, 'A guide for the development of palliative nurse education in Europe', proposes three levels of nursing knowledge acquisition. The decision about what constitutes each level remains the prerogative of each country, as does the number of hours associated with the educational preparation for each level (see Chapter 30 for a full account of the framework).

In the UK, NICE (2004) has recommended national guidelines for the preparation of a 'suitably trained workforce' to provide supportive and palliative care to patients with cancer including families and other informal care-givers. Such developments are significant in terms of their recognition of the need to prepare an effective and informed workforce at *all* levels rather than at just post-registration, which has been the traditional approach (Cunningham *et al.* 2006). However, it remains unclear the commitment to and extent to which UK Universities and Trusts have implemented these recommendations to meet the national education targets for cancer and palliative care (Cunningham *et al.* 2006).

In the USA, the End-of-Life Nursing Education Consortium (ELNEC) has launched a national initiative to improve and unify educational programmes in end-of-life care. Ferrell and colleagues have recently reported on an evaluation of this ELNEC project in which over 2,445 nurses representing all 50 states have received training and it is estimated that over the next few years, 'project leaders will touch the lives of 8.75 million people facing the end of life' (Ferrell *et al.* 2006: 269).

## Scarcity of resources and teaching staff with skills in general palliative care

In some palliative care units, there is a scarcity of resources to support learning, especially in the workplace. In many units, there are not the finances to establish a library and employ a librarian; nevertheless, careful thought should be given before the purchase of costly resources such as journal subscriptions and books. Journal subscriptions are an annual, costly expense yet are essential in education, training and lifelong learning of staff.

An additional constraint to the delivery of high-quality palliative care education appears to be lack of trained and experienced teachers to deliver educational programmes. While the appointment of full-time educators in palliative care from a number of disciplines has been a common feature in the UK for several decades, currently only the USA, Canada, Ireland, Australia and New Zealand are developed sufficiently in their education infrastructure to follow suit (Becker and Gamlin 2004). Although there has been numerous attempts at defining the baseline content of courses across the spectrum of subjects that encompass palliative care (see Chapter 30, Larkin), little attention has been paid to the requirements of the professionals who deliver educational programmes. Becker (2007) offers a useful framework for the development of core competencies for palliative care educators. Used judiciously the competency statements can assist palliative care educators with a benchmark for:

- Self-assessment of performance in relation to Individual Performance Review (IPR) and the development of a Personal Development Plan (PDP).
- The planning and development of career pathways.

For educational managers in the private, state or higher education sectors the framework has the potential to provide them with a robust system for:

- Informing future roles and responsibilities, job descriptions and person specification development.

- Assessing and monitoring ongoing competency as part of the IPR and PDP process.

(Becker 2007: 382)

# Delivering education in resource-poor countries

Whereas the number of palliative care services and clinical educational programmes are increasingly rapidly in Western industrialized countries (Centeno *et al.* 2006), the extent to which urgently needed clinical and educational palliative care programmes in the developing world remains at a critically low level (Bruera and Sweeney 2002; Clemens *et al.* 2007). Clemens *et al.* (2007) point out that, unfortunately, some clinical and education leaders in the developing world believe that palliative care is a luxury that cannot be afforded by countries that do not have the means to provide many of the basic curative interventions for their population. Students frequently travel to developed countries for their medical or nursing professional development. Unfortunately, many of these students choose to continue their careers in other countries because they find the system in their own country incompatible with what they have learned overseas (Clemens *et al.* 2007).

The key challenges facing palliative care in many developing countries are funding and the scarcity of trained personnel, although a number of writers draw attention to improvements due to innovative educational interventions (c.f. Dowling 2006; Hunt Chapter 33). Education is often described as an essential effective development aid because of its future-orientated and sustainable nature. According to Clemens *et al.* (2007) it is essential to design structured educational programmes that are innovative and linked to the national and regional health plans of the respective country. Moreover,

> the main challenge is to evolve training of two broad types: first, basic programmes should be widely available for doctors and nurses to empower the primary health care system to address common palliative care issues and second, courses to train future trainers and professionals to support referral units (specialist palliative care).

(Clemens *et al.* 2007: 174)

Less economically developed countries are confronted with the added difficulty of being perceived primarily as beneficiaries of palliative care education rather than adapting programmes to meet their local context. As Newell-Jones (2007) points out, the challenge of adapting both curriculum content and approaches to teaching and learning to local contexts is rooted in the historical origins of palliative care education in the UK and other Western, more economically affluent, countries. The need for more locally tailored educational programmes in India is identified by Kumar (2007) as a pressing issue. Similarly, Goh and Shaw (2007) give an excellent account of the problems of Western-trained staff being less able to assimilate into the local context. In short, the overall picture remains one of palliative care academics, educationalists and practitioners from Europe, North America and Australasia tending to engage in collaborative learning primarily with each other (Newell-Jones 2007). This in stark contrast to the situation in developing countries where the sharing of expertise is more unidirectional with the Western-trained staff cast as the experts. Becker (2004: 192–3) sums this up well:

> It is important to remember that the well-developed, university validated, academic, formal model of education based on western ethical values does not hold the moral high ground.

Development agencies are now learning that parachuting so called experts into developing countries to work for a limited time is, in the long term, futile. Rather, they have learned that to achieve sustainable change they must work long term with local people, building on their indigenous knowledge and helping them to develop the capacity to address their issues themselves (Graham and Clark 2005).

## The paucity of evidence to indicate the effect on practice of education

In considering the availability of palliative care education for nurses and other health care professionals, studies have broadly focused upon two perspectives: first, examining whether nursing curricula incorporate teaching about death and dying; and, second, exploring nurses' experience with dying patients (Copp 1994). In the USA, Quint's (1967) seminal work on the education of nurses to care for dying patients highlighted the considerable inadequacy of educational provision for nurses in this area. Quint's landmark study has gone on to profoundly influence the way in which these aspects of education have been incorporated and taught in schools of nursing throughout the developed world.

Although education is considered an integral part of the work of palliative care teams, there is little evidence to indicate the effect on practice of such education. Research examining the effectiveness of various education programmes on care of the dying has frequently revealed equivocal results. Studies evaluating education often lack a theoretical basis, few employ controlled experimental designs and are predominantly concerned with participants' perceptions or assessment of their knowledge base. One of the reasons for this could be that, in common with research in palliative care generally, such research presents methodological challenges. Issues relating to research in palliative care are discussed in Chapter 32 by Grande and Ingleton. They highlight the methodological challenges researchers face in conducting studies in palliative care and the reasons for these difficulties. However, if we subscribe to the view that perceptions of increased knowledge, self-confidence and attitude change are more reliable (and meaningful) than measurable differences, there is substantial evidence to support the effectiveness of education in palliative care (Kenny 2001; Dowell 2002).

## Distance, cost and access to effective programmes of education

Access to continuing education is a challenge for nurses who have work and family responsibilities, work shifts and may live a considerable distance from institutions of higher education. Factors mitigating against day release frequently include difficulty obtaining study leave; insecurity of funding for post-qualifying professional development; staff shortages; and late withdrawal or non-attendance at study days (O'Connor and Fitzsimmons 2005). Clearly, further work needs to be carried out to explain this lack of take-up of educational courses, which could relate to the difficulties nurses have in obtaining release from work to attend such programmes and/or lack of understanding of the need to undertake such specialist training if they work in non-specialist areas. However, it should be noted that attendance of staff members at educational courses and training does not necessarily ensure that palliative care practice will improve at an organizational level. If individual course members are to apply theory to practice, then certain organizational factors need to be in place: appropriate management and peer support, provision of financial resources and a collective commitment to developing practice (Froggatt 2000). In Chapter 33, Froggatt and Turner discuss the importance of the organizational context and organizational support needed in helping colleagues to improve palliative care practice.

Obstacles to accessing courses could be overcome with further development of more flexible modes of delivery, including providing work-based educational preparation, web-based learning, problem-based learning and through the promotion of inter-professional learning. These approaches are now discussed in turn.

### Work-based learning

The type of courses available and mode of delivery must adapt to changing professional expectations; work-based learning in professional practice is one way of responding to these changes. Work-based learning, in valuing learning that takes place outside of an educational institution, and in integrating practice with theory, offers an interesting alternative to purely academic university-based courses (Colquhoun and Munro 2007). Work-based learning embraces a number of learning and teaching strategies that take place outside educational institutions and in students' workplaces. One of the primary modes of work-based learning is through the use of on-line materials, such as web-based resources. These are increasingly being employed to overcome the traditional barriers to continuing education.

### Web-based learning

Developments in technology have allowed substantial progress to be made in the way educational opportunities are delivered, not least in the field of palliative care (Jones and Finlay 2007). Rural nurses practising in isolated settings face unique challenges in gaining education instruction.

Yu and Yang (2006) discuss the value of web-based learning for nurses, suggesting that nurses working in Taiwan at village health centres, removed from education bases, valued the access that the internet afforded them. They also identified that some nurses lacked the necessary computer skills to complete on-line courses. In order for nurses to be able to work with these computer-based systems, and to be able to support patients effectively they need, at the very least, to have the skills and knowledge to use information technology efficiently and safely (see Chapter 31 by Bath and colleagues). Nurses, however, have been found to have poor IT skills and are resistant to the introduction of IT (Timmons 2003). Student nurses had two priorities: one was developing the skills and knowledge they needed to be able to understand and use the available information, the other was access to equipment. In a comparative study of nurses in New Zealand and the UK, Bond (2007) found that nursing informatics was embedded in the pre-registration nursing curricula in New Zealand; basic IT skills were, however, not taught. Conversely, in the UK, nursing informatics expertise was not as well embedded, although programmes did include some basic IT skills. Nursing informatics expertise was found to be lacking in UK course teams (Murphy *et al.* 2004; Bond 2007).

### Problem-based learning

Problem-based learning (PBL) is a method of group learning that uses true-to-life problems as a stimulus for students to learn problem-solving skills. More specifically, teachers facilitate learning in student-led group tutorials, but do not provide specific content information. PBL aims to develop clinical reasoning skills and is of increasing interest in palliative care; and although it offers a valuable addition to the palliative education repertoire, some questions exist over its theoretical basis (Filbet and Larkin 2007). Reporting on a study to integrate PBL into clinical nursing education in Sweden, Ehrenberg and Haagblom (2007) found that to be successful in implementing PBL, information, training and support of students and preceptors is needed. However, many nurse preceptors were unfamiliar with PBL and lacked personal experience of this educational approach.

### Inter-professional learning

There has been much written about how changes in patterns of health care delivery and structure of services have impacted upon the development of the health professions globally. These changes have included calls for collaboration between professions in health and social care. Inter-professional education is seen as one way forward in promoting professional and proficient team-working. As this need for teamwork has been recognized, there is a need to change the way in which health care professionals are educated. The impetus for this has arisen, in part, from the belief that separate training encourages different health professional groups to hold on to their independence and autonomy, thereby detracting from effective teamwork. Cox and James explore the concept of boundaries and team-working in palliative care in Chapter 28. The need for change has also been accelerated in the developed world by the move towards shifting the balance from secondary to primary care and the need to use resources effectively and in a timely manner. Taken together, these changes have been instrumental in accelerating the growth and development of inter-professional learning in health care settings.

As Larkin points out in Chapter 30, in no other health care area is learning alongside different disciplines welcomed so readily as in the field of palliative care. It is postgraduate palliative care specialist education which has embraced the concept of inter-professional learning most enthusiastically, with many courses advertising themselves as having a multi-professional intake of students. This appears to reflect the holistic and team approach mirrored in palliative care practice, although how this multi-professional group is engaged in the teaching and learning process is largely unknown. The wide variety of approaches and levels of study at different institutions can make application and integration difficult when applying learning to practice. An additional challenge to applying and integrating inter-professional learning in practice is what is described by Fealy (2005: 319) *as the weight of history*. This includes the historical gender division of labour within disciplines; the hierarchical relationship between physicians and other health care workers; and the different traditions of professional training. The imperatives that exist for each individual professional discipline to meet the professional training requirements in respect of course content, minimum periods of instruction and supervision can also present a particular challenge. These legislative constraints notwithstanding, professional regulatory authorities are generally amenable to the principles and practice of shared learning among health care disciplines.

The crucial question that remains unanswered is how inter-professional learning affects professional practice in palliative care. As yet there are no answers to this question. What is clear from the evidence available in the wider research literature is that a fundamental approach to inter-professional learning is required, one that integrates the best external evidence with educational expertise and students' choices. This highlights the need for greater discussion from an early stage between educators, practitioners and students to determine basic requirements (Cooper *et al.* 2001).

Inter-professional approaches to teaching and learning are increasingly being used in the context of research training in palliative care, as attempts to strengthen the evidence base for the care and services provided to patients and their families continue. Although palliative care research is a growth activity with practitioners ever more involved in palliative care research as the field expands, this expanded contact with research is not without its pressures and problems, nor does this preclude the opportunity to build upon what has been already achieved. These problems and possible opportunities for advancing the contribution of nurses towards research activity in palliative care is the focus of the next section (see Box 27.2).

It is important to preface the following discussion by highlighting the difference in skills and knowledge which may be required by nurses, depending on their contribution towards research-based activity. The majority of clinical nurses are 'consumers of research'; they require appropriate access to research publications, libraries and sources of information to develop and implement evidence-based practice. Arguably, only a minority of nurses are 'research producers' and, as such, research methods skills, ethical knowledge and ability to disseminate findings are most relevant to their role. However, clearly research education should equip *all* nurses to critically assess those studies on which they plan to develop their practice.

# Nurses' access to and use of research-based knowledge

Nurses' access to and use of research-based knowledge is an essential element of proposals to enhance the quality of health care. Researchers at the Centre for Evidence Based Nursing at the University of York, UK (Thompson *et al.* 2001), conducted a study in which they hoped to identify the sources of information *actually* used by nurses, as well as those they *said* they used. Using a variety of data sources from 15 different clinical sites (none were specialist palliative care), three perspectives on information accessibility were identified. Human sources – that is, people – were perceived by nurses to be more accessible than text-based information. Clinical specialization was found to be associated with different approaches to information access and, in coronary care units, nurses were more likely to find local guidelines, protocols and on-line databases to be more accessible than colleagues in general medical and surgical wards. Perhaps the most worrying finding was how little of the available text-based evidence had a

---

**Box 27.2** Problems and opportunities for advancing the contribution of nurses towards research-based activity

- Nurses' access to and use of research-based knowledge
- Building research capacity
- Small-scale nature of studies conducted in palliative care
- Perceived dissonance between academic nursing and clinical practice
- Changes to ethical approval processes for research studies
- Promoting effective teamwork through leadership
- Expanding practitioner roles

research base, and how out of date the available textbooks were. In terms of what was *not* useful, no nurses viewed textbooks as a useful resource and equally the role of local information files was not found to be helpful. This was an important finding given that both of these resources were very much in evidence on the wards. More worryingly, perhaps, the internet, on-line databases and other library-based resources, such as the Cochrane Library, were not viewed as having much utility for practice. What emerged clearly from this study was that library skills and support to enable nurses to make the most of the often extensive resources available in each of the sites were seen as poorly developed. Physical access to research information is a significant barrier to research. There are parallels here with the findings relating to obstacles for nurses accessing continuing professional education for nurses, discussed above. Physical access to research information may present problems for specialist palliative care nurses who may not have the same facilities at their disposal as those offered to their counterparts employed in large acute units, attached to university departments. These findings resonate with findings from a more recent study conducted with Greek nurses. This study sought to explore their perceptions of the barriers to research utilization. Two key barriers related to 'availability' of research findings. Despite the nurses' willingness and desire for research implementation, major organizational barriers, lack of peer support, limited research accessibility and lack of knowledge hindered the process (Patiraki *et al.* 2004).

## Building research capacity

Building research capacity is recognized as a significant challenge worldwide (Segrott *et al.* 2003). In placing the concept of capacity building within an international context it is important to acknowledge that a large proportion of the published literature in this area originates in the UK (McCance *et al.* 2007). While some progress has been achieved within nursing research and development (see Chapter 32), building capacity and infrastructure remains an important challenge (Hartley 2005). The position on a European level presents a similar picture with findings from a European scoping report indicating that there is: 'a lack, for the most part, of nursing research career pathways that straddle clinical work and higher education and enhance the generation and utilisation of research in practice settings' (Moreno-Casbas 2005: 11). Arguably, the move of basic and post-basic nurse education into higher education institutions in most developed countries means that nurses are better equipped to conduct more advanced studies into areas of their practice. From an initial faltering start, the number of nurses undertaking doctoral level studies continues to grow (Kirkham *et al.* 2007) and this is a positive move towards providing an international network of nurses in key positions in practice and academia, though much work remains to be done.

Opportunities to date, however, have tended to target doctoral level preparation, with fewer directed to developing programmes at post-doctoral level. Findings from the European scoping report (Moreno-Casbas 2005) support this view, indicating that the vast majority of nurse researchers obtaining doctorates and doing post-doctoral work do so on a part-time, non-funded basis. Developing the required knowledge and skills to engage in research and development activity at different levels is fundamental to capacity building. Developing leaders at the highest level who can influence strategy and policy is crucial to the further advancement of the research and development agenda. While progress is evident in relation to building capacity for conducting research, further investment is required to move towards post-doctoral programmes that are multidisciplinary in their approach. Sadly, there appears to be clear messages within the literature that research and development activity is not always valued as part of everyday practice (Pravikoff *et al.* 2005).

## Small-scale nature of studies conducted by nurses in palliative care

Although the need for practice to be based on reliable evidence rather than anecdote has been recognized since the establishment of the modern hospice movement, much of the research undertaken to date has been limited and fragmented, with small-scale, single-centre studies being the norm. Grande and Ingleton delineate some of the explanations for this in Chapter 32. Similarly, much nursing research has been justly criticized as being small-scale, under-funded and locally based. This situation is mirrored in palliative care research more generally. In a selected review of journals and a pilot survey describing the status of palliative care research over the last two decades, Kaasa *et al.* (2006) found that the status of palliative care research is that it is in its infancy, relatively diverse and not very well developed. It would seem that while some countries are in the process of building up research activities, some formerly active countries have reached more of a plateau stage. For example, Kaasa found no national and/or regional possibilities for funding for palliative care research in Europe, except for the UK. Therefore, palliative care researchers have to compete on the 'open market' or rely on private foundations. Equally, there are few European research groups in palliative care reaching a critical size, which hampers the progress of large multi-centre studies.

Seymour *et al.* (2003) suggest that synthesizing data from studies with similar aims and designs highlights a methodological approach that may be valuable in palliative care research. They draw upon data on 37 patients' expectations and experiences of specialist palliative care services, as expressed in in-depth interviews across three evaluative studies of specialist palliative care services in the UK (Seymour *et al.* 2003). This approach provides an exemplar for synthesizing findings from small-scale qualitative studies and provides the possibility of demonstrating their applicability beyond local and specific contexts, while recognizing that caution must be shown in checking that methods of data collection and data analysis are comparable.

## Perceived dissonance between academic nursing and clinical practice

A predominant theme in the nursing literature is the dissonance between academic nursing and clinical practice. Some writers have suggested that the gap between the two sectors arises primarily because of the 'idealized' views of nursing held by academic nurses, that seem incompatible with the 'messy realities' of the practice world (Watson 2006). The continuing tensions between academic and clinical nursing has resulted in calls to develop models for minimizing these tensions and to enhance links between academic and clinical settings. Establishing joint appointments is one means suggested for addressing the ambivalent relationship that has existed between academic and clinical nursing. The introduction of clinical chairs, which are joint appointments at the professorial level with links to both the academic and clinical settings, is one means by which more active cooperation between stakeholders can be achieved.

Dunn and Yates (2000) conducted a study to describe the roles of chairs in clinical nursing in Australia. Eight clinical professors were interviewed using semi-structured telephone interviews. The participants highlighted the diversity of arrangements between university and health sector partners in establishing their respective roles. All roles included components of education, research and politics, but the relative contribution of each of these areas, and the viability of the posts, depended to a large extent on the ability of post holders to maintain sustainable income sources and to consolidate outcomes. Dunn and Yates conclude that although not a panacea, clinical professorial appointments do provide, perhaps, one of the best opportunities to bring together the major stakeholders in the nursing community: clinical, academic and professional.

Possibilities in promoting scholarship within clinical practice relate not only to the establishment of clinical nursing professoriates as described above, but also the establishment of dedicated nursing research wards and units, and maintaining the practice links of university-based nursing staff.

There are other models of scholarship emerging in the USA, such as the development of the National Center for Nursing Research, which emphasizes health care and promotion. In the light of continuing emphasis on evidence-based practice and clinical excellence, such a centre might provide an invaluable interface between evidence and practice.

# Changes to ethical approval processes for research projects

In many parts of the developed world, policy changes to the ways in which ethical approval is sought are under review. In the UK, professional organizations involved in health care research have now established research ethics committees (first at local level and then at regional level) within the past decade. More recently, governance frameworks for health and social care research and for research ethics committees (Department of Health 2002) have been developed in which it is made clear that attention to ethical issues are central to the whole research process from commissioning to dissemination (Seymour and Skilbeck 2002). These frameworks set out standards and mechanisms to protect and prioritize the well-being and safety of research participants, while at the same time creating an environment in which high-quality research is nurtured.

While this extra scrutiny can be seen as a positive move to academic excellence and rigorously conducted studies, it does present difficulties for some student projects or small-scale studies. The time frames for these projects need to be scrutinized to take into consideration any comments or changes required by research ethics committees and research governance frameworks. This may make such projects difficult to complete. Already, additional aspects of research governance in the UK, such as the need for project research staff to hold honorary NHS contracts, even when working on projects involving minimal or no actual presence on NHS premises, have added to the difficulties of conducting research.

Similar arrangements exist in Australia where the National Health and Medical Research Council (NHMRC) consider the ethical issues associated with research. Organizations in Australia that receive public funds administered by the NHMRC are required to establish another tier in the form of human research ethics committees to review research proposals involving humans. Lee and Kristjanson (2003), writing about human research ethics committees in Australia and the discomfort of the members of these committees who have no experience of palliative care, warn that committees may disallow access to palliative care patients and families as they perceive the notion of conducting research with this group as abhorrent. The authors, reflecting on 20 years' experience of presenting applications to human research ethics committees, call for a less adversarial approach to gaining ethics approval and an acknowledgement of the rights of palliative care patients, families and health care workers to choose to be involved in research.

Arguably, changes to research governance will have major implications for the type of research conducted in the future. Research projects involving staff members/professional groups have been the mainstay of undergraduate nursing and many postgraduate nursing projects. This has been a deliberate strategy to avoid the involvement of patients and to obviate the risk of their 'research fatigue' in research active environments (Watson and Manthorpe 2002). With the new difficulties in gaining ethical approval, this situation is likely to continue.

# Promoting effective teamwork through leadership

According to Junger *et al.* (2007) newly established palliative care teams are confronted with three different challenges: first, they are required to form relationships with new colleagues in order to build up an effective working group; second, they need to become attuned to a field of work with a high emotional burden (see Chapter 29); and, third, at the same time they have to bear the uncertainty of not having defined standards compared to other fields of health care (Payne 2001).

Junger *et al.* (2007) conducted a study to determine the factors which enhance both the success and outcome criteria of good teamwork from the perception of team members in a palliative care unit in Aachen. They found that factors crucial to cooperation in the team members' view were: close communication, team philosophy, good interpersonal relationships, high team commitment, autonomy and the ability to deal with death and dying. Moreover, close communication was by far the most frequently mentioned criteria for successful team working.

Although some writers point to the particular culture in palliative care teams which emphasize higher levels of autonomy, flat hierarchy, more realistic workloads and high levels of personal feedback by colleagues, patients and relatives, there is still a need to create an atmosphere which allows the team members to cope with the sometimes ambiguous nature of palliative care. Junger *et al.* (2007) propose a model which highlights the influencing factors with regard to multi-professional cooperation in a palliative care team.

Previous research on team functioning and development within hospice interdisciplinary teams has focused upon the study of high-functioning teams and job satisfaction. High-functioning teams are said to be characterized by clearly understood goals and a positive interpersonal climate that allows for trust, the ability to learn from mistakes and technical and emotional support (Wittenberg-Lyles and Parker 2007). However, the empirical evidence supporting the notion of interdisciplinary teams is not always positive. A meta-analysis found that the palliative care team approach, after accounting for the composition of the team, patient diagnosis, country of study and study design, resulted in benefits in the relief of pain and other symptoms. However, there were no significant effects for patient satisfaction therapeutic interventions (Higginson *et al.* 2003). As such, the assumption that interdisciplinary teams inevitably lead to greater patient satisfaction in non-palliative care settings is challenged (Hermsen and ten Have 2005) and the need for evidence that such teams are indeed necessary is highlighted (Zwarenstein and Reeves 2000; O'Connor *et al.* 2006).

Another potential conflict area in palliative care is the distinction between the philosophy of 'democracy' with a flat team structure, and the traditional medical model, which places physicians at the top of the health care hierarchy. Willard and Luker (2005) report an example that highlights these problems and challenges. These authors examined how specialist cancer nurses in the UK operated across several settings, including specialist palliative care. One of their findings highlighted medical staff as 'gate keepers' who asserted their power to block nurses' access to patients or relegated support care to a subordinate role.

Haward *et al.* (2003), reporting on a study on the interactions within an interdisciplinary breast cancer team, found that leadership style was a significant aspect of team functioning. Lack of clarity or conflict over leadership resulted in a less effective team, whereas a single leader had a negative effect on innovation. However, every team needs someone to coordinate the activities of its members. Effective leadership and functioning of palliative care interdisciplinary teams will not just occur; though developing future leaders in palliative care nursing is a challenge. Mahoney (2001) describes a leader as someone who, through interpersonal relationships, can influence people, is a recognized authority, is responsible for supporting others and giving assistance, has the ability to influence others to achieve their goals and has certain personality characteristics including being competent, confident, courageous and creative. A number of issues prohibit the development of leaders. Those who try to reform things can meet with hostility when they try to make changes (Lorentzon and Brown 2003). The fact that nursing across Europe does not have a collective vision is another barrier (Kearney and Molassiotis 2003). The creation of new specialist roles in nursing have the potential to create and nurture a new generation of leaders, but lack of role clarity and the different agendas they are called upon to take forward may affect its potential to do so.

## Expanding practitioner roles

Specialization within nursing has a long and well-documented history. Much of the early writings originate from the USA where the Clinical Nurse Specialists (CNS) roles first developed, the four major components of CNS practice being defined as expert practice, education, consultation and research. These descriptors have acted as the template for CNS practice internationally (Austen *et al.* 2006). As 'experts' CNS appear to be in a good position to promote evidence-based practice in health care settings internationally. During the past 20 years, there has been a significant expansion in the number of specialist nurses practising in many areas of patient and family care. The designation of 'specialist nurse' is currently conferred on individuals with a wide range of knowledge and skills, with very different roles, remits and titles, and with diverse backgrounds in terms of education preparation. Accompanying this trend is a growing international literature concerned with specialist nurses in palliative care (Colquhoun and Dougan 1997).

However, CNSs can encounter difficulties when trying to effect their role. A recent systematic review indicates that the facilitators and barriers to CNS practice have much in common throughout the world, and that positive working relationships are important to the success of their role (Lloyd Jones 2005).

As we have seen in Chapter 2, modern specialist palliative care services began earlier and have developed further in the UK than in other parts of Europe. One particular example of this is the number of palliative care clinical nurse specialists working in the UK, particularly those employed with initial support from the UK charity Macmillan Cancer Relief, normally referred to as 'Macmillan nurses'. These posts have been influential in the models of specialist palliative care nursing adopted in other countries. Macmillan nurse posts were first developed in the UK in the mid-1970s and have been established in both hospital and community settings. From being introduced as nurses with special responsibility for caring directly for terminally ill people and their families, the role of the Macmillan nurse has changed gradually to that of the clinical nurse specialist in which clinical, consultative, education, research and supportive functions are combined (Seymour *et al.* 2002). This evolution has, in part, occurred in response to the recognition that palliative care is a right for everyone with life-limiting illness. Although the work of Macmillan clinical nurse specialists in palliative care is now well established, there has been little research into a number of key areas of the role.

The extent to which Macmillan nurses can meet the ideals of specialist practice is little understood, although problems of role clarity and role overload have been linked to clinical nurse specialist posts more generally. As Skilbeck and Seymour (2002) point out, there is little evidence about the character of Macmillan nurses' clinical work with patients; most research has concentrated on specific aspects of their duties, such as work patterns, referral trends, levels of support and stress, or have been small-scale evaluations. The extent to which generic Macmillan nurses are adapting to these new demands was addressed as part of a major evaluation study of UK Macmillan nursing in 12 sites in the Trent and Thames regions of the UK, commissioned by the UK charity Macmillan Cancer Relief. As part of this evaluation, Seymour *et al.* (2002) examined the extent to which Macmillan nurses are adapting to new working practices and procedures brought about by policy initiatives (Department of Health 1999, 2002).

Drawing on data from semi-structured interviews with 44 Macmillan nurses and 47 of their key colleagues, the study found differences of expectation between Macmillan nurses and their managers about the appropriate focus of their work, which led to problems of role ambiguity and role conflict. Moreover, Macmillan nurses were found to lack resources with which to develop an educative and consultative role and that problems existed in co-working with newly appointed cancer site-specific nurses and palliative medicine colleagues (Seymour *et al.* 2002). The authors conclude by pointing to a need to clarify the nature and scope of the Macmillan nurse role, to attend to issues of team working and to improve the skills of non-specialist staff in palliative care.

As part of this evaluation and acknowledging that there has been little research into the organizational context in which these nurses operate and the implications for the services they deliver, data were also collected about the Macmillan nursing care mix, nature of interventions and organization of workloads. The results showed a wide variation in the intensity of input into care of individual patients by Macmillan nurses. For the majority of patients, one or two contacts were undertaken with the purpose of resolving a particular problem or need. This variety of input was observed in the context of a caseload in which two-thirds of patients died within 200 days of referral to the services (Skilbeck and Seymour 2002). The evaluation also showed wide variation in organization and management of their practice (Clark *et al.* 2002). It would appear that there is a need to clarify the Macmillan nurse's role to ensure that their expertise is used effectively and efficiently. Other literature highlights the need for clarity over lines of responsibility, strategic planning and adequate resource allocation. These are all essential factors for nurses to accommodate change effectively. Overlaying these elements is the changing landscape of expanding roles and policy directives surrounding nurses' practice. For example, in recent years a range of risk management strategies has been introduced into health care settings in response to growing litigation and a transfer of the associated costs to health care providers. Within this context, nursing is being primed to play a more effective and central role in care delivery by developing new ways of working and promoting quality care through the use of clinical protocols, or care pathways, as a means of delivering evidence-based practice. The final section of this overview will explore the ways in which care pathways are being used and whether they offer the potential to improve palliative care delivery for patients and families.

## Clinical protocols/Integrated care pathways

The development and use of clinical protocols, or integrated care pathways (ICPs) as they have come to be known, has attracted substantial international research interest. There are three main reasons for the drive to develop these protocols: risk management, the speedier integration of research into practice and the standardization of practice to provide a more cost-effective and efficient health care system.

Widely accepted and used in the North American health care system, ICPs are increasingly being used in the UK. In the USA, advocates of pathways have placed them within an overall strategy for managed care, arguing that they result in resource efficiency while *maintaining* quality and managing costs. In the UK, rather than emphasizing the resource efficiency aspect, pathways are seen as a tool to implement clinical governance which aims to *improve* the quality of care and ensure that clinical care is based on the latest research evidence (de Luc 2000).

Integrated care pathways (ICPs) are designed to bring evidence-based health care to the workplace and to audit compliance through analysis of reported variations from the care plan (Fowell *et al.* 2006). The Liverpool

Care Pathway (LCP) was developed by Ellershaw in the 1990s in order to provide a template of appropriate, evidence-based care for the last days and hours of life. It has evolved rapidly and to date in the UK 280 hospitals, 120 hospices, 484 primary health care teams and 371 care homes have registered their involvement with the LCP (Ellershaw 2007).

There is a need, however, to test its efficacy, rather than extending the ICP for the care of dying patients into more care settings. Although the best method of study would arguably be a randomized controlled trial of the ICP, this would not be feasible for ethical reasons. Shah (2005: 352) in a letter to the editor of *Palliative Medicine* suggests the following approach as a way forward in conducting a more robust appraisal of testing the efficacy of ICPs:

> More desirable under the circumstances would be an after-death analysis of the care of dying patients in units not implementing the pathway and clinicians in participating units trying to maximise efforts to anticipate death and record it, in order that patient groups could be further stratified into anticipated and unanticipated deaths.

In the context of primary care, The Gold Standards Framework for community palliative care (Thomas 2004) is a primary care led programme in the UK which is attracting increasing international attention (Murray *et al.* 2006). Although there has been some positive evaluative evidence of the framework (Munday *et al.* 2006; Thomas and Noble 2007), variations in how the programme has been implemented; differences in levels of commitment among professionals within individual practices; and the increased administrative burden have been highlighted as drawbacks.

Lawton and Parker (1999) conducted a study to investigate the perceptions of doctors, nurses, midwives and health service managers towards the proposed development and implementation of clinical protocols. Twenty-four focus groups were convened across three hospitals in the UK. The effect of 'proceduralization' on professional autonomy and on the working relationships among professional groups emerged as an important theme. Importantly, the study revealed that successful implementation of protocols/guidelines depends on achieving the right balance between standardizing practice and allowing professionals to use clinical judgement.

De Luc (2000) reported on a quasi-experimental case study of two care pathways developed within one NHS Trust. In this study, de Luc makes a comparison of clinical care delivered before and after the introduction of the two pathways and the views of staff involved in the development and operation of the two pathways. Overall, the conclusions from this study are mixed. The findings suggest that the development aspects of pathways offer the easiest and most immediate route for change, including the development of multidisciplinary team working, design of clinical documentation and updating of clinical practice. The author points out that a considerable ongoing commitment of time and effort is required in the operation of pathways once implemented to engender a culture of continuous monitoring and comparing the standards of care provided. While these elements are ascribed to by many advocates of ICPs, they are rarely reflected in the increasing descriptive literature on pathways.

More generally, however, few evaluations have looked at either costs of development and implementation or, importantly, the efficacy of care pathways in changing practice and improving outcomes. The need for systematic evaluations to measure the effectiveness of pathways has been cited by many writers in the international literature.

In the context of palliative care, critics of ICPs suggest that, left unchecked, there is a danger that the 'process of dying' may be reduced to a number of flow diagrams (algorithms as they were called in some palliative care journals) and a series of boxes ticked by professional carers instead of recognizing the importance of spontaneity and creativity in palliative care (Kelly 2003). Importantly, the question still remains as to whether the introduction of pathways results in the benefits ascribed to them by their supporters and whether they warrant investment in time and resources to develop them.

Ultimately, though, for ICPs to be successfully introduced into palliative care settings, an integrated multi-professional approach and an open, flexible and participative culture is required. Otherwise, they may be viewed as a 'paper exercise' and merely another type of clinical audit tool; an approach to care that does not seem to resonate with philosophical statements about the individuality of patient needs.

In the remainder of this overview, we introduce the nine chapters that form the final section of the book. The chapters are wide-ranging in character and set out contemporary issues in the rapidly changing field of palliative care.

## Overview of chapters in Part Four

Multi-professional working is said to be a key component of effective palliative care and it is generally recognized that the complex needs of patients and their families can best be met by a well-coordinated team of various professionals. In Chapter 28, Karen Cox and Veronica James explore the concepts of boundaries, roles and team working within which palliative care is delivered. They detail how, over the past 30 years, the palliative care team has changed considerably in both its constitution and complexity. These changes have stemmed, in part, from patients' and families' increasingly high expectations of health care provision, in terms of power sharing, improved information giving, increased choice and better patient-centred care. However, the authors make the very salient point that these expectations will continue to be mediated by the fundamental need for human warmth and attention at times of vulnerability, when the needs for support and the potential desires to opt out by adopting a 'sick role' may be heightened.

As palliative care professionals are asked to respond to demands to extend their work beyond a focus on cancer, it follows that there is either a need to spread the effort further with few additional resources, or that there is a need to pay greater attention to the allocation of resources to those most in need, however these needs may be defined. Either way, this can add increasing pressure and stress to the daily work of palliative care professionals. While occupational stress and 'burnout' are common phenomena across health care settings, and are certainly not unique to palliative care, there are some characteristics of palliative care as a specialty that require specific attention. While acknowledging the significant work undertaken on occupational stress and burnout in palliative care, Sanchia Aranda's chapter on occupational stress and coping strategies (Chapter 29) departs from influential work (most notably by Vachon) by exploring the relationship between the underlying philosophy of palliative care, what counts as 'stressful' and the meaning of this for nursing work in palliative care. Understanding how we perceive stress is critical to how the subject is approached. Aranda suggests that stress occurs at points of dissonance between the beliefs and values of the individual and their capacity to deliver care according to those values. Aranda concludes that it is critical that palliative care research moves beyond a description of stress in the working lives of palliative nurses and other health professionals to develop theoretically informed and rigorously tested interventions to ensure the retention of the workforce and the health of us all.

In Chapter 30, Philip Larkin considers current perspectives on palliative care education and scholarship within an international context. In doing so, he offers an overview of the wide variability in educational opportunity and career advancement for nurses working in palliative care. Looking to the future, he predicts that palliative care education in Europe will be dependent on evaluative empirical studies that can elucidate the benefits of education to health care and offer flexible learning and teaching solutions to engage with practitioners on their terms about the acquisition of new knowledge to benefit their practice. The use of information and communication technology (ICT) is central to achieving this goal and this is the subject of Chapter 31 by Peter Bath and colleagues. These authors explore how ICT is playing an increasing role in health, not only from the perspective of health care professionals but also for patients, their families and carers, and the general public. However, while innovations in ICT are not intended to remove the feelings of fear and anxiety, uncertainty, sadness and loss for the patient and their families, tailoring the access to information and support via ICT for individuals throughout the stages of palliative care can help reduce the impact of the illness on quality of life and on the dying process.

The development of a wide-ranging and multidisciplinary programme of palliative care research is crucial to a more evidence-based approach to care. Within the broad field of palliative care, nursing is beginning to emerge as an important focus. In Chapter 32, Gunn Grande and Christine Ingleton consider some of the main methodological challenges and opportunities in conducting and participating in palliative care research. Although they concede there is still a long way to go, Grande and Ingleton conclude that nurses are making a growing contribution to the wider palliative care research community. The challenge for the future will be to develop leaders at the highest level who can influence strategy and policy to the further advancement of the research agenda in palliative care nursing.

Practice development has a role to play in developing these future leaders and this is the focus of the next chapter by Katherine Froggatt and Mary Turner (Chapter 33). The authors outline some of the key features of practice development and describe a number of different development initiatives to support improvements in practice. However, they caution that for initiatives to be worthwhile and fully effective, there needs to be the commitment from both commissioners and provider services to continue to support and develop staff when the initial projects are over.

After 40 years of hospice, and the funding of nurse specialist posts, palliative care has important recognition in the UK policy agenda in the structure of health and social care. Jo Hockley (Chapter 34) suggests that despite this position, there are reports that reform is patchy and that nurses need to engage more comprehensively with health care policy in palliative care. She goes on to set out how nurses working in palliative care need to be aware of assessment tools to improve quality of life, the importance of needs assessment and user involvement, and the contribution that community can bring to policy to effect policy change.

Although the key components to delivery of palliative care have been articulated by the WHO (Clarke and Wright 2007) as policy, education, drug availability and implementation, this creates enormous challenges in resource-poor countries. In the final chapter of this book (Chapter 35), Jennifer Hunt considers some of these challenges namely in respect of: policy restrictions, particularly with regard to opioid drugs; monetary constraints; too few training institutions; lack of skilled human resources; and the overwhelming number of chronically ill and dying people. While lessons can undoubtedly be learnt and adapted from palliative care developments in resource-rich countries, Hunt reminds us that lessons can also be learnt from the challenges facing resource-poor countries.

# References

Austen, L., Luker, K. and Roland, M. (2006) Clinical nurse specialists and the practice of community nurses. *Journal of Advanced Nursing*, 54(5): 542–51.

Barclay, S., Wyatt, P., Shore, S., Grande, G. and Todd, C. (2003) Caring for the dying: How well prepared are general practitioners: A questionnaire survey. *Palliative Medicine*, 17(5): 355–9.

Becker, R. (2004) The use of competencies in cancer and palliative care. In: L. Foyle and J. Hostad (eds) *Innovations in Cancer and Palliative Care Education*. Oxford: Radcliffe Press.

Becker, R. (2007) The development of core competencies for palliative care educators. *International Journal of Palliative Nursing*, 13(8): 377–84.

Becker, R. and Gamlin, R. (2004) *Fundamental Aspects of Palliative Care Nursing.* Salisbury: Quay Books.

Bond, C. (2007) Nurses' requirements for information technology: a challenge for educators. Guest editorial. *International Journal of Nursing Studies*, 44(7): 1075–8.

Brajtman, S., Fothergill-Bourbonnais, F., Casey, A., Alain, D. and Fiset, F. (2007) providing direction for change: assessing Canadian nursing students learning needs. *International Journal of Palliative Nursing*, 13(5): 213–19.

Bruera, E. and Sweeney, C. (2002) Palliative care models: international perspective. *Journal of Palliative Medicine*, 5(2): 319–27.

Centeno, C., Clark, D., Roccafort, J., Flores, L.A. and Pons, J.J. (2006) The map of specific resources of palliative care in Europe. *Palliative Medicine*, 20: 316.

Clark, D., Ingleton, C. and Seymour, J. (2000) Support and supervision in palliative care research. *Palliative Medicine*, 14: 441–6.

Clark, D., Seymour, J., Douglas, H.R., Bath, P., Beech, N., Corner, J., Halliday, D., Hughes, P., Haviland, J., Normand, C., Marples, R., Skilbeck, J. and Webb, T. (2002) Clinical nurse specialist in palliative care. Part 2. Explaining diversity in the organisation and costs of Macmillan nursing services. *Palliative Medicine*, 16: 375–85.

Clark, D. and Wright, M. (2007) The International Observatory on End of Life Care: a global view of palliative care development. *Journal of Pain Symptom Management*, 33(5): 542–6.

Clemens, K.E., Bruera, E., Klaschik, E., Jaspers, B. and de Lima, L. (2007) Palliative care in developing countries: what are the important issues? *Palliative Medicine*, 21: 173–5.

Colquhoun, M. and Dougan, H. (1997) Performance standards: ensuring that the specialist nurse in palliative care is special. *Palliative Medicine*, 11: 381–7.

Colquhoun, M. and Munro, K. (2007) Work-based learning. In: B. Wee and N. Hughes (eds) *Education in Palliative Care: Building a Culture of Learning.* Oxford: Oxford University Press, 14: 127–37.

Cooper, H., Carlisle, C., Gibbs, T. and Watkins, C. (2001) Developing an evidence base for interdisciplinary learning: a systematic review. *Journal of Advanced Nursing*, 35(2): 228–37.

Copp, G. (1994) Palliative care nursing education: a review of research findings. *Journal of Advanced Nursing*, 19: 552–7.

Cunningham, S., Copp, G., Collins, B. and Bater, M. (2006) Pre-registration nursing students experience of caring for cancer patients. *European Journal of Oncology Nursing.* 10: 59–67.

de Luc, K. (2000) Care pathways: an evaluation of their effectiveness. *Journal of Advanced Nursing*, 32(2): 485–96.

Department of Health (1999) *Making a Difference.* London: HMSO.

Department of Health (2002) *Research Governance Framework for Health and Social Care.* London: HMSO.

Dickinson, G. (2006) End of Life issues in US nursing school curricula: 1984–2006. *Progress in Palliative Care*, 14(4): 165–7.

Dowell, L. (2002) Multi-professional palliative care in a general hospital: education and training needs. *International Journal of Palliative Nursing*, 8(6): 294–303.

Dowling, J. (2006) Palliative care and education in Uganda. *International Journal of Palliative Nursing*, 12(8): 358–61.

Dunn, S. and Yates, P. (2000) The role of Australian chairs in clinical nursing. *Journal of Advanced Nursing*, 31(1): 165–71.

Easom, L., Galatas, S. and Warda, M. (2006) End-of-life care: an educational intervention for rural nurses in south-eastern USA. *International Journal of Palliative Nursing*, 12(11): 526–34.

Ehrenberg, A. and Haagblom, M. (2007) PBL in clinical nursing education: Integrating theory and practice. *Nurse Education in Practice*, 7(2): 67–75.

Ellershaw, J. (2007) Care of the Dying: What a difference an LCP makes! *Palliative Medicine*, 21: 365–8.

Fealy, G. (2005) Sharing the experience. Interdisciplinary education and inter-professional learning. *Nurse Education in Practice*, 5: 317–19.

Ferrell, B., Viriani, R. and Malloy, P. (2006) Evaluation of the end-of-life nursing education consortium project in the USA. *International Journal of Palliative Nursing*, 12(6): 269–76.

Filbet, M. and Larkin, P. (2007) Europe. In: B. Wee and N. Hughes (eds) *Education in Palliative Care: Building a Culture of Learning*. Oxford: Oxford University Press, 8: 69–77.

Fowell, A., Johnstone, R., Russell, I. and Finlay, I. (2006) Reported symptoms in the last days of life: the need for robust research. *Palliative Medicine*, 20: 845–6.

Froggatt, K.A. (2000) Evaluating a palliative care education project in nursing homes. *International Journal of Palliative Nursing*, 6(3): 140–6.

Froggatt, K.A. (2004) *Palliative Care in Care Homes for Older People*. London: The National Council for Palliative Care.

Goh, C. and Shaw, R. (2007) Asia-Pacific. In: B. Wee and N. Hughes (2007) *Education in Palliative Care: Building a Culture of Learning*. Oxford: Oxford University Press, 6: 49–59.

Graham, F. and Clark, D. (2005) Addressing the basics of palliative care. *International Journal of Palliative Nursing*, 11(1): 36–9.

Hartley, D. (2005) Rural Health Research: Building capacity and influencing policy in the UK and Canada. *Canadian Journal of Nursing Research*, 37(1): 7–13.

Haward, R., Amir, Z., Borrill, C., Dawson, J., Scully, J., West, M. and Sainsbury, R. (2003) Breast cancer teams: the impact, constitution, new cancer workload and methods of operation on their effectives. *British Journal of Cancer*, 89(7): 15–22.

Hermsen, M.A., ten Have, H.A.M.J. (2005) Palliative care teams: effective through moral reflection. *Journal of Inter-Professional Care*, 19(6): 561–8.

Higginson, I.J., Finlay, I.G., Goodwin, D.M., Hood, K., Edwards, A.K.G., Cook, A., Douglas, H-R. and Normand, C.E. (2003) Is there evidence that palliative care teams alter end-of-life experiences of patients and their care-givers? *Journal of Pain and Symptom Management*, 25(2): 150–68.

Hughes, P., Parker, C., Payne, S., Ingleton, C. and Noble, B. (2006) Evaluating an education programme in general palliative care. *International Journal of Palliative Nursing*, 12(3): 123–32.

Jones, S. and Finlay, I. (2007) Distance Learning. In: B. Wee and N. Hughes (eds) *Education in Palliative Care: Building a Culture of Learning*. Oxford: Oxford University Press, 19: 179–201.

Junger, S., Pestinger, M., Elsner, F., Krumm, N. and Radbruch, L. (2007) Criteria for successful multi-professional cooperation in palliative care teams. *Palliative Medicine*, 21: 347–54.

Kaasa, S., Hjermstad, M.J. and Loge, J.H. (2006) Methodological and structural challenges in palliative care research: how have we fared in the last decades? *Palliative Medicine*, 20: 727–34.

Kearney, N. and Molassiotis, A. (2003) I have a dream . . . cancer nursing leadership. *European Journal of Oncology Nursing*, 7(4): 227–90.

Kelly, D. (2003) A commentary on 'An integrated care pathway for the last two days of life'. *International Journal of Palliative Nursing*, 9(1): 39.

Kenny, L. (2001) Education in palliative care: making a difference to practice. *International Journal of Palliative Care*, 7(8): 401–7.

Kirkham, S., Thompson, D., Watson, R. and Stewart, S. (2007) Are all doctorates equal or are some 'more equal than others'? *Nurse Education in Practice* 7: 61–6.

Kluster, T., Hoie, M. and Skar, R. (2007) Nursing students' career preferences: a Norwegian study. *Journal of Advanced Nursing*, 59(2): 155–62.

Kumar, S. (2007) India. In B. Wee and N. Hughes (eds) *Education in Palliative Care: Building a Culture of Learning*. Oxford: Oxford University Press, 9: 77–85.

Lawton, R. and Parker, D. (1999) Procedures and the professional: the case of the British NHS. *Social Science and Medicine*, 48: 353–61.

Lee, S. and Kristjanson, L. (2003) Human research ethics committees: issues in palliative care research. *International Journal of Palliative Nursing*, 9(1): 13–19.

Lloyd Jones, M. (2005) Role development and effective practice in a specialist and advanced practice roles: systematic review and meta-synthesis. *Journal of Advanced Nursing*, 49(2): 191–209.

Lloyd-Williams, M. and Field, D. (2002) Are undergraduate nurses taught palliative care during their training? *Nurse Education Today*, 22: 589–92.

Lorentzon, M. and Brown, K. (2003) Florence Nightingale as 'mentor of matrons'. *Journal of Nursing Management*, 11: 266–74.

Mahoney, J. (2001) Leadership skills for the 21st century. *Journal of Nursing Management*, 9: 269–71.

Mallory, J.L. (2003) The impact of a palliative care educational component on attitudes towards care of the dying in undergraduate nursing students. *Journal of Professional Nursing*, 19(5): 305–12.

McCance, T.V., Fitzsimmons, D., Keeney, S., Hasson, F. and McKenna, H. (2007) Capacity building in nursing and midwifery research and development: an old priority with a new perspective. *Journal of Advanced Nursing*, 59(1): 57–67.

Moreno-Casbas, T. (2005) *Nursing Research in Europe Scoping Report*. Madrid: Institute of Health, Carlos iii.

Munday, D., Mahmood, K., Agarwal, S., Dale, J., Koistinen, J., Lamb, K. and Thomas, K. (2006) Evaluation of the Macmillan Gold Standards Framework for palliative care: phases 3–6, 2003–2005. *Palliative Medicine*, 20: 134.

Murphy, K., Stramer, S., Clamp, P., Grubb, J., Gosland, J. and Davis, S. (2004) Health. *International Journal for Medical Informatics*, 73: 205–13.

Newell-Jones, K. (2007) Implications for global education. In: B. Wee and N. Hughes (eds) *Education in Palliative Care: Building a Culture of Learning*. Oxford: Oxford University Press, 12: 104–11.

NICE (2004) *Improving supportive and palliative care for adults with cancer*. London: National Institute for Clinical Excellence. www.nice.org.uk.

O'Connor, S. and Fitzsimmons, D. (2005) Embedding cancer care within pre-registration nurse education programmes: policy, practice and opportunity for change. *European Journal of Oncology Nursing*, 9(4): 347–51.

O'Connor, M., Fisher, C. and Guilfoyle, A. (2006) Interdisciplinary teams in palliative care: a critical reflection. *International Journal of Palliative Nursing*, 12(3): 132–7.

Patiraki, E., Karlou, C., Papadopoulou, D., Spyridou, A., Kouloukoura, C., Bare, E. and Merkouris, A. (2004) Barriers in implementing research findings in cancer care: the Greek registered nurses' perceptions. *European Journal of Oncology Nursing*, 8(3): 254–6.

Payne, S. (2001) Occupational stressors and coping as determinants of burnout in female hospice nurses. *Journal of Advanced Nursing*, 33: 396–405.

Pravikoff, D., Tanner, A. and Pierce, S. (2005) Readiness of US nurses for evidence-based practice. *American Journal of Nursing*, 105(9): 40–51.

Quint, J.C. (1967) *The Nurse and the Dying Patient*. New York: Macmillan.

Robinson, R. (2004) End-of-life education in undergraduate nursing curricula. *Dimensions in Critical Care Nursing*, 23(23): 89–92.

Royal College of Nursing (RCN) (2003) *A Framework for Adult Cancer Nursing*. RCN: London.

Seymour, J., Clark, D., Hughes, P., Bath, P., Beech, N., Corner, J., Douglas, H-R., Haviland, J., Marples, R., Normand, C., Skilbeck, J. and Webb, T. (2002) Clinical nurse specialists in palliative care, Part 3: issues for the Macmillan nurse role. *Palliative Medicine*, 16: 386–94.

Seymour, J., Ingleton, C., Payne, S. and Beddow, V. (2003) Specialist palliative care: Patients' experiences. *Journal of Advanced Nursing*, 44(1): 24–33.

Seymour, J. and Skilbeck, J. (2002) Ethical considerations in research user views. *European Journal of Cancer Care*, 11: 215–19.

Shah, S. (2005) Integrated care pathway for the last days of life. *Palliative Medicine*, 19: 351–3.

Skilbeck, J. and Seymour, J. (2002) Meeting complex needs: an analysis of Macmillan nurses' work with patients. *International Journal of Palliative Nursing*, 8(12): 574–82.

Takeda, F. (2002) Japan: Status of cancer pain and palliative care. *Journal of Symptom Management*, 24(92): 197–9.

Thomas, K. and Noble, B. (2007) Improving the delivery of palliative care in general practice: an evaluation of the first phase of the Gold Standards Framework. *Palliative Medicine*, 21: 49–52.

Thomas, K. (2004) *Caring for the dying at home*. Oxford: Radcliffe Medical Press.

Thompson, C., McCaughan, D., Cullum, N., Sheldon, T.A., Mulhall, A. and Thompson, D.R. (2001) Research information in nurses' clinical decision making: what is useful? *Journal of Advanced Nursing*, 36(3): 376–88.

Timmons, S. (2003) Nurses resisting information technology. *Nursing Inquiry*, 10(4): 257–69.

Vlieger, M., Gorchs, N., Larkin, P. and Porchet, F. (2004) Palliative nurse education: towards a common language. *Palliative Medicine*, 18: 401–3.

Wang, X.S., Tong-du, L., Gu, W. and Xu, G. (2002) China: Status of pain and palliative care. *Journal of Pain and Symptom Management*, 24(2): 147–51.

Watson, R. (2006) Is there a role for higher education in preparing nurses? *Nurse Education Today*, 26: 622–6.

Watson, R. and Manthorpe, J. (2002) Research governance: for whose benefit? (editorial). *Journal of Advanced Nursing*, 39(6): 515–16.

Wee, B. (2007) Bedside Teaching. In: B. Wee and N. Hughes (eds) *Education in Palliative Care: Building a Culture of Learning*. Oxford: Oxford University Press, 13: 115–27.

While, A. (2005) In defence of nursing and the generic nurse. Editorial. *International Journal of Nursing Studies*, 42(7): 715–16.

Willard, C. and Luker, K. (2005) Supportive care in the cancer setting: rhetoric or reality. *Journal of Palliative Medicine*, 19(4): 328–33.

Wittenberg-Lyles, E.M. and Parker Oliver, D. (2007) The power of interdisciplinary collaboration in hospice. *Progress in Palliative Care*, 15(1): 6–13.

Yu, S. and Yang, K. (2006) Attitudes towards web-based distance learning among public health nurses in Taiwan: a questionnaire survey. *International Journal of Nursing Studies*, 34(6): 767–74.

Zwarenstein, M. and Reeves, S. (2000) What's so great about collaboration? We need more evidence and less rhetoric. *British Medical Journal*, 320: 1022–3.

# 28

# Professional boundaries in palliative care

*Karen Cox and Veronica James*

---

**Key points**

- There are a multiplicity of palliative care settings and changing roles within the palliative care team.
- Teams need to reach out towards community, user, voluntary and social service, and wider professional networks and to understand the contexts within which they are working.
- Teams need to become reflexive in their practice and regularly review their functions and processes drawing on the 'broader team' (as in point 2 above) wherever feasible.
- Evaluations of teams are required that consider their effectiveness as well as the user perspective in order to develop future successful models of teams.

---

A boundary is a demarcation of some kind. Specialist palliative care is a small but important area in the growing complexity of bounded, community and acute care provision. It is an area which, with the patient and family seen as a whole unit, prides itself on the delivery of care through multidisciplinary teamwork. Thus, from the beginning, a tension arises. Patients and families want us to see them as a whole, and work in collaboration with them to meet a range of changing physical, psychological and domestic needs. They also want us to work with each other, seamlessly across the boundaries of general services and specialisms, acute and community, professions and organizations, without bands of fragmented specialists marching up the path. There is a danger that, despite a notion of teamwork, organizational fragmentation overrides the core purposes of palliative care – the central work with patients, or users, and families. Obviously, there must be a considerable number of people, often working part-time, involved in running any 24-hour service efficiently and effectively. Yet, the greater the number and types of professions and occupations, the greater the demarcations – and the greater the need for a team approach. So how should lay and professional expertise, community and inpatient organizations, and curative and palliative care intersect to focus on the family as the unit of care?

This chapter explores the concept of boundaries, roles and team working within which palliative care is delivered. We will first consider the definitions of team and teamwork. Both these terms conjure up images of positive working relationships and a shared common goal. However, teams are complex and the work of the team in palliative care needs to be centrally concerned with the patient (or user) and family as key team players, albeit with a variable interest in decision-making. Other members of the team, affected by funding, political and organizational agendas, contribute within the context of committed professional and occupational teams, intra- and inter-team boundaries, and external influences. The chapter explores these issues further by examining debates relating to the effectiveness of palliative care teams and considers the palliative care team within the overall perspective of patient and carer involvement in health and palliative care, taking account of new ideas of 'teams', their leadership and coordination.

## Background

Over the past 30 years the palliative care team has changed considerably. Traditionally, the focus of care delivery was within the setting of the hospice which meant that the professionals involved worked in close proximity and were bounded by the physical space within which they worked. In addition, the nature of health care delivery at that time with its medical domination meant that the health care professionals involved, such as nurses and doctors, had fairly well-defined roles and responsibilities. This combination of a relatively clear demarcation between the contribution made by each of the team members and the physical boundary of the hospice meant that the palliative care team was relatively easily defined and understood. There are now, however, a multiplicity of palliative care settings beyond the traditional cancer focus and a changing of roles within the palliative care team. The relatively straightforward concept of health care provision (institution-based care led by medical staff) has shifted with the growth of broader based public provision to a complex pattern of interrelated services (Payne 2000). Specialist teams for palliative care now do not simply reside in hospice settings. They can be found in acute or community settings, in public, voluntary or private care. Teams work across disciplinary divides and institutional boundaries and need to be able to liaise effectively between a range of health and social care agencies (Clark and Seymour 1999). Similarly shifts have occurred in relation to the roles and responsibilities of team members. Nursing in particular has undergone an enormous shift in terms of extended and advanced nursing roles and nurses are taking on tasks that were previously the preserve of their medical colleagues. Patients, users, consumers; family, lay and informal carers; inequality, difference; ethnic minorities, cultural diversity, cultural competence – these changes in terminology tell us something of the shifts occurring about role boundaries and the place of the patient as a team member since the modern hospice movement started in the 1960s. While variations in patient choice and involvement have always occurred as the result of different health insurance, funding and organizational systems, new movements to involve patients (Gillespie *et al.* 2002) mean that palliative care providers will want to look outward to broader health contexts, to see what patients and carers will be bringing with them to palliative care. The palliative care team of today is therefore a transformed and diverse entity. Finally, the policy context in relation to the provision of palliative and supportive care has also developed, with increasing emphasis being placed on these elements of care and service provision. In the United Kingdom the key document in this area, the 'NICE Guidance on Improving Supportive and Palliative Care for Adults with Cancer' (NICE 2004), highlights that those living at home with advanced cancer continue to be undersupported, have poorly coordinated care and little choice about where they die. Recommendations note that specialist palliative care advice should be available on a 24-hour, seven days a week basis and that community teams should be able to provide support to patients in their own homes, community hospital and care homes (p. 11). Recommendations also cover team members' expertise and communication between teams.

## The established view of teams and teamwork in palliative care

Palliative care teams are an interesting example of teamwork in the health care system. The National Council for Hospices and Specialist Palliative Care Services (NCHSPCS 1995) suggests that teamwork is a key element of specialist palliative care services. The trend towards interdisciplinary team working and collaboration has been identified as a particular strength of specialist palliative care services, with hospice teams being described as good examples of interprofessional work (Ajemian 1993). Interprofessional work in this instance refers to people with distinct disciplinary training within the health service working together for a common purpose, as they make different, complementary contributions to patient-focused care (Leathard 1994). Furthermore, writers in this area also note that team working in palliative care is essential as it provides mutual support in what can be emotionally draining work (in relation to caring for the dying) (Vachon 1987; Field 1989), as well as promoting enhanced clinical standards by facilitating exchange of knowledge, ideas and experience (Woof *et al.* 1998).

The established view of the palliative care team is invariably presented as a list of health and social care professionals from statutory and non-statutory services. Pick up any palliative care textbook from the 1980s and 1990s and it will talk about team members and their roles, providing lists of professionals and their potential input to the team (Corr and Corr 1983; Hull *et al.* 1989; Dunlop and Hockey 1990; Saunders 1990; Clark *et al.* 1997;

Faull 1998). Faull (1998), for example, provides a list of professionals and identify 'who does what'. This description of roles includes health care based services such as: medical roles (general practitioner, palliative care physician, hospital consultants), nursing roles (district nurse, specialist palliative care nurse, Marie Curie nurse, practice nurses, other nursing specialities), pharmacist, physiotherapist, occupational therapist, social worker, counsellor, clinical psychologist and dietician. Social services based roles include home help, meals on wheels and voluntary organizations. Other services include private agencies, spiritual advisors and complementary therapists, in addition to the proliferation of services such as art, music and pets for health. Other authors (for example, Hull *et al.* 1989; and Ingham and Coyle 1997) use diagrammatic representations to convey the vast array of professionals involved in palliative care teams. These tend to be presented in a circular fashion, presumably to get away from the idea of any hierarchy, with the patient and family in the centre.

As can be seen from the UK Hospice Information Directory 2005 not only are there national level teams of hospice leaders – Africa, Australasia, Europe, North America; and hospice administration, fund raising and management teams, but those delivering direct services have also divided into multiple, separate teams both within the hospice system, and drawing on an increasing range of medical and social care specialists from broader health and social care services, with the effect that there is now no such thing as a 'standard' team.

While the lists and diagrams many textbook authors devise to represent these teams are useful for the reader who requires an insight into the variety of potential provider roles in palliative care and an outline of their area of expertise, they leave us asking a number of questions. There are two main ones that we will concentrate on in this chapter. First, these lists identify a huge number of people potentially involved and one has to question if the resulting combination actually amounts to a palliative care 'team' or simply denotes anything from a network with varying degrees of collaboration to a loose reference to the multitude of specialist areas available within health, social care and voluntary services and beyond who may contribute to the care of any particular patient and their family. In addition, only limited reference is made to how professionals may or may not interact with each other or different agencies. Thus there is little attention given to issues such as ambiguity, overlap and conflict of roles, communication difficulties and leadership issues. Second, where is the patient in all this? The 'team', as presented in these texts, is invariably health care dominated with little reference made to the users of services playing a real part in the team even though they are now habitually claimed as 'central' to the palliative care philosophy. This critique has been partly addressed with the recent publication of Peter Speck's book on 'teamwork in palliative care', which attempts to present a more contemporary account of the realities and difficulties of current palliative care team working (Speck 2006). However, the concern remains that the user voice still remains under-represented in discussions about teams and team working in health care.

# Limitations of the established view of palliative care teams

The absence of any critique of the development of palliative care teams could be attributed to what Dunlop (1998) refers to as a 'culture of niceness' which has been identified in particular with voluntary hospices, as well as a natural reluctance on the part of the professionals within a team to expose their vulnerabilities. In effect what we are left with is a limited understanding of the dynamics that are at play in specialist palliative care teams. In addition, with the more recent development of palliative care specialists and specialist teams, for example in areas related to heart failure and chronic obstructive airways disease, our current understanding of palliative care teams is even more limited as these new teams and models of care are currently being evaluated and examined as part of the new focus on palliative and end-of-life care (for example, Boyd *et al.* 2004; Horne and Payne 2004; Segal *et al.* 2005). This is not to criticize those who to date have attempted to outline the various roles involved in delivering palliative care services. Rather, it is an attempt to draw attention to the limitations of such analyses and identify the complexity of teams and the plethora of agencies and professionals involved in the delivery of this particular aspect of health care. It is to raise the question of what, in this context, does teamwork actually mean? In order to explore this question further we need to refer to some of the theory on teams, team development and teamwork by social scientists and management theorists.

# Theories of teams and teamwork

More people than ever will find themselves working in a team and health care is no exception to this (Dechant *et al.* 1993). Indeed, many health service providers have embraced team-based organization in an attempt to create new modes of delivery (Manion *et al.* 1996). It is important then that we understand how teams grow and develop and the contributions that are required from individual team members in order for this to happen, involving the tacit order of teams as well as formal structures (Dechant *et al.* 1993; Hindmarsh and Pilnick 2002; Goodwin 2007). However, defining 'teamwork' is not straightforward. The meaning of 'team' and 'teamwork' is controversial (Payne 2000) and there is little empirical evidence of what is effective teamwork (Opie 1997, 2000).

A team is often defined as a group of people with diverse but related skills and knowledge who associate for the purpose of directing, coordinating and developing the separate parts as well as the sum total of their expertise (Pritchard and Pritchard 1994). In health care contexts, team working is often portrayed as a way to tackle the potential fragmentation of care, a means to widen skills, and an essential part of the complexity of modern care (Firth-Cozens 1998). However, while the terms themselves may conjure up images of positive working relationships and a shared common goal, there is more to building an effective team than simply putting together a group of people (Zollo 1999). Highly detailed empirical studies may offer insights into team-work but these are difficult to translate into strategic action (Carmel 2006).

Understanding teamwork and how it operates in health care delivery is complex. Health care teams have to contend with what Payne (2000) identifies as three paradoxes common to all types of teamwork. First, in the building of team relationships we may become more inward looking and yet, in care services, it is often also essential to build relationships with professionals in other agencies and teams. This is a common feature of many palliative care teams who have to look beyond their 'core' of staff in order to provide a comprehensive service for patients. Second, members of a team often value it for the mutual support it offers in the face of the institutional demands placed upon them, yet managers see teamwork as an instrument for carrying out the organization's objectives. Here again, this can be seen as an issue grappled with by many palliative care teams who work in a stressful and demanding world and who often need to find support in like-minded colleagues. Finally, Payne (2000) suggests, teamwork forces us to think about our interactions with colleagues, and yet in the current health care climate teams and the services they deliver should be responsive to users' needs. Again, we can draw parallels with palliative care teams in that the focus on teams and writing about teams comes from a professional perspective with professionals talking about other professionals in the team with limited reference to the users' perspective of the team and its workings. These three paradoxes mean that teamwork in health care settings is not straightforward as teams are often struggling with the tensions between their own needs and the needs of the organizations and consumers whom they are supposed to serve.

Teams in health care have been predicated on a division of labour in terms of complex tasks. They are made up of individuals who have their own area of expertise, traditions, professional interests, working practices and professional regulatory requirements. Not only are teams made up of multiple professions, individuals with their own experiences, agendas and ambitions, but they also function within a global organizational culture, which demands more for the health dollar. This places increasing demands upon teams in terms of efficiency and effectiveness and, as this is politically driven, often forces teams to operate on a short-term, quick-paced agenda. Miller *et al.* (2001), in their study of interprofessional and occupational practice in health and social care, identify organizational issues that influence team working. These are dependence and response to recent government policies, the importance of team-orientated structures and processes, the diversity of patient populations, and the opportunities for the team to work closely. With the growth in the number of diseases being brought under the palliative care umbrella (HIV/AIDS, respiratory, renal, heart disease), it is little wonder that teams, while often being seen as a positive part of the work of health care delivery, can also be a source of angst and stress. Helping a 'team' to understand what is influencing it and how to overcome conflict is vital if a 'team' is to survive and develop. Palliative care teams need to be aware of the many pressures that have shaped the way they have developed in the past and question whether those pressures continue to shape the way they deliver services appropriately or whether there are new pressures. Understanding how teams develop over time is crucial to this process, as is recognition of the inclusion of 'new stakeholders' as local practicalities and state and national policies interact.

In relation to clearly bounded teams, there are two main views about how teams come into being: developmental and situational. Developmental views argue that teams go through a process of building up towards being a team. There are two versions of this view. One – expressed by Brill (1976) – holds that a group naturally develops and ends up as a team and that the team-builder's work is to speed it on its way. The second is that team development requires team building to help overcome the barriers to effective team working (Shaw 1994). Probably the most cited and well-known developmental view is based on Tuckman's (1965) review of over 50 published papers on group development. He noted that groups go through four stages: forming (getting together), storming (rebellion and establishing roles), norming (agreement over the group work) and performing (getting on with the work) when they come together. Tuckman is careful to note that not all groups work through all of the stages, nor are the stages necessarily completed one after the other and in that order. Similarly, caution must be used when attempting to apply his findings in the real world of teamwork. The studies he reviewed were largely based on laboratory studies of small groups as opposed to situations where teams are together on a longer-term basis, have real tasks to deal with and are there as part of an organization, or multiple organizations, with their own distinct imposed structures and responsibilities. Subsequently work by Tuckman and Jenson in the 1970s revealed that a fifth stage, 'adjourning', should be added to the hypothesis relating to team development and recommended further empirical work (Tuckman and Jenson 1977). More recent work continues to draw on Tuckman's model as a framework in which to examine teams but suggests more attention is given to the structure, process, context and productivity of teams when assessing their development and effectiveness (Zeiss and Heinemann 2002).

Situational views (in contrast to developmental views) suggest that different kinds of team and teamwork are appropriate to different situations in which teams are placed. Team building in this view requires an understanding of the factors that the team face and involves designing a plan of action taking into account members' preferences, the type of work and the organization (Burrell and Lindström 1987). Situational views see team building as responding to and improving work environments.

## Building teams and teamwork in palliative care

In many respects elements of both approaches are necessary if we are to build teams to work in health care settings because of the demands of service delivery and the range of different disciplines, backgrounds and organizations involved. Payne (2000) presents an interesting alternative to the models of team development and team working set out above but which contains elements of both. He argues for open teamwork, which combines the established view of teamwork with the concept of networking. Payne suggests that teams cannot just be about interpersonal relations between professionals working together but require team members to reach out towards community, user and wider professional and volunteer networks, and to understand the contexts within which they are working. This concept of team working maps nicely onto palliative care where a core team may be required to interact with other teams, individuals and organizations, each with a different ethos, funding system and team values. We will return to this later.

Teamwork is also affected by members' roles and the way in which members interact with each other (interpersonal relations). Early research in this area typically concerned the role of individual team members as opposed to how they interacted with each other. For example, Benne and Skeats (1948) work refers to three types of group member; those who help the group to achieve its task, those who develop group cohesion and those concerned with personal needs. Later work focused on the effect of different personality types or behaviours on the functioning of the team (Brill 1976). A major advance on the understanding of member roles within a team came in the early 1980s. Based on research among management teams, Belbin (1981) identified eight roles as necessary for a successful team (company worker, chair, shaper, plant, resource investigator, monitor evaluator, team-worker, completer-finisher). Belbin suggests that a successful team will have all or most of these eight roles within it and that if significant roles are missing, the team will not function well. Most people, however, have both main and secondary roles, and therefore can contribute in multiple ways. Which roles they take on depends on other skills in the team (Payne 2000). Although Belbin's work has been highly influential there are a number of cautions which must be applied. First, people draw on a range of skills, knowledge and experience and the roles they take on may change over time, and in relation to who else is in the team. Second, Belbin's model suggests that only changing team membership achieves the desired roles, and thus does not offer an intervention that can help an existing team make progress (Clark 1994). Later work focuses on skills and competencies as the primary issues affecting the functioning of the team and refers to styles of the team members, such as contributors, collaborators, communicators and challengers (Parker 1990; Spencer and Pruss 1992; Margerison and McCann 1995). These kinds of role preferences are possibly more helpful than Belbin's team roles when considering the issue of teamwork in palliative care, where the team may be made up not only of individuals who work and meet together on a daily basis but may also contain elements of distant working across organizational and professional boundaries. It may be useful for readers to consider their own teams in this way and note which role preferences they take on as well as considering their colleagues. Understanding where each other is coming from and how to use the strengths of individual team members in particular circumstances can make for a more effective and responsive team.

Another issue facing palliative care teams is the changing nature of health care professional roles. Contributions within a team are often shaped by how people see themselves within the team and where they locate (see) the team's and their own boundary. For those involved in palliative care, the changing place and pace of care delivery, the increasingly vast array of individuals involved, and the changing roles and boundaries of health care professionals, mean that roles within the team are constantly changing. The place of the physician as the leader of the team is shifting and the rise of consumerism has secured the place of the patient and family at the centre of the team. Voluntary staff are also increasingly viewed as part of palliative care teams (Freeman *et al.* 1998). Nurses are increasingly seen as the leader or coordinator of care in the palliative care setting, primarily because of their close proximity to the patient and family (Ingham and Coyle 1997). Indeed nurses have pioneered new approaches to clinical care delivery and organization in palliative care; for example, nurse-led clinics for patients with breathlessness (Corner *et al.* 1995), managing ascites (Preston 1995), as well as in the area of prescribing (Latter *et al.* 2005) and heart failure (Grange 2005), with good evidence that nurse coordinators reduce the number of days patients spend in hospital (NICE 2004). This constant 'modernization' through new developments in palliative care introduces a further level of complexity around working across a range of boundaries in order to deliver palliative care across a range of disease sites.

This shift in professional boundaries – that is, with nurses incorporating and sometimes taking over elements from the traditionally clinically and organizationally medical led service – is likely to have an impact on the team dynamics in terms of its development and functioning.

Teamwork in palliative care (as in any area of health care) is multi-layered, delivered by a range of professionals, in a range of settings from a variety of perspectives. Different individuals will be more or less important at a particular point in time according to the needs of the patient and their family. The palliative care team may be better viewed as a kaleidoscope of roles, skills and knowledge, of teams within teams, of blurred boundaries and of sometimes overlapping roles, that will look different according to the needs and place of the individual and family they are caring for. This description does not fit neatly with the earlier descriptions of teams and teamwork, which present teams as fairly static entities. In contrast to the view that we have presented and Payne's (2000) concept of open teams, the older established view of teams took no account of the moving array of roles suggested here. Our kaleidoscope approach to viewing teams can, however, be disconcerting as it raises questions about overall responsibility and issues of coordination. As such it requires mutual respect, excellent communication, a clear understanding of each other's skills and abilities, and of what collaborative practice means – including conjoint problem solving, shared record keeping and shared accountability (Kedziera and Levy 1994), an ability to cross organizational and professional boundaries, and give up ownership of 'the patient'. This kind of teamwork requires members of the team to be more reflexive (Opie 1997). Being reflexive in this sense requires teams to review and critique their performance and move beyond familiar ways of working with each other (Opie 1997). Opie (2000) suggests that reflexive practice may be particularly important in complex cases or when the team believes that its work with the client is not progressing as well as it might.

## Patients and the palliative care team

We now turn to the second of our concerns around teams and teamwork as traditionally described in the literature, which relates to the place of the patient and family in the health care team. It is natural that health care practitioners and researchers consistently conceptualize their own work in terms which position 'the patient' at the 'centre' of their approach, and this can be seen in a number of the familiar models of the palliative care team referred to earlier in this chapter (Corr and Corr 1983; Hull *et al.* 1989; Dunlop and Hockey 1990; Saunders 1990; Clark *et al.* 1997; Faull 1998). However, if we wish to deliver the best possible palliative care services, it is surely crucial to ask whether patients really are so consistently at the 'centre' of palliative care teams in practice, and the best way to do so is to explore patients' own experiences of the team and their place in it.

As previously stated, palliative teams consist of a range of health and social care professionals who deliver care in a variety of different situations to patients with a range of diseases. In practice, however, individual patients and their families may not see the complete cast of characters which health care professionals regard as the 'team' or indeed perceive that they are in fact also part of this 'team'. In the course of their dying trajectory they may come across one or two leading players in each part of the care services (primary, acute, voluntary, social services), with other teams and individuals having bit parts. Professionals may be aware of all the others in the broader team and what is available; however, the patient is likely not to have any idea about the characters 'backstage' and the alternatives available to them. The patient's perspective of the team is likely therefore to be very different to the professionals'. Patients' and families' perspectives, as the users of palliative care services, are likely to throw a very different light onto our professional constructs of the palliative care team. It is important then for us to consider what the team looks like from the patient's perspective if the team is to have any meaning at all.

As a measure of how rapidly the field moves, a systematic review of the impact of specialist palliative care provision on consumer satisfaction, opinion and preference Wilkinson *et al.* (1999) identified only 83 studies relating to work undertaken in North America and Europe. The team noted that consumers were more satisfied with all types of palliative care, whether provided by inpatient units or in the community, than provided by general hospitals. However, the majority of the studies they reviewed were based on small-scale local studies which were mainly focused on a single hospice. There was little research in relation to home care or other forms of palliative community-based services. In addition, there was little reference to patients' and families' perceptions of the palliative care team, rather the focus was on comparing place of care, i.e. hospice versus hospital, the satisfaction with specialist community services, and preference for place of death. Further, it did not take account of those who were not offered or refused hospice care. The review concluded that there were few consistent trends in consumer opinion on and satisfaction with specialist models of palliative care.

The lack of a consumer perspective at that time may have been related to some of the methodological difficulties of collecting information at a vulnerable time in patients' and families' lives (Fakhoury 1998). However, while newer policies focus on how patient and carer voices can be incorporated into policy and practice development (Department of Health 2006), the World Health Organization (WHO) sponsored review of palliative care by Davies and Higginson (2004) struggled to convey the centrality of patients and carers as actively engaged. Yet this kind of information is invaluable to providers of palliative care services as it can present a unique perspective on the quality of the service, access to care provision, problem areas and service successes (Wilkinson *et al.* 1999). In examining consumer perceptions of teamwork, more consumer-oriented, qualitative approaches that take a longitudinal perspective may be one way to begin to uncover some of the experiences of being cared for by a palliative care team. This would allow for exploration of the concept of a team approach to care as perceived by the patient, as well as exploring who they perceive to be responsible for which aspects of their care at different points in their illness trajectory. This kind of information can be used to develop future, more successful models of palliative care teams and team practices. Work which addresses the shortcomings relating to consumer involvement in the evidence base is now beginning to be undertaken and disseminated as outlined below.

## The effectiveness of palliative care teams

We have noted earlier that various writers on interdisciplinary teams in palliative care suggest that such team working impacts positively on the quality of care received by dying patients and their carers, and that it is beneficial for staff (Vachon 1987; Hull *et al.* 1989; Hockley 1992; Opie 1997; Woof *et al.* 1998; NICE 2004; Speck 2006). There is little empirical evidence, however, to suggest that interdisciplinary teams improve patient outcomes (Opie 1997; Zwarenstein and Reeves 2000). The bulk of the literature presented earlier in relation to palliative care teams tends to be descriptive, focusing on team composition, team working and changing working practices but with little reference to whether these teams are effective or not. In addition, the growth of palliative care services has in the main been unplanned and unevaluated. Developments have largely been in response to local pressure, public demand and fundraising activities and while they are becoming an increasing part of mainstream provision, are often still situated in the voluntary and independent sectors (Faull 1998). As a result, there are now a wide variety of models and approaches to delivering palliative care. However, because of the haphazard approach to service development, there has been limited evaluation of the effectiveness of this kind of service provision. In the current health care climate it is no longer sufficient simply to claim that the service you are delivering is effective. Services now have to provide clear evidence to this effect. For palliative care teams this means being able to demonstrate clinical effectiveness, quality services, service-user involvement, collaborative working and cost-effectiveness. Questions on these issues are increasingly being asked of palliative care services and are a subject of debate among the palliative care community (NCHSPCS 2001).

Service level evaluations have not been able to demonstrate the superiority of specialist services over non-specialist services in palliative care (Robbins 1997). Indeed many of the basic comparative studies, taking into account outcomes, measures of performance, and cost, have not been carried out for palliative care services (Robbins 1997). A systematic review undertaken by Hearn and Higginson (1998), focusing on specific palliative care interventions, demonstrated improved outcomes for those cared for by specialist teams rather than standard care. In the 18 studies that they reviewed, they noted that effectiveness of the team was evidenced by an increased satisfaction on the part of patients and carers, better symptom control, reduction in the number of days per hospital stay, more time spent at home and an increased likelihood of patients dying in the place of their choice. On this basis Hearn and Higginson (1998) concluded that the palliative care approach does have an impact on the quality of care delivered. However, whether this was attributable to the fact that it was a team providing such interventions is debatable. It is notoriously difficult to identify which particular elements of the team or its approach are most effective. Similar work that has attempted to evaluate the impact of teamwork in specialist stroke services or breast care teams has identified analogous problems.

Measuring the effectiveness of health services is not straightforward. 'Effectiveness' itself is a multilayered concept that can be approached from numerous perspectives, although 'value for money' and 'health gain' often emerge as two of its essential elements. Evidence of what might constitute 'effectiveness' is also a matter of debate, since the significance of one patient's experience, as compared with evidence produced by a large-scale, multi-centre, randomized controlled trial of a large population, may be more or less appropriate and valuable to health care practitioners, depending upon the purpose and nature of the particular study. Health service research suggests that the complex and multifaceted nature of health care means that traditional experimental approaches may be inappropriate for certain kinds of enquiry (Fitzpatrick and Boulton 1994; Klein 1996; Campbell *et al.* 2000). Alternative approaches grounded in more naturalistic methods – such as pluralistic evaluation (Smith and Cantley 1985) or realist evaluation (Pawson and Tilly 1997; Pawson 2006) – may be more appropriate when outputs are less quantifiable and the process is also of importance. In addition, there is a real need to consider the user perspective in relation to the effectiveness of services. How do patients and families perceive the care they receive? What worked for them, what did not work as well? These how, what and why questions are important if we are to understand anything about the processes that are underway as palliative care is delivered and received. Simply relying on quantitative measurable outputs is not enough if we wish to be able to answer these more complicated in-depth questions. It seems that if we are to achieve any meaningful evaluation of palliative care teams, there is a need for a multi-method approach that embraces both quantitative and qualitative research data to help us identify how and why something is – or is not – effective.

Specialist palliative care teams pose another challenge for researchers. Specialist input in palliative care is invariably provided in addition to mainstream care. In some instances they work alongside the mainstream caregivers or may simply provide additional resource in terms of information, advice or equipment. The point is that it is very difficult to identify a 'pure effect'; that is, make any comparison between the specialist service and the routine services as the two are often so intertwined. In addition, patients who do not receive any input from the specialist team may receive care of the same standard from mainstream services provided by numerous practitioners who have received additional education and training in palliative care. In 1989, Seale pointed out that hospices were no longer providing care that was radically different to mainstream health services (Seale 1989). This extensive dispersal of palliative care knowledge has caused an interesting dilemma for palliative care teams. If professionals outside the specialist team are capable of providing the care and support traditionally within that team's domain, what is to become of the specialist team? In addition, if these same teams cannot provide evidence of their effectiveness, how can they defend the need for their presence?

Evaluating the effectiveness of specialist palliative care teams might appear then to be an impossible task. Yet palliative care teams, like all other branches of health service provision, need to be able to demonstrate their effectiveness in order to survive. They cannot continue simply on the basis of what has gone on in the past. What appears to be vitally important is that first and foremost there needs to be a clear definition of specialist palliative care teams (and this, as noted earlier, is notoriously difficult to achieve in the palliative care setting because of the plethora of professionals involved). Second, it seems important to identify which elements of the team can be meaningfully assessed in relation to concepts of 'effectiveness'. Only with a clear definition and an identification of the assessable elements can any progress be made towards examining the effectiveness or otherwise of the specialist team in palliative care.

This drive to articulate 'effectiveness' has resulted in a number of studies which have sought to provide evidence of the impact of palliative care services on patient outcomes and experiences. A focused review of the literature carried out by the authors in 2007 revealed recent studies which had sought to address this gap in the evidence base. A number of these studies identify an impact on patient experiences and outcomes after referral to palliative care teams. Bostrom *et al.* (2004), for example, note that after referral to palliative care patients reported significant improvement in their care, in particular pain control and feelings of security and continuity of care. Jack *et al.* (2004) noted that palliative care team input improved patients' understanding of their illness and in work reported in 2006 they noted that hospital-based patients receiving input from a palliative care team experienced significantly greater improvement in pain control than control. Similarly O'Mahoney *et al.* (2005), in an evaluation of a hospital-based inpatient palliative care team, noted from an audit of medical records that pain and other symptoms improved in 87 per cent of patients after team intervention and 95 per cent of family care-givers responding to a telephone survey said they were likely to recommend the service to others. Rabow *et al.* (2004) conducted a year-long controlled trial involving 90 patients split between control and intervention arms attending an out-patient clinic. Patients had congestive heart failure, chronic obstructive airways disease or cancer. The intervention group received palliative care team consultations, advanced care planning, psychosocial support and family care-giver training. Outcomes were assessed at 6 and 12 months. The researchers found that the intervention group had improved outcomes in dyspnoea, anxiety and spiritual well-being. They also had decreased primary care input and urgent care visits without an increase in emergency care visits. Other studies are less conclusive. In a systematic review of palliative day care services to December 2003, Davies and Higginson (2005) note there were insufficient studies to conclusively show improved symptom control or quality of life.

The problem of defining the most appropriate model for palliative care teams to operate from and identify their cost/benefit remains. Abernethy *et al.* (2006) identify the key barriers to efficacy and effectiveness studies which include recruitment, opposition to randomization, attrition, inconsistent interventions, ill-chosen outcome measures and difficulty estimating costs. Experimental designs testing palliative care interventions remain few in number and generalizability of results is weak (Bakitas and Lyons 2006). Researchers are now beginning to outline studies that may be able to transcend some of these criticisms. For example, Abernethy *et al.* (2006) outline a pragmatic factoral cluster, randomized controlled trial of educational outreach visiting and case conferencing in palliative care, and Higginson *et al.* (2006) has published a study protocol to evaluate a new palliative care service in a non-cancer setting which utilizes a randomized controlled trial design and draws on the Medical Research Council framework for the evaluation of complex interventions. We should all await the results of both these studies with interest.

# Conclusion

Patients and families have increasingly high expectations of health care provision and what services should offer. These include higher expectations of power sharing, improved information giving, increased patient choice, and better patient-centred care (Gillespie *et al.* 2002). These will continue to be mediated by the fundamental need for human warmth and attention at times of vulnerability, the family support and tension created by illness, and of a desire to adopt the 'sick role', with its version of opting out. Underpinning these changes, is the challenge to the idea of 'professional/expert' and 'lay' boundaries, which in turn cause us to think anew about 'team' inputs. As palliative care continues to face the call, started in the mid-1980s, for broader delivery beyond the traditional cancer focus, palliative care teams will continue to face the challenge of collaborative working. While users and families may welcome the different professionals who offer support, there is also the danger of intrusiveness as well as fragmentation. One thing remains certain, however: palliative care teams need to develop new models of practice and evaluations of that practice if the successes of their past are to be mirrored in their future.

# References

Abernethy, A.P., Currow, D., Hunt, R., Williams, H., Roder-Allen, G., Rowett, D., Shelby-James, T., Esterman, A., May, F. and Phillips, P. (2006) A pragmatic 2×2×2 factorial cluster randomised controlled trial of educational outreach visiting and case conferencing in palliative care-methodology of the palliative care trial. *Contemporary Clinical Trials*, 27: 83–100.

Ajemian, I. (1993) Interdisciplinary teamwork. In: D. Doyle, G. Hanks and N. Macdonald (eds) *Oxford Textbook of Palliative Medicine*. Oxford: Oxford Medical Publications.

Bakitas, M.A. and Lyons, K.D. (2006) Palliative care program effectiveness research: developing rigor in sampling design, conduct and reporting. *Journal of Pain and Symptom Management*, 31(3): 270–84.

Belbin, R.M. (1981) *Management teams: Why they succeed or fail*. Oxford: Heinemann.

Benne, K.D. and Skeats, P. (1948) Functional roles of group members. *Journal of Social Issues*, 4(2): 41–9.

Boyd, K.J., Murray, S.A., Kendall, M., Worth, A., Frederick Benton, T. and Clausen, H. (2004) Living with advanced heart failure: a prospective, community based study of patients and their carers. *European Journal of Heart Failure*, 6(5): 535–7.

Bostrom, B.M., Sandh, M., Lundberg, D. and Fridlund, B. (2004) Cancer patient's experiences of care related to pain management before and after palliative care referral. *European Journal of Cancer Care*, 13: 238–45.

Brill, N.I. (1976) *Teamwork: Working together in the human services*. Philadelphia, PA: Lippincott.

Burrell, K. and Lindström, K. (1987) *Teamview: a teambuilding programme* (original Swedish edn, 1985). Hove: Pavilion.

Campbell, M., Fitzpatrick, R., Haines, A., Kinmouth, A., Sandercock, P., Spiegelhalter, D. and Tyrer, P. (2000) Framework for the design and evaluation of complex interventions to improve health. *British Medical Journal*, 321: 694–6.

Carmel, S. (2006) Boundaries obscured and boundaries reinforced: incorporation as a strategy of occupational enhancement for intensive care, *Sociology of Health and Illness*, 28(2): 154–77.

Clark, D. and Seymour, J. (1999) *Reflections on palliative care*. Buckingham: Open University Press.

Clark, D., Hockley, J. and Ahmedzai, S. (1997) *New themes in palliative care*. Buckingham: Open University Press.

Clark, N. (1994) *Teambuilding: a practical guide for trainers*. London: McGraw-Hill.

Corner, J., Plant, H. and Warner, L. (1995) Developing a nursing approach to the management of dyspnoea in lung cancer. *International Journal of Palliative Nursing*, 1(1): 5–11.

Corr, C.A. and Corr, D.M. (1983) *Hospice care: principles and practice*. London: Faber and Faber.

Davies, E. and Higginson, I. (eds) (2004) *The Solid Facts: palliative care*. WHO Europe, www.euro.who.int/document/E82931.pdf (downloaded 27 August 2007).

Davies, E. and Higginson, I. (2005) Systematic review of specialist palliative day care for adults with cancer. *Supportive Care in Cancer*, 13: 607–27.

Dechant, K., Marsick, V.J. and Kasl, E. (1993) Towards a model of team learning. *Studies in Continuing Education*, 15(1): 1–14.

Department of Health (2006) *Patient and Public Involvement*. www.dh.gov.uk/en/Policyandguidance/Organisationpolicy/PatientAndPublicinvolvement/index.htm (downloaded 27 August 2007).

Dunlop, R.J. (1998) *Cancer: Palliative Care*. London: Springer.

Dunlop, R.J. and Hockey, J.M. (1990) *Terminal care support teams. The hospital-hospice interface*. Oxford: Oxford University Press.

Fakhoury, W.K.H. (1998) Satisfaction with palliative care: what should we be aware of? *International Journal of Nursing Studies*, 35: 171–6.

Faull, C. (1998) The history and principles of palliative care. In: C. Faull, Y. Carter and R. Woof. (eds) *Handbook of Palliative Care*. Oxford: Blackwell Science, pp. 1–12.

Field, D. (1989) *Nursing the dying*. London: Routledge.

Firth-Cozens, K.J. (1998) Celebrating teamwork. *Quality in Health Care*, (Suppl) S3–S7.

Fitzpatrick, R. and Boulton, M. (1994) Qualitative methods for assessing health care. *Quality in Health Care*, 3: 107–13.

Freeman, M., Ramanathan, S., Aitken, A., Dunn, P. and Aird, J. (1998) Rural palliative care volunteer education and support program. *Australian Journal of Rural Health*, 6(3): 150–5.

Gillespie, R., Florin, D. and Gillam, S. (2002) *Changing relationships: findings from the patient involvement project*. London: King's Fund.

Goodwin, D. (2007) Upsetting the order of teamwork; is 'the same way every time' a good aspiration, *Sociology*, 41(2): 259–75.

Grange, J. (2005) The role of nurses in the management of heart failure. *Heart*, 91: ii39–ii42.

Hearn, J.H. and Higginson, I.J. (1998) Do specialist palliative care teams improve outcomes for cancer patients? A systematic review. *Palliative Medicine*, 12(5): 317–32.

Higginson, I., Vivat, B., Silber, E., Saleem, T., Burman, R., Hart, S. and Edmonds, P. (2006) Study protocol: delayed intervention randomised controlled trial within the Medical Research Council (MRC) framework to assess the effectiveness of a new palliative care service. *BMC Palliative Care*, 5: 7.

Hindmarsh, J. and Pilnick, A. (2002) The tacit order of teamwork: collaboration and embodied conduct in anesthesia, *The Sociological Quarterly*, 43(2): 139–64.

Hockley, J. (1992) Role of the hospital support team. *British Journal of Hospital Medicine*, 48(3): 250–3.

Horne, G. and Payne, S. (2004) Removing the boundaries, palliative care for people with heart failure. *Palliative Medicine*, 18(4): 291–6.

Hull, R., Ellis, M. and Sargent, V. (1989) *Teamwork in palliative care*. Oxford: Radcliffe.

Ingham, J.M. and Coyle, N. (1997) Teamwork in end of life care: a nurse-physician perspective introducing physicians to palliative care concepts. In: D. Clark, J. Hockley and S. Ahmedzai *New themes in palliative care*. Buckingham: Open University Press, pp. 255–74.

Jack, B., Hillier, V., Williams, A. and Oldham, J. (2004) Hospital based palliative care teams improve the insight of cancer patients into their disease. *Palliative Medicine*, 18: 46–52.

Jack, B., Hillier, V., Williams, A. and Oldham, J. (2006) Improving cancer patient's pain: the impact of the hospital specialist palliative care team. *European Journal of Cancer Care*, 15: 476–80.

Kedziera, P. and Levy M. (1994) Collaborative practice in oncology. *Seminars in Oncology*, 21(6): 705–11.

Klein, R. (1996) The NHS and the new scientism: solution or delusion? *Quarterly Journal of Medicine*, 89: 85–7.

Latter, S., Maben, J., Myall, M., Courtenay, M., Young, A. and Dunn, N. (2005) *An evaluation of extended formulary independent nurse prescribing*. Southampton: University of Southampton. www.dh.gov.uk/assetRoot/04/11/40/86/04114086.pdf (accessed 19 May 2007).

Leathard, A. (1994) *Going Interprofessional*. London: Routledge.

Manion, J., Lorimer, W. and Leander, W.J. (1996) *Team-based health care organisations: Blueprint for success*. Gaithersburg, MD: Aspen.

Margerison, C.J. and McCann, D. (1995) *Team management: practical new approaches* (2nd edn). Oxford: Management Books.

Miller, C., Freeman, M. and Ross, N. (2001) *Interprofessional practice in health and social care. Challenging the shared learning agenda*. London: Arnold.

NCHSPCS (National Council for Hospice and Palliative Care Services) (1995) *Information Exchange No. 13*. London: National Council for Hospice and Palliative Care Services.

NCHSPCS (2001) *What do we mean by palliative care? A discussion paper*. London: National Council for Hospice and Palliative Care Services.

NICE (2004) *Improving supportive and palliative care for adults with cancer*. London: National Institute for Clinical Excellence.

O'Mahoney, S., Blank, A., Zallman, L. and Selwyn, P. (2005) The benefits of a hospital-based inpatient palliative care consultation service: preliminary outcome data. *Journal of Palliative Medicine*, 8(5): 1033–9.

Opie, A. (1997) Thinking teams thinking clients: issues of discourse and representation in the work of health care teams. *Sociology of Health and Illness*, 19(3): 259–80.

Opie, A. (2000) *Thinking teams thinking clients: Knowledge-based team work*. New York: Columbia University Press.

Pawson, R. and Tilley, N. (1997) *Realist Evaluation*. London: Sage Publications.

Pawson, R. (2006) Evidence based policy: A realist perspective. London: Sage Publications.

Parker, G.M. (1990) *Team players and teamwork: The new competitive business strategy*. San Francisco: Jossey-Bass.

Payne, M. (2000) *Teamwork in multi-professional care*. London: Macmillan Press Ltd.

Preston, N. (1995) New strategies for the management of malignant ascites. *European Journal of Cancer Care*, 4(4): 178–83.

Pritchard, P. and Pritchard, J. (1994) *Teamwork for primary and shared care: a practical workbook* (2nd edn). Oxford: Oxford University Press.

Rabow, M.W., Dibble, S., Pantilat, S. and McPhee, S. (2004) The comprehensive care team. A controlled trial of outpatient palliative medicine consultation. *Archives of Internal Medicine*, 164: 83–91.

Robbins, M. (1997) Assessing needs and effectiveness; is palliative care a special case? In: D. Clark, J. Hockley and S. Ahmedzai (eds) *New themes in palliative care*. Buckingham: Open University Press, pp. 13–33.

Saunders, C. (1990) *Hospice and palliative care. An interdisciplinary approach*. London: Edward Arnold.

Seale, C.F. (1989) What happens in hospices: a review of research evidence. *Social Science and Medicine*, 28(6): 551–9.

Segal, D., O'Hanlon, D., Rahman, N., McCarthy, D. and Gibbs, S. (2005) Incorporating palliative care into heart failure management: a new model of care. *International Journal of Palliative Nursing*, 11(3): 135–6.

Shaw, I. (1994) *Evaluating international training*. Aldershot: Avebury.

Smith, G. and Cantley, C. (1985) *Assessing health care: A study in organisational evaluation*. Milton Keynes: Open University Press.

Speck, P. (2006) *Teamwork in palliative care: Fulfilling or frustrating?* Oxford: Oxford University Press.

Spencer, J. and Pruss, A. (1992) *Managing your team: How to organise people for maximum results*. London: Piatkus.

Tuckman, B. (1965) Developmental sequences in small groups. *Psychological Bulletin*, 63: 384–99.

Tuckman, B. and Jensen, M. (1977) Stages of small group development. *Group and Organisation Management*, 2(4): 419–27.

Vachon, M.C.S. (1987) *Occupational stress in caring for the critically ill, the dying and the bereaved*. Washington, DC: Hemisphere.

Wilkinson, E.K., Salisbury, C., Bosanquat, N., Franks, P., Kite, S., Lorentzon, M. and Naysmith, A. (1999) Patient and carer preference for, and satisfaction with, specialist models of palliative care: a systematic literature review. *Palliative Medicine*, 13(3): 197–216.

Woof, R., Carter, Y. and Faull, C. (1998) Palliative care: the team, the services and the need for care. In: C. Faull, Y. Carter and R. Woof. *Handbook of Palliative Care*. Oxford: Blackwell Science, pp. 13–32.

Zeiss, A. and Heinnemann, D. (2002) *Team performance in health care: assessment and development*. New York: Kluwer Academic/Plenum Publishers.

Zollo, J. (1999) The interdisciplinary palliative care team: problems and possibilities.

In S. Aranda and M. O'Connor, *Palliative Care Nursing: a guide to practice*. Melbourne: Ausmed, pp. 21–37.

Zwarenstein, M. and Reeves, S. (2000) What's so great about collaboration? We need more evidence and less rhetoric. *British Medical Journal*, 320(7241): 1022–3.

# 29

# The cost of caring

Surviving the culture of niceness, occupational stress and coping strategies

*Sanchia Aranda*

---

**Key points**

- Stress is an inevitable consequence of undertaking palliative care work where work environments and the realities of care provision threaten our ability to provide the desired level of care for people who are dying and their families.
- The relationship between the values inherent in palliative care and our ability to make a difference in the lives of patients and families is a critical one for understanding what counts as stressful for palliative care nurses.
- Our goals in reducing stress in palliative care appear sensibly to lie in reducing dissonance between our values and the care we can provide either by enhancing care delivery or in recognizing the limits of what can be achieved while continuing to emphasize the difference palliative care nurses make in the lives of people at the end of life.
- Research is needed to test interventions that further these goals.

---

## Introduction

Palliative care nursing occurs in a context of significant human suffering, suffering in which nurses are both witness and participant. As palliative care nurses we deal everyday with people facing one of life's greatest challenges – people who are often distressed, in pain and struggling with questions of meaning. We are not immune to this suffering and, for most of us, our reason for working in this field is a desire to make a positive difference in the lives of dying people and their families.

We work in a setting that for the rest of health care is associated with the failure of modern medicine to hold death at bay. Our work is also often hidden from view in a social context where there is both a fascination with death and an avoidance of its proximity. We are lauded for the work we do because others see it as distasteful, yet the skill of our work is seen as hidden (Aranda 2001), innate rather than learnt. Nursing in palliative care is even described as the quintessential spirit of nursing (Bradshaw 1996) – potentially little more than attention to the basics. For me such beliefs minimize the complexity of our work and undermine its skill – a skill that is a combination of disease knowledge, clinical expertise and human compassion.

Believing that palliative nursing is natural rather than learned leads to what I consider to be a clear paradox in the self-perception of palliative care nurses – on the one hand, this is something everyone with a bit of humanity can do and, on the other, it is hard work and skilled practice. This paradox means we work in a constant balance between emphasizing the ordinariness of what we do and having to defend the need for skilled nurses in the delivery of palliative care. If nurses are to survive and even thrive in this context attention must be paid to the skills and support required to do this.

While occupational stress and burnout are common phenomenon across health care, and certainly not unique to palliative care, there are some characteristics of palliative care as a specialty that require specific attention. This chapter, while acknowledging the significant work undertaken on occupational stress in palliative care (e.g. Vachon 1987, 1995, 1999), seeks to depart from this work through an exploration of the relationship between the underlying philosophy of palliative care, what counts as stressful and the meaning of this for nursing work in palliative care. It is from an understanding of this relationship that I argue for greater emphasis on self-knowledge and reflective capacity, both within individuals and teams, as the key mechanism for surviving and thriving as a palliative care nurse.

## ▌ Stress in palliative care nursing

Stress in palliative care workers has received ongoing attention in the literature since the seminal work of Mary Vachon (1987). Terms associated with stress in health workers include compassion fatigue (Welsh 1999), burnout (Payne 2001) and chronic grief (Saunders and Valente 1994; Feldstein and Gemma 1995). Much of the descriptive work on stress in palliative care has focused on the identification of specific stressors and a summary of such stressors is presented in Table 29.1. While there is some evidence that levels of burnout are low in palliative care nurses and that stressors contribute to the burnout that does occur (Payne 2001), how we understand stress is critical to how the subject is approached.

### *Theoretical understandings of occupational stress and coping*

Vachon, the leading author on occupational stress in palliative care, utilizes the person-environment fit framework to understand work stress in palliative care. This framework works from the principle 'that adaptation is a

**Table 29.1**   Sources of stress

***Environmental factors***
- Working conditions
  - high workloads
  - staff shortages
- Inadequate preparation for work situation
- Inadequate preparation for care demands
- Lack of time to relax or grieve
- Poor or negative interrelationships between staff
- High levels of organizational change
- Lack of management support or appreciation
- Role conflict or lack of role clarity
- Role change
- High levels of uncertainty

***Patient factors***
- Role overlap with family members
- Nature of the patient's illness
- Patient's emotional state
- Family's emotional state
- Nature of the death

***Personal factors***
- Demographic variables often listed but relationship unclear
- Gaps between ideals
- Feelings of inadequacy
- Personality disorders
- Identification with the patient
- Provision of care that was not optimal
- Accumulated grief

function of the "goodness of fit" between the characteristics of the person and the work environment' (1999: 93). This framework requires an exploration of the needs of the person and the resources available to meet these within the environment and also a comparison between the abilities of the individual and the demands of the work environment. Essentially stress occurs when the demands of the environment exceed the abilities of the person or when the environment cannot meet the needs of the individual. This framework makes intuitive sense in considering occupational stress in palliative care because it acknowledges that this field is built on a set of values and beliefs, about the care of people who are dying, which must at some level be shared by individuals who choose this work. These beliefs and values include a valuing of each individual, a belief that dying can be a time of personal growth and that quality of life in dying is a central goal of care.

However, the person-environment fit framework is limited when attempting to understand the nature of stress in palliative care more specifically. While it is sometimes said that working with the terminally ill is stressful (McNamara *et al.* 1995), it is not necessarily more so than for other specialist areas of health care. Why do some situations cause stress for one individual and not another? Why is a certain type of situation more stressful for the same individual at one time than at another?

Lazarus and Folkman (1984) developed the transactional model of stress and coping that can help to answer such questions. They argue that individuals constantly appraise events in their environment in relation to the potential impact these events have for them. Stressful events are those that are appraised as indicating a threat, challenge or harm for the individual, thus it is the appraisal of the situation by the individual rather than an inherent characteristic of the situation that leads to stress as an outcome. Coping is anything the individual does 'to regulate the distress (emotion-focused coping) or manage the problem causing distress (problem-focused coping)' (Folkman 1997: 1216).

Benner and Wrubel (1989), drawing on Lazarus and Folkman's transactional model of stress and coping, argue that stress occurs in a context where things matter to the individual. Essentially when the things that you hold to be important are threatened or challenged, stress is the result. If we apply this to stress in palliative nursing we begin to see some of the daily stress facing nurses in this field. If what matters to you draws from palliative care philosophy, such as the ability to spend time with patients and families, the ability to alleviate symptoms, having the time to bring closure to a relationship with a patient by attending a funeral, then anything that reduces your capacity to do this is a potential cause of stress. While this may seem obvious it is rarely brought out in work on stress in palliative care.

McNamara *et al.* (1995) offer a sociological perspective on stress that is consistent with both the person-environment and transactional models but which allows a closer examination of how the philosophical basis of palliative care both sets up what counts as stressful and frames the mechanisms through which nurses and others deal with stress. Essentially their work draws from Saunders and Baines's (1983) contention that 'if we are to remain for long near the suffering of dependence and parting we need also to develop a basic philosophy and search, often painfully, for meaning even in the most adverse situations' (pp. 65–6). Thus the ability to work in palliative care in the long term is understood by these authors as residing in 'the development of a value system that supplies meaning and direction' (McNamara *et al.* 1995: 223). This shared value system becomes the group's work driver and is closely related to their sense of efficacy and of having done a good job. For McNamara *et al.* 'Perceptions of stress and strategies for coping, therefore, are not entirely idiosyncratic, but are grounded in a learned logic that is systematically shared' (p. 224). From this perspective, stress relates to threats to the practitioner's ability to deliver care according to these shared values and perhaps also to challenges to the shared strategies for dealing with such threats.

The values-based perspective on stress offered by McNamara *et al.* is afforded more theoretical strength by the recent work of Folkman (1997) on meaning-focused coping. Drawing on research with partners of men with HIV disease, Folkman argues that even in the event of an unfavourable resolution of a stressful event, such as a diagnosis of a terminal disease, individuals can modify the stress response through meaning-focused coping efforts. These efforts include positive reappraisal, revisited goals, spiritual beliefs and positive events. Significant similarities can be drawn here between the global way in which palliative care philosophy is an attempt to reappraise the negative outcome of death through emphasizing the growth possible in the face of death or acceptance of death and reconciliation of a life well lived (positive reappraisal); focusing on short- rather than long-term goals, such as living day to day to the maximum (revisited goals); belief in an afterlife or having made a contribution that will be remembered (spiritual beliefs); or making opportunities for positive events in an otherwise distressing situation, such as developing a memory book for a loved one (positive events). Thus stress in palliative care can be understood as intimately linked to the practitioner's capacity to personally engage in meaning-focused coping. I would argue also that the practitioner's experience of stress may also be related to the degree to which their clients engage in meaning-focused coping, as it is through such coping efforts that patients can be understood to directly assume the values inherent in the delivery of palliative care and where the practitioner gains tangible evidence of the difference their work makes in the lives of patients and families.

A further concept explored in the literature on health and stress is Antonovsky's sense of coherence theory arising from his work on factors that lead to resistance to stress and ill health. A sense of coherence is related to a global sense of confidence that there is consistency and predictability between a person's internal and external environments and a sense that overall things in life will work out well (Sullivan 1993). Concepts linked to a sense of coherence include a belief that life events make sense (comprehensibility), that the person is able to meet the demands imposed on them (manageability) and that challenges in life are worth the effort to overcome them (meaningfulness) (Sullivan 1993). These concepts are linked to others in the stress and coping literature that suggest a meditating role in stress through the achievement of meaning and a sense that the individual has the power to overcome difficulties. I would argue that a strong sense of coherence can equate to a nurse whose values and beliefs about their work are consistent with the daily reality of practice, where they feel able to manage the work demands in making a difference for the dying person and family and where overall a sense of meaningfulness in this work is retained as a motivator to continue.

# The tyranny of niceness

The importance of understanding the relationship between palliative care values and stress becomes critical if one accepts my previously argued view that the philosophical basis of palliative care suffers from a lack of critique and in many respects is ideological rather than rooted in reality

(Aranda 1998a). In this work I argued that values such as acceptance of the inevitability of death, the family as unit of care and excellence in pain and symptom management were often used in the language of palliative care but that little evidence existed to support the achievement of these values in practice (Aranda 1998a). More recently I have argued that indeed several tyrannies of palliative care act to reduce open critique and thus leave the field in danger of further ideological stagnation (Aranda 2001). What is important from this for a discussion of stress is that without this critique palliative care nurses are more at risk of stress as care systems develop increasingly in ways that threaten their value system but these systems are unable to be openly challenged. Aranda and Brown (2006) address the example of bodywork as an example of important nursing practices that are in danger of being ruled out of practice by policy frameworks that see 'basic nursing care' as able to be delegated to less qualified workers. If challenge to such system and policy change is not possible then nurses will experience a lack of fit with their environment, experience challenges to what matters to them or gives their work life meaning and in addition feel powerless to change their situation. Much of this lack of open challenge relates to what I have previously referred to as the tyranny of niceness (Aranda 2001).

The tyranny of niceness is referred to by Street (1995) as a culture which involves ' "being nice"; "not making a fuss"; "smiling a lot"; "speaking in a sympathetic voice even if you go away and complain about the person afterwards"; "not letting on that you think the other person is being unfair"; and "always putting the other person first even when you know they are a user" ' (Street 1995: 30). Street argued that for nurses in units where the tyranny of niceness operated there was a blurring between being nice and being caring such that to be genuinely caring meant always being nice and fitting in with the unit/service expectations. What she found in her research was that although everyone on the study unit described the environment and people within it as nice, very few nurses felt as if they were good enough to be a part of the team and did not see themselves as fitting in. Importantly, she described how the expectation of always being nice prevented constructive critique and debate with others.

Being nice or good is a central value in palliative care. This is in part linked to the strong historical links between palliative care and Christianity but also to the highly moral nature of palliative care philosophy. Thus one of the central, but perhaps unwritten, values of palliative care is being nice. Indeed people who work in palliative care often make a distinction between the good of their world and the bad of mainstream health care. For example, in McNamara *et al.*'s study (1994) one of the nurses said 'sometimes we live in a false world, everybody in hospice is so "nice". When you get outside of it, you find it's all a bit of a shock' (pp. 229–30). Added to this is the voice of believing palliative care to be work that is somehow unable to be understood by others or would be a burden to them. As another nurse from McNamara *et al.*'s study said, 'You know it's not arrogance that we don't confide in our families. What we do is special and only we can understand really what it's like. We don't want to burden them with something they don't need to know' (pp. 232–3).

Thus the pre-existing drive towards being nice in palliative care has the potential to exacerbate the tyranny of niceness in ways that cover over or even silence critical thought about organizational and practice issues. The increasing gap between what we value and what we do as a result of health care reforms, such as mainstreaming and increased economic pressures, increases the potential dissonance between our capacity to deliver care according to our core values and the reality of our practice world, a dissonance that is difficult to fight against while the tyranny of niceness is operant.

The value of being nice or good is lived out in palliative care through the central value of the good death and understanding the challenges to our ability to deliver the good death is critical to understanding stress in palliative care nursing.

## The good death

The good death is an ideal commonly associated with the efforts of palliative care practitioners to achieve positive outcomes in the lives of people who are dying and has received significant commentary in palliative care literature (e.g. McNamara *et al.* 1994; Payne *et al.* 1996). Elements of a good death vary but include open awareness of impending death, acceptance or adjustment to this, engaging in preparation for death, talking with others about death and making final farewells. Good death in this palliative care sense is in contrast to the use of the term within the euthanasia debate where the emphasis is on a quick, painless exit.

McNamara *et al.* (1995) present an excellent account of the relationship between stress in palliative care nursing and ideas about the good death. In the context of their study a good death referred to one where there was 'an awareness, acceptance and a preparation for death' undertaken by the person who was dying, characteristics I would argue that are centrally linked to Folkman's (1997) ideas about meaning-focused coping. Many of the nurses in their study recalled stories of deaths that reinforced their belief that 'there must be a better way to die' and precipitated a decision to become a palliative care nurse. Thus, an inherent part of becoming a palliative care nurse appears to be a commitment to achieving a good death for patients, often contrasted against previously encountered bad deaths. However, notions of a good death are largely ideological and it is common for patients to die deaths that may be in keeping with how they have lived their lives but might not fit with images of a good death. Patients may also not engage with attempts to portray their situation in a more positive light, becoming depressed and demoralized rather than actively embracing the growth palliative care portrays as possible at the end of life.

McNamara *et al.* (1995) articulated five threats to a good death that act as sources of stress for palliative care nurses. The five threats related to societal values and reactions, organization of the work environment, exchanges between nurses and the patients and families, exchanges between nurses and their families, friends and colleagues and personally facing death. Drawing on these threats I suggest that understanding the oppositions at the heart of these threats helps us to understand stress in palliative nursing as it relates to the good death. Centring on a simplistic binary split between good and bad these oppositions are:

- Dissonance between social reactions to death and the values of palliative care.

- Dissonance between the organization of the work environment and the values of care delivery.

While clearly binary oppositions overly simplify reality, they can be a helpful way of understanding the tensions that exist in practice.

### Dissonance between social reactions to death and the values of palliative care

The first and fourth threats articulated by McNamara *et al.* (1995) concern a dissonance between the values of palliative care and the values of society and social reactions to what palliative care nurses do, both in terms of the nurses' relationship to society as a whole and to individuals within their family and friendship group. The binary opposition is that society generally sees death as a negative experience, while palliative care nurses have adopted a value system that reappraises the meaning of death in a more positive light, a natural part of life and not inherently negative. This then leads to a perception of isolation within the field of palliative care and a sense of not being understood. McNamara *et al.* (1995) report that some nurses felt unable to speak openly about their work in situations outside of palliative care because people did not want to be confronted by death in social situations. They suggest that nurses 'perceive stress, in this context, to be related to "the general society's" non-acceptance of death and, implicitly, to the ensuing disregard for their system of values' (p. 229). These feelings extended for some nurses into not feeling able to confide in family and friends, turning instead for support to fellow workers.

Essentially these threats see the 'good' palliative care workers happily embracing death while bad society seeks to push it from view. Additionally, individuals within society are seen as lacking the capacity to understand or would be burdened by what palliative care nurses see and do. Indeed the sociologist Julia Lawton produces a powerful thesis arguing that society's inability to cope with the realities of dying is an important driver of the hospice movement. In her work Lawton (1998, 2000) argues that bodily disintegration resulting in incontinence and other forms of boundary loss are unacceptable to society, resulting in the sequestration of dying people within hospices. Palliative care nurses, particularly those who work in the hospice setting, can thus be understood as dealing with those aspects of death that society shuns. Obviously social attitudes to death and dying are not this simplistic. What is important though is that when palliative care nurses perceive themselves as isolated from society, family and friends through differences in values about dying and death, through their different life experience or through fears about not being understood, they become isolated from the very social environments that provide them with necessary time out from this potentially draining work.

Spending more and more time in the company of other palliative care nurses because of a shared value system may be counterproductive in other ways. McNamara *et al.* (1995) reveal that some nurses identify a 'level of dishonesty' or a 'conspiracy of silence' around admitting to feeling personal pain or struggles with their work. The meaning-focused coping inherent in palliative care approaches to death portray a positive reappraisal of a negative situation that is not always easy to sustain and workers are likely to feel pain as bonds with patients and families are broken through death or when they cannot achieve a 'good' death for the patient. Taking the moral high ground in relation to palliative care values may also mean a reluctance to admit that this work involves personal struggle. In my work with Mary (see Case study 29.1) she felt unable to talk about her struggles in caring for Lucy within the nursing team. While discussion sessions were held within this team to allow nurses to talk about their work, there was a perception that the team leader was holding back. This senior nurse was a nun and appeared to Mary to be trapped in a missionary approach to her work that meant her own needs were always secondary. In the team this resulted in role expectations that personal needs were always subsumed to the needs of the patient. Thus on the surface and in the rhetoric of the group this team understood itself as supportive, in reality much of each nurse's personal struggle was silenced.

---

**Case study 29.1**

Mary was an experienced home-based palliative care nurse who, at the time of her participation in a research project on nurse–patient friendship, had just re-entered nursing after an experience of professional burnout. During our first interview she recounted the story of her work with Lucy, a young woman with terminal cancer that had led to significant weight gain and quadriplegia. Lucy had been a model and found these alterations to her body very distressing. Her husband, David, also found the changes distressing and this led to less and less contact between them and little involvement in Lucy's physical care. Mary described how in caring for Lucy her efforts focused on maintaining feelings of worth and personhood in the face of such degrading tasks as enemas and faecal disimpaction. In addition, Mary recognized Lucy's loss of physical contact with David and tried to meet some of these needs through massage and touch. She found herself spending more and more time delivering care to Lucy, making her late for other clients and often providing less than her usual care to them in order to fill the enormous care needs of Lucy, even past the time when it would perhaps have been appropriate for Lucy to be in the hospice. When Mary raised her concerns over Lucy within the nursing team the response was usually one of giving her a break from the care, which served to silence Mary's concerns as she did not wish to be replaced or to stop caring for Lucy.

Mary's reflections on her situation were in contrast to another nurse from this team who also participated in the study. Jane's reflections showed a concerned team willing to assist Mary, however the nurse lacked the skills to know how to openly critique what was happening. The first interview for this study occurred many months after Lucy's death but resulted in a significant delayed grief response for Mary requiring several sessions of grief counselling to work through the many issues that had resulted in Mary's burnout experience. Mary's resolution of her experience was also aided by her continued participation in the research project, which provided extended opportunities for her to reflect on this and other experiences with patients who were dying. At the completion of the study Mary said that prior to this she probably had a built-in desire to rescue patients from their experiences (to provide a good death) and that she no longer felt this level of responsibility and was able to work to make a difference in their lives but understood that she could not make this happen always. (Anonymous case study taken from Aranda 1998b)

Nurses in a study of nurse–patient friendships in cancer and palliative care were asked to consider this issue of team openness to personal struggle and the provision of support when it was raised by Mary (Aranda 1998b). At the group meeting where this was first discussed, Tessa suggested that her team was safe and allowed everyone to discuss personal feelings. However, at the following meeting Tessa expressed a modified view. Her discussions with one of her nursing colleagues over the ensuing weeks revealed that one nurse felt censored in the team and this had led to her hiding her feelings and behaviours with patients from the group. Tessa identified that safety and support were conditional within their nursing team with conditions set around behaving in certain ways and premised on length of time in the team. While palliative care teams may indeed be supportive in general and aim for a degree of openness and support not usual in other team settings, achievement of this is hard work. The tyranny of niceness prevented the nurse in Tessa's workplace from disclosing her feelings because admitting them and thus criticizing the team for its lack of support for her would not be nice behaviour and would place her outside of the group. When we assume our teams to be supportive and fail to acknowledge the level of work required to create a supportive environment the end result can be a significant dissonance between what we say, do and feel, generating potential for individual and team stress.

### *Dissonance between the organization of the work environment and the values of care delivery*

Vachon (1987) argues that patients are not the major source of stress in palliative care and that the real problems are the work environment and the nurse's occupational role. The desire to assist the patient to achieve a good death is often thwarted by the work environment and role factors. Indeed, Tishelman *et al.* (2004) suggest that the most prominent source of tension in their study was between the care nurses wanted to provide and that which was actually possible. Work environment factors include the involvement in care of individuals who appear not to share the values of palliative care, such as medical specialists who continue to treat the cancer beyond what the nurse considers reasonable. Indeed attempts to avoid this source of stress are present in arguments that cancer treatments have no place in hospice settings, an argument that seeks to separate palliative care from mainstream health care, perhaps because of conflicting values (Biswas 1993).

Such arguments are based on a simplistic division between, for example, the 'bad' oncologist using yet more chemotherapy and the 'good' palliative care nurse wanting to protect the patient from harm. The patient is passive in the argument, ignoring both the patient's role in the decision and the complexity of balancing the side effects of cancer treatments against the benefits that might be gained in terms of pain and symptom relief. All too often there is no attempt to openly discuss the apparent conflict between the various practitioners involved, a discussion that could lead to mutual understanding and hopefully improved sharing of patient care. The absence of conflict resolution in such situations leaves the palliative care nurse to deliver care in ways that are not consistent with their value system as the patient's acceptance of ongoing treatment is understood as indicating a lack of acceptance of death. While clearly patients can still be accepting of the inevitability of death while continuing to seek treatments that will either lengthen life or reduce symptoms, such choices are not always well accepted in palliative care.

Similarly, the work environment in palliative care is becoming increasingly mainstreamed, adding new pressures of workload that threaten the provision of time – a highly valued aspect of the palliative approach to care and a key factor in ensuring a good death. Palliative care is asked to respond to criticisms about being a form of deluxe dying for the few (Johnston and Abraham 1995) and to demands to extend their work beyond a focus on cancer (Clark and Seymour 1999). This means either spreading the effort further with few additional resources or greater attention to the allocation of resources to those most in need, however this is defined. Ultimately either outcome can add increasing pressure to the daily work of palliative care nurses. In the Australian environment in the 1980s a community palliative care nurse undertook a direct care role providing holistic care to about four patients a day, leaving sufficient time for prolonged visits with patients who needed this. Today this same nurse is more likely to be sharing care with a generalist community nurse, have a role that is more case management than direct care and will visit six to eight patients in one day. The case management role also reduces the level of direct physical care that is provided and on observation this significantly reduces delivery of many of the comfort elements of palliative care such as extended touch through massage (Brown 2007). Reductions in the real government funding for palliative care, for example down to 32 per cent in 2006 in the United Kingdom (www.helpthehospices.org.uk), severely limit the resources available locally, force role changes and add to the stress for palliative care nurses. Chapter 35 by Jennifer Hunt considers this issue in relation to resource-poor countries.

Similarly, in Australia acute palliative care units focusing more on acute symptom management than care of the dying are gradually replacing in-patient hospices. Length of stay is reducing, patients may be receiving treatments such as intravenous antibiotics and patients who are not immediately dying may be transferred to nursing homes or go home when this might not be considered ideal. This reality threatens ideas about a good death by reducing the time spent with the patient, fracturing holistic care and reducing the palliative nursing role to monitoring of outcomes of acute treatments such as intensive pain management. The result is greater dissonance between the shared values of palliative care and the daily reality of nursing work, a dissonance that threatens the meaning of our work and thus is likely to result in greater stress.

A further area of dissonance between the work environment and the values of palliative care is an increasing social acceptance of euthanasia as an end-of-life option. The modern hospice movement is significantly influenced by Christian values and the field's public position is thus overtly anti-euthanasia. Nurses want to see patients achieve a good death, yet the palliative definition of a good death rules out both euthanasia and physician-assisted suicide. Opting for a quick exit through euthanasia is seen to portray a life without meaning, while a significant part of palliative care work is about helping patients to obtain meaning in the face of death. Work stress can result when caring for patients with differing values about end-of-life decisions, when caring for patients who refuse to engage in a search for meaning in their death or when the nurse is not personally opposed to euthanasia.

Our earlier work around palliative care nurses' attitudes to euthanasia showed that not all were opposed to hastening death (Aranda and O'Connor 1995), demonstrating a potential dissonance between the nurse and the value system operant in the organization. In addition, at least three nurses in this study believed that they had been involved in euthanasia in the workplace. Leaving aside the more complex legal concerns this raises, from a stress perspective there are palliative care nurses who believe they have contributed to a patient's death but work in situations where these issues are rarely discussed in open and frank ways.

The philosophy of palliative care and its anti-euthanasia position makes it very difficult for palliative nurses to hold views even moderately supportive of attempts to hasten death, let alone to discuss these in the workplace. However, it is possible for people with a desire for assisted death to be cared for within a palliative care environment (Aranda *et al.* 1999) by encouraging an open dialogue with patients that is respectful of their wishes and desires but reinforces the legal constraints and value position of the palliative care system.

# The good nurse

The nurse's role in a good death is one of involvement, provision of effective symptom control to allow the person to live as fully as possible until death, death that is pain free and provision of an environment that allows death that is peaceful and dignified (McNamara *et al.* 1995: 234). A significant part of achieving this involves assisting patients to gain meaning in their lives at this time. Good palliative care nurses are skilled in symptom management because a patient with few symptoms can live their remaining life more fully. Good palliative care nurses are also willing to help patients talk about their deaths, helping them to resolve issues in their lives and thus find meaning in their deaths. Good palliative care nurses are also those who assist the patient to find meaning through their relationships with others, facilitating family discussions, helping patients create legacies such as letters for those they will leave behind, and bringing in others who can assist with issues like spiritual conflict and psychological distress.

Living up to this image is not always easy and a significant component of stress in palliative care nursing can be linked to not achieving a good death, *vis-à-vis*, not being a good palliative care nurse.

# Reducing stress in palliative care

Strategies for dealing with stress in palliative care nursing are frequently discussed (e.g. Pearce 1998; Barnes 2001; Payne 2001). Significantly, coping efforts in palliative care are understood in the literature as a shared responsibility between the individual and the work setting. Nurses describe palliative care environments as more supportive than was their experience in other settings (Newton and Waters 2001), although there is little comparative research to support this.

The literature on reducing workplace stress in nursing and palliative care tends towards helpful lists of strategies that make sense intuitively (Rokach 2005) but have not been empirically tested. Suggested strategies include 'developing realistic perspectives' about the work (Byrne and McMurray 1997) and seeing the bigger picture (Vachon 1998). A recent review of approaches to enhancing psychosocial well-being in oncology nurses as a means of avoiding burnout and enhancing retention suggested the need to focus on supportive relationships in the workplace, the normalization of grief experiences among nurses and the design of strategies to empower nurses (Medland *et al.* 2004). Again few of the recommended strategies are backed up with rigorous research. Many of these approaches appear time and resource intensive (van Staa *et al.* 2000) and while they help to create a general sense of well-being, such as in the study by Mackereth *et al.* (2005), there is no measurement of intended outcomes such as burnout, retention rates or job satisfaction.

Some significant attempts to investigate structured approaches to reducing stress in nurses and others who work in palliative care are beginning to appear in the literature. For example, von Klitzing (1999) studied the development of reflective learning in a psychodynamic group of general nurses although the reflections predominantly focused on the care of people who were terminally ill. Practice reflection is frequently cited as an important means of coping with the demands of palliative care work (Rokach 2005) but with little evidence to suggest that reflection alone mediates stress. However, von Klitzing found that nurses could develop reflective capacity in this supported process, with these reflections becoming increasingly high level when about the patient. Of concern was that the level of reflection about the nurse herself decreased over time, suggesting perhaps that this level of self-work may need specific emphasis over time. A critical next step is to determine if the development of reflective capacity improves the ability of nurses to cope with workplace stress.

A popular self-awareness or reflective strategy employed by disciplines such as social work and psychology is clinical supervision. Hopkins (2004) has advocated clinical supervision from a management perspective. Use of clinical supervision in nursing was, until recently, largely confined to the psychiatric setting. One of the possible reasons for this is that nursing was largely understood as a collective profession while clinical supervision focuses on the issues arising from dyadic relationships between an individual practitioner and an individual patient. An interesting study from Sweden (Palsson *et al.* 1994) explored the use of group clinical supervision in cancer care in terms of its effect in handling difficult situations. While caution must be exercised in generalizing this qualitative study, the findings show enhanced capacity to gain relief from distressing situations through the clinical supervision process. In addition, the nurses felt their professional roles and self-perceptions confirmed through the group with signs of increased knowledge, greater sense of well-being and enhanced self-confidence. The Palsson *et al.* (1994) study was theoretically based on Antonovsky's sense of coherence theory and offers one of the few well-theorized approaches to interventions for stress reduction in nursing. A further area receiving some attention in the research literature is mindfulness or a therapeutic approach that focuses on purpose and experience. A small pilot study of a mindfulness intervention with nurses and nurses' aides suggests that enhanced attention to personal and interpersonal reflection might improve symptoms of burnout, enhance relaxation and improve life satisfaction (Mackenzie *et al.* 2005), although further testing is required.

A further intervention strategy proposed in recent literature is the application of Frankl's logotherapy as a meaning-centred therapy to enhance job satisfaction and reduce burnout in palliative care (Fillon *et al.* 2006). While still in progress, this randomized controlled trial aims to assist palliative care nurses to 'find meaning in their work and better cope with emotional stress and suffering' (p. 342). The findings of this study will be of interest to us all as it promises to be a rare example of a rigorous research design and strong theoretical base applied in the area of work-related stress in palliative care.

# Conclusion

The over-riding premise of this chapter is that stress occurs at points of dissonance between the values and beliefs of the individual and their capacity to deliver care according to these values (see Table 29.2). The absence of a strong evidence base to preventing and managing the impact of this dissonance on work stress means that palliative care services need to foster a flexible and varied approach to the provision of support in the workplace, and to encourage nurses to identify their personal approach to stress as an overt part of professional development.

However, it is clear from the literature that in palliative care a sense of meaning in the work, of making a contribution and of helping the person to die a good death, when not idealized, are fundamental to professional well-being. The capacity to maintain a balance between making a difference and

**Table 29.2** Strategies for managing stress

*Within the palliative care unit*
- Teamwork and team cohesiveness
- Selecting staff to ensure environment-person fit
- Professional development/education programme
- Clinical supervision made available

*By the individual*
- Seek counselling
- Attend a support group
- Attend regular clinical supervision
- Change roles or take time out from role
- Undertake more education
- Establish outside interests
- Balance work and home life
- Exercise
- Religious beliefs
- Understand personal boundaries
- Having a sense of mastery
- Finding meaning in work
- Distancing
- Caring for the self

accepting the limitations of what can be achieved requires a significant level of self and team awareness. There is some evidence that this awareness can be promoted through processes such as clinical supervision and structured reflection. However, this reflection requires moving beyond the tyranny of niceness to an open and penetrating critique of what we do, how we do it and the effects of our work on both our patients and ourselves.

There are also important beginnings to intervention research consistent with the theoretical premise that meaning is important in the working lives of palliative care nurses. It is critical that palliative care research moves beyond a description of stress in the working lives of nurses and other health professionals to develop theoretically informed and rigorously tested interventions to ensure the retention of the workforce and the health of us all.

# References

Aranda, S. (1998a) Palliative care principles: masking the complexity of practice. In: J. Parker and S. Aranda (eds) *Palliative Care: Explorations and Challenges*. Rosebery: MacLennan and Petty Pty Ltd, pp. 21–31.

Aranda, S. (1998b) *A Critical Praxis Study of Nurse-Patient Friendship*, Unpublished doctoral thesis. Melbourne: La Trobe University.

Aranda, S. (2001) Guest Editorial: The Tyrannies of Palliative Care, *International Journal of Palliative Nursing*, 7(12): 572–3.

Aranda, S. and O'Connor, M. (1995) Euthanasia, nursing and care of the dying: Rethinking Kuhse and Singer, *Australian Nursing Journal*, 3(2): 18–21.

Aranda, S., Bence, G. and O'Connor, M. (1999) Euthanasia: A perspective from Australia, *International Journal of Palliative Nursing*, 5(6): 298–304.

Aranda, S. and Brown, R. (2006) Nurses must be clever to care. Chapter 8 in: S. Nelson and S. Gordon. *The complexities of care: Nursing reconsidered*. New York: ILR Press, An Imprint of Cornell University Press.

Barnes, K. (2001) Staff stress in the children's hospice: causes, effects and coping strategies, *International Journal of Palliative Nursing*, 7(5): 248–54.

Benner, P. and Wrubel, J. (1989) *The Primacy of Caring*. Menlo Park: Addison-Wesley Publishing Company.

Biswas, B. (1993) The Medicalization of Dying. A Nurse's View. In: D. Clark (ed.) *The Future for Palliative Care: Issues of Policy and Practice*. Buckingham: Open University Press.

Bradshaw, A. (1996) The Spiritual Dimension of Hospice: The Secularisation of an Ideal, *Social Science and Medicine*, 43: 409–20.

Brown, R. (2007) *Exploring 'bodywork': An ethnographic study of palliative care nursing*, unpublished Master of Nursing (research) thesis. Melbourne: Melbourne University.

Byrne, D. and McMurray, A. (1997) Caring for the dying: nurses' experiences in hospice care, *Australian Journal of Advanced Nursing*, 15(1): 4–11.

Clark, D. and Seymour, J. (1999) *Reflections on Palliative Care*. Buckingham: Philadelphia.

Feldstein, M.A. and Gemma, P.B. (1995) Oncology nurses and chronic compounded grief, *Cancer Nursing*, 18(3): 228–36.

Fillon, L., Dupuis, R., Tremblay, I., De Grace, G. and Breitbart, W. (2006) Enhancing meaning in palliative care practice: A meaning-centered intervention to promote job satisfaction, *Palliative and Supportive Care*, 4: 333–44.

Folkman, S. (1997) Positive Psychological States and Coping with Severe Illness. *Social Science and Medicine*, 45(8): 1207–21.

Hopkins, M. (2004) Leading and managing nurses in a changing environment. In: S. Payne, J. Seymour and C. Ingleton (eds) *Palliative Care Nursing*. Maidenhead: Open University Press.

Johnston, G. and Abraham, C. (1995) 'The WHO objectives for palliative care: to what extent are we achieving them?' *Palliative Medicine*, 9: 123–37.

Lawton, J. (1998) Contemporary hospice care: the sequestration of the unbounded body and 'dirty dying'. *Sociology of Health and Illness*, 20(2): 121–43.

Lawton, J. (2000) *The Dying Process: Patients' experiences of palliative care*. London: Routledge.

Lazarus, R.S. and Folkman, S. (1984) *Stress, Appraisal and Coping*. New York: Springer.

Mackenzie, C.S., Poulin, P.A. and Seidman-Carlson, R. (2005) A brief mindfulness-based stress reduction intervention for nurses and nurses aides. *Applied Nursing Research*, 19(2): 105–9.

Mackereth, P.A., White, K., Cawthorn, A. and Lynch, B. (2005) Improving stressful working lives: complementary therapies, counseling and clinical supervision for staff. *European Journal of Oncology Nursing*, 9: 147–54.

McNamara, B., Waddell, C. and Colvin, M. (1994) The institutionalization of the good death. *Social Science and Medicine*, 39(11): 1501–8.

McNamara, B., Waddell, C. and Colvin, M. (1995) Threats to the good death: the cultural context of stress and coping among hospice nurses. *Sociology of Health and Illness*, 17(2): 222–44.

Medland, J., Howard-Ruben, J. and Whitaker, E. (2004) Fostering psychosocial wellness in oncology nurses: addressing burnout and social support in the workplace. *Oncology Nursing Forum*, 31(1): 47–54.

Newton, J. and Waters, V. (2001) Community palliative care clinical nurse specialists' descriptions of stress in their work. *International Journal of Palliative Nursing*, 7(11): 531–40.

Palsson, M.E., Hallberg, I.R. and Norberg, A. (1994) Systematic clinical supervision and its effects for nurses handling demanding care situations. *Cancer Nursing*, 17(5): 385–94.

Payne, N. (2001) Occupational stressors and coping as determinants of burnout in female hospice nurses. *Journal of Advanced Nursing*, 33(3): 396–405.

Payne, S., Langley-Evans, A. and Hillier, R. (1996) Perceptions of a 'good' death: a comparative study of the views of hospice staff and patients. *Palliative Medicine*, 10(4): 307–12.

Pearce, S. (1998) The experience of stress for cancer nurses: a Heideggerian phenomenological approach. *European Journal of Oncology Nursing*, 2(4): 235–7.

Rokach, A. (2005) Caring for those who care for the dying: Coping with the demands on palliative care workers. *Palliative and Supportive Care*, 3: 325–32.

Saunders, C. and Baines, M. (1983) *Living with Dying: The Management of Terminal Disease*. Oxford: Oxford University Press.

Saunders, J.M. and Valente, S.M. (1994) Nurses' grief. *Cancer Nursing*, 17(4): 318–25.

Street, A. (1995) *Nursing Replay: Researching Nursing Culture Together*. Melbourne: Churchill Livingstone.

Sullivan, G.C. (1993) Towards clarification of convergent concepts: sense of coherence, will to meaning, locus of control, learned helplessness and hardiness. *Journal of Advanced Nursing*, 18: 1772–8.

Tishelman, C., Berhardson, B-M., Blomberg, K., Borjeson, S., Franklin, L-L., Johansson, E., Levealahti, H., Sahlberg-Blom, E. and Ternestedt, B-M. (2004) Complexity in caring for patients with advanced cancer. *Journal of Advanced Nursing*, 45: 420–9.

Vachon, M. (1987) *Occupational Stress in the Care of the Critically Ill, the Dying, and the Bereaved.* New York: Hemisphere Publishing Corporation.

Vachon, M. (1995) Reflections on the History of Occupational Stress in Hospice/Palliative Care. *The Hospice Journal*, 14(3/4): 229–46.

Vachon, M. (1998) Caring for the Caregiver in Oncology and Palliative Care. *Seminars in Oncology Nursing*, 14(2): 152–7.

Vachon, M. (1999) Staff stress in hospice/palliative care: a review. *Palliative Medicine*, 9: 91–122.

van Staa, A.L., Visser, A. and van der Zouwe, N. (2000) Caring for caregivers: experiences and evaluation of interventions for a palliative care team. *Patient Education and Counseling*, 41: 93–105.

von Klitzing, W. (1999) Evaluation of reflective learning in a psychodynamic group of nurses caring for terminally ill patients. *Journal of Advanced Nursing*, 30(5): 1213–21.

Welsh, D.J. (1999) Care for the Caregiver: Strategies for Avoiding 'Compassion Fatigue'. *Clinical Journal of Oncology Nursing*, 3(4): 183–4.

# 30

# Education and scholarship in palliative care

## A European nursing perspective

*Philip Larkin*

---

**Key points**

- Education and scholarship are not mutually exclusive entities but based on an inter-relationship with practice.
- Technical-rational knowledge should not overshadow the artistry of palliative nursing.
- Higher academic learning is key to the articulation of palliative care.
- Reciprocity is a vital element of the future direction for palliative education.

---

# Introduction

The purpose of this chapter is to consider current perspectives on palliative nursing education and to set this within a wider international context of nursing scholarship. Themes arising from this chapter are generated from a critical review of current European developments in palliative care and their impact on professional nursing practice. Applying a European context offers an overview of the wide variability in educational opportunity and career advancement for nurses working in palliative care. However, there are complexities in defining the entity of Europe. The economic partnership model of a European Union (EU) offers only a limited description, given the dynamics of EU expansion (Filbet and Larkin 2007). At the time of writing, the EU comprises 27 member states, with three candidate countries waiting for ratification (Croatia, Former Yugoslav Republic of Macedonia and Turkey). A particularly valuable tool for interpreting palliative care education challenges across Europe is provided by Centeno *et al.* (2007) in their European Association for Palliative Care (EAPC) Atlas of Palliative Care in Europe. In mapping the current status of palliative care service provision across 42 countries based on the World Health Organization regional classification of Europe, the Atlas demonstrates how strong political infrastructure and economic stability are key to the success of both service developments and education initiatives. The Atlas presents wide variation in terms of access, funding, workforce capacity and specialist accreditation. What is clearly noticeable is that for every country in the project, the promotion of education and scholarship pose key challenges for the development of palliative care services. Many lack academic leadership, higher education opportunities beyond basic level programmes and limited resources to foster academic and workplace learning. These challenges raise the following questions for palliative care educators:

- What does the emphasis on palliative care as a 'speciality' mean for education?
- How do we enable practitioners to seek higher academic learning (where such developments are clearly aspirational)?
- How is learning translated into practice?
- Has palliative nursing knowledge been lost?

It is also important to consider these questions in relation to important issues identified in the first edition of this book for the advancement of palliative care education:

- The philosophy of palliative care must be clearly evident in specialist palliative care education.
- Generic curricula are an important way to set standards and benchmarks for best practice.
- Education is only effective through partnership.
- Education needs to be innovative and collaborative.

(Sneddon 2004)

Some of these questions have already been addressed in the international literature and provide a context for discussion. In this chapter, I will consider each of the above issues in light of the key questions posed and make specific reference at the end of each section to the impact of these challenges for palliative care nursing education. To begin, I ask what exactly is meant by the terms education and scholarship and if there is a difference between them?

# Education and scholarship, is there a difference?

### *Considering education*

It is suggested that palliative education should 'mirror' palliative care through integration rather than imposition of knowledge (Sheldon and Smith 1996). James and Macleod (1993) offered one of the first academic appraisals of palliative care education and suggested a number of reasons why such education was problematic. These included the problems of providing learning to meet the needs of a disparate multidisciplinary group, limited understanding of symptom management and conceptual problems in describing palliative care. Fifteen years later, it may be fair to suggest that current descriptions of palliative care remain conceptually frail (Ilhardt 2001), and multidisciplinary learning still poses problems for educators in planning mutually beneficial programmes. Contemporary end-of-life education needs to strike a balance between the effective application of technical skills and the effective ability to respond incisively to a fellow human being (Sneddon 2004). For adult learners, education is not always about an outcome (such as certification) but rather a process of life-long learning which does not have a discrete end in sight but which requires an integration of theoretical knowledge with personal fulfilment and personal growth (Peters 1979). Education embraces a broader and more holistic definition to learning than the 'training' many nurses associate with their first experiences of gaining professional knowledge. However, there is an increasing emphasis on palliative education being a measurable commodity in order to determine if outcomes and objectives are reached to prepare people for practice (Smith 2003; Morrison *et al.* 2007). Although this is a valuable strategy for the evidence base of palliative care, the focus would appear to be on instilling the learner with a package of skills from which to draw on. Yet, the role of the educator is not only to impart theoretical knowledge, but to enable the learner to understand how they can access personal resources derived from life experiences when faced with clinically challenging scenarios. Dying, after all, is a global human experience and not just a clinical outcome. There is clear evidence from research into communication skills training that the failure to attend to personal attitudes on death and dying does not reduce blocking behaviours if patients choose to disclose (Booth *et al.* 1996; Heaven and Maguire 1996). Palliative education, therefore, must be based on a mutual and reciprocal relationship between the educator and learner, where the former guides the latter to seek knowledge for themselves. Such ideals underpin many of the learning strategies currently seen in palliative education practice, such as reflection, clinical supervision, evidence-based learning (EBL) and distance-learning initiatives (Adriaansen and Frederiks 2002; Heaven *et al.* 2006).

### Considering scholarship

Arising from the need to strengthen the evidence base for palliative care nursing, the ideal of scholarship has placed an onus on practitioners and educators to seek greater understanding of practice through higher education and research (Humphreys *et al.* 2000; Royal College of Nursing 2001). The essential elements of scholarship are well explored by Ingleton and Davies (2004), based around principles of critical appraisal and interpretation, judgement, synthesis of ideas and the ability to communicate those ideas in a logical and coherent fashion (Kitson 1999). There is a need to determine how scholarship is shaped in relation to a practice-based profession such as nursing and, in as much as education is at risk of focusing solely on measurable outputs, scholarship must overcome the inherent risks of being measured in terms of publications and impact factors (Burgener 2001; Ramcharan *et al.* 2001). Ingleton and Davies (2004) argue that the success of palliative nursing scholarship is dependent on a creative practice setting supported by expert scholars acting in a mentorship or role model capacity. Palliative nursing scholarship cannot develop within a vacuum and dialogue with scholars from other disciplines who represent the broader academic influences on palliative care (for example, political science, sociology, anthropology, etc.) is essential to further refine the knowledge base of palliative nursing. In terms of difference, there is always potential for confusion when boundaries become increasingly blurred. Education which views clinical competency as its summative outcome may result in skilled technicians, rather than therapeutic practitioners who embrace a more fluid definition of caring at end of life. Scholarship which judges achievement by theoretical knowledge fails to appreciate that palliative care knowledge (beyond its individual disciplines) is really about responding to the immediate needs of people whose lives are ending and finding ways to make that end less onerous for them. To put this in context, both a philosophy student and a palliative care student may study the nature of suffering in the classroom. For the philosophy student, studying the nature of suffering will enhance their knowledge of the living world. For the palliative care student, to understand the nature of suffering is not simply a theoretical exercise but a way to engage responsively with real people living the reality of their suffering in their own world.

## What does the emphasis on palliative care as a 'speciality' mean for education?

In reality, the idea of palliative care as a speciality in clinical practice applies to only a small number of European countries (notably the UK, Ireland and Norway). As Centeno *et al.* (2007) show, most European countries do not perceive palliative care as a speciality in its own right, but rather a sub-speciality of another discipline (such as neurology or internal medicine). For historical reasons of social exclusion, palliative care as a descriptor of enhanced life quality is favoured over the term hospice (Ventafridda 1998). Palliative care has embraced a new language of clinical intervention and reversibility of symptoms which needs careful consideration in relation to people at end of life (Praill 2000; Appleton and Corboy 2005; Seymour 2005; Foggo 2006).

These perspectives pose certain challenges for the development of curricula in terms of what should be taught, to whom and when. The shift in the World Health Organization (2002) definition of palliative care from *speciality* to *approach* evidently suggests that practitioners need to develop transferable principles of care to meet the diverse needs of a wider clinical population beyond the original cancer remit of practice. Palliative care knowledge needs to be disseminated across a broad spectrum of client groups for whom the benefits of such knowledge is vital; chronic ill health, the elderly and critical care. Yet, confusion exists regarding the current place of palliative care in the illness trajectory, blurred by competing and essentially different goals and philosophical positions regarding end-of-life care (Van Kleffens *et al.* 2004). An implied adherence to a biomedical model of linear progression towards death seeks to create false boundaries between the facets of living and dying (curative, palliative and terminal care, for example) and at the same time, frames the aims and objectives of palliative care practice within a more integrated structure of 'supportive care'. This provides a complex language to interpret for palliative care education.

Across Europe, shifting language complicates matters even further, given that there are 230 indigenous languages. However, English remains the '*lingua franca*' of most educational resources, a problem for nurses who may not have had the same opportunity to learn the language in comparison to their medical colleagues. To emphasize this problem for educators, the term 'palliative care' in English has no lexical equivalent in many European languages. Usually, a direct translation is used (*cuidados paliativos* in Spanish, or *cure palliative* in Italian, for example) but its meaning in terms of practice may differ greatly from its English interpretation (Larkin *et al.* 2007). The description of palliative care in German as *palliativmedizin* (palliative care in its multidisciplinary context beyond medicine) is distinguished from *palliativepflege* (emphasis towards nursing care). However, Austrian German may use the English language term (Becker *et al.* 2007). I use these examples merely to emphasize the multifaceted nature of defining palliative care in terms of speciality (Filbet and Larkin 2007). How does this impact on education in Europe?

Arising from the recommendations of an education network chaired by Professor Derek Doyle in 1992, the European Association for Palliative Care endeavour to foster education and scholarship across Europe in order to:

> promote the implementation of existing knowledge; train those who at any level are involved in the care of patients and families affected by incurable and advanced disease, and promote research.
>
> (EAPC 2005)

In 1997, there was a call for national palliative care associations to establish minimal palliative care education recommendations and appropriate training skills for palliative care educators (De Vlieger *et al.* 2004). Although there remains limited international agreement to date on minimum standards for curricula, the EAPC has produced a set of recommendations for palliative nursing education and more recently, for undergraduate medicine (De Vlieger *et al.* 2004). The nursing recommendations reported here have been utilized in a number of European nursing curricula and cited in clinical competency and curriculum development literature (Scottish Partnership for Palliative Care and the NHS Executive for Scotland 2007).

**Table 30.1**   Levels of palliative education (adapted from De Vlieger *et al.* 2004, p. 9)

| Level A | | Level B | Level C |
| --- | --- | --- | --- |
| *Basic (undergraduate)* | *Basic (postgraduate)* | *Advanced (postgraduate)* | *Specialist (postgraduate)* |
| Future health care professionals during their initial training. | Qualified health care professionals working in a general health care setting, who may be confronted with situations requiring a palliative care approach. | Qualified health care professionals who either work in specialist palliative care, or in a general setting where they fulfil the role of resource person.<br><br>Qualified health care professionals who are frequently confronted by palliative care situations (e.g. oncology, community care, paediatrics and elderly care). | Qualified health care professionals who are responsible for palliative care units, or who offer a consultancy service and/or who actively contribute to palliative education and research. |

In proposing a three-tiered structure of cumulative learning for education (Table 30.1), programme development should be relative to the stage of service development. Further, it should not assume that everyone starts from the same place in academic terms, nor that speciality is the '*sine qua non*'.

This tri-partite approach suggests that some degree of palliative care learning (Level A) should be evident in all generic training programmes, appropriate to the multiplicity of other learning that general students need (Adriaansen and Achterberg 2002). For those deployed to act as a resource for palliative care clinical knowledge within their own non-specialist work (Level B), additional levels of education are required. Specialist levels of education (Level C) need university-based programmes in tandem with clinical exposure to the specialist clinical setting. Already, there are calls to include non-professional and public education initiatives as well. Even though the overall benefits to palliative education need to be rigorously evaluated, there is evidence that Level B training is seen as the primary target of education at this time. This is appropriate, given the magnitude of services outside of a specialist remit that would benefit from palliative care education. This also means that educators need to work effectively to avoid duplication in curricular content and to develop innovative ways to share learning. One example of this is cited in Box 30.1.

The EAPC is not alone in moving towards generic curricula in palliative

---

**Box 30.1** Innovative learning

The 'synchronicity' in practice between palliative care nurses and mental health nurses has been documented (Cutcliffe *et al.* 2001). As part of respective postgraduate courses in palliative care and mental health nursing, students from both disciplines come together to take a module on interdisciplinary collaboration. Through an evidence-based learning format (EBL), students use clinical cases, tutorials and self-directed learning to explore the dynamics of care for patients at end of life with mental health problems. Students gain skills in information retrieval, assessment of evidence, group dynamics and presentation skills. Practitioners in the field present a multidisciplinary case in a round-table discussion facilitated by the programme directors to enable students to debate team interactions and the rationale for respective professional decision-making.

---

care. Weissmann *et al.* (2007) report on developing palliative care curricula for resident physicians working in a variety of clinical specialities. What is evident here is that specialization should not be a 'holy grail' to be sought and educators need to influence the dynamic which places palliative care speciality as a linear process of achievement, rather than a hierarchical process of attainment.

## How do we enable practitioners to seek higher academic learning?

Given that specialist education needs to have a strong academic base, it is important to review how well academic learning prepares practitioners for practice. At a specialist level, Copp *et al.* (2007) demonstrated that didactic education was insufficient to prepare newly qualified health care professionals for oncology practice and that real 'learning' came from supportive professionals in the field. Yet, the assessment of clinical skills in practice seems to attract a low priority (Hale *et al.* 2006). For educators, this raises the issue of competency. The mobility of the workforce across Europe necessitates some criteria by which to judge if a practitioner from one jurisdiction has requisite skills and knowledge to practise in another. There is limited evidence about the transferability of skills, even though there is an 'open-door' policy which enables EU citizens to move freely and work in Member States (Cowan *et al.* 2007). France, for example, allows Spanish nurses and German doctors to practise in the state without further training. However, mismatch between professional roles, skills and knowledge can cause considerable problems. Some autonomous roles (such as clinical nurse specialist or advanced nurse practitioner) are not evident outside the UK and Ireland (with the possible exception of the *infirmière clinicienne* in France), although degrees of autonomous practice are variable. Many EU palliative care teams are more likely to have a clinical psychologist undertaking grief work than a social worker. There has been particular interest in the issues of competence in nursing (Norman *et al.* 2002; Redfern *et al.* 2002; Cowan *et al.* 2005). There are also notable examples of developing methods to assess competence in a multidisciplinary palliative care context and particularly in relation to the socio-spiritual dimension of care (AHPCC 2003; MCCC 2003; Gordon and Mitchell 2004; Gwyther *et al.* 2005; Morrison *et al.* 2007; Scottish Partnership for Palliative Care and the NHS Executive for Scotland 2007). The complexity in defining competency for palliative care (and indeed other disciplines) is noted: 'We believe that the struggle between breadth and depth, between consciousness and completeness is an intrinsic challenge in competency development' (Morrison *et al.* 2007: 328).

Tools and frameworks for the development of competency are helpful only if the assessor is able to draw a balance between reasonable expectation and a gold standard. Gwyther *et al.* (2005) identify that competency frameworks offer guidance to assist in assessing quality, not guarantees. Key to success is a strong liaison between the academic centre and service provider (De Vlieger *et al.* 2004; Hale *et al.* 2006). It is, however, an imperative that academic centres are clear about the benefits of what higher level education can offer the practitioner. There are suggestions that lengthy academic courses which focus on accredited learning are being promoted over shorter, clinically based programmes (Gould *et al.* 2004, 2007). This can only be challenged if service providers are provided with categorical proof of the benefits of higher learning. On their part, this means clear delineation of roles and functions of the specialist nurse (clinical nurse specialist, nurse practitioner, advanced nurse practitioner and latterly nurse consultant) to prevent competing agendas (Roberts-Davis and Read 2001). Educators need to provide courses that are sensitive to the life needs of adult learners and which promote measurable learning outcomes for practice. Sound theoretical preparation and the continued contribution of palliative nursing to a research agenda will further the clinical-academic links.

In terms of future developments, the doctoral preparation of palliative care nurses warrants further attention. There is clear evidence that nursing is beginning to seek the value of a doctorally prepared profession, not only its academics but also its practitioners (Kirkman *et al.* 2007). There are clearly pros and cons to the various methods of obtaining a doctorate, either through the traditional route of original research and preparation of a thesis, through to a doctorate which emphasizes a taught or professional element to its content. These latter options would appear to have found some increased interest in nursing and it would be important that potential candidates understand the differences (Ellis 2005; Yam 2005). However, the professional or taught doctorate has been criticized for lacking the independent development of theoretical work which marks a PhD and is therefore considered to be essentially lacking in merit. Ellis' (2005) mapping study into the range of development of professional doctorates revealed a dichotomy in so far as educators extolled the virtue of such programmes in bridging theory and practice, while at the same time holding reservations about their academic merit. Given the noted challenges of competency and the diverse nature of palliative care, the benefit of the professional taught doctorate may enhance rather than inhibit scholarship in the discipline. Yam (2005) provides a succinct description of the benefits of the professional doctorate in terms of collegiality, policy development and practice-orientated research, all of which are meaningful in contemporary palliative care. Further work is necessary to establish national and international academic programmes which enhance the academic credibility of palliative nursing.

# How is learning translated into practice?

Undoubtedly, there is a need for rigorous mechanisms to assess the impact of training on practice. Adriaansen and Achterberg's (2007) comprehensive review of the content and effects of palliative care courses for nurses determine that the most appropriate type of course, which can demonstrate transferability to practice, is one involving an array of didactic teaching methods across a range of topics, in tandem with practical experience. Meeting diverse multiprofessional needs in palliative care is a key principle of palliative care education. Although multidisciplinary learning is a corner-stone for palliative care practice (Koffman 2001), accreditation of learning for a diverse group of health care professionals answerable to a variety of legislative bodies for their practice is another matter. The production of a programme which frames palliative care practice (caring, empowering, advocating, healing) in a multidisciplinary context is both an art and a science. Palliative education should seek to extol commonality and welcome diversity in setting the boundaries of curricula. There are significant weaknesses in the transition from classroom to practice. Morita *et al.* (2007) describe a validation study in which nurses were provided with a five-hour workshop on better supportive care for patients to address meaningless in their lives, and then asked to complete self-assessment tools to judge the effect of that learning. The results demonstrated only modest improvements in confidence and skill to address the issue. Further, a telephone survey of students, physicians and educators in the United States revealed inequity in end-of-life educational provision, despite attempts to revise medical curricula and a subsequent inability to respond to patients' fears or deal with issues of death and dying following graduation (Sullivan *et al.* 2003). The emphasis on subjective scales and self-report questionnaires indicate a need for more robust measures to be developed to interpret if education truly meets perceived clinical need and to close the ever-present theory–practice gap. This said, it is equally argued that the success or failure of the transfer of knowledge to practice should not be assessed by objective methods alone, since the best judge of the impact is the individual themselves (Sheldon and Smith 1996; MacDougall *et al.* 2001). Continuing professional education (CPE) or continuing professional development (CPD) for nurses is particularly noted in the United Kingdom and is deemed a key factor in retention of staff (Gould *et al.* 2007). It is far less evident outside the United Kingdom since funding of services and education is variable. There are notable exemplars (the Cataluña project in Spain, for example), where a dyad of education and practice learning has transformed a health system into focusing on the needs of end-of-life patients across a whole autonomous region of Spain.

There are limitations in CPE, notably what appears to be an omission in meeting the personal needs of mature staff with life commitments (Shields 2002; Kevern and Webb 2005). It may appear to staff that the needs of the service outweigh the needs of the individual (Gould *et al.* 2007). As the body of evidence which can demonstrate that education can inform practice is currently weak, it is essential to promote the idea of work-based learning through interface between academics and educators (Birchenell 1999). Limited understanding of classroom learning and knowledge may lead team members to question what is being taught in multidisciplinary learning scenarios about shared working practices (Bliss *et al.* 2000; Seymour *et al.* 2002; Sasahara *et al.* 2003). Box 30.2 gives an example of one innovative practice designed to promote greater understanding within the multidisciplinary team and enhance CPE opportunities for them.

The exemplar given here highlights that the effectiveness of education is relative to the degree of 'buy-in' from the clinical area. The greater the degree of shared working, the more likelihood of being able to develop clinically focused and cost-effective courses that have the potential to inform practice.

# Has the art of palliative nursing been lost?

In this final section, I consider a somewhat philosophical question about the art and science of palliative nursing knowledge. The shift away from

---

**Box 30.2**   Care of the body at the end of life

As part of a postgraduate module exploring dimensions of palliative care nursing, students were required to visit a crematorium to witness the disposal of remains. The purpose of the visit was to enable students to understand the social context of death in the community. Cremation is relatively rare in the Republic of Ireland and one multidisciplinary team was unclear of the learning gained for the student (their colleague) by such a visit. To consolidate the experience, three staff members (the hospice doctor, social worker and senior nurse) were invited to accompany the student to the crematorium. The opportunity was useful for the team to acknowledge their limitations and gain new knowledge which would inform practice. For the student, the visit gave her the possibility to demonstrate the technical knowledge she had gained in the class regarding the process of cremation and so supplement the knowledge base of her team.

specialization raises this question in so far as palliative care nurses need to articulate what they contribute to care above and beyond any other nurse who cares for people at the end of life. The fact that advances in symptom management seem to favour biomedical and technical-rational knowledge above all other types of learning challenges nurses to think carefully about their contribution to the care, the team and the discipline. Reflecting back on the work of De Vlieger *et al.* (2004), the dimensions of learning (Figure 30.1) required of a nurse far surpass the biomedical rationality which shapes clinical advancements. The ability to engage with the patient, family and team effectively, and be cognizant of the impact of the health system and society on their respective interpretations of this palliative care scenario is the hallmark of expert nursing practice. This is not to say that biomedical advancements are not worthy and, given the possibility to improve the quality of someone's life, quite possibly justifiable. However, it is incumbent on the palliative care nurse and those responsible for their education to ensure that the contextual nature of palliative nursing knowledge is not lost. The language of caring should mirror the ideals of palliative care and address those aspects of the 'total pain' dimension which good palliative nursing practice embraces; comfort, presence and intuition. Connell Meehan's (2003) concept of 'careful nursing', although in need of further conceptual refinement for palliative nursing practice, would resonate with the artistry which ostensibly makes palliative nursing unique. Intuitive knowledge, valued as 'personal knowing', thus complements empirical science, aesthetics and moral knowledge as a framework for interpreting the rigour of palliative nursing (Carper 1978).

Given the shift towards evidence-based practice and the holistic

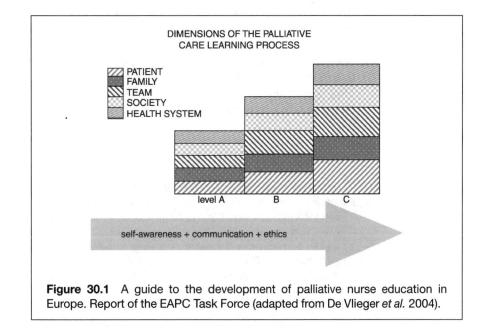

**Figure 30.1** A guide to the development of palliative nurse education in Europe. Report of the EAPC Task Force (adapted from De Vlieger *et al.* 2004).

approach to care cherished by palliative care nurses, it is surprising that more research into intuition in palliative nursing has not been explored. Naturally there are counter-arguments against intuition on the grounds that intuitively based decisions cannot be made explicit and therefore limit transparency (Lamond and Thompson 2000). Yet, Seymour (2004) argues that where the observable and measurable is valued above that which is sensed or felt, the very 'doing' of palliative nursing risks becoming inferior to rational science. Hence, palliative nurses have a responsibility to respond at the personal as well as professional level and this is only possible by blending intuitive and empirical ways of knowing.

To create education to meet the art as well as the science of palliative nursing is based around the creativity and expertise of the educator to enable an academic and personal process to grow together. The sand tray exercise (Box 30.3), as a tool to explore the psychodynamic processes which impact on who we are as nurses who care for dying people, is a way in which the technical-rational can be balanced against the creative-intuitive aspects of practice and demonstrate to the learner the flux of palliative care knowledge.

## Defining future directions for palliative care education

The United Kingdom remains a beacon of palliative care learning, offering not only theoretical but clinical learning opportunities which are less readily available in many European countries and which are essential to the translation of theory to practice. The international education programme run through St Christopher's Hospice in London gives a sense of the importance that centres of academic excellence play in the expansion of palliative care learning for European practitioners. Yet, in terms of sustainability and the best use of resources, are there even more innovative ways, through e-learning and distance education, that learning can be shared? The changing face of the European Union will challenge palliative care educators to be sensitive to cultural diversity in interpreting end-of-life care, particularly

---

**Box 30.3**   The sand tray

In silence, the group collect a small bag and enter a room where there are many different objects laid out – small toys, beads, feathers, cards, etc. They choose a selection and then sit in front of a tray filled with sand, obscured from other members of the group. Under the supervision of the facilitator, the learner is invited to place the objects in the sand to tell the story of their journey into palliative care. The learner is then invited to share their story with the group, explaining the reasons for the choice and why certain objects are placed in a particular way. At the end, each tray is revealed and the total shared experience of the sand tray is revealed to the whole group.

when faced with learners who are themselves immigrant to the host culture.

Whittaker *et al.* (2006) have explored the particular complexities of palliative education for nurses outside of the specialist framework. This is most appropriate given the fact that nursing homes are seen as a key target for improving general end-of-life care (Komaromy *et al.* 2000; Froggatt and Hoult 2002; Nolan *et al.* 2003). They confirm contemporary studies (Mallory 2003) which highlight that 'nurse education lacks an effective and efficient approach to educating nurses about end-of-life care' (Whittaker *et al.* 2006: 507). Educators need to meet this challenge through sharing of resources and skills. Particularly in smaller countries, decisions need to be made about strategic planning for education which highlight particular strengths and avoid duplication and expensive courses which do not meet service planning needs. Accreditation of programmes across jurisdictions not only increases workforce capacity but raises the benchmark by which education is judged. Further, innovative measures for education should heed the resource limitations of some countries and, although the IT revolution has contributed greatly to the expansion of knowledge, more simple measures may be just as effective. The Open Society Institute's (a George Soros Foundation) palliative care newsletter initiative for Eastern Europe is one example.

There is evidence of progress in palliative care education across Europe (Dowell 2002; Dowling and Broomfield 2002), although it would seem that criticism of inadequate opportunity for education is more prevalent than the assessment of its potential effect. The future of palliative care education in Europe will be dependent on evaluative empirical studies which can explicate the benefits of education to health care providers and offer flexible and person-centred solutions to engage with practitioners on their own terms about the acquisition of new knowledge to benefit their practice.

# Conclusion

In this chapter, I have explored some of the challenges for palliative nurse education and suggest that modest evidence is available that some of these issues and questions raised here are being addressed. Palliative nursing is beginning to contribute effectively to scholarship (Corner and Bailey 2002) and palliative care nursing itself has been subject to study (Lawton 1998). There is no doubt that an increasing evidence base is valuable for the advancement of palliative nursing, but should be judiciously managed so that the essence of nursing is not overwhelmed by scientific endeavour. It is incumbent on European palliative care educators to devise ways of preparing education that extols the uniqueness of collaboration, summed up in the EAPC motto, 'One Voice – One Vision'.

# References

Adriaansen, M.J.M. and Achterberg van, T. (2007) The content and effects of palliative care courses for nurses: a literature review. *International Journal of Nursing Studies*, doi.10.1016/j/ijnurstu.2007.01.016.

Adriaansen, M.J.M. and Frederiks, C.M.A. (2002) Design of a post graduate course in palliative care. *Journal of Continuing Nurse Education*, 15: 279–82.

AHPCC (2003) *Standards for hospice and palliative care chaplaincy.* Help the Hospices, London: Association for Hospice and Palliative Care Chaplains.

Appleton, M. and Corboy, K. (2005) When palliative medicine is not palliative care. *American Journal of Hospice and Palliative Medicine*, 22: 169–70.

Becker, G., Momm, F., Gigl, A., Wagner, B. and Baumgartner, J. (2007) *Competency and educational needs in palliative care.* Wiener Klinische Wochenschrift, 119(3–4): 112–16.

Birchenell, P. (1999) Editorial. Developing a work-based learning philosophy. *Nurse Education Today*, 19: 173–4.

Bliss, J., Cowley, S. and While, A. (2000) Interprofessional working in palliative care in the community: a review of the literature. *Journal of Interprofessional Care*, 14(3): 281–90.

Booth, K., Maguire, P., Butterworth, T. and Hillier, V.F. (1996) Perceived professional support and the use of blocking behaviour by hospice nurses. *Journal of Advanced Nursing*, 24: 522–7.

Burgener, S.C. (2001) Scholarship of practice for a practice profession. *Journal of Professional Nursing*, 17(1): 46–54.

Carper, B.A. (1978) Fundamental Patterns of Knowing in Nursing. *Advances in Nursing Science*, 1: 13–23.

Centeno, C., Clark, D., Lynch, T., Rocafort, J., Greenwood, A., Flores, L.A., De Lima, L., Giordano, A., Brasch, S. and Praill, D. (2007) *EAPC Atlas of Palliative Care in Europe.* Houston: IAHPC Press.

Connell Meehan, T. (2003) Careful nursing: a model for contemporary nursing practice. *Journal of Advanced Nursing*, 44(1): 99–107.

Copp, G., Caldwell, K., Atwal, A., Brett-Richards, M. and Coleman, K. (2007) Preparation for cancer care: perceptions of newly qualified health care professionals. *European Journal of Oncology Nursing*, 11: 159–67.

Corner, J. and Bailey, C. (2002) *Nursing research in palliative care.* Paper delivered to the Royal Society of Medicine conference, London, November.

Cowan, D.T., Norman, I.J. and Coopamah, V.P. (2005) European health care training and accreditation network. *British Journal of Nursing*, 14: 613–17.

Cowan, D.T., Wilson-Barnett, J., Norman, I.J. and Murrells, T. (2007) Measuring nursing competence: Development of a self-assessment tool for general nurses across Europe. *International Journal of Nursing Studies*, doi:10.1016/j/ijnurstu.2007.03.004.

Cutcliffe, J.R., Black, C., Hanson, E. and Goward, P. (2001) The commonality and synchronicity of mental health nurses and palliative care nurses: closer than you think? *Journal of Psychiatry and Mental Health*, 8(1): 53–9.

De Vlieger, M., Gorchs, N., Larkin, P.J. and Porchet, F. (2004) A guide to the development of palliative nurse education in Europe. *Report of the EAPC Task Force.* September 2004.

Dowell, L. (2002) Multiprofessional palliative care in a general hospital: education and training needs. *International Journal of Palliative Nursing*, 8(6): 294–303.

Dowling, S. and Broomfield, D. (2002) Ireland, the UK and Europe: a review of undergraduate medical education in palliative care. *Irish Medical Journal*, 95(7): 215–16.

Ellis, L.B. (2005) Professional doctorates for nurses: mapping provision and perceptions. *Journal of Advanced Nursing*, 50(4): 440–8.

European Association for Palliative Care (2005) www.eapcnet.org/Congresses/Aachen2005.htm

Filbet, M. and Larkin, P. (2007) Palliative Care Education in Europe. In: B. Wee and N. Hughes (eds) *Palliative Care Education: Building a Culture of Learning*. Oxford: Oxford University Press, pp. 69–76.

Foggo, B.A. (2006) Hospice: A place to die or just passing on? *Progress in Palliative Care*; 14: 109–11

Froggatt, K.A. and Hoult, L. (2002) Developing palliative care practice in nursing and residential care homes: the role of the clinical nurse specialist. *Journal of Clinical Nursing*, 11(6): 802–8.

Gordon, T. and Mitchell, D. (2004) A competency model for the assessment and delivery of spiritual care. *Palliative Medicine*, 18: 646–51.

Gould, D., Drey, N. and Berridge, E-J. (2007) Nurses' experiences of continuing professional development. *Nurse Education Today*, 27: 602–9.

Gould, D.J., Kelly, D., White, I. and Glen, S. (2004) The impact of commissioning processes on the delivery of continuing professional education for cancer and palliative care. *Nurse Education Today*, 24: 443–51.

Gwyther, L.P., Altilto, T., Blacker, S., Christ, G., Csakai, E.L., Hooyman, N., Kramer, B., Linton, J.M., Raymer, M. and Howe, J. (2005) Social work competencies in palliative and end-of-life care. *Journal of Social Work in End-of-Life and Palliative Care*, 1(1): 87–120.

Hale, C., Long, T., Sanderson, L., Carr, K. and Tomlinson, P. (2006) An evaluation of educational preparation for cancer and palliative care nursing for children and adolescents: Issues in the assessment of practice arising from this study. *Nurse Education Today*, 26: 528–37.

Heaven, C.M. and Maguire, P. (1996) Training hospice nurses to elicit patient concerns. *Journal of Advanced Nursing*, 23: 280–90.

Heaven, C., Clegg, J. and Maguire, P. (2006) Transfer of communication skills training from workshop to workplace: the impact of clinical supervision. *Patient Education and Counseling*, 60(3): 313–25.

Humphreys, A., Gidman, J. and Andrews, M. (2000) The nature and purpose of the role of the nurse lecturer in practice settings. *Nurse Education Today*, 20(4): 311–17.

Ilhardt, F.J. (2001) Scope and demarcation of palliative care. In: H. ten Have and R. Janssens (eds) *Palliative care in Europe: concepts and policies*. Amsterdam: IOS Press, 109–16.

Ingleton, C. and Davies, S. (2004) Research and Scholarship in palliative care nursing. In: S. Payne, J. Seymour and C. Ingleton *Palliative Care Nursing: Principles and Evidence for Practice*. Buckingham: Open University Press, 35: 676–96.

James, C.R. and Macleod, R.D. (1993) The problematic nature of education in palliative care. *Journal of Palliative Care*, 9(4): 5–10.

Kevern, J. and Webb, C. (2005) Mature women's experiences of pre-registration nurse education. *Journal of Advanced Nursing*, 45: 297–306.

Kirkman, S., Thompson, D.R., Watson, R. and Stewart, S. (2007) Are all doctorates equal or are some 'more equal than others'? An examination of which ones should be offered by schools of nursing. *Nurse Education in Practice*, 7: 61–6.

Kitson, A. (1999) The relevance of scholarship for nursing research and practice. *Journal of Advanced Nursing*, 29(4): 773–5.

Koffman, J. (2001) Multiprofessional palliative care education: past challenges, future issues. *Journal of Palliative Care*, 17(2): 86–92.

Komaromy, C., Sidell, M. and Katz, J.T. (2000) The quality of terminal care in residential and nursing homes. *International Journal of Palliative Nursing*, 6(4): 192–200.

Lamond, D. and Thompson, C. (2000) Intuition and Analysis in Decision Making and Choice. *Journal of Nursing Scholarship*; 32(3): 411–14.

Larkin, P.J., Dierckx de Casterlé, B. and Schotsmans, P. (2007) Translation in qualitative research: reflections on a metaphorical process. *Qualitative Health Research*, 17: 468–76.

Lawton, J. (1998) Contemporary hospice care: the sequestration of the unbounded body and 'dirty' dying. *Sociology of Health and Illness*, 20(2): 121–43.

MacDougall, G., Mathew, A., Broadhurst, V. and Chamberlain, S. (2001) An evaluation of an interprofessional palliative care education programme. *International Journal of Palliative Nursing*, 7(1): 24–9.

Mallory, J.L. (2003) The impact of a palliative care educational component on attitudes towards care of the dying in undergraduate nursing students. *Journal of Professional Nursing*, 19(5): 305–12.

MCCC (2003) *Spiritual and religious care competencies for specialist palliative care.* London: Marie Curie Cancer Care.

Morrison, L.J., Opatik Scott, J. and Block, S.D. (2007) Developing initial competency-based outcomes for the hospice and palliative medicine sub-specialist: Phase I of the Hospice and Palliative Medicine Competencies Project. *Journal of Palliative Medicine*, 10(2): 313–30.

Morita, T., Murata, H., Hirai, K., Tamura, K., Kataoka, J., Ohnishi, H., Akizuki, N., Kurihara, Y., Akechi, T. and Uchitomi, Y. (2007) Meaninglessness in terminally ill cancer patients: a validation study and a nurse education intervention trial. *Journal of Pain and Symptom Management*, 34(2): 160–70.

Nolan, M., Featherston, J. and Nolan, J. (2003) Palliative care philosophy in care homes: lessons from New Zealand. *British Journal of Nursing*, 12(16): 974–9.

Norman, I.J., Watson, R., Murrells, T., Calman, L. and Redfern, S. (2002) The validity and reliability of methods to assess the competence to practice of pre-registration nursing and midwifery students. *International Journal of Nursing Studies*, 39: 133–45.

Peters, R.S. (1979) *The Concept of Education.* London: Routledge and Kegan Paul.

Praill, D. (2000) Editorial: Who are we here for? *Palliative Medicine*, 14: 91–2.

Ramcharan, P., Ashmore, R., Nicklin, L. and Drew, J. (2001) Nursing scholarship within the British University system. *British Journal of Nursing*, 10(3): 196–201.

Redfern, S., Norman, I.J., Calman, L., Watson, R. and Murrells, T. (2002) Assessing competence to practise in nursing: a review of the literature. *Research Papers in Education*, 17(1): 51–77.

Roberts-Davis, M. and Read, S. (2001) Clinical role clarification using the Delphi method to establish similarities and differences between nurse practitioners and clinical nurse specialists. *Journal of Clinical Nursing*, 10: 33–43.

Royal College of Nursing (2001) *Charting the challenge for nurse lecturers in higher education.* London: RCN.

Sasahara, T., Miyashita, M., Kawa, M. and Kazuma, K. (2003) Difficulties encountered by nurses in the care of terminally ill cancer patients in general hospitals in Japan. *Palliative Medicine*, 17(6): 520–6.

Scottish Partnership for Palliative Care and the NHS Executive for Scotland (2007) *A guide to using palliative care competency frameworks.*

Seymour, J., Clark, D., Bath, P., Beech, N., Corner, J., Douglas, H-R., Halliday, D., Haviland, J., Marples, R., Normand, C., Skilbeck, J. and Webb, T. (2002) Clinical nurse specialists in palliative care. Part 3. Issues for the MacMillan Nurse role. *Palliative Medicine*, 16(5): 386–94.

Seymour, J. (2004) What's in a name? A concept analysis of key terms in palliative care nursing. In: S. Payne, J, Seymour and C. Ingleton, *Palliative Care Nursing: Principles and Evidence for Practice*. Buckingham: Open University Press, 3: 55–74.

Seymour, J.E. (2005) Using technology to help obtain the goals of palliative care. *International Journal of Palliative Nursing*; 11: 240–1.

Sheldon, F. and Smith, P. (1996) The life so short, the craft so hard to learn: a model for post-basic education in palliative care. *Palliative Medicine*, 10: 99–104.

Shields, P. (2002) Commissioning post-registration education programmes for health care professionals. *Nurse Education Today*, 22: 285–92.

Smith, S.A. (2003) Developing and utilizing end of life nursing competencies. *Home Health Care Management and Practice*. Downloaded 30 June 2007 at http://hhc.sagepub.com/cgi/content/abstract/15/2/116.

Sneddon, M. (2004) Specialist professional education in palliative care. How did we get here and where are we going? In: S. Payne, J. Seymour and C. Ingleton (eds) *Palliative Care Nursing: Principles and Evidence for Practice*. Buckingham: Open University Press, 33: 636–54.

Sullivan, A.M., Lakoma, M.D. and Block, S. (2003) The status of medical education in end-of-life care. A national report. *Journal of General Internal Medicine*, 18: 685–95.

Van Kleffens, T., Van Baarsen, B., Hoekman, K. and Van Leeuwen, E. (2004) Clarifying the term 'palliative' in clinical oncology. *European Journal of Cancer Care*, 13: 263–71.

Ventafridda, V. (1998) Ten years on in EJPC. *European Journal of Palliative Care*, 5: 140.

Weissman, D.E., Ambuel, B., Von Gunten, C.F., Block, S., Warm, E., Hallenbeck, J., Milch, R., Brasel, K. and Mullan, P.B. (2007) Outcomes from a national multispecialty palliative care curriculum development project. *Journal of Palliative Medicine*, 10(2): 408–19.

Whittaker, E., Kernohan, W.G., Hasson, F., Howard, V. and McLaughlin, D. (2006) The palliative care education needs of nursing home staff. *Nurse Education Today*, 26: 501–10.

World Health Organization (2002) downloaded 21 July 2005 at http://www.int/cancer/palliative/definition/en/.

Yam, B.M.C. (2005) Professional doctorate and professional nursing practice. *Nurse Education Today*, 25: 564–72.

# 31

# Information and communications technology (ICT) in palliative care

*Peter Bath, Barbara Sen and Kendra Albright*

---

**Key points**

- The use of information and communications technology (ICT) in health has increased dramatically in recent years.
- ICTs have the potential to improve palliative care for patients, families, carers and health care professionals at all stages of the palliative care pathway.
- The advent of the world wide web (www) and Web 2.0 technologies have provided opportunities for better communication and exchange of information within and among these groups.
- The development of electronic records for patient care and systems to support them could enable better access to patient information for health care professionals, as well as to patients receiving palliative care and their families and carers.

---

# Introduction

The past ten to fifteen years has seen an increase in the use of information and communication technology (ICT) within health and medicine, and the emergence of health informatics as a discipline. Health informatics can be considered to be an extension of medical informatics: while medical informatics focused predominantly on the development and use of computing applications in clinical medicine, health informatics has emerged to include the use of ICTs by other health professions in addition to clinical medicine, as well as by the patients and the general public.

We describe recent and current developments in ICT in health and medicine and examine the potential they offer to palliative care. We consider this from the perspective of the health care professionals, the patients receiving palliative care and their families through the different stages of palliative care: from pre-diagnosis, through diagnosis, treatment and management, continuing illness to death or bereavement.

Palliative care can be supported by combining the use of ICT with the care given by multidisciplinary teams of health and social care workers and those who give psychological or spiritual support in providing day-to-day care to patients and carers in their homes, and in hospitals or hospices. In this sense, palliative care aims to:

- affirm life and regard dying as a normal process
- provide relief from pain and distressing symptoms
- integrate the psychological and spiritual aspects of patient care
- offer support to help patients live as well as possible till death
- offer a support system to help the family cope during the patient's illness and in bereavement (NICE 2004, http://guidance.nice.org.uk/csgsp/guidance/pdf/English).

Any use of information and communications technology (ICT) should align with these aims, not be in conflict with them. When conflict arises patients can experience negativity. This can give support to the argument against the use of technology, which can be invasive, a situation where technology fails to co-exist appropriately with dignified dying (Seymour 2003). However, there are strong arguments for the use of technology in health care which can bring huge benefits, improve patient safety and quality of life and support better health care decision-making (Connecting for Health 2007). Thus, technological advances can be helpful in alleviating the suffering of many dying patients (Tinnelly *et al.* 2000).

The lives of people coping with terminal illness have complicated and sometimes competing priorities. Their needs extend beyond medical interventions to include the social, emotional and spiritual aspects of life that are important in maintaining quality of life throughout the palliative care process. Where ICT is applied in the palliative care setting, it should be used in a holistic way, sensitive to the best interests of the patient and with consideration for their wishes and their beliefs. Throughout the whole cycle of illness there are ways in which developments in ICT are helping patients, and those who care for them.

Figure 31.1 provides a rich picture to illustrate the types of issues and needs that may arise: this chapter discusses how advances in ICT may help at the various stages of palliative care. Currently, the United Kingdom (UK) government is investing heavily in ICT with a view to modernizing the National Health Service (NHS), potentially bringing efficiencies throughout the NHS. We describe both general developments in ICT, e.g. the world wide web (www) and Web 2.0 technologies, and particular initiatives, such as NHS Direct and the National Programme for IT (NPFIT) in the UK together with developments in other countries, as examples of ICT supporting people receiving or giving palliative care.

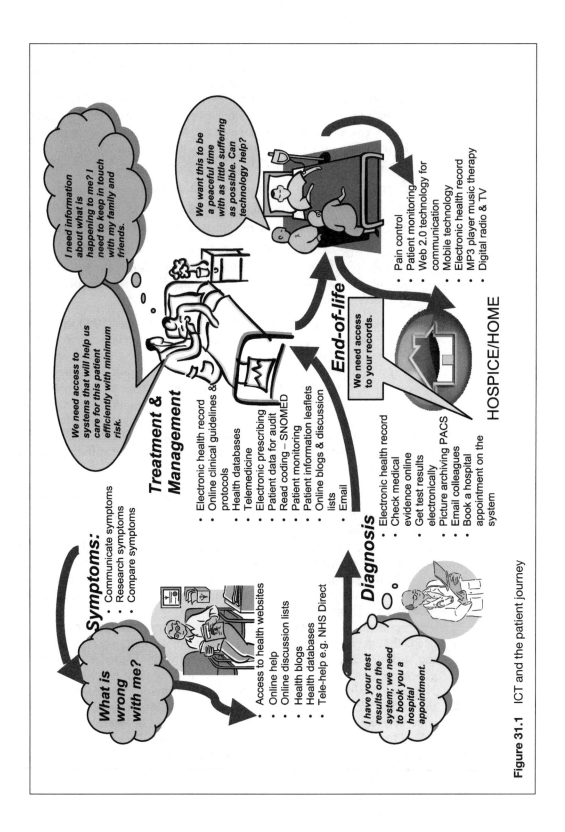

**Figure 31.1** ICT and the patient journey

# Role of ICT

The advent of the world wide web in the 1990s led to the development of a huge resource of information previously unimaginable. The increasing availability of computers and accessibility to the internet (www) has expanded our capabilities for communication and information in everyday life, including health. The provision of health information through web-sites has meant that the internet has become a major information resource for health globally. More recently, the advent of Web 2.0 has led to greater information sharing and communication.

Since 1997 in the UK, there has been major investment in information technology (IT) within health care, following Information for Health (Burns 1998) and more recently the National Programme for IT (NPFIT). While there have been major problems with the implementation of these programmes (Protti 2002), the developments offer opportunities to access better quality information for both health professionals and patients, supporting better quality health care for patients.

The development of health information on the internet and of electronic health records has led to the concept of e-health, and palliative care may benefit from this. While the underlying technology is important in facilitating communication and access to information, we concentrate on describing facilities and services that have been developed and their impact on patient care.

# Symptoms and pre-diagnosis

When a person first notices a change in their health, i.e. the development of one or more symptoms, they may look to a variety of information sources before, or in parallel with, seeking medical opinion from a doctor, usually the family doctor or general practitioner (GP).

Information on the internet can be retrieved using a search engine such as Google, Yahoo!, Ask Jeeves, by typing in keywords describing their symptoms or suspected condition to find relevant websites. Patients have searched Google in this way and come to a diagnosis themselves, and presented this to their doctor (Tang and Ng 2006). The concept of the 'expert patient' has emerged and such patients can assist doctors in diagnosis and encourage patient participation in health care decision-making, facilitating the doctor–patient relationship. However, disadvantages to patients accessing information on health via the internet include health professionals feeling threatened and patients accessing incorrect information.

People can access the internet 24 hours a day, seven days a week, at times when their health care professional might not be available, for example weekends. While a person with an obvious clinical emergency is likely to utilize Accident and Emergency services, a person with symptoms that are not urgent or immediately life-threatening might use the internet to search for information rather than wait until their health care professional is available. The internet also provides information for individuals who suspect that something is wrong but would prefer reassurance from a less formal, confidential source rather than seeking professional help.

A disadvantage of information on the internet is the variable quality of information (Purcell *et al.* 2002). Anyone with access to a computer and the internet can set up their own website and post information there. The danger is that individuals will find and use wrong or misleading information to make decisions: this could adversely affect their own health and well-being. Therefore, although authoritative organizations such as the National Health Service in the UK, or health charities (e.g. Breast Cancer Care, Macmillan Cancer Support) can provide valuable, credible information, other organizations/individuals may provide information that is potentially harmful.

Two methods of trying to ensure high quality health care information is found on the internet have been developed:

- portals, or web gateways providing links to specific sites that have been checked and certified by health or information professionals, e.g. *Intute* (2006) (formerly OMNI) in the UK provides access to over 31,000 evaluated web resources in health and life sciences; and the National Library for Health (formerly the National Electronic Library for Health), a portal providing access to approved sites.

- tools to evaluate the quality of information on the internet (Purcell *et al.* 2002). A wide range of instruments have been developed to evaluate the quality of information on the internet (Gagliardi and Jadad 2002). Although these assess the validity and reliability of information, e.g. whether the website authors' details are present, how recently the website has been updated, there are relatively few tools developed to assess how well the websites meet the information needs of patients, carers and family members (Bath and Bouchier 2003; Bouchier and Bath 2003; Harland and Bath 2007).

Numerous organizations in different countries provide websites that provide information to individuals before they receive a diagnosis (e.g. BACUP, Breast Cancer Care, European Association for Palliative Care). This information should be used to *supplement* medical advice and care rather than to replace it. In particular, NHS Direct, a telephone help service in the UK, and NHS Direct online, a web-based service, provide information and advice to members of the public.

General practitioners may also use the internet to access information portals, such as the National Library for Health (see section on Treatment and management) to help make a diagnosis, as well as to provide care and support for the patient. One study showed that searching Google was helpful to doctors in making diagnoses on difficult conditions (Tang and Ng 2006). Using 26 cases from the *New England Journal of Medicine*, the authors made 15 correct diagnoses (58 per cent) by performing a Google search for each case.

## Diagnosis

Health care professionals may use the internet to obtain information that can help in the diagnosis and subsequent treatment and management of a patient (see below). At diagnosis, patients and family members may have diverse, and conflicting, information needs. Some patients want as much information as possible to cope with the diagnosis, whereas others do not want any information, and actually avoid information, for example after being diagnosed with cancer (Rees *et al.* 1998). Although patients may avoid information, family members may actively seek as much information as possible. Health care professionals need to be sensitive to the unique information needs of individual patients and family members, and offer information at a time and in a way that is appropriate for each person, for example answering questions verbally or providing patient information leaflets (PILs). Electronic information resources offer an additional source of information that patients and family members can access.

After diagnosis, the patient and/or family members may search the internet for information about their condition or for specific organizations (e.g. Cancer BACUP, MS Society). These websites can provide useful information about all aspects of a particular condition, including symptoms, treatments, side effects, and support available, in a variety of languages. An important advantage of using these online resources is that the individual can access them at a convenient time, print information to keep, or return to the online source.

Patients and family members may also use other web resources including discussion boards and web logs (often called blogs, see the section on Treatment and management). Discussion boards, operated by organizations such as Breast Cancer Care, enable people to post messages to the website and share information or experiences or give emotional support. Other people can view and respond to these or they may have professionals who respond to queries from people or act as a moderator to check messages for appropriateness and etiquette, for example removing messages that may cause offence or might reveal the author's identity. 'Asynchronous' communication, using discussion boards/blogs, enables people to post information at one particular time and other people to respond to it at a different time; they do not have to be online simultaneously.

Organizations may also provide opportunities for 'synchronous' (i.e. simultaneous) communication. For example, chat rooms, which allow people to communicate in real time, and instant messaging. This requires more intensive moderation to ensure that the content remains appropriate, potentially inflammatory messages are dealt with immediately, and emotive issues are discussed in an appropriate way to limit offence or to avoid upsetting people who might be emotionally vulnerable.

Through the internet, patients can also gain access to medical and health bibliographic databases and journals, such as the PubMed version of Medline, produced by the National Library of Medicine (NLM) in the

United States (US), BioMed Central, as well as the online version of the *British Medical Journal*. This provides patients and the general public with ready access via the internet to health and medical research literature about their condition.

Another potentially useful technology for patients at diagnosis, and implemented through the UK National Programme for IT (NPFIT), is the *Choose and Book* system, which enables patients to select hospital services and book an appointment at a time and place that is convenient to them. If a patient is in a consultation with a GP and the patient needs secondary care, for example a biopsy in a hospital, the GP can log into Choose and Book from their desktop PC to find out what services are available locally. The patient can select which service they wish to use and select an appointment from those available. The rationale is that by customizing appointments to the needs of patients, fewer appointments will be missed resulting in a more efficient and effective service. The previous system where the GP wrote to the local hospital requesting an appointment led to problems and appointments being missed or left vacant. Despite the potential benefits of Choose and Book, there have been considerable delays with implementation, uptake and usage of the system, and to date there has not been an independent evaluation of the service.

# Treatment and management

At this point, the aim is not to use technology to treat the illness with invasive procedures, but to use technology to treat and alleviate distressing symptoms in a way that will allow the patient to have as reasonable a quality of life as possible. Examples of how technology can be employed are in consultation and management of the case, patient monitoring, pain relief, patient support, and the management of patient data.

### Access to health care databases

Health care professionals need access to the best evidence available to support clinical decision-making and, as mentioned above, in the UK, the National Library for Health (NLH) provides professionals with access to evidence via health care databases and other validated resources (www.library.nhs.uk).

The NLH provides timely health care news and tracks the underlying research. A wide range of nationally procured datasets are available including premier resources such as Medline, Cinahl, Psychinfo, AMED and the Cochrane Library. There are also links to the National Institute for Health and Clinical Excellence (NICE) clinical guidelines, health protocols and Clinical Knowledge Summaries. The emphasis is on reliable, quality evidence for health care professionals with links to sources specifically for patients. NLH also provides a range of specialist information sources, one of which is the *Palliative and Supportive Care Specialist Library* (Figure 31.2).

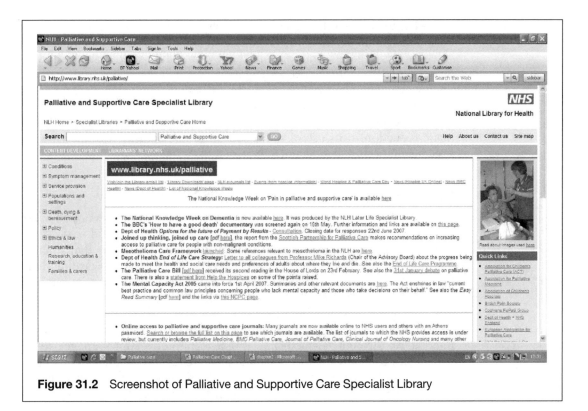

**Figure 31.2**   Screenshot of Palliative and Supportive Care Specialist Library

(www.library.nhs.uk/palliative). In the USA, the National Library of Medicine (www.nlm.nih.gov) performs a similar role.

### Telemedicine

Technology also plays a supportive role during medical consultations. Telemedicine is one example of how ICTs can support palliative care. Wooten (2001) defines telemedicine as 'an umbrella term that encompasses any medical activity involving an element of distance' (p. 557). Telemedicine can be used for education and training, teleconsultations, and communication. It can also incorporate the use of medical call centres such as NHS Direct. An example of a telemedicine project is the St David's Foundation Hospice Care in Wales, the UK's largest provider of community-based palliative care (Saysell and Routley 2003). The project was developed to address a shortage of consultants in palliative care and proved successful in developing closer working relationships between specialist palliative care, acute and primary care staff.

Benefits of telemedicine include sharing of knowledge and expertise, building relationships, costs saved in time and travel, and access to a wider range of expertise. Special consideration should be given to people's ability to feel comfortable, and engage, with the technology, and the need for effective planning, preparation and management of the telemedicine sessions.

Telemedicine developments offer potential for patients to stay at home during their final stages of life. Through the use of webcams, computers and videophones, patients can be supported by providing virtual access to doctors, nurses and other specialists based remotely in a hospital, hospice or practice. The potential benefits are particularly valuable in rural areas throughout the world where access to health care is limited (Smith *et al.* 2005). The Royal Flying Doctor Service in rural Australia has seen a dramatic reduction in its use of radio consultations, parallel with increases in teleconsultations and videoconferencing (RFDS 2006).

### Picture Archiving and Communications Systems (PACS)

PACS is another use of images and technology that is being developed in the UK through NPFIT. PACS enables images such as x-rays and scans to be captured, stored, distributed and displayed electronically, so that doctors and other health professionals can make effective decisions regarding diagnosis and treatment. PACS technology removes the need to print on film and manually file or distribute images. It eliminates costs associated with hard film and provides valuable space used for storage. An image can be made available to different clinicians, in different places, simultaneously via the internet or through telemedicine. PACS technology allows images to be stored electronically in the patient's care record. The first PACS implementation was in the USA in the early 1980s, which led to developments in European countries including Belgium, Austria, Germany, France and the UK.

### Electronic prescribing

ICT developments are also aimed at improving and streamlining the process of prescribing medications. In England, the Electronic Prescription Service and Electronic Prescribing (e-Prescribing) programme is facilitating the development of systems to improve patient safety by reducing prescribing and administration errors. e-Prescribing systems will enable medications and other prescribed therapies to be managed electronically, and facilitate reductions in paperwork, audit and communication. For patients coping with illness at home, they do not need to visit the surgery for repeat prescriptions, the drug information is input once and transferred electronically between the prescriber, the pharmacist and the reimbursement agency.

### Patient monitoring and patient data for audit

At each stage of managing the patient's care, patient data is needed for effective case management and the audit of health care provision. A recent development central to effective management of the patient is the electronic health care record (EHR). In the UK the development of an EHR is part of the NPFIT programme and similar initiatives are being developed in other countries such as Australia's Health *Connect* and Canada's Health Infoway

(Detmer 2006). An EHR enables the electronic collection and storage of patient data that can be communicated across networks to health care providers, providing health care professionals with information to support decision-making either about individual patients or broader health care planning.

EHRs have the potential to improve end-of-life care by giving better access to patients so that they could be continually informed as to their health situations. In addition, patients could record their end-of-life wishes with regard to issues such as treatment, resuscitation and regarding death and dying. This could aid decision-making for ICU or palliative care professionals and reduce ethical dilemmas (Pang 2003; Seymour 2003; Gustafson 2007; Menezes *et al.* 2007).

### SNOMED CT® read coding

SNOMED CT® is a clinical terminology, a common computerized language that will be used on all computers in the NHS to facilitate communications between health care professionals. A clinical terminology is a structured list of terms for use in clinical practice. These terms describe the care and treatment of patients and cover areas like diseases, operations, treatments, drugs and health care administration. By using the terminology and the computer system, the clinician can record patient information in a consistent way. Clinical data can be communicated efficiently between health care workers, for example, prescribing, referrals and hospital discharges.

### Patient access to information

Patients and their families need access to information during treatment. The internet is a source of patient empowerment (Meier *et al.* 2007), regardless of the vast amount of dubious content found on it. Web 2.0 is the second phase of development on the internet, which has been called the 'social web' (Boulos 2007) because users can easily generate content, enabling a more socially-connected environment than previously possible. The human element enabled by Web 2.0 technology makes it particularly useful for social interaction within a health care setting. Web 2.0 offers flexibility and collaboration for patients, health care professionals and students of health studies. Some of the most popular applications for Web 2.0 technology in the health care setting include:

- Enabling professional communities of practice to share information and discuss professional issues.
- Patient support:
  - through access to health professionals from all over the world
  - through shared information and experiences with those undergoing similar health problems
  - enabling contact with friends and family who may be unable to be physically close.

- Therapy: enabling access to music, photos and pictures that are beneficial for patients in stressful situations.

The internet offers opportunities for patient support through the sharing of information and experiences through websites, blogs, wikis, online mailing or discussion lists, patient education, therapeutic benefits (e.g. writing, online diaries or therapeutic music downloads) and the opportunity to communicate with health professionals through email (e.g. NHS Direct's email enquiry service, www.nhsdirect.nhs.uk/ask).

A blog is a simple way to publish an online diary with links to other sources of interest (see, for example, www.pallimed.org and www. thecancerblog.com). Blogging is increasingly popular and opens new channels of communication. Wikis are similar to blogs but are more useful for collaboration (see www.wikicancer.org). They can be public (open to anyone) or private (limited to a defined group of users). Critical evaluation of information content on blogs and wikis is essential as many have no health professional input.

Podcasts are digital files (audio – podcasts or video – vodcasts) that can be downloaded and transferred to a portable player such as an iPod or other MP3 player and can be listened to or watched later. They can be used for educational purposes or leisure and can be copied to other laptops or desktops. Podcasts could be downloaded from websites and used for patient information, education for health care professionals, or therapy in a palliative care setting.

Web gateways such as *Intute* (2006), mentioned earlier, can be used to access validated information from a wide range of quality health resources. Eventually one such gateway, Healthspace, will enable patients to access their electronic health care record. Healthspace (www.nhs.uk/healthspace) is currently being developed as a secure website where patients can store their personal health information online, such as height, weight and blood pressure. This site will form the basis for communication by email to health care professionals to discuss such things as symptoms, medication and appointments.

Social bookmarking allows online bookmarks to be shared; social bookmarking sites can be searched by topic by using keywords. Examples of social bookmarking sites include http://del.icio.us/ and www.rekommend. com. Social search tools allow for searches across blogs, newsfeeds and podcasts. Users can subscribe on these sites to receive updates automatically according to their search preferences, for example www.feedster.com and Google Co-op (http://google.com/coop/) allows users to build their own search engine, specific to their needs and interests. Other applications and sites (for example, www.myspace.com) allow groups of people with common interests to connect have enabled social networking, through which users can form links with people through friends and colleagues.

The internet is one example of how technology can equip patients and families to deal with stressful issues regarding palliative care, treatment, death and dying. It will be increasingly valuable as it becomes more widely available on wards and in hospices in providing access to health care information for patients and their families (Gustafson 2007). Future developments of ICTs in health care may allow clinicians to have the information they need wherever they are via computers, laptops, hand-helds, smartphones, thereby enabling them to make timely and accurate decisions and reduce risk for the patient. The use of ICTs will allow the patient to participate in their own health care management and decision-making from pre-diagnosis to end of life.

# End-of-life care

Most research on palliative care does not distinguish between the stages of progressive illness and there has been very little research on the use of ICTs in the end stages of palliative care. However, different approaches are necessary as a patient moves from being seriously ill to dying. There is a shift in the efforts required for managing illness to providing as much comfort as possible and allowing the person to experience 'a good death'.

A good death is defined as 'one that is free from avoidable suffering for patients, families and caregivers in general accordance with the patients' and families' wishes' (http://books.nap.edu/html/approaching/1.html). Palliative care first came about because of concerns that medical technology was dehumanizing health care and the treatment of the dying (Tinnelly *et al.* 2000). The use of ICTs in end-of-life care must be decided on an individual basis, where there are clear benefits to the patient. Health care professionals can guide the patient in using ICTs by addressing the potential advantages and appropriate uses.

The end-of-life stage in palliative care presents particular considerations for patients that need to be taken into account. Patients have physical, mental, social and spiritual health requirements that are often complicated by limited stamina (Chang *et al.* 2007). This creates barriers to information that do not exist in earlier stages of palliative care. As patient mobility is reduced, access becomes more constrained by the physical requirements of technological interaction. The careful selection and appropriate uses of ICTs at the end of life offer emotional and spiritual support by providing additional means of communication, comfort and pain management.

Emotional and spiritual support comes through communication between patients and their families and carers. ICTs that facilitate the opportunity to communicate with distant relatives and carers may be useful. Emotional and spiritual support may include a review of one's life and memories, including photographs and stories from loved ones that could be sent via ICTs directly to the patient's room. Access to art and music therapy as well as prayer programmes could be provided via ICTs including radio and television, iPods and MP3, and internet distribution. Allowing patients to interact with reminders of their lives can help to 'create personal meaning out of the circumstances of their terminal illness and develop an enriched repertoire of coping strategies' (Tinnelly *et al.* 2000).

ICTs can also be used as part of an overall system for managing patient information as the patient is dying. Patient information that includes medical information, pain management and other changes can be monitored from a distance for rapid response and reassurance to patients and carers. Lind and Karlsson (2003) reported the use of digital pens in pain management. The patient uses the pen on digital paper to rate their pain and record their pain levels up to three times per day, transferring their records digitally over a global satellite mobile (GSM) network to the hospital where they are stored in a database. This allows the patient's medical staff to monitor their pain symptoms and follow up on treatment for pain management. The system also allows the carers to track pain management treatments by recording administration of analgesics.

Family carers often provide practical and emotional support for patients with terminal illness who may be facing difficult decisions towards the end of life. Communication between patients and their families is important, particularly with those who are nearby and can be involved in the face-to-face meetings necessary for making important decisions. For distant family members, telephone and conference calls may be useful. Email and web-based communications can also help to keep distant relatives informed, although their asynchronous nature may limit participation in decision-making. The use of communication technologies, however, may increase the potential for breaches of privacy for patients or confidentiality in patient–physician communications and should be used carefully (Rabow *et al.* 2004).

ICTs can help health care professionals care for dying patients, for example in answering patients' questions or helping with issues of depression, anxiety, decision-making and pain management. Health care provision and particularly palliative care is by no means delivered consistently across the globe. Different cultures demand different sensitivities to end-of-life care. In developing countries, such as many African nations, robust infrastructures may not be in place for supportive strategies and technologies. There is a lack of information regarding dying. Without this information it is difficult to develop global initiatives to improve end-of-life experiences. Singer and Bowman (2002) call for organizations like WHO to do much more information specific research in end-of-life experiences globally.

The process of dying requires a different approach to other stages of palliative care and consideration should be given to whether the use of ICTs is appropriate at all. The culture of modern medicine is to provide life-saving treatment based on 'the belief that doing something is always better than doing nothing' (Maxwell 2004). Patients facing imminent death may decide to prolong it as long as possible by requesting additional medical intervention. Invasive medical interventions and technologies may, therefore, already be present and the addition of ICTs may add to the confusion and reduce the comfort of patients and their families.

# Future developments in ICTs and implications for palliative care

Finally, what does the future hold, and how might further developments in ICT support the palliative care of patients? As the advent and impact of the world wide web in information and communication could not have been foreseen in the 1980s, we do not try to second guess new technologies here; rather, we can consider how the different ICTs and their interfaces might converge to help improve quality of life, a 20/20 vision for patients experiencing palliative care.

We can imagine a world in which a person can measure and monitor their own health, continually receiving regular updates on their well-being: reminders could be sent to a mobile device to undertake specific exercise or for a health scan. A change in body functioning, for example increased blood pressure, weight loss, might alert the person to visit their GP, offering the person particular times for this, matching the appointments available at the surgery with gaps in the person's electronic diary. Meanwhile, specific symptoms could be entered automatically into a search that identifies relevant information that the patient can bookmark and could be added to the electronic record for health care professionals to discuss with the patient during the consultation.

Following consultation and discussion with the GP, which could be audio recorded for the patient to replay later to remind them of details, and online booking of a hospital appointment, the person could be linked to information and support groups and other people in similar circumstances through their mobile device, for them to access as and when they felt they needed this information and support. The specificity of the information provided could be modified upon diagnosis, linking the person and their family members to information on their condition, the types of treatment available, the results of clinical trials of particular interventions, and links to other people at different stages of the care pathway to share experiences. Through the treatment and management of the disease the patient and their family would be able to access relevant information as they needed it, and the person concerned would have the relevant information recorded and monitored remotely, prompting additional input and support from appropriate health care professionals.

For a person entering the terminal stages of an illness, monitoring and support would change to ensure that the person's quality of life was maintained as much and as long as possible, adjusting the information that was made available depending on the individual circumstances and needs, and helping the person to prepare for death. For the family the final stages and time of death and bereavement could be accompanied by access to additional sources of information and support, for example information on legal requirements, funeral arrangements and preparation and bereavement support groups.

# Conclusion

In this chapter, we have discussed the benefits that ICTs can bring to the people involved in the palliative care pathway; however, ICTs must be developed and used with the individual patient's well-being in mind. ICTs can only be used to supplement and enhance, and not to replace, the personal care provided by professional and informal carers. The development of ICTs to record and transfer information about the health of individuals does raise ethical concerns regarding the security, privacy and confidentiality of personal data. Although there is an understanding that sharing health information about individuals among members of the multi-disciplinary health team is beneficial, if not essential, for effective health care, there are concerns about the use of the internet to transfer information. If patients and the public are to trust the systems with their personal health data, they have to have confidence that their information is safe, and an understanding of the extent to which the data might be shared. While we have not explored these issues in detail in this chapter, the current developments and future impact they will have on the patient's care have to be considered in parallel with the ethical issues that are raised.

Developments in ICTs can support patients, their families and carers, and health care professionals throughout the palliative care process. From the time when a person first suspects there might be something wrong, through diagnosis, treatment, management and end-of-life care, there are opportunities for patients to become better informed and utilize the diverse range of information resources and communication facilities available on the internet. Families and carers can use these resources to find out the information and to gain the support they need, both for themselves and to fulfil their role as family member or care-giver. Developments in electronic records and new ways to transfer information about patients will help health care professionals to provide better care for patients through information being available in the right time and in the right place.

While innovations in ICT are not intended to remove the feelings of fear and anxiety, uncertainty, sadness and loss for the patients, their families and carers, tailoring the access to information and support via ICTs for individuals throughout the stages of palliative care can help to reduce the impact of the illness on quality of life and on the dying process.

# References

Bath, P.A. and Bouchier, H. (2003) Development and application of a tool designed to evaluate websites providing information on Alzheimer's Disease. *Journal of Information Science*, 29(4): 279–97.

Bouchier, H. and Bath, P.A. (2003) Evaluation of websites that provide information on Alzheimer's Disease. *Health Informatics Journal*, 9(1): 17–32.

Boulos, M.N.K. (2007) The emerging Web 2.0 social software: an enabling suite of sociable technologies in health and health care education. *Health Information and Libraries Journal*, 24(2): 2–23.

Burns, F. (1998) *Information for health: an information strategy for the modern NHS 1998–2005*. A national strategy for local implementation. Leeds: NHS Executive. Available from: www.dh.gov.uk/en/index.htm (accessed 5 July 2007).

Chang, C.H., Boni-Saenz, A.A., Durazo-Arvizu, R.A., DesHarnais, S., Lau, D.T. and Emanuel, L.L. (2007) A system for interactive assessment and management in palliative care. *Journal of Pain and Symptom Management*, 33(6): 745–55.

Connecting for Health (2007) London: The National Health Service. www.connectingforhealth.nhs.uk (accessed 28 June 2007).

Detmer, D. (2006) *Learning from abroad: Lessons and questions on personnel health records for national policy*. Washington, DC: American Medical Informatic Association.

Gagliardi, A. and Jadad, A.R. (2002) Examination of instruments used to rate quality of health information on the internet: chronicle of a voyage with an unclear destination. *British Medical Journal*, 324: 569–73.

Gustafson, D.H. (2007). A good death. *Journal of Medical Internet Research*, 9(1): e6. www.jmir.org/2007/1/e6 (accessed 27 June 2007).

Harland, J.A. and Bath, P.A. (2007) Assessing the quality of websites providing information on multiple sclerosis: evaluating and comparing websites. *Health Informatics Journal* (in press).

*Intute* (2006) London: Intute Consortium. www.intute.ac.uk (accessed 28 June 2007).

Lind, L. and Karlsson, D. (2003) Symptom assessment in home healthcare using digital pens. *AMIA Symposium Proceedings*, 914. www.pubmedcentral.nih.gov/picrender.fcgi?artid=1480067&blobtype=pdf (accessed 2 July 2007).

Maxwell, T. quoted in Margaret Hawke (2004) From cure to comfort in the ICU. *Nursing Spectrum*. www.community.nursingspectrum.com/Magazine Articles/article.cfm?AID=11206 (accessed 5 July 2007).

Meier, A., Lyons, E.J., Frydman, G., Forlanz, M. and Rimer, B.K. (2007) How cancer survivors provide support on cancer-related Internet Mailing lists. *Journal of Medical Research*, 9(2): e12. www.jmir.org/2007/2/e12 (accessed 27 June 2007).

Menezes, A., Esplen, P., Bartlett, P., Turner, B., Keel, M., Etherington, V., Conisbee, E., Plant, A., Haslam, V. and England, J. (2007) A system of electronic records developed by a children's hospice. *International Journal of Palliative Nursing*, 13(5): 237–42.

National Institute for Clinical Excellence (NICE) (2004) *Supportive and Palliative Care: The Manual*. London: NICE. http://guidance.nice.org.uk/csgsp/guidance/pdf/English (accessed 28 June 2007).

Pang, S.M. (2003) Medical technology, end-of-life care and nursing ethics. *Nursing Ethics*, 10(3): 236–7.

Protti, D. (2002) *Implementing information for health: even more challenging than expected?* Available at: www.hinf.uvic.ca/archives/Protti.pdf (accessed 5 July 2006). Published by the Department of Health: London.

Purcell, G.P., Wilson, P. and Delamothe, T. (2002) The quality of health information on the internet. *British Medical Journal*, 324: 557–8.

Rabow, M.W., Hauser, J.M. and Adams, J. (2004) Supporting family caregivers at the end of life: 'They don't know what they don't know'. *The Journal of the American Medical Association*, 291(4): 483–91.

Rees, C.E., Bath, P.A. and Lloyd-Williams, M. (1998) The information concerns of spouses of women with breast cancer: Patients' and spouses' perspectives. *Journal of Advanced Nursing*, 28(6): 1249–58.

Royal Flying Doctor Service (RFDS) (2006) *Annual report*. Available at www.flyingdoctor.net/pastannual.htm (accessed 22 August 2007).

Saysell, E. and Routley, C. (2003) Telemedicine in community-based palliative care: evaluation of a videolink teleconference project. *International Journal of Palliative Nursing*, 9(11): 489–95.

Seymour, J. (2003) Technology and 'natural death': a study of older people. *Zeitschrift für Gerontologie und Geriatrie*, 36(5): 339–46.

Singer, P.A. and Bowman, K. (2002) Quality end-of-life care: A global perspective. *BMC Palliative Care*, 1(4). Available at www.biomedcentral.com/1472-684X/1/4 (accessed 21 August 2007).

Smith, A.C., Bensink, M., Armfield, N., Stillman, J. and Caffery, L. (2005) Telemedicine and rural health care applications. *Journal of Postgraduate Medicine*, 51(4): 286–93.

Tang, H. and Ng, J.H.K. (2006) Googling for a diagnosis – use of Google as a diagnostic aid: internet based study. *British Medical Journal*, 333: 1143–5.

Tinnelly, K., Kristjanson, L.J., McCallion, A. and Cousins, K. (2000) Technology in palliative care: steering a new direction or accidental drift? *International Journal of Palliative Nursing*, 6(10): 495–500.

Wooten, R. (2001) Telemedicine. *British Medical Journal*, 323(7312): 557–60.

## Suggestions for further reading

Hersh, W.R. (2003) Information retrieval: a health and biomedical perspective (2nd edn) New York, NY: Springer, ISBN 0387955224.
This book provides an excellent introduction to the theory and application of information retrieval in health and biomedicine. For a comprehensive description and preview of the book, plus a review, search Google using the terms 'Hersh' and 'Information Retrieval'.

Kiley, R. (2003) *Medical Information on the Internet: A Guide for Health Professionals*. Published by Elsevier Health Sciences. ISBN: 0443072159.
As the title suggests, this book provides a very useful introduction to the internet and world wide web for health professionals, including descriptions of specific resources available on the web. For a comprehensive description and preview of the book, plus a review, search for 'Medical Informatics' in Google books.

Shortliffe, E.H. and Perreault, L.E. (eds) (2002) *Medical Informatics: Computer Applications in Health Care and Biomedicine*. Published by Springer-Verlag New York Inc.; 2nd revised edn. ISBN: 0387984720.
This text provides an extensive introduction to health and medical informatics, largely from a US perspective, but with useful consideration of general principles and applications of computerized medical records.

# 32

# Research in palliative care

*Gunn Grande and Christine Ingleton*

---

**Key points**

- Within the broad field of palliative care research, nursing is now emerging as an important focus.
- Many interlinking factors shape the research agenda, including: government, international trends, demographic and cultural change, pressure groups and charities, legislation and user views.
- Palliative care research poses particular methodological challenges owing to its complex nature and the vulnerability of the patient population.
- Palliative care research needs to be flexible and sensitive to ensure responsiveness to fluctuations in patients' ability to contribute, preservation of their privacy, and to enable participants to distance themselves from the research, if they wish.
- Despite the difficulties in conducting research in palliative care, it can be a deeply rewarding activity.

---

# ▎ Introduction

In the current climate of health care, practitioners are accustomed to working within a constantly changing environment, and palliative care is no exception. Changes in government health policy within many industrialized countries are generally aimed at raising standards of care and service delivery within a cost-constrained environment, while ensuring that health care practice is based on research evidence wherever possible.

Within the broad field of palliative care research, nursing is now emerging as an important focus (Seymour *et al.* 2005b). Palliative care is a challenging and expanding area of nursing, with major developments in service organization and the creation of new nursing roles (Seymour *et al.*

2002; Skilbeck *et al.* 2002; Corner *et al.* 2003). Such initiatives require ongoing systematic evaluation, demanding skills in research capability and capacity in the form of dedicated research posts, access to funding and a supportive infrastructure. Within this chapter, we begin with a brief overview of the current status of palliative care nursing research and its contribution to the future direction of palliative care research. We then consider some of the main methodological challenges and opportunities in conducting and participating in palliative care research and evaluation, particularly in relation to:

- factors that influence the palliative care research agenda;
- selecting approaches that are both methodogically appropriate and ethically sensitive;
- capacity building to support research and evaluation in palliative care enquiry;
- getting research and evaluation findings into the public domain in order to influence practice, service development and policy.

# The contribution of nursing to palliative care research to date

Research in palliative care has been influenced by a number of traditions and disciplines. Historically, early research in pain management was influential in establishing the specialty of palliative medicine (Saunders 1958; Twycross and Lack 1983; Hanks and Justins 1992) and involved clinical studies of the effectiveness of treatment, particularly the treatment of pain. More recently, nurses have been active in shaping research in this important area of work (Seymour *et al.* 2005b). Alongside these clinical studies, research adopting sociological and psychosocial perspectives has explored experiences of death and dying (Glaser and Strauss 1965; Quint 1967; Field 1989), with bereavement and communication studies emerging as important and influential themes (Kubler-Ross 1969; Murray Parkes 1970; Faulkner 1992). Cartwright *et al.* (1973) added a public health perspective by investigating patterns in the UK of symptoms, needs and care in the year before death. These early studies were crucial in establishing the specialty of palliative care and provided important data on care of the dying person. In her review of research in palliative care published from 1966 onwards, Corner (1996) found that pain and symptom control accounted for 21 per cent of the work, studies of health workers for 17 per cent and studies evaluating patient care 9 per cent. A review by Wilkes (1998) that focused on nursing research 1987–1996 found a slightly different emphasis where 22 per cent of studies considered professional issues, 19 per cent patient care services and 16 per cent psychosocial issues, while 15 per cent considered pain and symptom control. A more recent review of medical and nursing journals by Kaasa *et al.* (2006) reports that symptom control and management remains the most common topic (36 per cent), followed by service delivery and development (27 per cent). While these were the two main topics both for nursing and medical journals, nursing journals contained a smaller proportion of studies on symptom control and management (27 per cent versus 37 per cent of papers). Furthermore, they were more likely to contain studies on education (12 per cent versus 3 per cent) and less likely to report studies of assessment and methodology (1 per cent versus 13 per cent) than medical journals.

Corner (1996) found that early palliative care studies were characteristically descriptive, employing survey methods, retrospective views of patients' case notes and reviews of admissions to hospices and palliative care. Correspondingly, early nursing research commonly used surveys for quantitative research, but Wilkes (1998) also reported a large proportion of qualitative studies. Kaasa *et al.* (2006) similarly show nursing journals to contain considerably more qualitative studies than medical journals (27 per cent versus 9 per cent of papers). They also contain fewer (quantitative) descriptive and retrospective studies (6 per cent versus 22 per cent), prospective and comparative studies (1 per cent versus 15 per cent), and more comment and review papers (31 per cent versus 18 per cent) than medical journals. Overall, randomized controlled trials (RCTs) represent a very small proportion of palliative care research both in medicine and nursing (4 per cent Kaasa *et al.* 2006).

While nursing in general makes a very small contribution to UK NHS research compared to its contribution to care (Rafferty *et al.* 2004), palliative care is an area where the discipline is particularly strong in terms of quality research (Rafferty and Traynor 2006). Nurses represent the largest single group of the research workforce (34 per cent) and a high number of research groups with ten or more research staff are led by nurses (four of nine, NCRI 2004). Nursing appears in particular to make an important contribution to qualitative research in palliative care. Nearly half (48.6 per cent) of qualitative papers relating to palliative care published between 1990 and 1999 were from nursing journals (Bailey *et al.* 2002). Wilkes (1998) found that the UK was the origin of the highest number palliative nursing research publications, ahead of the USA, Australia and Canada.

## Factors that influence the future palliative care research agenda

Many interlinking factors shape the research agenda, including: government, NHS and international trends, demographic and cultural change, pressure groups and charities, legislation and user views. For instance, in the UK, government and cancer research funding bodies combined efforts to review the current state of palliative care research and provide directions for the future (National Cancer Research Institute (NCRI) 2004; National Institute of Clinical Excellence (NICE) 2004). This highlighted areas of

---

**Box 32.1**   Strong and weak evidence as defined by NICE (2004)

**Strong evidence**
Identifying patient needs and
problems

Face-to-face communication
(including training)
Information giving
Psychological support
Specialist palliative care

**Weak evidence**
How to address patient needs and
problems

Coordination and integration of care
User involvement
Social care
Spiritual support
General palliative care
Rehabilitation
Complementary therapies
Support for families and carers
Bereavement support

---

importance to cancer patients and their carers where the evidence is already strong and areas where more research is required (Box 32.1). The NCRI (2004) review has led to the establishment of two national research collaboratives to build research capacity and take the research agenda forward (Bailey *et al.* 2006).

Tools to support care promoted under the NHS End of Life Care Programme are furthermore likely to form part of future evaluation (Thomas and Noble 2007; Lhuisser *et al.* 2007), likewise the development of new professional roles (Seymour *et al*, 2002; Ryan-Woolley *et al.* 2007). The increasing proportion of older people in developed countries pose new challenges for palliative care (Davies and Higginson 2004), suggesting future research will focus on challenges of frail old age, increased cognitive impairment and co-morbidities, increased care-giver burden and care home provision (Hockley and Froggatt 2006; Kite 2006). The increasing proportion of people living alone will require further investigation into the feasibility of supporting care at home, while an increasingly multicultural society requires understanding of culture sensitive delivery of palliative care. Internationally, service user views are increasingly likely to influence research topics (Wright *et al.* 2006). Taken together, researching these diverse issues will present many methodological challenges (see Box 32.2). We will now discuss these methodological challenges in turn.

---

# Challenges faced by palliative care researchers

## *Multi-method approach*

Palliative care poses particular challenges for research due to its complex nature and the vulnerability of the patient population. Palliative care is holistic and multidisciplinary, encompassing control of pain and other

---

**Box 32.2**   Challenges faced by palliative care researchers

- Multi-method designs
- Defining samples
- Loss of participants and data
- Establishing outcome measures
- Understanding interventions
- Comparing interventions
- Conducting ethically sensitive research

---

symptoms, psychological, social and spiritual problems and addressing the needs of both patients and carers (Higginson 1997). The needs and journeys of patients and carers and the interventions required to address them are complex. Palliative care therefore requires multi-method research approaches to tackle that complexity. The recent review of palliative care (NICE 2004) recognizes how both qualitative and quantitative research needs to be incorporated into the hierarchy of evidence. Each approach can capture something that cannot be captured by the other (Ingleton and Davies 2007).

Qualitative approaches are valuable in capturing what matters to people, their experiences, the dimensions and variations of complex phenomena, processes, systems and contexts (Payne 2007). Quantitative approaches are valuable in capturing the prevalence and degree of phenomena, identifying overall patterns, associations, antecedents and consequences (Bennett 2007). Quantitative approaches benefit from qualitative input to ask the relevant questions, understand what is behind the numbers and patterns, and why something works. Qualitative approaches benefit from quantitative input to establish wider patterns, generalizability of findings, the strength of relationships or trends and the relative contribution of different factors. For instance, quantitative studies show that older patients are consistently less likely to be referred to palliative care than younger patients (Grande *et al.* 1998), a pattern that would have been difficult to discover through qualitative research. However, in order to understand fully why this pattern occurs and its potential solutions, we need to draw on more qualitative approaches.

The need for multi-method approaches requires palliative care researchers to have a good understanding of the contribution of each approach and to work collaboratively to combine research skills and perspectives to address important research topics effectively. Nursing may in particular hold strengths in qualitative research, although the quality of some this research may still be improved. For a more detailed consideration of the problems in evaluating quality in research, see Crookes and Davies (2004).

### Defining the patient sample

Difficulties in defining who is a palliative care patient pose problems both for palliative care research and providers (Addington-Hall 2002). This definition is difficult regarding cancer patients and even more so when considering patients with other diagnoses. While in its broadest definition any patient facing problems of life-threatening illness may come under the umbrella of palliative care, palliative care patients have been defined on the basis of limited prognosis, care switching from curative to palliative or having palliative care needs. All these definitions are broad and open to subjective judgement. For instance, professionals differ considerably in their assessment of who has palliative care needs (e.g. Gott *et al.* 2001).

Reluctance by professionals to attach a palliative care label to patients may mean that patients are not referred to interventions and studies until they are too ill. Conversely, a desire by gatekeepers to protect patients may mean that they only allow access to patients who are doing well physically and psychologically (Ewing *et al.* 2004). Therefore, while the population of palliative care patients is diffuse and heterogeneous due to problems with definition, any given study may contain a very small and selective sample of patients. This makes study findings difficult to generalize and compare as different patient groups may have different needs and respond differently to interventions.

Solutions include placing more emphasis on understanding and describing the patient sample in any given study, more longitudinal research to improve our understanding of needs and preferences of patients at different stages of illness (NCRI 2004), better prognostication and clearer recruitment criteria (Maltoni and Tassinari 2004; Steinhauser *et al.* 2006). More representative samples have been obtained in studies using more participatory approaches (Hopkinson *et al.* 2005) and with greater emphasis on establishing patient rapport and involvement (Steinhauser *et al.* 2006), and further development of such approaches offer promising directions for the future.

### Loss of participants and data

Regardless of any improvements through participatory approaches, the nature of palliative care means that research often represents the experiences of the patients that are least ill (Hanks *et al.* 2002; McPherson and Addington-Hall 2003). A study by Rathbone *et al.* (1994) found that even when patients were involved in research, only 79 per cent were able to answer three simple questions in their last three weeks of life, 57 per cent in their last two weeks and 29 per cent in their last week. Palliative care studies have therefore often used proxies to speak for the patient; normally a family carer or a health professional, to minimize patient burden, reduce loss of information and represent more patients in studies. Data may be collected prospectively, while the patient is alive. However, many studies have used retrospective data collection after the patient's death, normally from the patient's next of kin (Cartwright *et al.* 1973; Addington-Hall *et al.* 1998a and b). As it is difficult to identify many patients with potential palliative care needs until death, this is sometimes the only means of gaining insight into the palliative care of some patient groups, particularly for other diagnoses than cancer (McPherson and Addington-Hall 2003). However, the views of proxies may not always represent patients' views, and may rather reflect carers' own distress (Addington-Hall and McPherson 2001). A review by McPherson and Addington-Hall (2003) concluded that proxies can reliably report on the quality of services and on observable symptoms. However, they are less accurate on subjective aspects of the patient's experience, such as pain, anxiety and depression. Again, to get a complete picture we need to use a range of approaches, to sensitively gain patients' own views from those able and willing to contribute, and to gain some insight, albeit vicariously, into the experiences of the whole patient population and the later stages of terminal illness.

### Outcome measures

Palliative care poses particular challenges in designing outcome measures that are sensitive and relevant to patients. When evaluating how palliative care impacts on patients, common outcome measures of mortality, morbidity and survival do not apply, as the inevitable outcome is death. Physical deterioration is a natural part of the process, and palliative care 'aims neither to hasten, nor to postpone death' (www.who.int/cancer/palliative/definition/en). Many palliative care outcome measures have been designed to measure aspects of quality of life, but rarely cover all domains important to palliative care (Hearn and Higginson 1997, 1999) and lengthy measures are inappropriate for most patients. Developing a core measure that can be supplemented with smaller modules that are appropriate and sensitive to particular aspects/situations may be a solution (Echteld *et al.* 2006). Recent reviews (NCRI 2004; NICE 2004) stress the need to develop and use consistent and sensitive outcome measures to build up the evidence base in palliative care, noting a need to 'develop measures for less tangible, patient-centred outcomes, e.g. hope' (NCRI 2004). This suggests we need to work more closely with patients themselves in the development of such measures while acknowledging that it is not possible (or desirable) to measure all outcomes using quantitative approaches.

### Understanding interventions

Palliative care is by its nature holistic, tailored to the individual and multidisciplinary in nature. Palliative care interventions are therefore not simple and cannot easily be standardized without threatening the ethos of palliative care. Consequently, when evaluating such interventions we need to gain a far better understanding of the intervention itself than would be the case for drugs trials, for example. Correspondingly, evaluations of palliative care require more work in the developmental phases (MRC 2002; NCRI 2004). That is, to understand how and why palliative care interventions work, we need a better understanding of external influences (including organizational constraints and responses to the intervention), the components of the intervention and their interaction, its likely active ingredients, and how the intervention may need to be adapted for different groups (MRC 2002). Palliative care interventions need to be flexible and adaptable to local circumstances, and new approaches are required to enable systematic evaluation of such variation (Hawe *et al.* 2004). There is growing recognition for the need to combine qualitative approaches such as interviews, focus groups and case studies with more traditional quantitative approaches to understand the processes, people and context of complex interventions within health service evaluation (Bradley *et al.* 1999; Campbell *et al.* 2000) and the challenge is to develop such an approach.

### Comparing interventions

Review of palliative care research highlights the need for more evaluation and comparative studies to improve the evidence base (NCRI 2004; NICE 2004). As this normally involves comparing patients who receive different care, this can pose ethical dilemmas because we want all patients to have the best possible care, and a new service is often presumed to be better even if its value is not proven. This is particularly difficult within RCTs which are seen by some as the gold standard for evaluation. One trial arm is normally seen as better than the other, therefore the principle of equipoise between the two arms is not perceived to apply, except perhaps when comparing two versions of the same intervention (MRC 2002), or services to facilitate utilization of existing services (Addington-Hall *et al.* 1992). Resource limitations are commonplace in health care, and it may under some circumstances be acceptable to use randomization as a means to allocate patients to scarce resources (Grande *et al.* 1999). A promising way forward for palliative care evaluations may be the use of cluster randomized trials (Jordhoy *et al.* 2000; Fowell *et al.* 2006), whereby for example, teams, practices or geographical areas are randomized to an intervention rather than individual patients. Nevertheless, randomization will often be difficult to achieve within palliative care evaluation, and reviews suggest that a well-designed, non-randomized comparative study may provide better evidence than a small, poorly designed and exclusive RCT (Britton *et al.* 1998). Precisely because of considerable local variation in provision, palliative care lends itself to quasi-experimental studies. For instance, new initiatives such as the Gold Standards Framework (Thomas and Noble 2007), the Liverpool Care Pathway (Ellershaw *et al.* 1997) or the Preferred Place of Care Document (NHS 2006) are rolled out at different times, in different locations and offer opportunities for rigorous comparison studies. With such an approach we cannot assume that differences between intervention and control groups are due to the intervention with the same certainty as for RCTs. However, both qualitative investigation of local context and quantitative control for baseline differences can help us assess whether outcomes are likely to be due to the intervention or to confounding factors. The future direction of comparative studies is likely to involve multi-site evaluation. This again emphasizes the need for future palliative care to promote teamwork and collaboration.

### Conducting ethically sensitive research

Ethics in health care research involves achieving an appropriate balance between the desire to extend knowledge and the rights of the research participants (Robbins 1998). Such tensions are exacerbated when research involves particularly vulnerable people, such as the terminally ill and their families. Concerns include the burden imposed on participants, the preciousness of the limited time they have left, patients' unease with criticizing care on which they are dependent, and lack of tangible benefits to participants from the research (Addington-Hall 2002; Seymour *et al.* 2005b). While quantitative research may place considerable energy and time demands on participants, qualitative research may be more intrusive and prompt difficult emotions (Wilkie 1997; Dean and McClement 2002). Although not unique to palliative care such ethical challenges are often more acute in this context. Concerns about the ethics of involving people who are dying in research have consequently been widely expressed and debated (de Raeve 1994; Wilkie 1997; Field *et al.* 2001). The argument that research is an ethical imperative to ensure improved quality of care has been placed against the view that palliative care research places too great a demand on people who are very ill (Field *et al.* 2001). When patients themselves are asked, their view of research appears overwhelmingly positive (Dean and McClement 2002) and Hopkinson *et al.* (2005) argue that excluding palliative care patients from research removes their autonomous choice and right to decision-making. Terry *et al.* (2006) found that patients felt that research gave a valued opportunity to give something back, to be seen as something more than just a dying person, and to gain reassurance that palliative care is considered sufficiently important to warrant research to optimize care.

Any palliative care research requires thorough consideration of research ethics. Researchers must ensure that research questions are relevant and the research design rigorous to reduce burden to a minimum and make optimal use of data collected (Field *et al.* 2001: 78). This includes careful piloting to establish the appropriateness of the design and materials (Robbins 1998, Addington-Hall 2002) and user involvement in the development where possible (Hopkinson *et al.* 2005). For instance, when hospice patients were asked about design in one study (Terry *et al.* 2006), they wanted to be approached about participation by a health professional involved in their care, to have researchers who understood their situation and the issues of dying, to have health professionals take responsibility for explaining the research to families, and to receive verbal explanations rather than having to read documents.

Palliative care research needs to be flexible and sensitive to ensure responsiveness to fluctuations in patients' ability to contribute, preservation of their privacy, and to enable participants at times to distance themselves from the research if necessary (Robbins 1998, Seymour *et al.* 2005b). Sensitivity also has to be exercised in preserving patients' level of awareness of their prognosis, as it cannot be assumed that all patients have a similar degree of awareness (Addington-Hall 2002; Seymour *et al.* 2005b). Careful thought should be given to potential researcher role conflict and guidelines for action if anything arises that may require intervention (Dean and McClement 2002).

Both the patient's circumstances and their view of their participation may change considerably during the course of palliative care research, posing problems for informed consent (Lawton 1998). For some studies consent may need to be renegotiated at regular intervals (Robbins 1998; Addington-Hall 2002). Ethics suggest erring on the side of caution if there are unclear messages about willingness to participate (Seymour *et al.* 2005b). Any concerns about cognitive impairment may suggest screening for cognitive deficits before recruitment to ensure consent is truly informed (Addington-Hall 2002; Dean and McClement 2002).

## Building research capacity and capability

In many respects, palliative care nursing research is still in its infancy and requires a sustained programme of investment if nursing practice in palliative care is to be underpinned by a sound and well-constructed knowledge base. While the UK NCRI (2004) review noted several strengths of nursing research within palliative care, many problems were also uncovered. Nursing research typically involved single-site small-scale studies and was often not taken seriously enough by other disciplines for true collaboration. The report noted a lack of academic career structure, the long time it took to become a researcher, fixed-term research contracts and a pronounced clinical/academic split causing researchers to become isolated from the clinical setting. While Rafferty and Traynor (2004) note improvements in productivity and quality for nursing in general, they also highlight that a very high proportion of published research in nursing remains unfunded, a low output of publications overall and a low number of PhDs.

To improve the research base for nursing there is a need to build capacity through training and protected time, combined with funding for infrastructure and research (Dean and McClement 2002). The UK Clinical Research Collaboration has outlined the steps it believes are required to achieve such capacity building within nursing in a five-year programme (UKCRC 2006). This includes introducing dedicated nursing award schemes for Masters, PhD and post-doctoral career development to develop the skill base. Furthermore, there is a need to improve career flexibility through introduction of sessionally based contracts to enable balancing of clinical and research commitments and provide protected time for research. Finally, there needs to be a mentoring system for aspiring researchers and better careers advice. These developments are conjoint with the UK Department of Health Capacity Development Programme, aiming to strengthen research capacity of all NHS health professionals (DOH 2006) and the National Information Services in Australia (Albert and Mickan 2002). Although research capacity building has been recognized internationally as important (c.f. Farmer and Weston's work in Australia 2002 and the North American Primary Care Research Group 2002), there is currently little evidence on how to plan and measure progress in research capacity building, or agreement to determining activities. Traditional outputs in peer reviewed journals, and successful grant capture may be the easy and important outcomes to measure, but they do not necessarily address issues to do with the usefulness of research, professional outcomes, or on measuring health gain. A useful framework is provided by Cooke (see Box 32.3), which could form the basis by which measuring the impact of research capacity building could be achieved, shaped around six principles of research capacity building, and which includes four structural levels on which each principle can be applied.

---

**Box 32.3** Examples of research capacity development indicators

| PRINCIPLE | INDICATOR |
|---|---|
| Skills development | Evidence and use of research secondments opportunities. |
| Infrastructure | Evidence of resource investment from the organization to support pump-priming of research, e.g. research support sessions, pump-priming money for pre-protocol or pilot work. |
| Close to practice | Number of projects that have user involvement built into them. |
| Linkages | Evidence of links with regional research and development units. |
| Dissemination | The organization has a searchable database of projects and findings. |
| Sustainability | Evidence in the strategy of year-on-year commitment to research development. |
| Leadership | There is a director of R&D within the organization. |
| Research culture | Achievements in research have a high profile and are celebrated, e.g. in newsletters, showcase events, praise and rewards. |
| Research activity | Level of research activity hosted by the organization. |

Reproduced with permission of author, Jo Cooke

## Gaining access to funding and support for palliative care research

The first step in preparing a successful proposal is in knowing where to apply for funding. There are many types of potential funders for palliative care research (see Box 32.4) and many types of grant opportunities available for would-be researchers to access. These range from explicit invitations to tender to undertake a clearly specified project to a more flexible and open agenda in which funding agencies invite researchers to develop their own ideas within broad parameters.

Developing funding proposals and accessing sources of funding are skilled and time-consuming activities. For nurses who want to become involved in research, collaboration on projects with experienced researchers is a good way to get started. When moving on to independent research, it is important to start small with pilot studies and then build on these to develop larger studies (Dean and McClement 2002). Linking with academic colleagues and securing appropriate mentorship and supervision is important throughout the development of your own research (see Ingleton and Davies 2004). The palliative care collaboratives under NCRI, for instance, aim to facilitate such linking and mentorship (Bailey *et al.* 2006). However, nursing still suffers from a lack of doctorally prepared nursing professionals to meet the growing need for supervision of new researchers (Ingleton *et al.* 2001). It is important to ensure emotional support is available alongside academic mentorship and supervision to help researchers deal with the emotional challenges of palliative care research (Sque 2000) including potential role conflicts of researcher and clinician in the face of patient and carer need (Dean and McClement 2002).

### Getting research findings into the public domain in order to influence practice and service development

Unfortunately, dissemination of findings is something that is usually thought about at the conclusion of the project rather than at the outset. This

---

**Box 32.4**   Potential funding sources

- Government and state funded health and social care research agencies
- Research councils
- Health care and disease specific charities
- Professional organizations
- Pan national organisations
- Institutional funding
- Partnerships with industry

is part of the research process that is frequently allowed little or no time; it must be somehow fitted alongside other commitments.

There may be a number of conflicting pressures that have to be reconciled at the dissemination stage of the research project. For example, projects that relate to new products and treatment interventions may be tentative about reporting findings due to constraints by commercial sponsors. Commissioned research, in particular evaluation studies, undertaken for government departments, health authorities and trusts, or major evaluations, may be subject to contractual clauses that restrict or control the process of dissemination.

Although publication in peer reviewed journals is often advocated by academic departments to ensure positive research assessment exercise ratings, such journals may not be those to which nurses working in palliative care and cancer care subscribe, and so the impact of evidence upon practice may be limited (Richardson *et al.* 2001).

There is also the question of how others will react to the work itself. The mechanisms of peer review, external examination of research degrees and conference presentations act as quality control mechanisms to some extent. Citation indexes provide some evidence of whether the research appears to have contributed to knowledge, changed attitudes, or influenced policy or practice.

# Conclusion

Despite the many challenges that exist in conducting research in palliative care, it can be a rewarding experience. Research in palliative care nursing has come a long way in the past 30 years. Nurses are making a growing contribution to the wider palliative care research community in terms of publications in international academic and professional journals and presentations at interdisciplinary conferences but there is still some way to go. Designated research and practice units now exist and greater resources and effort are being put into both, synthesizing the evidence in the form of systematic reviews and producing evidence relevant to practice. Nurses already possess the many strengths and skills necessary to foster research collaboration and find a clear and distinct position within the mainstream of interdisciplinary effort. Looking to the future, joint initiatives between clinical and academic centres may enhance the relevance and timeliness of research and so reduce the much discussed theory–practice gap. Likewise, the development of collaborative research groups within and between academic and service organizations and user groups are further mechanisms for creating working partnerships. Developing leaders at the highest level who can influence strategy and policy is crucial to the further advancement of the research and development agenda in palliative care nursing.

# References

Addington-Hall, J.M. (2002) Research sensitivities to palliative care patients. *European Journal of Cancer Care*, 11: 220–4.

Addington-Hall, J.M. and McPherson, C. (2001) After death interviews with surrogates/bereaved family members: some issues of validity. *Journal of Pain and Symptom Management*, 22: 794–9.

Addington-Hall, J.M., MacDonald, L.D., Anderson, H.R., Chamberlain, J., Freeling, P., Bland, J.M. and Raftery, J. (1998a) Randomised controlled trial of effects of coordinating care for terminally ill cancer patients. *British Medical Journal*, 305: 1317–22.

Addington-Hall, J.M., Walker, L., Jones, C., Karlsen, S. and McCarth, M. (1998b) A randomised controlled trial of postal versus interview administration of a questionnaire measuring satisfaction with and use of services received in the year before death. *Journal of Epidemiology and Community Health*, 52: 802–7.

Albert, E. and Mickan, S. (2002) Closing the gap and widening the scope. *Australian Family Physician*, 31: 1038–41.

Bailey, C., Froggatt, K., Field, D. and Krishnasamy, M. (2002) The nursing contribution to qualitative research in palliative care, 1990–1999. *Journal of Advanced Nursing*, 40(1): 48–51.

Bailey, C., Wilson, R., Addington-Hall, J., Payne, S., Clark, D., Lloyd-Williams, M., Molassiotis, A. and Seymour, J. (2006) The Cancer Experiences Collaborative (CECo): building research capacity in supportive and palliative care. *Progress in Palliative Care*, 14(6): 265–70.

Bennett, M. (2007) Principles of designing clinical trials. In: J. Addington-Hall, E. Bruera, I. Higginson and S. Payne (eds) *Research Methods in Palliative Care*. 2: 13–26. Oxford: Oxford University Press.

Bradley, F., Wiles, R., Kinmonth, A-L., Mant, D. and Gantley, M. for the SHIP Collaborative Group (1999) Development and evaluation of complex intervention in health services research: case study of the Southampton heart integrated care project (SHIP). *British Medical Journal*, pp. 711–15.

Britton, A., McKee, M., Black, N., McPherson, K., Sanderson, C. and Bain, C. (1998) Choosing between randomised and non-randomised studies: a systematic review. *Health Technol Assessment*, 2(13).

Campbell, M., Fitzpatrick, R., Haines, A., Kinmonth, A-L., Sandercock, P., Spiegelhalter, D. and Tyrer, P. (2000). Framework for design and evaluation of complex interventions to improve health. *British Medical Journal*, 321: 694–6.

Cartwright, A., Hockey, L. and Anderson, J.L. (1973). *Life before death*. London: Routledge & Kegan Paul.

Corner, J. (1996) Is there a research paradigm for palliative care? *Palliative Medicine*, 10: 201–8.

Corner, J., Halliday, D., Haviland, J., Douglas, H.R., Bath, P., Clark, D., Normand, C., Beech, N., Hughes, P., Marples, R., Seymour, J., Skilbeck, J. and Webb, T. (2003) Exploring nursing outcomes for patients with advanced cancer following intervention by Macmillan specialist palliative care nurses. *Journal of Advanced Nursing*, 41(6): 561–75.

Crookes, P. and Davies, S. (eds) (2004) *Research into practice; essential skills in interpreting and applying research for nursing and health care*. London: Bailliere Tindall.

Davies, E. and Higginson, I. (2004) *Better palliative care for older people.* WHO Report.

Dean, R.A. and McClement, S.E. (2002) Palliative care research: methodological and ethical challenges. *International Journal of Palliative Nursing*, 8(8): 376–80.

Department of Health (DoH) (2006) *Best Research for Best Health – a new national health strategy.* London: DoH.

de Raeve, L. (1994) Ethical issues in palliative care research. *Palliative Medicine*, 8: 298–305.

Echteld, M.A., Onwuteaka-Philipsen, B., van der Wal, G., Deliens, L. and Klein, M. (2006) EORTC QLQ-C15-PAL: the new standard in the assessment of health-related quality of life in advanced cancer? *Palliative Medicine*, 20: 1–2.

Ellershaw, J., Foster, A., Murphy, D., Shea, T. and Overill, S. (1997) Developing an integrated care pathway for the dying patient. *European Journal of Palliative Care*, 4(2): 203–7.

Ewing, G., Rogers, M., Barclay, S., McCabe, J., Martin, A. and Todd, C. (2004) Recruiting patients into a primary care based study of palliative care: why is it so difficult? *Palliative Medicine*, 18: 452–9.

Farmer, E. and Weston, K. (2002) A conceptual model for capacity building in Australian primary care research. *Australian Family Physician*, 31: 1139–42.

Faulkner, A. (1992) The evaluation of training programmes for communicating skills in palliative care. *Journal of Cancer Care*, 4: 175–8.

Field, D. (1989) *Nursing the dying.* London: Routledge/Tavistock.

Field, D., Clark, D., Corner, J. and Davis, C. (eds) (2001) *Researching Palliative Care.* Buckingham: Open University Press.

Fowell, A., Johnstone, R., Finlay, I.G., Russell, D. and Russell, I.T. (2006) Design of trials with dying patients: a feasibility study of cluster randomisation versus randomised consent. *Palliative Medicine*, 20(8): 799–804.

Glaser, B. and Strauss, A. (1965) *Awareness of Dying.* Chicago: Aldine.

Gott, M.C., Ahmedzai, S.H. and Wood, C. (2001) How many inpatients at an acute hospital have palliative care needs? Comparing the perspectives of medical and nursing staff. *Palliative Medicine*, 15: 451–60.

Grande, G.E., Todd, C.J., Barclay, S.I.G. and Farquhar, M.C. (1999) Does hospital at home for palliative care facilitate home death? A randomised controlled trial. *British Medical Journal*, 319: 1472–5.

Grande, G.E., Addington-Hall, J.M. and Todd, C.J. (1998) Place of death and access to home care services: are certain patient groups at a disadvantage? *Social Science and Medicine*, 47(5): 565–79.

Hanks, G.W. and Justins, D.M. (1992) Cancer pain: management. *Lancet*, 339: 1031–6.

Hanks, G.W., Robbins, M., Sharp, D., Forbes, K., Done, K., Peters, T.J., Morgan, H., Sykes, J., Baxter, K., Corfe, F. and Bidgood, C. (2002) The imPaCT study: a randomised controlled trial to evaluate a hospital palliative care team. *British Journal of Cancer*, 87: 733–9.

Hawe, P., Shiell, A. and Riley, T. (2004) Complex interventions: how 'out of control' can a randomised controlled trial be? *British Medical Journal*, 328: 1561–3.

Hearn, J. and Higginson, I.J. (1997) Outcome measures in palliative care for advanced cancer patients: a review. *Journal of Public Health Medicine*, 19(2): 193–9.

Hearn, J. and Higginson, I.J. on behalf of the Palliative Care Core Audit Project Advisory Group (1999) Development and validation of a core outcome measure for palliative care. *Quality in Health Care*, 8: 219–27.

Higginson, I. (1997) *Palliative and Terminal Care*. Health Care Needs Assessment, Second Series. A. Stevens and J. Raftery (eds) Abingdon: Radcliffe Medical Press.

Hockley, J. and Froggatt, K. (2006) The development of palliative care knowledge in care homes for older people: the place of action research. *Palliative Medicine*, 20(8): 835–43.

Hopkinson, J.B., Wright, D.N. and Corner, J.L. (2005) Seeking new methodology for palliative care research: challenging assumptions about studying people who are approaching the end of life. *Palliative Medicine*, 19(7): 532–7.

Ingleton, C., Ramcharan, P., Ellis, L. and Schofield, P. (2001) Introducing a professional doctorate in nursing and midwifery. *British Journal of Nursing*, 10(22): 1469–76.

Ingleton, C. and Davies, S. (2004) Research and scholarship in palliative care. In: S. Payne, J. Seymour and C. Ingleton (eds) *Palliative Care Nursing: Principles and Evidence for Practice*, 35: 676–97. London: McGraw-Hill.

Ingleton, C. and Davies, S. (2007) Mixed methods for evaluation research. In: J. Addington-Hall, E. Bruera, I. Higginson and S. Payne (eds) *Research Methods in Palliative Care*, 12: 191–207. Oxford: Oxford University Press.

Jordhoy, M.S., Fayers, P., Saltnes, T., Ahlner-Elmquist, M., Jannert, M. and Kaasa, S. (2000) A palliative care intervention and death at home: a cluster randomised trial. *Lancet*, 356: 888–93.

Kaasa, S., Hjermstad, M.J. and Loge, J.H. (2006) Methodological and structural challenges in palliative care research: how have we fared in the last decades? *Palliative Medicine*, 20(8): 727–34.

Kite, S. (2006) Palliative care for older people. Editorial. *Age and Ageing*, July issue: 1–3.

Kubler-Ross, E. (1969) *On Death and Dying*. London: Tavistock.

Lawton, J. (1998) Contemporary hospice care: the sequestration of the unbounded body and 'dirty dying'. *Sociology of Health and Illness*, 20(2): 121–43.

Lhussier, M., Carr, S.M. and Wilcockson, J. (2007) The evaluation of an end of life integrated care pathway. *International Journal of Palliative Nursing*, 13(2): 74–81.

Maltoni, M. and Tassinari, D. (2004) Prognostic assessment in terminally ill cancer patients, from evidence-based knowledge to a patient-physician relationship and back. *Palliative Medicine*, 18(1): 77–9.

McPherson, C.J. and Addington-Hall, J.M. (2003) Judging the quality of care at the end of life: can proxies provide reliable information? *Social Science & Medicine*, **56**(1): 95–109.

Murray Parkes, C. (1970) Seeking and finding a lost object: evidence from recent studies of reaction to bereavement. *Social Science and Medicine*, 4: 187–201.

Medical Research Council (MRC) (2002) *A framework for development and evaluation of RCTs for complex interventions to improve health*. London: MRC.

National Cancer Research Institute (NCRI) (2004) *Supportive and palliative care in the UK: Report of the NCRI Strategic Planning Group on Supportive and Palliative Care*.

National Health Service (2006) The End of Life Care Programme. www.endoflifecarenhs.uk or www.eolc.cbcl.co.uk/eolc

NICE (2004) *Guidance on Cancer Services Improving Supportive and Palliative Care for Adults with cancer*. Oxford: NICE.

North American Primary Care Research Group (2002) What does it mean to build research capacity? *Family Medicine*, 34: 678–84.

Payne, S. (2007) Qualitative methods of data collection and analysis. In: J. Addington-Hall, E. Bruera, I. Higginson and S. Payne (eds). *Research Methods in Palliative Care*, 9: 139–59. Oxford: Oxford University Press.

Quint, J.C. (1967) Institutional practices of information control. *Psychiatry*, 28: 119–32.

Rafferty, A.M. and Traynor, M. (2004) Context, convergence and contingency: political leadership for nursing. *Journal of Nursing Management*, 12: 258–65.

Rafferty, A.M. and Traynor, M. (2006) Assessing research quality. *Journal of Advanced Nursing*, 56(1): 2–4.

Rathbone, G.V., Horsley, S. and Goacher, J. (1994) A self-evaluated assessment suitable for seriously ill hospice patients. *Palliative Medicine*, 8(1): 29–34.

Richardson, A., Miller, M. and Potter, H. (2001) Developing, delivering and evaluating cancer nursing services: Building the evidence base. *Nursing Times Research*, 6(4): 726–35.

Robbins, M. (1998) *Evaluating palliative care: establishing the evidence base*. Oxford: Oxford University Press.

Ryan-Woolley, B.M., McHugh, G.A. and Luker, K.A. (2007) Prescribing by specialist nurses in cancer and palliative care: results of a national survey. *Palliative Medicine*, 21(4): 273–7.

Saunders, C. (1958) Dying of cancer. *St Thomas's Hospital Gazette*, 56(2): 37–47.

Seymour, J., Clark, D., Hughes, P., Bath, P., Beech, N., Corner, J., Douglas, H-R., Halliday, D., Haviland, J., Marples, R., Normand, C., Skilbeck, J. and Webb, T. (2002) Clinical nurse specialists in palliative care. Part 3. Issues for the Macmillan Nurse role. *Palliative Medicine*, 16(5): 386–94.

Seymour, J., Clark, D. and Winslow, M. (2005b) Pain and palliative care: the emergence of a new speciality. *Journal of Pain and Symptom Management*, 29(1): 2–13.

Skilbeck, J., Corner, J., Bath, P. *et al.* (2002) Clinical nurse specialists in palliative care (1): a description of the Macmillan nurse caseload. *Palliative Medicine*, 16: 285–96.

Steinhauser, K.E., Clipp, E.C., Hays, J.C., Olsen, M., Arnold, R., Christakis, N.A., Lindquist, J.H. and Tulsky, J.A. (2006) Identifying, recruiting, and retaining seriously-ill patients and their caregivers in longitudinal research. *Palliative Medicine*, 20(8): 745–54.

Sque, M. (2000) Researching the bereaved: an investigator's experience. *Nursing Ethics*, 7(1): 23–34.

Terry, W., Olson, L.G., Ravenscroft, P., Wilss, L. and Boulton-Lewis, G. (2006) Hospice patients' views on research in palliative care. *Internal Medicine Journal*, 36: 406–13.

Thomas, K. and Noble, N. (2007) Improving the delivery of palliative care in general practice: an evaluation of the first phase of the Gold Standards Framework. *Palliative Medicine*, 21(1): 49–53

Twycross, R.G. and Lack, S.A (1983) *Symptom control in Far-Advanced Cancer: Pain Relief*. London: Pitman.

UK Clinical Research Collaboration (UKCRC) (2006) 'Developing the best research professionals'. Qualified graduate nurses: recommendations for preparing and supporting clinical academic nurses of the future. Draft report of the UKCRC Sub Committee for Nurses in Clinical Research (Workforce).

Wilkes, L. (1998) Palliative care nursing research trends from 1987–1996. *International Journal of Palliative Nursing*, 4(3): 128–34.

Wilkie, P. (1997) Ethical issues in qualitative research in palliative care. *Palliative Medicine*, 11: 321–4.

Wright, D.N., Hopkinson, J.B., Corner, J.L. and Foster, C.L. (2006) How to involve cancer patients at the end of life as co-researchers. *Palliative Medicine*, 20(8): 821–7.

# 33

# Practice development in palliative care

*Katherine Froggatt and Mary Turner*

---

**Key points**

- Practice development is a process that enables changes in health and social care provision to be undertaken in order to improve the quality of care people receive.
- Practice development, while having common elements to staff development, education, audit and research, differs from them all and has the potential to bring about change in both individual practitioners and organizational practices.
- Sustainable practice development requires practitioners to be aware of the following elements: the knowledge they use to base their justification for change; the context within which they seek to bring about change; and the way they bring about the change.

---

# Introduction

An important emphasis within palliative care is to ensure that people dying with any condition receive high-quality end-of-life care. This has led to a need for the palliative care speciality to engage with ways that can help palliative care practitioners improve the quality of the care they provide. In this chapter, we address the following issues:

- a brief introduction to practice development comparing it to other organizational and staff development activities;
- we consider three dimensions of practice development that require attention if practice development is to be successful and sustained:
  - the knowledge used to justify and shape the changes introduced;

○   the context within which the practice development initiative is to occur; and

○   the way in which change is brought about through technical or emancipatory processes.

Practice development initiatives can be promoted on a range of different scales and examples of local, organizational and national initiatives are provided. While there may be innovative practice development activity being undertaken within palliative care settings and by palliative care practitioners, there is a lack of published literature concerning these initiatives. Consequently, some of the examples presented here are drawn from other nursing specialities, and offer potential models for palliative care nursing to emulate.

# What is practice development?

Practice development is a relatively new concept and, as a term, encompasses a broad range of approaches that seek to support changes to the provision of health and social care (McCormack *et al.* 2007a). Practice development has some of its roots in the nursing development units established in the early 1990s. With a growing recognition of the importance of multidisciplinary working, practice development units (PDUs), which moved beyond nursing as their sole focus, were established in many care organizations. These units have been supported by processes of accreditation and education (Gerrish *et al.* 2000). PDUs still exist in hospitals and primary care organizations worldwide (Cambron and Cain 2004) but latterly, there has been a further expansion. Practice development is increasingly used as a term to describe a process of change rather than being linked to specific units in any one organization. Despite this recent practice development work, there is little consensus on what it means and how to do it. This is both problematic and liberating. While a lack of agreed definitions can lead to difficulties in knowing what is counted as practice development, this openness creates a space for creativity and inclusivity in terms of how to bring about changes that improve practice. Practice development has at its core an engagement with the real world of care delivery with its contingencies and constraints. Consequently, pragmatic considerations of what works in particular care settings is possibly more important than justifying if a specific approach is in or out of the practice development fold.

The processes of care improvement can be addressed in various ways, aside from practice development, some of which are addressed in more detail elsewhere in this book (see Chapter 27). Here we briefly compare practice development with these other approaches to see how they differ (Table 33.1).

*Quality assurance* and more specifically *audit strategies* are similar to practice development in that all these approaches seek ultimately to ensure the best care for patients. However, as audit sits within wider systems of clinical governance the focus of the process is to gather data about current services and their quality, using predetermined standards. Usually audit focuses on very specific elements of the care provided, for example pressure sore prevalence. There is no consideration of the nature of the evidence gathered or its appropriateness and a narrow understanding of knowledge is used within the approach, as focused on measurement, which predefines what can be audited. Staff involvement in the audit process may be minimal as external personnel may undertake this activity, or they may be required to collect data within their normal role. Audit is usually seen as an ongoing process that will enable areas for improvement to be identified and to then measure that improvement once changes have been made, which should ultimately impact upon the care patients receive.

*Research* appears initially to have fewer features in common with practice development (Table 33.1). With an aim to generate generalizable new knowledge, the link between research and improvements in the quality of care provision is more distant. While there is an association, it is more contingent upon the extent to which dissemination and utilization of research findings is promoted. Research itself covers a broad spectrum of approaches (see Chapter 32), and some are more akin to practice development than others. Quantitative studies that seek to test hypotheses or establish the efficacy of clinical interventions are not concerned with the actual utilization of the intervention in practice. Qualitative studies that seek to understand people's experiences may make recommendations about the care people should receive on the basis of the research, but again the actual 'how to do this' is not addressed within the remit of these types of studies. However, more participatory approaches to research, such as action research, do specifically address the generation and utilization of new knowledge (often practical knowledge) within specific situations and settings (McCormack *et al.* 2007b). The relationship between participatory research approaches and the emancipatory approaches within practice development, which we discuss shortly, warrants further consideration.

Another approach used to improve the standard of care provided is through *staff development*, which is concerned with the development of an individual practitioner's knowledge skills and, possibly, values. Within the care home sector two broad approaches for staff development concerning palliative care have been identified (Froggatt 2001), which can also be applied for staff development with respect to palliative care in all care settings. The first approach focuses on the provision of formal *education and training* for staff. For example, in the long-term care setting, education has long been seen as an important means of ensuring change with respect to the provision of good palliative care in the setting (Maddocks 1996; Ersek *et al.* 1999). Educational intervention studies for staff in long-term care facilities have been undertaken and evaluated (e.g. Froggatt *et al.* 2000; Williams *et al.* 2002; Strumpf *et al.* 2004). Evaluations of these educational programmes have indicated positive benefits in terms of the staff knowledge and confidence. However, in some instances they have relied on self-report (Froggatt *et al.*

**Table 33.1** Comparison of practice development, audit and research

| Key features | Practice development[1] | Audit[2] | Research[2] |
|---|---|---|---|
| **Aim** | To improve the delivery of good quality patient care | To improve clinical practice by establishing if a service reaches a predetermined standard | To derive generalizable new knowledge |
| **Drivers** | Educational and credential Policy initiatives Practice experiences | Clinical governance strategies | Need for an evidence base for clinical decision-making and care delivery |
| **Focus** | Development of staff knowledge and skills Bringing about specific clinical changes | Specific elements of clinical care identified as requiring review and monitoring | Addresses clearly defined questions, aims and objectives in a wide range of clinical, patient and service provision areas Studies can generate and/or test hypotheses |
| **Breadth of clinical focus** | Addresses complexity of care provision | Uni-issue focused | Usually uni-issue focused unless specifically research addresses wider system |
| **Methods** | Technical Emancipatory | Measures current provision against a standard Analysis of existing clinical and service data with some additional simple data collection | Quantitative, qualitative and participatory methods of research are undertaken, all using systematic methods of data collection and analysis |
| **Knowledge** | Works with current evidence and generates new knowledge Different types of knowledge embraced | A narrow understanding of knowledge used, as focused on measurement and standard | Knowledge engaged with will reflect the research question and research methods adopted |

| | | | |
|---|---|---|---|
| **Role of clinical staff** | Integral to the process, as they are a key focus and deliverer of change | May administer audit tools and collect audit data within normal role | May assist with recruitment of patients<br>In a study about staff, will be participants |
| **Time frame** | Can be a defined period or ongoing | Ongoing and continuous | Usually an endpoint with a defined duration |
| **Impact on care provision and services** | Potential to improve specific clinical care/services provided | Identification of areas for improvement | Immediate impact may be negligible<br>Impact dependent on dissemination activities following study |
| **Impact on clinical staff** | Use of time to engage with change processes, reflection and learning<br>Potential to empower practitioners in their ways of working | Possible use of time to administer measurement tools<br>May ultimately lead to changes in ways of working to better meet the required standard | Possibly use of time to recruit participants, administer research tools or participate<br>Limited impact on current practice unless a participatory approach |
| **Impact on organization** | Potential to change cultures and ways of working | Ensures organization meets clinical governance targets | Usually minimal unless participatory research undertaken |

1 Adapted from McCormack et al. 2007a and b

2 Information about research and audit adapted from the NHS Ethics Consultation E-Group (downloaded from www.nres.npsa.nhs.uk/docs/guidance/Audit_or_Research_table.pdf on 14 August 2007)

2000; Williams *et al.* 2002). The efficacy of education to bring about changes in practice is generally debated (Hutchinson 1999) and has also been questioned with respect to education in palliative care (Kenny 2001).

A second way to develop staff skills and knowledge involves *consultation services*, with an implicit role to develop staff through clinical encounters. Consultation services often use designated specialists (usually nurses) to ensure clinical need is met in particular care settings, and are usually focused on the specific care of individuals. Research on the role of clinical nurse specialists in palliative care in the UK (Clark *et al.* 2002; Seymour *et al.* 2002) identified that the education and consultation roles of the clinical nurse specialist are often neglected, in response to more pressing clinical needs. There are competing demands placed upon palliative care clinical nurse specialists to be both a clinical expert and an agent of change. A similar picture is seen in the UK with the work of clinical nurse specialists in palliative care with care homes to support the residents living there. This work was generally reactive and focused mainly upon symptom control (pain management) issues for specific residents (Froggatt and Hoult 2002; Froggatt *et al.* 2002).

In staff development activities with care home staff, an impact upon the working practices of individual nurses and care assistants and the subsequent care of residents and their relatives has been identified (e.g. Froggatt 2000). However, these initiatives are less successful at influencing practice at an organizational level and this constrains the extent of the changes individual practitioners may make. Practice development offers a way to move beyond regarding the provision of education or a consultation service as an activity sufficient in itself. Education and consultation services can then be regarded as tools that may help in the process of developing practice, rather than ends in themselves.

## How can practice development be undertaken?

Practice development is concerned with the ways in which practitioners engage with, and create knowledge in order to develop both their understanding and practice of care for patients (Clarke and Wilcockson 2001). We present three dimensions of practice development that concern knowledge, the context within which this activity is occurring and the processes of change used. These dimensions are congruent with the elements of effective implementation of evidence-based practice first articulated by Kitson and colleagues (Kitson *et al.* 1998; McCormack *et al.* 1999; Harvey *et al.* 2002). They proposed in their model that there is the interaction of three elements – evidence, context and facilitation. They suggest that each of these elements need to be addressed if effective change and the successful implementation of a new initiative is to occur. In this model, not only is knowledge required about the initiative (evidence), but there is also recognition that the environment within which the initiative is to be implemented (context) and the way in which the change is brought about (facilitation) are equally important. Each of these factors are present on a spectrum from weak to strong (Table 33.2) and the authors argue that the extent to which these factors are strongly present will influence the extent to which practice can be changed. We consider each of these dimensions in turn.

# Knowledge

Within nursing there has been for many years a recognition that different types of knowledge and ways of knowing exist, as exemplified by work by Carper (1978) on different forms of knowledge in nursing (empiric, aesthetic, moral and personal knowing) or Liaschenko and Fisher (1999) on professional knowledge which can be typified as case, patient and person knowledge. Underpinning these different types of knowledge are systems of knowing which McNiff and Whitehead (2002) categorize as propositional and dialectical systems of knowing.

The propositional system is dominant in Western society and is based on abstract formal logic. This system assumes a static model of reality that can be understood intellectually. Knowledge is seen as external to the knower, an objective commodity that can be understood, as in facts and figures, what McNiff and Whitehead would call 'know that' knowledge. This is exemplified in the health care world in the identification and use of a form of knowledge called 'evidence' and the related promotion of evidence-based care. Many Western countries seek to promote the use of particular types of evidence as a foundation for all care delivery. In order to do this, they define a hierarchy of knowledge generated through research, where some forms of

**Table 33.2**  Dimensions of practice development

|  | *Weak* | *Strong* |
|---|---|---|
| **Evidence** | | |
| Research | Anecdotal/descriptive | RCT/Systematic reviews |
| Clinical experience | Divided expert opinion | High levels of consensus |
| Patient preference | No patient involvement | Partnerships |
| **Context** | | |
| Culture | Unclear values | Agreed prevailing values |
| Leadership | Traditional; command and control | Transformational |
| Evaluation | No/limited feedback processes | Multiple feedback to individual, team and system |
| **Facilitation** | | |
| Purpose | Task | Holistic |
| Role | Doing for others | Enabling others |
| Skills | Task/doing for others | Holistic/enabling others |

(Adapted from Kitson *et al.* (1998))

knowledge (evidence) are rated more highly than others. For example, a randomized controlled trial or a systematic review is rated as strong as opposed to descriptive information which is weak. An example of this hierarchy of knowledge was used to develop a palliative care approach in Australian residential aged care facilities, and is presented in Box 33.1.

Kitson *et al.*'s (1998) model, too (Table 33.2), rates certain types of research evidence more highly than others identifying what they view as strong and weak evidence.

While not disputing the need to have a sound basis for the decisions made about the treatments and care delivered within health care, an evidence-based practice approach can be very constraining. The evidence-based practice movement has narrowly defined the meaning of 'valid' evidence, in order to evaluate their credibility and to support rational decision-making (Sackett *et al.* 1997). The highest confidence is placed in one type of evidence – that obtained through the conduct of randomized controlled trials, as illustrated in Box 33.1. Arising from a contemporary response to the control of risk in a culture of increasing managerialism and audit (Trinder 2000), evidence-based practice is seen to be a product of its time. The evidence-based health care movement emphasizes the importance of particular forms of knowledge such as 'technical-rational' knowledge. This aspiration is not without challenge, through other voices such as the user movement (see Chapter 3) and recognition that other types of knowledge are present and increasingly valued (Blomfield and Hardy 2000).

In contrast, McNiff and Whitehead (2002) describe a dialectical system of knowing that is fluid and based on relational forms of knowing. Reality is not 'out there' but something we are all part of. Other forms of knowledge need to be acknowledged and there is a wide spectrum of knowledge that can potentially contribute to the development of practice. In McNiff and Whitehead's discussion they identify 'know how' and personal knowledge. 'Know how' is procedural knowledge that is not fixed and external but rather is about capabilities and practical knowing. This type of knowledge is often linked to skills and competency and is present in the implicit practices of palliative care delivery. This form of knowledge is often the focus of educational interventions and training. Personal knowledge is equated with Polanyi's tacit knowledge (Polanyi 1958). It is subjective knowledge held by a person, gleaned through experience and how it is known cannot be rationally articulated. These and other forms of knowledge have been identified within the practice development movement (Kitson *et al.* 1998) (Table 33.2), in the form of clinical expertise and patient preference.

The dialectical approach to knowledge allows contradictions and paradoxes to be held in a dynamic embodied practice of knowing, and may reflect better the messiness of care delivery and interactions with people with life-limiting illnesses and their families. A dialectical approach is also more inclusive than the propositional system and can still hold with the need for 'evidence', regarding it as another form of knowledge that helps us understand and engage with the world of practice, but does not regard this as the only form of knowledge, as described in the propositional perspective.

**Box 33.1**   Guidelines for a palliative approach in residential aged care (Australian Government Department of Health and Aging 2006)

Evidence-based guidelines have been developed in Australia to support the development of a palliative approach in residential aged care facilities (long-term care facilities for older people). The guidelines address the following aspects of care:

- A palliative approach
- Dignity and quality of life
- Advance care planning
- Advanced dementia
- Physical symptom assessment and management
- Psychological support
- Family support
- Social support, intimacy and sexuality
- Aboriginal and Torres Strait Islander issues
- Cultural issues
- Spiritual support
- Volunteer support
- End-of-life (terminal) care
- Bereavement support
- Management's role in implementing a palliative approach

The guidelines were developed after a systematic review of the literature and each piece of relevant literature was graded by the level of evidence it provides. Based upon a categorization developed by the Australian National Health and Medical Research Council, the following hierarchy was used:

Level I      A systematic review of all relevant randomized controlled trials (RCT).
Level II     At least one properly designed RCT.
Level III-1  Well-designed pseudo-RCTs
Level III-2  Comparative studies with concurrent controls and allocation not randomized, case controlled studies, or interrupted timer series with a control group.
Level III-3  Comparative studies with historical control, two or more single-arm studies, or interrupted time series without a parallel control group.
Level IV     Case series, either post-test or pre-test and post-test.

Qualitative evidence was also considered, but the evaluation framework was less prescriptive.

# Context

In undertaking practice development work, there needs to be an awareness of the context for this change. We use the term context to consider the people involved in a practice development initiative, the environment in which the work is being undertaken and the culture of care. The people involved in practice development in any situation may range from practitioners of one discipline, for example a hospice at home nursing team; or practitioners from a range of disciplines, for example a multidisciplinary palliative care team; or a wider organizational team that incorporates managers, service users and external agencies.

The scale of the activity may also vary from practice development within a single clinical unit, for example a specific ward, a nursing home for older people (see Box 33.2), to larger scale foci within services, for example a palliative care home care team or an organization such as a hospice or a hospital (see Box 33.3). As outlined in the model proposed by Kitson *et al.* (1998), the context, culture and leadership of the care setting where the developments are being introduced can vary (Table 33.2). While a consideration of culture often focuses on the clinical unit or service or organization where the initiatives are being introduced, there is also a broader level of culture to be considered, such as the culture of nursing. As is described in Boxes 33.4 and 33.5, nursing practice development initiatives can be undertaken across whole nations and even internationally, to address the culture of care in nursing.

Culture and its impact on the practice development process also needs to be considered in terms of national cultures (Walsh and Moss 2007). In bicultural societies, such as New Zealand, how practice development is undertaken reflects cultural ways of working as well as utilizing known methods of change processes.

---

**Box 33.2**   Introducing a remembrance book in a care home for older people

During one winter period a care home for older people in the UK was experiencing a larger than expected number of deaths of their residents. Staff became concerned that they did not acknowledge the death of the person who had died before they had to move on to caring for the next person. In staff meetings, the staff talked about the difficulties they experienced in finding a space to deal with their emotional responses when someone has died. In a newly established staff development group they identified that there was a need to find a way to remember the individual residents, as currently the care home did nothing specific to mark a resident's death. In the discussion they together proposed creating a 'remembrance book'. In this book the photograph of each resident who had died would be placed, with space for staff and other residents to write in. This might be personal memories of the person who died, or a goodbye. A book was purchased by the manager and immediately the photos of the residents who had recently died were inserted and staff began writing their responses on the accompanying pages. The remembrance book was also explained to residents attending the residents' meeting, for them to look at if they wished.

## Processes of change

To understand further the 'how' of practice development, three elements will be described (McCormack *et al.* 2007a). These concern how learning occurs, how change happens and how knowledge is used in the development process. Two differing approaches to bringing about change within practice development have been identified (McCormack *et al.* 2007a). Each approach has its own values with respect to the nature of change and how it is best promoted. Although these approaches and the examples given are discretely described, there is overlap and we recognize that people do draw on more than one approach in their work.

A *technical* approach to practice development is concerned with achieving good quality patient-focused care and does this by developing the knowledge, skills and values of the people who provide the care (Mallet *et al.* 1997). There are great similarities between this approach and the features of staff development described earlier, as learning occurs through a training model, on issues specific to the project focus. It is therefore an instrumental utilization of knowledge that occurs in this approach. Change happens in a more controlled way, with direction from those with authority in the setting. One example that utilizes aspects of the technical approach is illustrated in the development of evidence-based practice in a hospital setting, as exemplified by Gerrish and colleagues in Sheffield, UK (Box 33.3).

Another example of a practice development initiative, on a larger scale,

---

**Box 33.3** Organizational practice development (Gerrish and Clayton 2002; Palfreyman *et al.* 2003)

**Aim**
To implement evidence-based practice for nurses and allied health professionals using a bottom-up approach.

**Methods for practice development**

- Hospital-wide evidence-based council established with representatives from clinical areas, nursing and allied health professionals and co-opted representatives. 27 members in total.
- Started journal clubs in each directorate at ward or department level.
- Provision of education and training in evidence-based practice.
- Coordinated by designated facilitator.

**Examples of products**
A focus on nutrition identified local evidence, examples of good practice and areas for future work. Development of a research proposal is underway.

**Scope**
Within one acute hospital in the UK.

that draws upon many elements of the technical approach is the Joanna Briggs Institute in Adelaide, Australia (Box 33.4). This institute seeks to improve health care provision through a systematic attempt to address the use of knowledge in practice.

Great emphasis is placed in the Joanna Briggs Institute work on the generation of high quality evidence, through systematic reviews of literature. A broad perspective on the types of evidence used in their reviews is adopted. Some attention is paid to the processes of how the evidence is introduced in

---

**Box 33.4**   The Joanna Briggs Institute model of evidence-based health care (Pearson *et al.* 2005)

**Aim**
To promote evidence-based practice that arises from clinical decision-making which uses the best available evidence.

**Elements of model**
Four components are identified:

- Health care evidence generation
- Evidence synthesis
- Evidence knowledge transfer
- Evidence utilization

There is a concern to address the feasibility, appropriateness, meaningfulness and effectiveness of health care practices.

**Implementing the model**
The Joanna Briggs Institute aims to facilitate evidence-based health care globally through leading work in the synthesis, transfer and utilization of evidence.
    Activities undertaken include:

- Systematic reviews and analysis of research literature.
- Dissemination of information through the development of guidelines.
- Establishment of collaborating centres across the world, in at least 13 countries.
- Education and training in evidence-based methods of engaging with evidence.

**Examples of products**
Systematic reviews, e.g. factors associated with constructive staff/family relationships in the care of older adults in the institutional setting.
    Best practice information sheets, e.g. topical skin care in aged care facilities.

**Scope**
International seeking to improve global health.

Website: http://www.joannabriggs.edu.au/about/home.php

---

the practice domain, but in a technical manner, through the use of clinical guidelines.

An *emancipatory* approach to practice development was originally developed in the UK by the Royal College of Nursing (McCormack *et al.* 1999). The purpose of this approach to practice development is increased effectiveness in person-centred care. The way this is achieved is through the development of practitioners' knowledge and skills, with the specific aim of changing the culture and context of care. A reflective model of learning is adopted. Skilled facilitation and a systematic continuous process of emancipatory change is proposed, which also empowers the practitioners as well as incorporating the views of services users (Garbett and McCormack 2002). The knowledge used in this approach is both inductively and deductively derived from the setting and also from wider literature. This approach goes beyond the technical definition defined earlier where the change is focused on the individual rather than the individual in the wider context.

An example of a practice development initiative which draws upon many of these principles of the emancipatory approach is the Caledonian model used to promote good practice within gerontological nursing in Scotland (Box 33.5). Although the processes used and values drawn upon are emancipatory and participatory, there is still a place in this model for evidence-based guidelines to be developed and used.

An important aspect of the way in which any of the practice development initiatives described are undertaken concerns the facilitation process used. Facilitators may be either based internally to the unit where the change occurs or externally and may have a clinical, education, research or practice development background or role. For example, we referred earlier to the change agent aspect of the clinical nurse specialist in palliative care role, which has to be balanced with their clinical work. How facilitators are introduced to the setting either by invitation, negotiated entry or by imposition will shape how the change process is experienced by the members of the setting involved in the change. This also reflects a more fundamental orientation of the practice developer about their approach to this work: is the model of working underpinned by a 'working on' or a 'working with' stance?

# Conclusion

The development of palliative care practice is a complex matter and draws upon a variety of sources for its energy and momentum. We have outlined here some key features of practice development and described a number of different practice development initiatives that have been developed within nursing to support the improvement of practice. These have been used in a variety of ways illustrating the flexibility that adopting a practice development approach offers to individual practitioners and managers. We have identified that the knowledge that underpins the practice development

---

**Box 33.5**   The Caledonian model of practice development (Tolson *et al.* 2006)

**Aim**

To develop an evidence-based approach to promoting best practice in gerontological nursing.

**Elements of model**

- Knowledge described as the integration of the *scholarship of practice* – combines what nurses know from practice and what older people themselves know and want from nursing services.
- *Scholarship of inquiry*, which is knowledge ascertained as a result of research and critical thinking.
- Recognition that as knowledge changes over time with new research and evaluation of ongoing practice.
- Creation of a community of practice helps integrate the scholarship of practice and inquiry.
- This community is supported by the establishment of a virtual practice development college.
- Evidence-based practice in the clinical setting is directed by the development of best practice statements in identified areas.

**Examples of products**

Best practice statements include:

- Maximizing Communication with Older People with Hearing Disability
- Nutrition for Physically Frail Older People

**Scope**

National initiative across Scotland.

Website: www.geronurse.com/en/caledonian-practice-development-model

---

process can be understood in a narrow or broad way, the latter offering a more inclusive approach to the forms of knowledge that are valued and incorporated into the work. There is a need to be aware of the context, its scale and culture, in order to develop initiatives that engage with practitioners and involve them. Both technical and emancipatory approaches to practice development are adopted, and each approach is concerned with learning change and the use of knowledge in practice.

Looking beyond palliative care, to gerontology for example, we can identify that when a broader systems approach is adopted, different types of knowledge can be used and integrated to identify best practice in specific aspects of care. Through appropriate facilitation this new knowledge can then used in the care settings. Unfortunately, in many areas palliative care facilitators or mentors are provided on a short-term basis as part of specific projects or initiatives, which creates particular challenges in relation to sustainability. A great deal of time and effort is often spent in developing and delivering training and education for clinical staff, only for the enthusiasm and momentum to be lost when the project comes to an end. For initiatives to be worthwhile and fully effective there needs to be the commitment from both commissioners and provider services to continue to support and develop staff when the initial projects are over.

The palliative care speciality is a small enough world to be able to come together and address the process of practice development. We could work across the boundaries and organizations to create a virtual community of learning. If this can be done within gerontology why not palliative care? Is there the potential to develop a virtual palliative care practice development community? This could support individual practitioners working in hospices and specialist palliative care units to develop their own palliative care practice. It could be a resource to palliative care nurses with a specific remit for change work, such as clinical nurse specialists, who could have access to knowledge, and a place to review and synthesize different types of knowledge. There is a challenge here for those of us who consider ourselves to be committed to the delivery of high-quality palliative care to look at the methods by which we develop our own practice and the practice of the clinicians and practitioners we support through education and other means. A practice development focus would enhance and take us beyond what we already achieve.

# References

Australian Government Department of Health and Aging (2006) *Guidelines for a Palliative Approach in Residential Aged Care. Enhanced Version.* Canberra: Rural Health and Palliative Care Branch, Australian Government Department of Health and Aging.

Blomfield, R. and Hardy, S. (2000) Evidence-based nursing practice. In: L. Trinder and S. Reynolds (eds) *Evidence-Based Practice. A Critical Appraisal.* Oxford: Blackwell Science, pp. 111–37.

Cambron, B. and Cain, L. (2004) Practice development: What we learn with our British partners, *Creative Nursing*, 2: 14–15.

Carper, B.A. (1978) Fundamental patterns of knowing, *Advances in Nursing Science*, 1(1): 13–23.

Clark, D., Seymour, J., Douglas, H-R., Bath, P., Beech, N., Corner, J., Halliday, D., Hughes, P., Haviland, J., Normand, C., Marples, R., Skilbeck, J. and Webb, T. (2002) Clinical nurse specialists in palliative care. Part 2. Explaining diversity in the organization and costs of Macmillan nursing service, *Palliative Medicine*, 16: 375–85.

Clarke, C.I. and Wilcockson, J. (2001) Professional and organisational learning: analysing the relationship with development of practice, *Journal of Advanced Nursing*, 34(2): 264–72.

Ersek, M., Kraybill, B.M. and Hansberry, J. (1999) Investigating the educational needs of licensed nursing staff and certified nursing assistants in nursing homes regarding end-of-life care, *American Journal of Hospice and Palliative Care*, 16(4): 573–82.

Froggatt, K.A. (2000) Evaluating a palliative care education project in nursing homes, *International Journal of Palliative Nursing*, 6(3): 140–6.

Froggatt, K.A. (2001) Palliative care and nursing homes: where next? *Palliative Medicine*, 15: 42–8.

Froggatt, K.A., Hasnip, J. and Smith, P. (2000) The challenges of end of life care, *Elderly Care*, 12(2): 11–13.

Froggatt, K.A. and Hoult, L. (2002) Developing palliative care practice in nursing and residential care homes: the role of the clinical nurse specialist. *Journal of Clinical Nursing*, 11: 802–8.

Froggatt, K.A., Poole, K. and Hoult, L. (2002) The provision of palliative care in nursing homes and residential care homes: A survey of clinical nurse specialist work, *Palliative Medicine*, 16: 481–7.

Garbett, R. and McCormack, B. (2002) A concept analysis of practice development, *NT Research*, 7(2): 87–99.

Gerrish, K. and Clayton, J. (2002) Promoting evidence-based practice: an organisational approach, *Journal of Nursing Management*, 12: 114–23.

Gerrish, K., Ferguson, A., Kitching, N. and Mischenko, J. (2000) Developing primary care nursing. *Journal of Clinical Nursing*. 14(6): 8–14.

Harvey, G., Loftus-Hills, A., Rycroft-Malone, J., Titchen, A., Kitson, A., McCormack, B. and Seers, K. (2002) Getting evidence into practice: the role and function of facilitation, *Journal of Advanced Nursing*, 37(6): 577–88.

Hutchinson, L. (1999) Evaluating and researching the effectiveness of educational interventions, *British Medical Journal*, 318: 1267–9.

Kenny, L. (2001) Education in palliative care: making a difference to practice, *International Journal of Palliative Nursing*, 7(8): 410–17.

Kitson, A., Harvey, G. and McCormack, B. (1998) Enabling the implementation of evidence based practice: a conceptual framework, *Quality in Health Care*, 7: 149–58.

Liashenko, J. and Fisher, A. (1999) Theorising the knowledge that nurses use in the conduct of their work, *Scholarly Inquiry for Nursing Practice: An International Journal*, 13: 29–40.

Maddocks, I. (1996) Palliative care in the nursing home, *Progress in Palliative Care*, 4(3): 77–8.

Mallett, J., Cathmoir, D., Hughes, P. and Whitby, E. (1997) Forging new roles. Professional and practice development, *Nursing Times*, 93(18): 38–9.

McCormack, B., Manley, K., Kitson, A., Titchen, A. and Harvey, G. (1999) Towards practice development – a vision in reality or a reality without vision? *Journal of Nursing Management*, 7: 255–64.

McCormack, B., Wright, J., Dewar, B., Harvey, G. and Ballantine, K. (2007a) A realist synthesis of evidence relating to practice development: Methodology and methods, *Practice Development in Health Care*, 6(1): 5–24.

McCormack, B., Wright, J., Dewar, B., Harvey, G. and Ballantine, K. (2007b) A realist synthesis of evidence relating to practice development: Findings from the literature analysis, *Practice Development in Health Care*, 6(1): 25–55.

McNiff, J. and Whitehead, J. (2002) *Action Research Principles and Practice*. Abingdon: Routledge Falmer.

Palfreyman, S., Tod, A. and Doyle, J. (2003) Learning from experience: Promoting evidence-based practice, *Practice Development in Health Care*, 2(2): 87–98.

Pearson, A., Wiechula, R., Court, A. and Lockwood, C. (2005) The JBI model of evidence-based healthcare, *International Journal of Evidence-Based Health Care*, 3(8): 207–15.

Polanyi, M. (1958) *Personal Knowledge*. London: Routledge and Kegan Paul.

Sackett, D., Richardson, L., Rosenberg, W.S. and Haynes, R.B. (1997) *Evidence-Based Medicine: How to Practice and Teach EBM*. New York: Churchill Livingstone.

Seymour, J., Clark, D., Bath, P., Beech, N., Corner, J., Douglas, H-R., Halliday, D., Haviland, J., Marples, R., Normand, C., Skilbeck, J. and Webb, T. (2002) Clinical nurse specialists in palliative care. Part 3. Issues for Macmillan Nurse role, *Palliative Medicine*, 16(5): 386–94.

Strumpf, N.E., Tuch, H., Stillman, D., Parrish, P. and Morrison, N. (2004) Implementing palliative care in the nursing home, *Annals of Long-Term Care*, 12(11): 35–41.

Tolson, D., Schofield, I., Booth, J., Kelly, T.B. and James, L. (2006) Constructing a new approach to developing evidence-based practice with nurses and older people, *Worldviews on Evidence-Based Nursing*, 3(2): 62–72.

Trinder, L. (2000) Introduction: the context of evidence-based practice. In L. Trinder and S. Reynolds (eds) *Evidence-Based Practice. A Critical Appraisal*. Oxford: Blackwell Science, pp. 1–16.

Walsh, K. and Moss, C. (2007) Practice development in New Zealand: Reflections on the influence of culture and context. *Practice Development in Health Care*, 6(1): 82–5.

Williams, A., Montelpare, W., Wilson, S., Cheng, S., Tremelling, K. and Wells, C. (2002) An assessment of the utility of formalized palliative care education: a Niagara case study, *Journal of Hospice and Palliative Nursing*, 4(2): 103–10.

# 34

# Policy and palliative care

*Jo Hockley*

---

**Key points**

- Policy is a moving target that has no closure.
- The World Health Organization (WHO) advocate a public health model for translating palliative care knowledge and skills into evidence-based, cost-effective interventions that can reach a population.
- The WHO define population needs as a basis to palliative care reform.
- International collaborative policy groups help support evolving policy initiatives in poorly resourced countries.

---

> Palliative care has developed through a strong sense of specialist mission. It may well be difficult to share this mission with a wider audience, yet the gains in patients' quality of life would be great. Past investment in palliative care has created a resource that is local rather than exceptional. The challenge is how to use this resource so that all patients, including those with non-cancer diagnoses, can benefit from access to better care. In an era of financial constraints, new alliances are needed for shared care if the full promise of palliative care is to be realised.
>
> (Bosanquet 1997)

This quote from a professor of health policy in the UK stresses the importance of partnership between palliative care and policy in order to improve care for all patients during the last months/year of life and the support given to their families. Over the past 40 years, palliative care services across the world have developed in different ways: through the charity/voluntary sector; the secular sector with monies from governments such as the NHS in the UK, Medicare in the USA; and the private sector. The original focus of the hospice movement in the UK was the unmet needs of people dying from cancer. This has now extended to those dying from advanced, progressive non-malignant disease including older people in care homes, those with end-stage chronic organ failure and those with a learning disability facing the end of life.

This diffuseness of need challenges policy in more ways than one. As Liao and Arnold (2006: 730) highlight, 'this is a critical and exciting time for palliative (care), as demographic, economic, medical and political factors collide'. As professionals we need to find our voice within the strategic planning of palliative care in order that high-quality care is delivered to our patients with end-stage disease and their families, wherever they choose to be cared for.

This chapter introduces the subject of health care policy 'as a moving target' and the difficulties associated with policy as something that never has closure. It addresses the evaluation of the quality of palliative care within whole populations. It highlights the WHO public health model for palliative care integration, and explores the policy cycle. We will see during this chapter how research and policy are very much intertwined; how one can impact on the other, and vice versa; how 'tensions' occur around new health policies; and how finances being made available to develop palliative care are often tied into different policy initiatives. The commissioning of new initiatives is part of policy, however implementing effective and efficient programmes must be part of that process too if cultures are to be changed.

Although this chapter has been written mostly from a UK perspective, an effort has been taken to illustrate the impact of health care reform and palliative care more globally with exemplars from richly resourced countries, such as the USA, Canada and Australia, as well as those that are more poorly resourced, such as the countries of central and eastern Europe (Wright *et al.* 2004).

# Policy – a moving target

One of the difficulties of engaging with health and social policy in general, and policy involving palliative care in particular, is that policy has the effect of continually moving on. As Mathew *et al.* (2003: 271) detail, 'policy is developmental in nature and incorporates the notion of a continuing process without closure'.

The speed with which policy can change and move on is illustrated in a recent review of the health improvement plans (HImPs) from English strategic health authorities during the period 1999–2003 (Seymour *et al.* 2002). The authors found that health authorities' awareness of government recommendations for the development of cancer and palliative care services were often out of date.[1] They report that 71 per cent of the HImPs cited the Calman-Hine report of 1995 as a framework for service development despite more recent local and national edicts from government in 1997/1998 for the development of action plans and guidance manuals for purchasers on improving palliative care outcomes. Seymour *et al.* (2002) do not dispute the important impact that the Calman-Hine report as a framework has had for cancer services and the formation of palliative and supportive care networks within the community, but their paper highlights how quickly new policies are generated.

# Defining palliative care need

Even though policies are rapidly changing, our awareness and/or involvement as professionals in health policy reform is very important in today's political climate if we want to improve palliative care services.

Addressing important goals in relation to *quality of care, needs assessment, accessibility* and *funding* underpin general health care policy; these are relevant to the field of palliative care in order to see if we are 'making the grade' (Lorenz *et al.* 2006). International and national health policy demand that the quality of services is assessed in order to inform policy developments and shape clinical care (Avis *et al.* 1995).

## Evaluating the quality of palliative care

Evaluating the quality of palliative care services is an enormous subject and space only allows for a brief overview in this section. Quality improvements, the setting of standards, peer review, PDSA circles are just a few of the strategies that have been employed to improve quality of care. 'Structure, process and outcome' (Donabedian 1980) has been highlighted as a conceptual framework for improving end-of-life care in whole communities (Byock *et al.* 2001). Byock *et al.* (2001) describe structure as referring to:

- access of services across such communities, organization of care and the physical environment where care is carried out;
- process of care involves the clinical care given, including information giving, and appropriate communication with patient and family involved;
- outcomes relate to satisfaction of care in relation to both patient and family and the quality of the dying experience.

There has been considerable emphasis on measuring the outcome of palliative care. Measurement should reflect palliative care goals in relation to quality of life. Much attention has been given to clinical assessment tools of various kinds, such as: the 'Palliative Care Outcome Scale – POS' developed by Higginson in the UK (Aspinal *et al.* 2002) or the 'Palliative Care Assessment – PACA' (Ellershaw *et al.* 1995) and others (Hearn and Higginson 2002). In Canada four standardized assessment tools including the 'Edmonton Symptom Assessment Scale – ESAS' are used routinely for all patients admitted to a regional palliative care service (Bruera and Sweeney 2002). The Liverpool Care Pathway for the Dying (www.lcp-mariecurie.org.uk) has been developed as an evidence-based tool to guide the care in the last days of life. However, it can also be used very effectively as an audit tool to evaluate the *process* of care.

Ovretveit (1992) highlights the importance of seeking opinions about quality of care from three personal perspectives – client, professional and management. Within palliative care the VOICES questionnaire (Addington-Hall *et al.* 1998) has been successful in gathering the opinion of bereaved relatives. Although more difficult, there is increasing realization of the importance given to the lived experience of patients and carers and their needs at the end of life (Worth *et al.* 2006). Satisfaction surveys are popular to measure the quality of care but, because of the differing expectations between patients and families, there is some controversy as to whether the theoretical basis that underpins the concept of satisfaction is relevant when using it to evaluate health care (Aspinal *et al.* 2003). Some have argued that we need to take 'a pragmatic approach in using satisfaction as a tool to measure quality and do the best we can while at the same time increasing clarity in the conceptualisation and the measurement of satisfaction' (Bond 2003: 534). Within the context of evaluation research, Corner *et al.* (2003) report on a technique using a narrative-based approach to assess satisfaction; patients' and carers' stories are analysed for their spontaneous reports of 'instances' of care by which outcomes of satisfaction might be assessed.

### Needs assessment

With the evolving nature of evaluating the quality of care in populations, growing attention has been given to the importance of needs assessments. Needs assessment has been defined as 'the process of exploring the relationship between health problems in a community and the resources available to address those problems in order to achieve a desired outcome' (Pickin and St Leger 1993: 6). But, *how* needs are defined and then measured is pivotal to the effectiveness of such a tool (Clark and Malson 2002). Jordan *et al.* (2002) undertook a survey of public health doctors in order to ascertain themes involved in health care needs assessment including initiating factors, methods and outcome. They came up with certain criteria (see Box 34.1) but added 'our findings suggest that, although methodological and analytical quality are necessary characteristics of effective health needs assessment, they are not sufficient without a favourable political environment'. When meeting such criteria as described in Box 34.1, needs assessment has the potential of making a significant impact on strategy, planning and service improvement (Mirando 2004).

The policy behind needs assessment is that 'need is inextricably linked first with service provision, and secondly with the ability to *benefit* from health or social care' (Clark and Malson 2002: 147). Clark and Malson (2002) raise important questions around components and methods of undertaking a needs assessment in palliative care. They highlight that limited financial resources and the grey areas around the conceptualization of complex psychosocial, spiritual and physical needs in palliative care do not make the undertaking of a needs assessment in palliative care that straightforward.

**Box 34.1**    Criteria for needs assessment to potentially impact on policy (Jordan *et al.* 2002)

- Careful design
- Methodological rigour
- Decisive leadership
- Good communication
- Involvement and ownership from relevant stakeholders
- Appreciation of the local political situation
- Engagement with local priorities
- Availability of resources
- An element of chance

They press for an inclusive approach and one that is constructed in such a way as to allow previously unidentified and unanticipated needs to be identified. Including service users, such as patients/clients/residents and their carers, as stakeholders within the assessment process alongside purchasers and planners is an important part of any evaluation/needs assessment.

### *Accessing palliative care*

A further complication occurs in evaluating services in relation to those people with palliative care needs who do not access specialist palliative care. An integral component of palliative care policy is that it is accessible to all people who are dying. There has been considerable concern both in the USA and in the UK that ethnic minorities are less likely to access palliative care. This has been for differing reasons. In the USA, Lorenz *et al.* (2006) report on several studies demonstrating this lack of access as a result of: lack of a primary care-giver,[2] not having a regular physician, and language barriers effecting the discussion on end-of-life care matters. They call on specialist palliative care services to address these barriers.

In the UK it is believed that the lack of uptake of specialist palliative care services by ethnic minorities has been due partially to how palliative care evolved within the middle classes in Britain. Interestingly, a recent small qualitative study of ethnic minority patients attending a day hospice, found that those ethnic minority patients who have managed to fit in with dominant cultures express basic human needs rather than specific cultural needs (Diver *et al.* 2003). However, there is evidence to suggest that there are cultural issues in the assessment and management of pain of people from ethnic minorities that include the under-assessment of pain in African American and Latino patients (Lorenz *et al.* 2006).

In Australia, the UK, the USA and Canada accessibility to specialist palliative care services and/or advice for those people with advanced non-malignant co-morbidities in old age is now being highlighted. Currently, in the UK there are many residents in care homes who have no access to specialist palliative care services. In a survey of 72 nursing homes only 4 per cent of nursing home managers regularly accessed specialist palliative care (Hockley *et al.* 2004). Currow *et al.* (2006) stress the importance of studying whole populations of people with life-threatening illness in any one area in order to define unmet need. They describe a novel approach of using a state-wide survey that could be developed further to improve the understanding of the characteristics and needs of those with life-limiting diseases.

Rawlings *et al.* (2006) describe an evaluation project where improving access to palliative care for people facing the end of life, including older people, in rural and remote communities is being rolled out in eight pilot sites across the whole of Australia. In Australia's rural and remote areas there is not the luxury of local tertiary hospitals or hospices. Here is an important example of where research and policy go hand-in-hand in order strategically to develop palliative care services across a country. It is an enormous undertaking but perhaps emphasizes Australia's commitment to reach out to one of the most vulnerable groups in their society with the financial backing to improve care.

### Funding services

The funding of end-of-life care services is currently a major concern because of the demographically older population in Western cultures is forecast to increase (Lynn and Adamson 2003; Lorenz *et al.* 2006). Efficiency emphasizes weighing the goals of quality of care and accessibility with cost in order to achieve a socially desirable balance (Lorenz *et al.* 2006).

There is no doubt that there will always be issues to do with the funding of health care over which group of people benefit from a larger portion of the financial cake. In the UK in the mid-1960s, the NHS system was not *offering* palliative care and that is why the hospice movement came in to being (Clark and Malson 2002; Clark 2004). Forty years on have attitudes within the NHS changed? It would appear that generally across the UK the NHS has adopted a number of aspects of care first promoted by the hospice movement. For example, there is considerably more attention across the NHS to multidisciplinary working, patient-focused care, attention to pain assessment and management that was being promoted by the hospice movement in the 1970s. Within UK oncology departments the influence has probably been more dramatic with a conscious effort to promote palliative care and work alongside local hospice units. Palliative care nurse specialists originally funded by the charity Macmillan are now fully funded by the NHS. More recently in England and Wales, the establishment of the End of Life Strategy (www.endoflifecare.nhs.uk), as a subcommittee of the Department of Health, has made important strides to promote end-of-life care across the health service.

Despite this swell of encouragement in the UK, those involved in the policy drive for 'palliative care for all' believe that the government still need to pay a higher proportion of the cost of hospice provision (Finlay 2006; Praill 2006). An alternative could be that general staff should have enhanced skills in palliative care to deal with their own patients better. Unfortunately, it could be argued that there has been a 'de-skilling' (Dunlop and Hockley 1998) of staff within general palliative care as a result of a lack of real empowerment by palliative care specialists.

In the USA there is concern that good care will not arise out of better education or even better behaviour of professional staff but by increased funding (Goldstein and Lynn 2002). Currently there is a range of different mechanisms for the financial provision of end-of-life care in the USA: Medicare, Medicaid, private insurance and the Veteran's Health Administration (Raphael *et al.* 2001). However, reimbursement is complex with many people being required to pay for care in advance of reimbursement (Lorenz *et al.* 2006). Funding of palliative care services may not be the only issue for patients and their families in order to benefit. In the USA, those patients able to get specialist advice still experience difficulties obtaining medication prescribed by their doctors because of lack of funding (Lorenz *et al.* 2006). Gee (2003) reports that 'patient inability to afford medications', 'lack of insurance' and 'lack of medication benefit' were three out of six categories that prevented patients from getting medication to treat symptoms in advanced cancer. Out of these six categories, 60.9 per cent of palliative care experts cited 'inability to afford medications'.

In resource-poor countries levels of funding for basic palliative care services are negligible. Many rely on international collaborative networks to contribute to the development of sustainable palliative care services (Callaway *et al.* 2007). Even if there has been development of clinical services and palliative care education, more often than not palliative care policy lags behind (Muszbek 2007). Despite this, enormous strides are continuing to occur.

## Engagement of health policy and palliative care

Addressing a global audience, Stjernsward *et al.* (2007) believe that a public health strategy offers an important approach for 'translating new knowledge and skills into evidence-based, cost-effective interventions that can reach everyone in the population' (p. 496). In addressing both richly resourced and poorly resourced countries he advocates the WHO public health model. This model highlights four important issues for the coverage of palliative care:

- appropriate policies in palliative care
- adequate drug availability
- education of policy makers, health care workers and the public
- implementation of palliative care services at all levels throughout the society.

Taking the UK as an example, the stages of integration of palliative care such as the above model advocates can be reviewed.

In the UK, St Christopher's Hospice, London was the first teaching/ research-based hospice that opened in 1967. Pain control using morphine delivered four-hourly underpinned its holistic model of care highlighting the importance of drug availability. However, it was to be over ten years before the first official government circular regarding palliative care (or rather terminal care as it was then known) was issued encouraging health authorities to lead the strategic planning for patients requiring hospice-type care (Seymour *et al.* 2002). There is no doubt that during this time a huge amount of effort was being put into individual palliative care services but there was little effective national strategy for the development of palliative care as a whole. Health authorities were being encouraged to think strategically but hospice units and their community teams were still most often set up in areas where there was passion for a service and where there was an expectation of charitable giving. Hospital palliative care teams were emerging but on an ad hoc basis (Dunlop and Hockley 1998).

An important 'landmark' came in 1987 when, after a considerable amount of debate, palliative care was recognized as a specialty by the Royal College of Physicians (www.rcplondon.ac.uk/specialty/Palliative.asp). Medical students were now formally examined about their knowledge of palliative care as part of their education, and consultant posts in palliative medicine were established within NHS hospitals. Care of the dying had always been a subject included in nursing curricula but now many hospices joined with local universities to have their palliative care courses validated at degree level. As a result clinical nurse specialist posts in palliative care both in the community and hospitals have been established.

The National Council for Hospice and Specialist Palliative Care Services (NCSPCS) now called the National Council for Palliative Care for England, Wales and Northern Ireland (NCPC) and their sister organization in Scotland (Scottish Partnership for Palliative Care – SPPC) encouraged the collective influence of clinicians and academics to come together to address policy issues within palliative care across the UK. Occasional papers were first published in the early 1990s giving guidance on outcome measurements, definitions of palliative care, and more recently advising on the commissioning of palliative care services for diseases other than cancer. Both organizations are well respected in the UK, not only in their role highlighting the needs of people with advanced disease (NCHSPCS and SPPC 2000; NCPC 2006) but also in the development of policy issues relating to palliative care through cross-party working (SPPC 2006).

More recently there has been strengthening links between the palliative care community and the bureaucracy of the NHS, mostly due to palliative care services working alongside mainstream cancer services. The Calman-Hine Report (DoH 1995) galvanized this work in a vision for cancer services within the community and developed the idea of supportive and palliative care networks (NICE 2004). At the close of the twentieth century, palliative care policy documents reveal an increasing recognition of extending beyond a focus on cancer services and terminal illness (Mathew *et al.* 2003).

Finally in 2006, 40 years after the inception of the New Hospice Movement, the Department of Health invested £12 million in an End of Life Care Strategy 'to improve the quality of care at the end of life for all patients and enable more patients to live and die in the place of their choice' (www.endoflifecare.nhs.uk). In preparation for the introduction of systems to help improve palliative care, primary care teams/local authorities are encouraged to perform a baseline review of current end-of-life care services. The baseline review will supply information to government to enable stronger evidence for commissioners in their role of working with the variety of service providers (DoH 2007). This programme has the remit to develop the end-of-life care strategy that will ensure 'choice, quality of care, equity of access and value for money'. The strategy board includes chief executives of leading charities, senior clinicians and managers from the NHS and social care. Five working groups carry out major aspects of the strategy, they include: measuring the quality of care; the care pathway for someone approaching the end of life and the services required to meet their needs; care homes; analysis and stronger commissioning of services; and workforce and development.

# Principles, policies and palliative care reform

As can be seen by the above example, the integration of palliative care into a national health care policy requires both a 'top-down' and 'bottom-up' change occurring at a local, regional and national level (Liao and Arnold 2006). As health care professionals within palliative care, it is vital that we are aware of the policy cycle (see Box 34.2) and are actively involved at the appropriate level at which we practise; this might be through management, education or at a clinical level. In this section exemplars are taken from different countries to highlight different aspects of policy and palliative care reform.

All countries striving to promote palliative care need to adopt national standards in order for care to be regulated. NHS Scotland (2002) have

---

**Box 34.2**   Policy cycle (Mathew *et al.* 2003: 272)

Policy formation:
* how policy is constructed, by whom and with what agenda

Policy implementation:
* where initiatives are transmitted into programmes, guidance and directives

Policy accountability:
* where policy is mature and the question of evaluation and outcomes are considered

written national standards that include access to specialist palliative care services, key elements of care, managing people and resources, professional education and communication (both interprofessional and between patients/ carers). Each standard is explored through a written 'standard statement', the 'rationale' behind the statement (including being referenced), and the 'criteria' (both essential and desirable) by which the standard will be audited. These specialist palliative care standards have been used by NHS Quality Improvement Scotland (NHSQIS 2004) in a formal process of peer review in palliative care services across Scotland, UK. See Box 34.3 for the review process.

The IAHPC website (www.hospicecare.com/standards) reports national palliative care standards from different countries around the world and

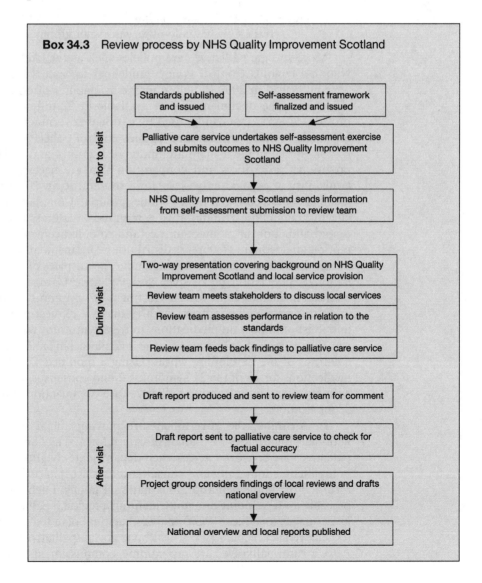

**Box 34.3**   Review process by NHS Quality Improvement Scotland

includes standards written by professionals caring in less well-resourced countries such as Hungary and Moldova. Romania is an example of how effective national standards in palliative care are being created:

> In 2002, national standards in palliative care were developed in a partnership project between the *Romanian Association for Palliative Care* and the *National Hospice and Palliative Care Organization* in the USA. These standards were developed in an attempt to maintain the quality of care by providing some basic requirements, and also to serve as an evaluation tool in the process of contracting funds. These standards are now part of a Ministry of Health White Paper that will define the palliative care services for Romania and present the strategy for development of services at a national level. This document is the first attempt to develop clear standards for palliative care services in Romania.
>
> (IOELC: www.eolc-observatory.net/global_analysis/index.htm)

More specific palliative care policies such as the 'Achieving Balance in National Opioids Control Policy: guidelines for assessment' (WHO 2000) were published in 2000 to help improve availability of opioids in countries worldwide. The document is now available in 22 different languages and provides 'criteria that can be used by national governments and health professionals to assess the national opioids control policies and their administration to determine if there are undue restrictions, and if they contain the provisions, procedures and cooperation that are necessary to ensure the availability of opioid analgesics' (Joranson and Ryan 2007: 529). However, members of the pain and policy studies group in Canada believe that a more effective communicative initiative is required to address fears in relation to opioid addiction in many countries and so enhance availability and set in motion an adequate system for distribution (Joranson and Ryan 2007).

De Lima *et al.* (2007), working under the auspices of the IAHPC (International Association of Hospice and Palliative Care), have drawn up an essential medicines guide for the treatment of symptoms in advanced cancer in poorly resourced countries. As a result of a request from the WHO, an initial list of important medications to treat symptoms was created. This list was then surveyed online and sent to 112 physicians and pharmacists in 77 countries of the developing world. Using a modified Delphi technique, 48 medications for 18 of the 21 symptoms found consensus. Further discussion with representatives from 26 palliative care organizations finalized a list of 33 medications.

In Australia, the government are moving ahead with a number of national programmes for palliative care reform. They are creating regional palliative care consortia across each departmental health region (consisting of inpatient, community and consultation services) in order to create a platform for the implementation of a national policy. Each consortium is responsible for developing and implementing a regional palliative care plan and given suggestions (i.e. SWOT analysis, regional plan templates, etc.) on how to achieve such a plan (www.health.vic.gov.au/palliativecare/strategy.htm). Also, a rural palliative care programme, commissioned by the Department of Health and Ageing in Australia, is being implemented in eight pilot sites across the country (Rawlings *et al.* 2006). The enormity of such a high leverage project is realized when the authors detail that one of the project sites is the size of Spain. One of the pilot areas has formed a 'governance committee' to direct, guide and implement the project. The committee is multidisciplinary and made up of local stakeholders including: executive officer from general practice, project manager, GP advisor, community health services, palliative care nurse consultant, director of nursing from acute services, director of nursing from a local residential aged care facility and a community representative.

In the USA, as in most developed countries, 'an ageing population, increasing diversity and changing patterns of death and disability are driving demand for changes in the way (end-of-life) care is financed as well as how it is provided' (Raphael *et al.* 2001: 459). One of the major concerns is the way end-of-life care is currently financed by 'prognosis' rather than being provided on a basis of disease severity and functional disability. The recent defining of three dying trajectories (cancer; organ failure such as heart failure, renal failure, etc.; frailty/dementia in older people) by Lynn and Adamson (2003) is one of those high-leverage opportunities for reform that might contribute to such a policy. The care of older people at the end of life forms a particular challenge to governments of richly resourced counties. It is often said that the mark of a civilized society is how it treats its most vulnerable citizens. There can be many cases cited as to whom might be the most vulnerable dependent on one's specific interest. However, the frail older person with multiple co-morbidities including advanced dementia has to be one such group. It is important to acknowledge that in the past ten years, the care of this group of people is being championed at a policy, academic and clinical level in Australia (The National Palliative Care Program 2004), in Canada (Fisher and Ross 2000), the UK (Froggatt 2004) and the USA (Lynn and Adamson 2003).

National palliative care standards and policy are less well-defined within social care across most countries. Until recently, palliative care policy has been placed within the context of health. However, the increased needs of older people at the end of life suffering from multiple co-morbidities and being cared for in care homes has meant that there has been greater working with social care networks. National practice statements for general palliative care in adult care homes (SPPC 2006) have been produced and are being used by the regulating body for care homes in Scotland. There is an expectation that the palliative care approach is to be adopted by care homes as a way of delivering care to their residents and families.

### Bringing about change

Proposing action through policy is important. However, often not enough time and therefore funding is given in order to embed new policies into areas where there is the need for substantial culture change.

Introducing new strategies and systems and managing that change is complex, especially in cultures where resistance from complacency and lack of up-to-date education are embedded. Iles and Sutherland (2001) review strategies for organizational change as part of the National Co-ordinating Centre for NHS Service Delivery and Organization. Currently, there is an emphasis on evidence-based care and the adoption of systematic tools to guide and monitor care such as those being recommended by the Department of Health's End of Life Strategy group mentioned in the previous section. However, an important aspect that has been the flagship of the hospice movement is the valuing, support and ongoing education of all staff working with and caring for patients and their families. Systems such as the Liverpool Care Pathway for the Last Days of Life are important but of *equal* importance and emphasis when implementing change across an organization is the inclusion of those people involved in the day-to-day care and management of services (Mortimer *et al.* 2004; Hockley 2006). Facilitating an opportunity for a 'communicative space' (Kemmis 2001) that spans traditional boundaries within organizations and across regions enables collaboration in the change process. Some of the work being done by the IOELC exemplifies such a concept.

### International palliative care reform

In October 2003 the Open Society Institute in USA commissioned the International Observatory on End of Life Care (IOELC: www.eolc-observatory.net) to facilitate a palliative care policy development conference for delegates from 12 resource-poor countries of central and eastern Europe. The IOELC worked with facilitators from seven countries with specific aims to share their experiences of integrating palliative care into national health care programmes in order to influence policy (Wright *et al.* 2004). As a result of debating the various issues in relation to policy development at the conference, each of the poorly resourced countries were encouraged to identify three realistic goals in policy development they wanted to take forward. These included: integrating palliative care into national health care policies and the necessary financial changes; addressing specific policies and standards for palliative care; educational programmes for health care professionals.

Palliative care nurse educators across Europe, under the auspices of the European Association for Palliative Care, have worked to provide guidance for the development of palliative nurse education in European countries (De Vlieger *et al.* 2004). The chair of the Palliative Nursing Education Task Force pulled together the experience of over 80 nurses using five different languages, a feat which only strengthens the contribution.

## ▌Tensions in relation to palliative care policy

In embracing the twenty-first century, changes in palliative care policy in the UK have created a tension for some when holding on to the roots of hospice/

palliative care. Long gone is the definition of 'terminal care', although one still sees it referred to in some articles; instead, there is an increasing use of 'end-of-life' and 'supportive care' (see Introduction) in an attempt to make palliative care more inclusive for those with diseases other than cancer. In questioning this new terminology, Praill (2000) cautions the hospice care community as to whether they are in danger of becoming 'death denying'. In revising the terminology and trying to accommodate pressures in health care practice, he wonders whether the palliative care community are in danger of weakening their identity with those people who are imminently dying. Are we witnessing what Kearney (1992) feared – that the focus on symptom control would take precedence over the specific care given to dying people and their families? Speaking about death and dying will always be difficult but the skilled communication and care in relation to death and dying was something that was pioneered by the hospice movement. The irony is that with the wider application of palliative care reform across health and social care, and in particular with older people in care homes, whatever terminology is being used might open up the communication around death and dying in our societies in a way that has not happened before.

There is also tension in relation to funding. Many argue that, in order for palliative care funding to be sustained, it needs to be integrated within mainstream health services. However, even when a country's health care system has integrated such a policy, services can still be vulnerable to major economic changes. Uganda is an important example of such a scenario (Sepulveda *et al.* 2002). In situations where a charitable model has been used as a basis for funding this too can be demanding on local communities especially poorer ones (Praill 2006).

Then there is the tension caused by general health care policy having an adverse impact on areas of palliative care that require reform in order to accommodate the new policy. A particular example has been the effect of recent policy changes to 'out-of-hours care' by general practitioners (GPs) in the UK. In the past individual general practices have taken part in being 'on-call' for emergencies (including palliative care issues) for their patients during the night and weekends. However, as a result of new government policies in the late 1990s, the relationship of GPs and the NHS changed. GPs are now contracted by the government to provide services, so 'out-of-hours' care is now contracted out through cooperatives across a much wider area. GPs have positively evaluated the cooperatives; but, because the emphasis of these new cooperatives is on acute medical care rather than palliative care, considerable barriers have been experienced by palliative care patients and their families, causing increased distress when trying to access advice and care (Worth *et al.* 2006).

## Professional/public divide and the discourse of death and dying

Whatever the efforts of policy by specialist palliative care, has Western society's opinion towards denial of death and dying been changed? Zimmerman and Rodin (2004) argue that there has been little influence, and others in the past have argued that there has been little public reform other than an increased routinization and medicalization of dying (Biswas and Ahmedzai 1994).

Raising community awareness is a major goal of the National Palliative Care Strategy in Australia (Rawlings *et al.* 2006). The project coordinators of the Adelaide Hills Palliative Care project publish a community-focused newsletter about the work twice a year. The newsletter is distributed in surgeries, libraries, community centres, clubs and local organizations with special 'expos' being organized with participation from local and state organizations. Posters advertising how the palliative care services can support patients and their families to live well are also displayed in 35 surgeries across the state.

Personal advocacy and public activism outside the specialist palliative care agenda is highlighted by Blacksher and Christopher (2002) as an opportunity for reform being addressed in the USA. They highlight the Community-State Partnerships to Improve End-of-Life Care programme that has been convening citizens since 1999. These programmes now operate in 21 states across the USA. The Community-State Partnerships have provided opportunities to gather information regarding barriers to good end-of-life care directly from contacting the public through meetings such as rotary clubs, church groups and town hall meetings. Blacksher and Christopher (2002) report on a number of the programmes and highlight how the coalitions have provided opportunities to educate the public and empower them to be able to seek appropriate quality of care at the end of life for themselves or their loved ones, and have been instrumental for the strengthening and building of community awareness in end-of-life care. The groups are also encouraged to help reform policy. Many different public groups lobby Capitol Hill (Goldstein and Lynn 2002) but one public group in particular, the AARP (American Association of Retired Persons), have announced an initiative to address long-term care and end-of-life care over the next ten years.

Another initiative in engaging the public in education around end-of-life care has been the use of drama. 'A Time To Go' (Hunsaker *et al.* 1995) is a publication of three prize-winning one-act plays highlighting issues on advance directives. The plays, each with their commentary, are performed at local community centres in order to educate the public on issues such as advance directives. Ensuring that there is both a bottom-up approach as well as a top-down approach to palliative care reform at a regional and national level can help make reform more robust.

# Conclusion

I began this chapter with a quote from Professor Bosanquet who in 1997 felt that previous investment in palliative care had created a local resource rather than one that was exceptional. In this chapter I have tried to demonstrate a global palliative care community who are now making considerable strides, through policy and the public health agenda, towards greater equity and accessibility for all those people and their families who face a far-advanced, progressive and incurable disease.

For those in the resource-poor countries of central and eastern Europe, goals are being set to establish the importance of palliative care education for all professionals and to bring palliative care into mainstream health care. In countries where palliative care is more developed, we see more detailed policies such as the importance of creating baseline data on which to plan palliative care services; greater 'user involvement' in assessing the quality of services; the use of assessment tools to improve quality of life; and the importance of educating the public how to access palliative care and their contribution to policy issues.

In the UK, after 40 years of hospice and the funding of nurse specialist posts, palliative care has some recognition in the policy agenda on the structure of health and social care (Seymour *et al.* 2002). It is through the hard work of policy organizations and practitioners that it has come thus far. However, we cannot afford to be complacent. There are still reports that reveal that reform is patchy and a recent personal account of the death of the father of a professor of health service research in the UK highlights this (Bowling 2000).

This chapter has highlighted the important role that people in both practice and research have in establishing palliative care policy. All members of the multidisciplinary team need to encourage colleagues to engage with health care policy – and particularly policy in relation to palliative care. The move to partnerships across boundaries both national and international, between health and social care, can offer opportunities for considerable reform. Although policy is a moving target, nonetheless the very fact that it never keeps still brings a dynamism of its own that is alive and challenging.

# Notes

1  Even since this article was published, there has been further policy change with the abolition of health authorities in England and the formation of Primary Care Teams (PCTs) who are given the charge to work with local authorities and other agencies that provide health and social care (Mirando 2004). PCTs are now answerable to strategic health authorities.

2  Having a carer supporting the patient at home is one of the criteria laid down by

Medicare reimbursement in order that a cancer patient can receive hospice home care.

# References

Addington-Hall, J.M., Walker, L., Jones, C., Karlson, S. and McCarthy, M. (1998) A randomized controlled trial of postal versus interviewer administration of a questionnaire measuring satisfaction with use of services received in the year before death. *Journal of Epidemiology and Community Health*, 52: 802–7.

Avis, M., Bond, M. and Arthur, A. (1995) Satisfying solutions? A review of some unresolved issues in the measurement of patient satisfaction. *Journal of Advanced Nursing*, 22: 316–22.

Aspinal, F., Hughes, R., Higginson, I.J. *et al.* (2002) *A Users Guide to the Palliative Care Outcome Scale*. London: Palliative Care and Policy Publications.

Aspinal, F., Addington-Hall, J., Hughes, R. and Higginson, I.J. (2003) Using satisfaction to measure the quality of palliative care: a review of the literature. *Journal of Advanced Nursing*, 42(4): 324–39.

Biswas, B. and Ahmedzai, S. (1994) The Medicalization of Dying. In: D. Clark (ed.) *The Future of Palliative Care: issues of policy and practice*. Buckingham: Open University Press.

Blacksher, E. and Christopher, M. (2002) On the road to reform: advocacy and activism in end-of-life care. *Journal of Palliative Medicine*, 5(1): 13–22.

Bond, S. (2003) Responses to: 'Using satisfaction to measure the quality of palliative care: a review of the literature': letter. *Journal of Advanced Nursing*, 43(5): 533–4.

Bosanquet, N. (1997) New challenge for palliative care. *British Medical Journal*, 314: 1294.

Bowling, A. (2000) Research on dying is scanty (letter). *British Medical Journal*, 320: 1205–6.

Bruera, E. and Sweeney, C. (2002) Palliative Care Models: international perspective. *Journal of Palliative Medicine*, 5(2): 319–27.

Byock, I., Norris, K., Curtis, J.R. and Patrick, D.L. (2001) Improving End-of-Life Experience and Care in the Community: a conceptual framework. *Journal of Pain and Symptom Management*, 22(3): 759–72.

Callaway, M., Foley, K.M., De Lima, L., Connor, S.R., Dix, O., Lynch, T., Wright, M. and Clark, D. (2007) Funding for Palliative Care Programs in Developing Countries. *Journal of Pain and Symptom Management*, 33(5): 509–13.

Clark, D. (2004) History, gender and culture in the rise of palliative care. In: S. Payne, J. Seymour and C. Ingleton (eds) *Palliative Care Nursing: principles and evidence for practice*. Buckingham: Open University Press.

Clark, D. and Malson, H. (2002) Key issues in palliative care needs assessment. In: D. Field, D. Clark, J. Corner and C. Davis (eds) *Researching Palliative Care*. Buckingham: Open University Press.

Corner, J., Halliday, D., Haviland, J., Douglas, H.R., Bath, P., Clark, D., Normand, C., Beech, N., Hughes, P., Marples, R., Seymour, J., Skilbeck, J. and Webb, T. (2003) Exploring nursing outcomes for patients with advanced cancer following intervention by Macmillan specialist palliative care nurses. *Journal of Advanced Nursing*, 41: 561–74.

Currow, D., Abernethy, A.P., Shelby-James, T.M. and Phillips, P.A. (2006) The impact of conducting a regional palliative care clinical study. *Palliative Medicine*, 20: 735–43.

De Lima, L., Krakauer, E.L., Lorenz, K., Prail, D., MacDonald, N. and Doyle, D. (2007) Ensuring Palliative Medicine Availability: the development of the IAHPC list of essential medicines for palliative care. *Journal of Pain and Symptom Management*, 33(5): 521–6.

De Vlieger, M., Gorchs, N., Larkin, P.J. and Porchet, F. (2004) *A Guide for the Development of Palliative Nurse Education in Europe*. Report of the European Association for Palliative Care (EAPC) Task Force. www.eapcnet.org/download/forTaskforces/NurseEducationGuide.pdf.

Diver, F., Molassiotis, A. and Weeks, L. (2003) The palliative care needs of ethnic minority patients attending a day-care centre: a qualitative study. *International Journal of Palliative Nursing*, 9(9): 389–96.

Department of Health (DoH) (1995) *A Policy Document for Commissioning Cancer Services*. London: HMSO.

Department of Health (DoH) (2006) dh.gov.uk/en/Policyandguidance/Organisationpolicy/Endoflifecare/index.

Department of Health (DoH) (2007) *Operating Framework 2007–2008: PCT baseline review of services for end of life care*. www.dh.gov.uk (accessed 16 June 2007).

Donabedian, A. (1980) *The definition of quality and approaches to its assessment*. Ann Arbor, MI: Health Administration Press.

Dunlop, R. and Hockley, J. (1998) *Hospital-based palliative care teams: the hospital-hospice interface* (2nd edn). Oxford: Oxford University Press.

Ellershaw, J.E., Peat, S.J. and Boys, L.C. (1995) Assessing the effectiveness of a hospital palliative care team. *Palliative Medicine*, 9: 145–52.

Finlay, I. (2006) The continuing challenge of palliative care. *British Journal of General Practice*, 56: 3–4.

Fisher, R., Ross, M.M. and MacLean, M.J. (eds) (2000) *A guide to end-of-life care for seniors*. Ottawa: University of Toronto and University of Ottawa.

Froggatt, K. (2004) *Palliative Care in Care Homes for Older People*. London: National Council for Palliative Care.

Gee, R. (2003) Barriers to pain and symptom management, opioids, health policy and drug benefits. *Journal of Pain and Symptom Management*, 25(2): 101–2.

Goldstein, N.E. and Lynn, J. (2002) The 107th Congress' legislative proposals concerning end-of-life care. *Journal of Palliative Medicine*, 5(6): 819–27.

Hearn, J. and Higginson, I.J. (2002) Outcome measures in palliative care for advanced cancer: a review. *Journal of Public Health Medicine*, 19(2): 193–9.

Hockley, J. (2006) *Developing high quality end-of-life care in nursing homes: an action research study*. Unpublished PhD: University of Edinburgh.

Hockley, J., Watson, J. and Dewar, B. (2004) *Developing quality end-of-life care in eight independent nursing homes through the implementation of an integrated care pathway for the last days of life*. Available from: www.stcolumbashospice.org.uk/professional.

Hunsaker Hawkins, A. and Ballard, J.O. (1995) *Time to Go: three plays on death and dying*. Philadelphia: University of Pennsylvania Press.

Iles, V. and Sutherland, K. (2001) *Managing Change in the NHS – organisational change: a review for health care managers, professionals and researchers*. National Co-ordinating Centre fro NHS Service Delivery and Organisations Research & Development. Available from: NCCSDO, London School of Hygiene & Tropical Medicine, London WC1E 6AZ.

Joranson, D.R. and Ryan, K.M. (2007) Ensuring Opioid Availability: methods and resources. *Journal of Pain and Symptom Management*, 33(5): 527–32.

Jordan, J., Wright, J., Ayres, P., Hawkings, M., Thomson, R., Wilkinson, J. and Williams, R. (2002) Health needs assessment and needs-led health service change: a survey of projects involving public health doctors. *Journal of Health Service Research and Policy*, 7(2): 71–80.

Kearney, M. (1992) Palliative medicine – just another speciality query. *Palliative Medicine*, 6(1): 39–46.

Kemmis, S. (2001) Exploring the Relevance of Critical Theory for Action Research: Emancipatory Action Research in the Footsteps of Jurgen Habermas. In: P. Reason and H. Bradbury, *Handbook of Action Research: participator inquiry and practice*. London: Sage Publications, pp. 91–102.

Liao, S. and Arnold, R.M. (2006) Influencing physician behaviour: the reason to engage in health policy (editorial). *Journal of Palliative Medicine*, 9(3): 729–30.

Lorenz, K.A., Shugarman, L.R. and Lynn, J. (2006) Health care policy issues in end-of-life care. *Journal of Palliative Medicine*, 9(3): 731–48.

Lynn, J. and Adamson, D.M. (2003) *Living Well at the End of Life: adapting health care to serious chronic illness in old age*. Rand Health White Paper WP-137: Centre for Palliative Care Studies. www.medicaring.org (accessed 16 September 2003).

Mathew, A., Cowley, S., Bliss, J. and Thistlewood, G. (2003) The development of palliative care in national government policy in England, 1986–2000. *Palliative Medicine*, 17: 270–82.

Mirando, S. (2004) Palliative care needs assessment. *International Journal of Palliative Nursing*, 10(12): 602–4.

Mortimer, R.H., Sewell, J., Roberton, D., Thomson, N., Leigh, J. and Long, P. (2004) Lessons from the Clinical Support Systems Program: facilitating better practice through leadership and team building. *Medical Journal of Australia*, 180: S97–S100.

Muszbek, K. (2007) Enhancing Hungarian Palliative Care Delivery. *Journal of Pain and Symptom Management*, 33(5): 605–9.

NCHSPCS (1995) *Specialist Palliative Care: a statement of definitions*. London: National Council for Hospice and Specialist Palliative Care Services.

NCHSPCS and SPPC (2000) *Positive Partnerships: palliative care for adults with severe mental health problems*. Occasional paper 17. London: National Council for Hospice and Specialist Palliative Care Service.

NCPC (2006) *Changing Gear: guidelines for managing the last days of life in adults*. London: The National Council for Palliative Care.

NHS Scotland (2002) National care standards: hospice care. Available from: www.scotland.gov.uk/Publications/2002.

NHSQIS (2004) *NHS Quality Improvement Scotland National Overview – Specialist Palliative Care*. Available from: www.nhshealthquality.org.

NICE (2004) *Improving supportive and palliative care for adults with cancer*. London: National Institute for Clinical Excellence. www.nice.org.uk.

Ovretveit, J. (1992) *Health Service Quality: an introduction to quality methods of health services*. Oxford: Blackwell.

Pickin, C. and St. Leger, S. (1993) *Assessing Health Need Using the Life Cycle Framework*. Buckingham: Open University Press.

Praill, D. (2000) Who are we here for? *Palliative Medicine*, 14(2): 91–2.

Praill, D. (2006) Keeping up the pressure: pushing palliative and hospice care higher up the political agenda. *International Journal of Palliative Nursing*, 12(2): 81–2.

Raphael, C., Ahrens, J. and Fowler, N. (2001) Financing end-of-life care in the USA. *Journal of Royal Society of Medicine*, 94: 458–61.

Rawlings, D., Hatton, I. and McDonald, K. (2006) Implementation of the Adelaide Hills Palliative Care Project. *International Journal of Palliative Nursing*, 12(10): 478–83.

Sepulveda, C., Marlin, A., Yshida, T. and Ullrich, A. (2002) Palliative Care: The World Health Organization's Global Perspective. *Journal of Pain and Symptom Management*, 24(2): 91–6.

Seymour, J., Clark, D. and Marples, R. (2002) Palliative care and policy in England: a review of health improvement plants for 1999–2003. *Palliative Medicine*, 16(1): 5–11.

SPPC (2006) Making good care better. Scottish Partnership for Palliative Care: Edinburgh. www.palliativecarescotland.org.uk.

Stjernsward, J., Foley, K.M. and Ferris, F.D. (2007) Integrating Palliative Care into National Policies. *Journal of Pain and Symptom Management*, 33(5): 514–20.

The National Palliative Care Programme (2004) *Guidelines for a Palliative Approach in Residential Aged Care*. Prepared by Edith Cowan University. www.nhrmc.gov.au (accessed 24 June 2007).

WHO (2000) *Achieving Balance in National Opioids Control Policy: guidelines for assessment*. Geneva: World Health Organization.

Worth, A., Boyd, K., Kendall, M., Heaney, D., Macleod, U., Cormie, P., Hockley, J. and Murray, S. (2006) Out-of-hours palliative care: a qualitative study of cancer patients, carers and professionals. *British Journal of General Practice*, 56(522): 6–13.

Wright, M., Clark, J., Greenwood, A., Callaway, M. and Clark, D. (2004) Palliative care policy development in Central and Eastern Europe and Central Asia: an Open Society Institute initiative. *Progress in Palliative Care*, 12(2): 71–5.

Zimmerman, C. and Rodin, G. (2004) The denial of death thesis: sociological critique and implications for palliative care. *Palliative Medicine*, 18: 121–8.

# 35

# Palliative care in resource-poor countries

*Jennifer Hunt*

---

**Key points**

- Accessibility to pain-relieving medicines is problematic in resource-poor countries and there is minimal professional health support.
- Poverty, nutritional needs and lack of transport determine the models of palliative care.
- Home-based care is the most common delivery of palliative care in these settings.
- Family carers look after the sick with support from community volunteers.
- Palliative care needs to be integrated into mainstream health systems to be sustainable.

---

# Introduction

The definition of 'resource-poor' countries relates to an economic classification with accompanying social and cultural implications. Wright (2003) combines the five indices of gross domestic product, the human development index, health expenditure, overall health system achievement, and morphine consumption to identify resource-poor countries in relation to health care. In essence, these indices describe the potential of a country to provide comprehensive health support to its citizens, the prioritization of health care, and the possibility of effective provision of pain control for the chronically ill and dying. These indices have guided the selection of countries for inclusion in this chapter. Consequently, industrially developed countries such as Russia and India are considered resource-poor in provision of health care for the chronically ill and dying and will be referred to in this chapter along with several African countries.

Statistics relating to resource-poor countries can paint a dismal picture. In particular, those relating to health services and the implications of living with cancer, HIV or any other life-limiting progressive illness in such settings are conclusively depressing. For example, sub-Saharan Africa has twice as many deaths per 1,000 head of population annually as that of North America, yet has only 1.5 per cent of global palliative care resources compared to 55 per cent in North America (*Global Health Council Newsletter* 2007). While HIV/AIDS has received unprecedented coverage and recent financial support, it is worth noting that 12.5 per cent of all deaths in resource-poor countries are caused by cancer. This is more than the total percentage of deaths caused by HIV/AIDS, tuberculosis and malaria (*Global Health Council Newsletter* 2007). In 2004 the UK Prime Minister, Tony Blair, described Africa as 'the only continent to become poorer in the last 25 years', where world trade has halved in recent years and where direct foreign investment has diminished to less than 1 per cent (Wright and Clark 2006). The continent has become inextricably associated with poverty, malnutrition, corruption and AIDS, all factors that worsen conditions for the dying.

As there are many different beginnings of palliative care in resource-poor countries, this chapter will start with a brief history of the development of palliative care in southern Africa and India as examples of springboards for the diversity that has followed in many resource-poor settings. There are several literary resources that provide comprehensive insights into the issues pertaining to palliative care in resource-poor countries (O'Neill *et al.* 2002; Foley *et al.* 2003; Wright 2003; Stjernsward and Clark 2004) and readers of this chapter are encouraged to refer to them. A synthesis of the main points will be provided as an entry into the chapter. A brief overview is given of recent initiatives promoting palliative care in resource-poor countries to explain how services have grown rapidly despite poor national health support. Questions emerge relating to the sustainability of services established in these conditions. These are discussed using examples from selected countries, with an analysis of challenges and successes. Innovative services in India and South Africa show palliative care in resource-poor settings at their creative best. Such services may differ substantially from palliative care as it is known in resource-rich countries. Palliative care in Zimbabwe, its progress threatened by economic and political instability, exemplifies the challenges of providing care for the dying in settings where health budgets are woefully inadequate. The chapter concludes with a summary of lessons learned and a tentative preview of what may lie ahead.

## Development of palliative care in Africa and India

Modern palliative care began in England in response to the failure of post-World War II health services to provide adequate care for the dying. The hospice movement founded by Dame Cicely Saunders spread rapidly in various parts of the world and transferred preferentially to ex-British colonies that tended to replicate its health system. Programmes often initially reflected the background and experience of their founders until they evolved into systems that were more local and appropriate. While a hospice service had been established in Zimbabwe in 1979 and hospices were developing in South Africa in the 1980s, they were primarily for cancer patients and depended on the support and funds of families and affected communities. It took the HIV/AIDS pandemic in sub-Saharan Africa to attract the attention and financial support of the international community to consider alternative approaches of care of the dying in large numbers usually in dire poverty. In the past decade proposals have been urgently submitted to donor agencies for the funding of projects to begin countering the devastating effects of HIV/AIDS. Strategies have been devised to cope with overwhelming numbers of seriously ill in settings where health facilities are few and far between. Services that are free or inexpensive have characterized the development of palliative care initiatives in Africa. Similarly, palliative care in India has drawn on the expertise of the British hospice model but combines this with a home-grown community palliative care model in some settings, which is better suited to responding to the needs of so many. A clear model of home-based care (HBC) has emerged with medical back-up provided by a few specialist health personnel, clinic staff and community volunteers.

## Review of issues specific to palliative care in resource-poor countries

Common themes have been identified as issues that affect the development and effective implementation of palliative care in resource-poor countries. These form the foundation upon which this chapter is based, and from which to expand some of the issues by way of selected examples. A synthesis of issues and illustrations is presented in Table 35.1 (O'Neill *et al.* 2002; Foley *et al.* 2003; Wright 2003; Stjernsward and Clark 2004).

## Initiatives and funding

The push for palliative care in Africa especially has been driven by the HIV/ AIDS pandemic and significant funding is derived from several quarters. Although the greater focus is on the prevention and treatment of HIV/ AIDS, with the risk of ART side-tracking the need for quality palliative care, international awareness, commitment and financial investment in palliative care has never been so high. There still remain convincing reasons why palliative care is relevant and necessary in the care of people living with HIV. The side effects associated with ARV treatments themselves are disabling and demotivating and respond to palliative care management. Co-morbidities and other life-limiting illnesses are emerging, such as end-stage liver failure, cerebrovascular disease and malignancies, for which palliative care is required. The prevalence of distressing symptoms throughout the HIV/AIDS disease trajectory is high. Pain, dermatological problems, gastrointestinal problems, sexual dysfunction, and depression (Help the Hospices 2007) can all benefit from palliative care. People with HIV disease are still more likely to die earlier compared to the uninfected and need quality end-of-life care. Good quality terminal care is required too for all those who still die from this illness. Nearly 3 million deaths were reported globally from AIDS in 2006 (*Global Health Council Newsletter* 2007).

The World Health Organization (WHO) supports community-based palliative care through Ministries of Health in five African countries. The most recent WHO guidance on palliative care, symptom management and end-of-life care (the Integrated Management of Adult Infections training package) uses a public health approach. This emphasizes the decentralized delivery of an integrated package of essential HIV/AIDS services and has become the gold standard of palliative care implementation in resource-poor countries. The World Bank's multi-country AIDS programme (MAP) aims to accelerate community-based prevention, treatment and care initiatives, although proposals do not specify support for palliative care. The Global Fund provides extensive funding for those home-based care organizations that wish to deliver palliative care services but may not be practising this according to the WHO definition. The USAID-administered President's Emergency Plan for AIDS Relief (PEPFAR) has made the most significant recent impact on the funding of palliative care. Through its broad and controversial definition of palliative care, PEPFAR supports prevention and treatment of tuberculosis (TB), gender issues, human capacity development, policy development (such as opioid policy development) and supply chain management as components of palliative care. The Open Society Institute provides grants for specific projects related to palliative care. The Diana, Princess of Wales Memorial Fund has supported several palliative care initiatives in nine African countries. Links between palliative care services in resource-rich and resource-poor countries have been encouraged by the Foundation for Hospices in sub-Saharan Africa (FHSSA), now a part of the National Hospice and Palliative Care Organization in the USA (Wright and Clark 2006; Harding *et al.* 2007). These often take the form of twinning arrangements and support in kind. Numerous smaller donors contribute to this extraordinary upswing in palliative care training and provision.

Outside of Africa, dependence on international funding appears less integral to palliative care initiatives. A successful community-based initiative in southern India, the Neighbourhood Network in Palliative Care (NNPC), derives the majority of its funding from small community donations. The Mallapuram Initiative in one district raises 95 per cent of its operating capital from small contributions from its residents. Russia, despite its harsh economic climate, has managed steady progress in palliative care through a combination of state, business, charitable and non-commercial funding.

**Table 35.1** Main issues affecting palliative care development in resource-poor countries

| Issue | Example |
|---|---|
| Scarce monetary, nutritional and human resources affecting the care environment. | In Zimbabwe many people living with HIV/AIDS are rural dwellers dependent on crop production and community agricultural support. The decimation of many healthy young villagers due to HIV/AIDS, and the amount of time spent in caring for ill people means that fields are neglected and crop production is severely reduced. The nearest clinic is likely to be up to 40 km away and any palliative care expertise or medication is available only in provincial hospitals or in an urban setting. Rampant inflation has eroded the ability of many to seek medical care and treatments. Numbers of trained health personnel have dwindled due to emigration in search of better salaries. |
| Cultural and ethical sensitivity and country-specific adaptation, including preference of place of death, truth-telling, disclosure, information sharing and sustainable technologies. | Russia's culture of care has privileged state allegiance rather than patient rights. There are also strong taboos surrounding death and cancer that inhibit truth-telling (Wright 2003). The idea of discussing preference of place of death has been foreign. Physicians have tended to focus exclusively on curative care. Communication with patients was governed by an ethic of duty, prohibiting the disclosure of a terminal condition. The multidisciplinary teamwork associated with palliative care was unknown (Wright and Clark 2004). In India, a strong extended family system continues to believe that it is better for the patient not to be told of a life-limiting diagnosis.[1] |
| Low priority of cancer and AIDS prevention, treatment and care in national health budgets. | Uganda is alone in Africa in making palliative care for patients with AIDS and cancer a priority in its National Health Plan. Morphine is provided free of charge by the government and palliation was acknowledged as 'essential care' in 1998, a move that has accelerated palliative care development in that country. No other country in Africa has prioritized treatment and care for people living with cancer or AIDS in health budgets. |
| Stigma and isolation surrounding HIV/AIDS and cancer, the two main illnesses associated with palliative care in these countries. | In Russia most cancer patients receive no medical help once the terminal prognosis is known, and no attempt is made to support the patient or family during this time (Wright 2003). In India, hospice services have developed almost entirely to cater for the needs of cancer patients who continue to face stigma and rejection by families and communities. Secrecy, shame and refusal to accept the stigmatizing condition HIV contribute to the delayed acknowledgement of the threat of AIDS in India. Consequently, provision for HIV is limited to information, prevention and anti-retroviral treatments, rather than palliative care.[2] |
| The extent of the HIV epidemic, life expectancy and projections for budgeting, including anti-retroviral therapy (ART). | Swaziland is one of the countries worst affected by the HIV/AIDS epidemic in the world, with a prevalence rate of 39.2 per cent in 2006 among the 15–49 year age group (Swaziland Ministry of Health 2006). Life expectancy in Zimbabwe has dropped significantly in recent years due to the epidemic and in 2004 stood at 37.7 for males and 38 for females (Wright and Clark 2006). In Russia, life expectancy is currently 58.9 for males and 72.3 for females but has been declining since the 1980s. Deaths currently exceed births by 60 per cent, an unprecedented rise in mortality in an industrialized nation (Wright and Clark 2004). |

| | |
|---|---|
| Lack of national palliative care policy, including integrated community and home-based care policies. | In Tanzania the national health policy is under review and stakeholders agree that palliative care should be included. Scale-up of palliative care is dependent on the increased accessibility to morphine, the development of the national health policy to include palliative care, and the grafting of palliative care on to existing home-based care services but these are still to be implemented (Harding et al. 2007). Until 2006 Vietnam had no formal palliative care policy to guide development. A report on scaling up universal access to HIV/AIDS services that year did not mention palliative care even as a care and support option (Harding et al. 2007). India's palliative care activists continue to pressurize government to design and implement a national palliative care policy.[3] |
| Lack of education of health care professionals, family care-givers and the public in palliative care, leading to attitudinal change surrounding illness, death and bereavement. | Talking of death and illness remains taboo in many African countries, with witchcraft seen as the reason for an incurable illness. Although education is identified by the World Health Organization (WHO) as a key component in the development of palliative care (Powell et al. 2007), the numbers of trained practitioners remain pitifully low. |
| Drug availability (including cost and accessibility) for pain control, symptom management and anti-retroviral treatments (ARVs or ART), as well as the prescriber–patient ratio for morphine. | Access to medicines, including opioids, is one of the major barriers to palliative care scale-up. Morphine is largely unavailable in Africa and south-east Asia. Vietnam's restrictive opioid regulations permit a small number of urban-based physicians to prescribe limited doses for up to seven days. For decades, the only morphine available in India was injectable and used for post-operative pain. Only in 1998 were all state governments encouraged to apply for an improved extended licence and only ten have done so since. It is estimated that less than 3 per cent of cancer patients in India have adequate pain relief.[4] |
| Support for palliative care-givers, in particular women who are the main care-givers. | In the Zimbabwean rural home female carers are mainly responsible for the care of the dying. They may also be coping with household chores, subsistence farming or other employment, and looking after children, elderly people and other dependants. Most carers may have HIV themselves and their own health may be deteriorating. Elderly carers often lack the necessary resources, knowledge and support to provide effective care for the sick (HelpAge Zimbabwe 1992). |
| Need for national palliative care associations to establish country-specific standards. | The African Palliative Care Association (APCA), established in 2004 to promote and support palliative care across the continent, encourages the development of national associations within countries and works closely with them to develop appropriate palliative care services in-country. Countries in Africa, such as Lesotho and Namibia, that have elements of palliative care in practice, have struggled for integration into mainstream health systems without an active national association to facilitate this and to support and guide them. |

Twinning links with British hospices have successfully increased training and education opportunities. While support for palliative care development in Russia has come from the wider international community, local initiatives are driven by dedicated nurses and doctors with the support of city authorities.[5]

## Developing new ways

Care for the dying in resource-poor countries requires considering hospice and palliative care from a broader perspective. There are several examples of emerging palliative care programmes in resource-poor countries that are re-shaping themselves from a Western hospice model into services better suited to local conditions. This metamorphosis can result in a service delivery that is unrecognizable by Western standards. Focus on food support, assisting clients to establish income-generating projects and vegetable gardens, and integrating ARVs alongside palliative support all indicate different priorities to resource-rich countries. The WHO's preliminary survey in 2001 in five African countries to establish the needs of the terminally ill and their care-givers confirmed this (Sepulveda *et al.* 2003). For example, the most common problems experienced by patients and carers in Tanzania included economic hardships caused by unemployment, financial constraints and lack of time to do other chores. A survey in Zimbabwe found that agri-cultural output declined by nearly 50 per cent among households affected by HIV/AIDS (Ministry of Health and Child Welfare 2004), escalating the descent of many families into poverty. Ugandan families noted that food needs were one of their greatest concerns and that HIV/AIDS caused a dramatic decline in income as less time could be spent tending crops as the patient became progressively more ill. A recent evaluation of a palliative care provider in Swaziland showed that the major problems faced by patients and families were lack of food and money for transport and medication. Prob-lems in relationships and pain were listed after those (Mataure and Mavu 2007). Consequently, enlisting nutritional support from the World Food Programme, churches and other donors is a common feature of palliative care in Africa.

In India, a burgeoning palliative care movement is increasingly attend-ing to large numbers of dying poor using a variety of models. The hospital-based Pain and Palliative Care Clinic in Calicut has been recognized by WHO for its pioneering work in bringing pain relief to the poor and needy. The success of its HBC programme led to the formation of the NNPC, a dynamic community-led network of professionals who supervise and sup-port a network of volunteers and clinics throughout Kerala. Both projects emphasize community services and public participation. They draw on a primary health model involving volunteers from the community to increase coverage and sustainability in areas where there is a low ratio of health workers to patients. Advocacy from local palliative care practitioners resulted in the state government simplifying the drug licensing process, making oral morphine widely accessible to palliative care programmes. In Delhi, CanSupport has been offering quality home-based support for cancer patients since 1997 and continues to expand its mobile teams and day care centre. Locally-based clinics and improved links with local general practitioners who can provide continuity of patient care appear to be the preferred option in this setting. Elsewhere, as in Bangalore, inpatient hospice units offer respite care and a place for patients to be referred when families feel unable to cope. Twenty-three inpatient hospices have been identified in India that cater for the needs of cancer patients from marginalized groups, such as the destitute, homeless and those with offensive wounds rejected by families.[6]

In sub-Saharan Africa, a variety of palliative care approaches have grown over the past three decades. Examples of best practice are Uganda and South Africa, both of which work closely with their Ministries of Health and training institutions to guide the development of policies, standards and training. Opioids are mainly available, although not necessarily in rural areas, education and accredited training courses have been ratified by national associations, and policies have been implemented. Success has been achieved in linking palliative care providers with community hospitals and clinics to offer a continuum of care throughout the illness trajectory. A combination of inpatient units, day care centres and home-based care characterize palliative care in these countries.

The South African integrated care model includes recruiting, training and providing support and supervision to community care workers with close links to health facilities for support and guidance. The Hospice Palliative Care Association of South Africa (HPCA) has further promoted the community-based model of care through a mentorship programme which builds palliative care capacity in partner home-based care organizations. Another pilot programme employs one professional palliative care nurse to provide the support and supervision of care workers in a number of community home-based care organizations in one health sub-district, demonstrating effective use of scarce human resources. HPCA and the South African Department of Health have developed a strong partnership to facilitate the integration of palliative care into home-based care services and state health care facilities.

# Palliative care or home-based care?

In several African countries a groundswell of home-based care groups, often faith-based, have responded to the challenge of providing care to the dying in their communities, made possible with funding from international donors, and where necessary guided with technical assistance by organizations such as the APCA. Basic training of community home-based care volunteers in Zimbabwe, Kenya, Lesotho, Swaziland and Namibia includes facts about HIV/AIDS, management of AIDS-related conditions, some home nursing skills, environmental health, nutrition, reproductive health, psychosocial and spiritual support. Additional training in pain assessment and management, care of the dying, signs of approaching death, bereavement and expanded communication skills with adults and children by palliative care experts enhances knowledge of pain and symptom control and holistic care. A cascade model of training is used to impart this information from health workers to family carers. Strengthening the capacity of families to care for the dying is an approach that resonates with hospice care but it is becoming clear that without the support of professional expertise in regions that have minimal skilled human resources, it is unrealistic to refer to this as palliative care. Attention is most often paid to practical needs, such as basic patient care, hygiene and sometimes sourcing nutritional supplements. Accessing effective pain relief is difficult in all but a few settings. Although psychosocial support is reputedly provided by home-based care providers, the care in reality is overwhelmingly social, with emotional support limited to compassion, prayer and advice-giving.

Questions arise whether such community responses do in fact offer quality palliative care. Gupta (2004) in India and Hunt (2004) in Africa explored in parallel what model of palliative care is needed for resource-poor settings. Both acknowledge the tension between perceiving palliative care as a specialty skill and an approach that family members and community volunteers can perform with minimal training. An intensely individualized service performed by specialist palliative care staff has severe limitations when applied to a resource-poor environment where health workers are usually a scarce resource. This is exacerbated by serious limitations in training capacity, support services and medical resources to impart knowledge and skill to the family level (Graham and Clark 2005). More importantly, serious paucity of skilled manpower means little to no appropriate supervision, modelling and mentoring that could consolidate learning and practice *in situ*. This means that a much diluted version of palliative care, often no more than basic supportive care, is provided by family carers.

Such discourse has led to the need for a systematic framework to define palliative care in resource-poor settings. For the mapping of palliative care development in Africa, Wright and Clark devised a systematic categorization of four groups of palliative care development. The typology distinguishes between countries where there is no known activity, to where capacity building is evident, developing to localized provision of services, and finally expansion of palliative care where services are approaching integration and there is general awareness of palliative care (Wright and Clark 2006). Out of the 47 countries within Africa this typology categorized 21 in 2006 as having no known palliative care activity at all. Eleven countries had the beginnings of capacity building in place, and another 11 could be described as having established localized provision. Only four countries, namely Uganda, Zimbabwe, South Africa and Kenya, could be described as approaching integration. This meant that these countries had established capacity and local palliative care provision, as well as several other indicators, including a range of services and providers, a measure of integration with mainstream providers, established education centres, a broad awareness of palliative care, awareness of impact on policy and a national association. The process of categorization continues and adjustments are likely in the face of the refinement of the typology and dynamic changes in the socio-political conditions affecting health in some countries. While palliative care is developing rapidly in many resource-poor countries, it is salutary to remember that palliative care cannot operate in isolation. Box 35.1 offers a detailed vignette on Zimbabwe to illustrate the decline of palliative care services in the face of economic upheaval.

## Moving forward

A common theme that affects effective delivery of palliative care in resource-poor countries is opioid availability. Persistent advocacy, partnerships and a national organization representing all providers are proven to make an impact on policy change as shown in the example of Zambia given in Box 35.2.

---

**Box 35.1** Economic impact on palliative care delivery in Zimbabwe

Zimbabwe's deteriorating economy since 2000 has had far-reaching effects on palliative care service delivery. As the first hospice service in Africa in 1979, Island Hospice Service's home-based care programme initially delivered specialized care for a relatively small number of people suffering from cancer. It later became more community based, responding to the HIV/AIDS epidemic. Highly qualified nurses and social workers trained health workers and volunteers in the principles and practice of palliative care and bereavement to disseminate the care-load. Selection and supervision procedures to manage the army of trained volunteers were implemented according to quality standards. By 1996 a training department had been created and relationships established with the Ministry of Health, medical school and non-governmental organizations to extend knowledge and expertise countrywide. At the time of writing however, services are severely compromised by a serious depletion of skilled staff that has sought employment out of the country to counter hyper-inflation. Support services are increasingly provided by volunteers who are often HIV-positive themselves and who are struggling with the difficult living conditions in the country. Numbers of patients seen by Island Hospice Service have risen sharply, partly due to a clinic-based system introduced in highly populated urban areas. This enables many sick people to receive at least some components of palliative care, but does not allow for the in-depth holistic care the service used to be able to offer (Maasdorp 2007). Fuel shortages, erratic drug supplies, lack of policy implementation and ever-increasing numbers of needy ill underserved by inadequate mainstream health services all jeopardize the dream of palliative care being received by all who need it. As one of only four countries categorized as approaching integration in 2006, it is likely in 2007 that Zimbabwe can only claim to offer localized provision.

> **Box 35.2**   Integrating palliative care into the Zambian national health system
>
> The Zambian Dangerous Drugs Act allows the Ministry of Health to appoint health-related professionals outside of the Ministry to prescribe, dispense and supply opioids. This window of opportunity was recognized in early 2007 by a non-governmental organization supporting the Palliative Care Association of Zambia, and permission for this was granted by the Ministry of Health in June 2007. A secondary benefit has been the request by the Ministry to roll out training to district and provincial hospitals and health care professionals nationwide, which has the potential to dramatically increase palliative care skills in the mainstream health sector (*Worldwide Hospice and Palliative Care Online* 2007).

Website developments in recent years have made a significant impact on information accessibility for and about resource-poor countries. Besides the APCA website's[7] free download of its *Clinical Guide to Supportive and Palliative Care for HIV/AIDS in Sub-Saharan Africa*, clinical guidelines for palliative care appropriate for use in resource-poor countries are available to download free of charge in the Palliative Care section of the Institut Pasteur (INCTR) website.[8] Committed to improving the delivery of good quality cancer palliative care in developing countries, these guidelines were developed in Nepal and have been implemented in India and Tanzania.

Organizations developed within resource-poor countries for resource-poor countries are beginning to address the obstacles that have delayed rapid and acceptable progress in palliative care. The APCA has grown rapidly since its inception in 2004 to become a main player in the promotion, coordination and support of palliative care in the continent. It has enormous potential to ensure development of sustainable palliative care at a standard that is internationally recognized yet culturally appropriate within African countries. The Indian Association of Palliative Care, created in 1994, plays a key role in lobbying for morphine availability nationwide, and assists the development of palliative care through education and training.

The African Organization for Research and Training in Cancer (AORTIC) facilitates research and training and provides relevant and accurate information on the prevention, early diagnosis, treatment and palliation of cancer (*AORTIC* 2006).

# Emerging gaps

In the fast-moving environment of palliative care in resource-poor countries, the common issues earlier identified provide a comprehensive synopsis of known problems and opportunities. Yet, new areas of concern continue to be exposed as services are subject to increasingly rigorous review. Bereavement support is an example. The WHO definition of palliative care includes bereavement support but how this translates in reality varies widely and little research has been undertaken into this area of palliative care. With concurrent and multiple deaths due to AIDS in resource-poor countries, no longer can this aspect of palliative care be regarded simply as a postscript to the main body of patient care. Meaningful emotional support of both the patient and their family cannot ignore the impact of several close losses that the patient and family may have experienced in recent years. Having the opportunity to process other unresolved losses in life before the patient dies is implicit in the palliative care holistic approach, yet health workers, community volunteers and family carers equipped with only basic communication skills training find this a painful and emotional topic to explore with patients. Finding ways to normalize bereavement within the cultural context and to capitalize on helpful community and family responses will be more productive in resource-poor countries than attempting to train volunteers in Western bereavement counselling methods (Hunt *et al.* 2007)

For many countries in the process of developing palliative care services, energy and limited resources are almost entirely geared towards adult care leaving paediatric palliative care grossly underserved. There is no specific UNICEF policy on palliative care for children affected by HIV/AIDS, although reference is made in campaigns and frameworks to strengthening the capacity of families to provide psychosocial support and mobilizing community-based support to care for children (UNICEF 2004). A joint initiative between WHO and UNICEF identifies the need to address a lack of essential medicines for children, and WFP is coordinating with UNICEF on nutritional support. Training of health professionals and volunteers pays only cursory attention to the needs of sick and dying children and while attention and funds have been drawn to the plight of many children left orphaned and vulnerable due to the AIDS pandemic, this is overwhelmingly social in nature with few programmes integrating paediatric palliative care into the services they offer. Even fewer are equipped to support children emotionally who are struggling with losing parents, siblings and other relatives. Yet there are some initiatives that can demonstrate good practice in different settings. The Mildmay Centre's Jajja's Home in Uganda is a day care service for children and adolescents infected and affected by HIV. Some inpatient beds facilitate residential terminal care and training. Children and adolescents receive pain and symptom control for severe and persistent symptoms, and are fed an energy-rich diet. In South Africa, paediatric palliative care teams are beginning to be established. In Zimbabwe, a bereaved children's group work programme, established in 1992 at Island Hospice, has been expanded with donor funding to attend to the needs of young carers who are in the front line of providing care for dying parents and siblings.

An issue that seriously hinders palliative care development in resource-poor countries is lack of human resources but it is becoming clear that this obstacle is more complex than merely training more health professionals. Salaries of nurses in resource-poor countries are notoriously low and sometimes erratic. A massive investment in health services is needed, not only for drugs and supplies. Better wages for more nurses will probably have more effect on how many dying people receive palliative care than marginal decreases in the prices of ARV drugs, and this needs to be the focus of international advocacy. Voluntarism, upon which palliative home-based care depends, is urgently in need of review in settings where community volunteers are unemployed, living in poverty, often ill themselves and unable to afford transport to see clients or to meet with supervisors. Payments in kind or stipends are common and may well be a motivating factor for volunteering. The issue of payment repeatedly arises as one of the biggest problems for volunteers in many African countries (Coughlan 2006). In contrast, the NNPC project in Kerala capitalizes upon the numbers of community volunteers who carry the client work of the organization for no payment or reward. This model owes its extraordinary success to high levels of unpaid voluntarism, yet this approach is not easily replicated elsewhere in India or indeed all parts of Kerala.

# Conclusion

The key components to delivery of quality palliative care have been articulated by WHO as policy, education, drug availability and implementation (Powell *et al.* 2007). In resource-poor countries this creates enormous challenges. High density populations, significant geographical distances and the poverty of patients and families have determined the character of services that can be offered to the dying in these countries. Policy restrictions, especially with regard to opioid drugs, monetary constraints, too few training institutions, lack of skilled human resources and the overwhelming number of chronically ill and dying, are just some of the obstacles to effective provision of care for all who need it. Although there is a clear trend in resource-poor countries to deliver palliative care through a home-based care model, it has been argued that this is insufficient unless it exists within an informed public health model that embraces palliative care. Where this commitment is lacking, weak or sporadic, implementation of palliative care at country level results in unsustained and poor quality care (Harding *et al.* 2007). Varied developments across a range of resource-poor countries have demonstrated too that palliative care need not be accommodated entirely by home-based care. Obtaining resources to manage alternative models such as hospital-based care, day centres and inpatient units is possible as shown in the examples above. Lessons continue to be learnt and adapted from palliative care developments in resource-rich settings. Undoubtedly lessons can be learnt too from the particular challenges facing palliative care in resource-poor countries. Far from painting a picture of homogenous struggle and decline, the story of palliative care in these settings can indeed inspire and inform practice elsewhere.

# Notes

1  www.eolc-observatory.net/global_analysis/india_current_services
2  www.eolc-observatory.net/global_analysis/india_current_services
3  www.eolc-observatory.net/global_analysis/india_current_services
4  www.eolc-observatory.net/global_analysis/india_current_services
5  www.eolc-observatory.net/global_analysis/russia_pc_history.htm
6  www.eolc-observatory.net/global_analysis/india_current_services
7  www.apca.co.ug
8  www.inctr.org/projects/palliative.shtml

# Further reading

Foley, K., Aulino, F. and Stjernsward, J. (2003) Palliative Care in Resource-Poor Settings. In: J. O'Neill, P. Selwyn and H. Schietinger (eds) *A Clinical Guide to Supportive and Palliative Care for HIV/AIDS*. Rockville: US Dept. of Health and Human Services.

O'Neill, J., Romaguera, R., Parham, D. and Marconi, K. (2002) Practicing Palliative Care in Resource-Poor Settings. *Journal of Pain and Symptom Management*, 24(2): 148–51.

Stjernsward, J. and Clark, D. (2004) Palliative Medicine – A Global Perspective. In: D. Doyle, G. Hanks, N. Cherny and K. Chalman (eds) *Oxford Textbook of Palliative Medicine*, 3rd edn. Oxford: Oxford University Press, 21: 1196–224.

Wright, M. and Clark, D. (2006) *Hospice and Palliative Care in Africa*. Oxford: Oxford University Press.

# References

*African Organization for Research and Training in Cancer (AORTIC) News* (email version) (2006), Cape Town, 7(7).

Coughlan, M. (2006) *Trip Report on Technical Consultancy to USAID Regional HIV/AIDS Programme*.

Foley, K., Aulino, F. and Stjernsward, J. (2003) Palliative Care in Resource-Poor Settings. In: J. O'Neill, P. Selwyn and H. Schietinger (eds) *A Clinical Guide to Supportive and Palliative Care for HIV/AIDS*. Rockville: US Dept. of Health and Human Services.

*Global Health Council Newsletter*, 14 May 2007.

Graham, F. and Clark, D. (2005) Addressing the Basics of Palliative Care. *International Journal of Palliative Nursing*, 11(1): 36–9.

Gupta, H. (2004). How Basic is Palliative Care? *IJPN*, 10(12): 600–1.

Harding, R., Pahl, N., Goh, C., Hunt, J., Collins, K., Dickinson, C. and Morris, C. (2007) *Draft Review of Global Policy Architecture and Country Level Practice on HIV/AIDS and Palliative Care*. London: DFID.

HelpAge Zimbabwe (1992) *Support for Elderly, Rural Women Looking after AIDS Sufferers and Children Orphaned by AIDS*. (Research Reports), Harare.

Help the Hospices (2007) *Notes from symposium on palliative care for HIV/AIDS patients.*

Hunt, J. (2004). Questions for Hospice in Resource-Poor Settings. *Progress in Palliative Care*, 12(4): 1–6.

Hunt, J., Andrew, G. and Weitz, P. (2007) Improving Support for the Bereaved Within Their Communities. *Bereavement Care*, 26(2).

Maasdorp, V. (2007) Personal communication, 11 June.

Mataure, P. and Mavu, J. (2007) *Draft report on Swaziland Hospice at Home (SHAH) Palliative Care Assessment.* Unpublished.

Ministry of Health and Child Welfare, National AIDS Council (2004) *The HIV and AIDS Epidemic in Zimbabwe.* Harare.

O'Neill, J., Romaguera, R., Parham, D. and Marconi, K. (2002) Practicing Palliative Care in Resource-Poor Settings. *Journal of Pain and Symptom Management*, 24(2): 148–51.

Powell, R., Mwangi-Powell, F., Ddungu, H. and Downing, J. (2007) *Pain Assessment and Management in sub-Saharan Africa: An Overview and Way Forward.* HIV Implementers' Meeting, Kigaili, Rwanda.

Sepúlveda, C., Habiyambere, V., Amandua, J., Borok, M., Kikule, E., Mudanga, B., Ngoma, T. and Solomon, B. (2003) Quality Care at the End of Life in Africa. *British Medical Journal*, 327(7408): 209–13.

Stjernsward, J. and Clark, D. (2004) Palliative Medicine – A Global Perspective. In: D. Doyle, G. Hanks, N. Cherny and K. Chalman (eds) *Oxford Textbook of Palliative Medicine*, 3rd edn. Oxford: Oxford University Press, 21: 1196–224.

Swaziland Ministry of Health (2006) *UNICEF* (2004) *The Framework for the protection, care and support of orphans and vulnerable children living in a world with HIV and AIDS.* Swaziland Ministry of Health, Swaziland.

*Worldwide Hospice and Palliative Care Online* (*WHPCO*) e-newsletter 4 June 2007.

Wright, M. (2003) *Models of Hospice and Palliative Care in Resource-Poor Countries: Issues and Opportunities.* London: Hospice Information.

Wright, M. and Clark, D. (2004) Hospice care in Russia. *Progress in Palliative Care*, 12(1): 27–9.

Wright, M. and Clark, D. (2006). *Hospice and Palliative Care in Africa.* Oxford: Oxford University Press, p. 5.

# Useful websites

www.inctr.org/projects/palliative.shtml
www.apca.co.ug
www.eolc-observatory.net/global_analysis/india_current_services
www.eolc-observatory.net/global_analysis/russia_pc_history.htm

# Conclusion
*Sheila Payne, Jane Seymour and Christine Ingleton*

As we have read through these chapters we have been witness to the diversity of palliative care and the important contribution made by nurses to this endeavour. We have explored palliative care from many different perspectives, with a view to providing those who work in the field with a broad and critical understanding of the issues surrounding the care of people facing life-limiting illness and their companions. We now face the task of having to draw some conclusions: a daunting task given the complexity of the material that precedes these final words. We propose to proceed by asking some questions and trying to identify the factors that must be taken into account in moving towards the formulation of the answers to them.

Of course, the first question must be, 'Do we know what palliative care is?' In asking this, we have moved full circle, since we set out in the Introduction to define palliative care. We do not intend to repeat that discussion, but rather to tease out some of the tensions and common themes that have emerged. Of these, the most obvious tension is that between 'specialist' and 'general' palliative care. This tension is played out clearly in nursing, where debates seem set to continue about the remit, roles and boundaries of specialist nurses in palliative care, their different levels of specialism and exactly what is the 'added value' of specialist nursing care (see, for example, Corner 2003). As Corner notes, nurses in palliative care prioritize emotional and supportive care in their work and these aspects of care are likely to be highly valued by patients and their companions. However, there is no room for complacency: in spite of arguably widespread awareness of the core goals of palliative care and knowledge about how to reach them, too many nurses find it difficult to balance competing priorities and conflicting demands on their time, and work in poorly resourced organizations where these essential aspects of caring continue to be devalued and poorly articulated (Payne *et al.* 2007). Nor should we be deceived into thinking that 'specialists' in palliative care somehow have a monopoly on the skills and attributes that are required to provide good care to people with palliative care needs. Humility and a willingness to collaborate and learn from others, many of whom are experts and specialists in their own fields, can only enhance the quality of palliative and end-of-life care (Seymour *et al.* 2005). Chapter 35 highlights the challenge for nurses working in resource-poor countries where there are few 'specialist' palliative care nurses, and that arguably their role needs to focus on education and leadership rather than direct patient care.

The issue of teamwork emerges as a further theme within the book (see Chapter 28 by Cox and James), and the potential demands of hospice ideology and how they impact on nurses' welfare are explored further by Aranda (Chapter 29). Mount (2003) draws our attention to the two goals of caring in clinical practice: *hippocratic*, in which the controlling of disease from an objective standpoint is paramount; and *askelepian*, in which the care-giver tries to enter the experience of suffering for the patient and his family, and focuses on preparing a space of safety and security for them (Kearney 2000; Mount 2003). With advances in medical technology, the boundaries between palliation and curative treatment are increasingly blurred, and both of these goals may remain intertwined in the care and treatment of patients at the most advanced stages of disease. Without a highly developed sense of team-work, and in which the patient and his or her family is included as part of the team, the inevitable tensions between these two goals of caring cannot be resolved. Indeed, as Mount (2003) has observed so acutely and with charac-teristic humour: 'Whole person care requires a caregiver who is whole: until one comes along, use a team!' (p. 42). Teamwork is thus essential to high-quality palliative care. However, as we have seen in this book, a lack of atten-tion to team dynamics means that nurses, doctors and other members of the 'multidisciplinary team' will tend to work in parallel and from their own somewhat insular and well-defended disciplinary perspectives, rather than jointly and from a position of shared understanding about the objectives of care (Corner 2003).

In discussing the problem of teamwork, Corner (2003) develops a tax-onomy of cross-disciplinary working in which 'transdisciplinary working' is the ultimate goal. This model of teamwork involves developing a shared conceptual framework and working out together how to address common problems of patient care. In many health care settings, this may seem almost unattainable. Huntington's (1981, 1986) work with social workers and gen-eral practitioners demonstrated that difficulties lay within the social struc-tures of the organizations rather than being attributable to individual professionals. So while current rhetoric emphasizes multidisciplinary team-working, professional groups might seek to sustain power by developing and maintaining occupational cultures that emphasize differences and each pro-fession's 'uniqueness' (Loxley 1997). Problems that need to be addressed to achieve efficient teamworking are: inadequate organizational support; lack of training in teamwork; lack of interprofessional trust; lack of clear goals; lack of continuity among team members; the dominance of particular dis-courses; and the exclusion of others (Opie and Bernhofen 1997). An evalu-ation of a major programme of community nurse education in palliative care which was designed to increase home death rates and enhance primary care team skills and knowledge in England in the early 2000s, indicated worsening relationships with general practitioners and no change in death rate (Addington-Hall *et al.* 2006). The authors attributed the findings to a lack of interdisciplinary education which heightened divisions and failed to foster greater understanding in the team, although individual nurses benefited.

One approach to understanding these common difficulties may be by analysing the complex dynamics of institutional cultures, professional encul-turation and territoriality. For example, specialist palliative care providers may have to work across statutory and charitable organizations, across primary, secondary and tertiary health care services, and across health and social care services. Using a specific example from the UK, a community-based clinical nurse specialist providing care to a specific patient and family may have to work with NHS-funded general practitioners, a charitably funded hospice, a cardiologist or oncologist at a local general hospital, a radiologist at a distant regional cancer centre, a local authority-funded occupational therapist (to get adaptation to the home and obtain specialist equipment) and a social work team. The task of coordinating and managing the delivery of appropriate and timely care is formidable. It requires skills in liaison, management, planning and an understanding of how each of these very different organizations and professional groups operate. Analysis of these fundamental aspects of organizational work undertaken by nurses would benefit from further research.

In this book we have deliberately set out to highlight palliative care as a key issue for all health and social care professionals and, indeed, for all societies as a major public health issue (Foley 2003). How will changing patterns of disease and dying influence the nature of hospices, specialist palliative care services and general health care services? The population structure is changing with increasing longevity creating challenges in the care of increasing numbers of older people in many resource-rich regions such as Japan, North America and most of Europe. In comparison, in parts of Africa life expectancy has fallen in recent years, due to the combined impacts of war, famine, political mismanagement, poverty and diseases such as HIV/AIDS, seriously impacting upon end-of-life care provision (Wright and Clark 2006). Even in Europe, great diversity in the configuration and provision of palliative care services has been revealed in a recent mapping exercise (Centeno *et al.* 2007). For example, Jaramillo (2003) has painted a bleak picture of palliative care provision in Colombia, where political violence, high drug-related crime rates and poverty have conspired to create fatalism in the population and limited access to adequate health care for the majority of the population, and virtually none for those living in rural and remote areas. Public fears about morphine use, combined by tight control on morphine availability, mean that pain control is not readily available or affordable, except for the wealthy elite. Seymour *et al.* (2005) have drawn attention to wider international issues about the availability, regulation, marketing, pricing, prescription and delivery of opioids that seriously impact on pain relief for many people. Initial work has started in mapping and categorizing the global provision of palliative care and highlighting where no services exist (Wright *et al.* in press). Such activity challenges us to look critically at the transferability of models of palliative care developed predominantly in the UK and North America, and to think about some taken-for-granted assumptions we hold. Most obviously, the possibilities for palliative care must be understood in relation to the demography, epidemiology, politics, social and health care policies, economics and cultures of particular societies. One size certainly does not fit all. Changing patterns of disease and dying are likely to present new challenges not only to the technical aspects of medical and nursing care, but to the organizational aspects of provision.

Thinking of palliative care as a public health issue brings us to a further question that has emerged from the book: 'How is place of care and place of dying associated with delivering palliative care?' As well as marked differences between different societies and regions, we have seen throughout the book a concern to identify how 'places' impinge on palliative care and the whole experience of giving and receiving care. The technical and environmental qualities of particular places may limit or enhance possibilities surrounding 'quality' care and the degree of comfort that may be achieved for a dying person; and different types of place may engender particular types of care practice and interpersonal relationships that influence fundamentally the experience of mortal illness, death and bereavement (Volicer *et al.* 2003). In palliative care, 'home' is often accepted as the ideal place in which to give care to a dying person and for death to occur. However, this assumption is beginning to come under critical review in recognition that this is a culturally contingent preference not necessarily shared by all (Seymour *et al.* 2007). For example, in a study of older persons' views about home as a place of care at the end of life conducted in the UK, Gott *et al.* (2004) report that older people do not always have access to the material or care resources that make care at home either possible or rewarding and that they worry about the possibility of dying alone, invasion of their privacy by visiting staff, and being a burden to their adult children, spouses and other family members and friends. Likewise, Uwimana and Struthers (in press) argue that in Rwanda, civil war and genocide destroyed family traditional structures to such an extent that there were few care-givers available in the home and, consequently, hospitals are the preferred place of care at the end of life. Of course, places of care do not remain static: ill people move from place to place, often having to travel long distances between these to access the treatment they need. Moreover, places of care have symbolic value (such as the home) as well as practical aspects. In summary, we would argue that a fundamental principle is that people have a right to expect attention to their comfort, dignity, safety and respect for their wishes, wherever they die.

## Persons who give and receive care

In North America and some other Western cultures, personal choice and autonomy are held in high esteem. The cultural values placed on these aspects of personhood fundamentally influence the relationship of individuals to each other, and also their relationship with society as a whole (as explored in Chapter 17). For example, they underpin different ethical positions in respect of end-of-life choices, the notion of a 'right to die' and euthanasia (see Chapter 20). Health technologies make possible the re-engineering of death and dying, such as in the use of organ transplantation, artificial body parts, implantable defibrillation devices and heart pace-makers. Technological devices such as syringe driver pumps, Percutaneous Endoscopic Gastronomy (PEG) tubes and intravenous infusions make possible the delivery of medication, nutrition and fluids in ways that may sustain life and arguably prolong the dying process (Graham and Clark 2005a). These technological and medical developments raise important questions about what it means to be 'dying' and how that social and medical status is recognized and conferred on people. An emerging literature has focused on the classification of characteristic 'trajectories of dying' (e.g. Lunney *et al.* 2002) to assist in the allocation of palliative care services. However, the uncertainty of dying trajectories in late old age and for those with co-morbidities, in particular the phenomenon of 'bounce back', means that individuals may experience a number of episodes where they may be perceived to be dying but survive. The prognostication of 'dying' that is known to be unreliable and difficult for professionals, and widely resisted by both professionals and patients (Christakis 1999).

In North America, Australia and in the UK, advance care planning in the form of advance directives and 'living wills', or less structured advance statements of preferences, are becoming increasingly popular as discussed by Seymour and Ingleton in the Overview chapter to Part Two and in many countries, legislative changes mean that professionals have a duty to act upon them (Cartwright 2007). In these documents, people express their preferences for the types of life-sustaining interventions they would wish to be employed on their behalf, and record their advance refusal of life-sustaining interventions, if they were unable to express their views at the time they are needed. Enshrined in these documents is the right that individuals have to reject or refuse to be cared for. It is this notion that many family members and health professionals find difficult to contemplate. While these initiatives are compatible with notions of choice and autonomy, they are based on assumptions that everyone can access and afford a range of high-quality health care and they also assume that choices remain stable – in other words, that people do not change their mind as they adapt to functional decline. They are generally predicated on an assumption that it is possible for people to have 'preferences' about end-of-life care, a desire to contemplate their own death and a wish to communicate with others. Recent research indicates there are wide cultural, age-related and individual differences in the engagement with discussion of these topics in British (Vandrevala and Hampson 2002; Vandrevala *et al.* 2006) and Chinese people (Payne *et al.* 2005). Who makes choices about how death is managed, and how these choices are realized in practice, remain a difficult and under-researched topic.

In this book, we have emphasized the important role played by patients' families, friends, neighbours and other companions. We have also argued that the collective term 'carers' may be understood in rather different ways by those supporting a dying person and health and social care workers. Much of the research evidence suggests that their role is largely unrecognized and insufficiently valued by many societies (Harding and Higginson 2003). In the past, carers were predominantly women, either spouses or children of the dying person. Demographic trends with increased longevity, increased marital breakdown, geographical mobility and more dependence upon female income generation are all likely to impact on the availability of women to offer continuing (unpaid) care to family members. We know little about how people without immediate family members manage to make choices about provision of care and place of dying. A greater integration between health and social care than is currently the case in many countries is likely to be required in the future. In future, palliative care systems need to be seen as part of a wider approach to building services within communities to encourage greater social cohesion and thereby access alternative forms of support, rather than merely relying on kinship networks (Kellehear 2005). For example, in Sierra Leone palliative care services largely deal with patients dying from HIV/AIDS and their model of care has to take account of orphaned and vulnerable children whose parents die in the hospice (Kwaka 2006).

'So, who will provide care?' This book has predominantly been focused on the activities of nurses, but palliative care services in many countries are heavily reliant on unpaid labour – volunteer workers – who may or may not have professional qualifications. Like carers, the contribution of this group of workers largely goes unresearched and unacknowledged. What evidence there is suggests that the employment of volunteers may be mutually beneficial for organizations and the individuals concerned (Field and Johnson 1993; Field *et al.* 1997; Payne 2002). In resource-rich countries volunteer workers have tended to be recruited from middle-aged, middle-class women who have the time, motivation and sufficient economic means to donate their labour to hospices and specialist palliative care services. Economic pressures to earn more and changing patterns of female employment may mean that new categories of people will need to be recruited or that services will need to employ more paid workers. For example, in one part of India, an innovative programme of volunteer support is enabling very poor people to be cared for at home (Graham and Clark 2005b).

Nursing shortage is an increasing problem worldwide (Stordeur *et al.* 2006), resulting from increased demand due to population growth, an ageing population, technological advances and higher patient expectations. In the past two decades there has been a decline in the number of young people entering the nursing profession as job opportunities outside of nursing have expanded. With a lack of new recruits and an ageing nursing population, the current nursing shortage has important implications for employers and policy makers globally. The next generation of workers in their twenties and thirties has different expectations of their working life. They are more likely to be computer literate, adaptable and eager to advance. Moreover, they are a group of people who will wish for a balance between home and work life. This group of workers also may choose to develop a variety of useful skills by expanding their experience quickly and not staying with one employer for long periods. This generation is looking for performance-based rewards and, if these expectations are not met, they are more likely to change careers leaving a gap in the already depleted workforce. In many countries, health care settings face difficulty in the recruitment and retention of nursing staff.

This problem has two origins: the nursing shortage and staff turnover. Organizational determinants of nurse turnover have been extensively studied (Stordeur *et al.* 2006). Direct predictors of turnover include overload and work stress (see Aranda Chapter 29), whereas a supportive nursing management and favourable work-group climate that promotes job satisfaction and member cohesiveness have been found to be negative predictors of nursing turnover (Campion *et al.* 1996). Promotional opportunities and organizational characteristics, associated with empowerment and autonomy, have also been found to decrease the likelihood of leaving. Reasons for leaving that were common to nurses in the USA, Canada, England, Scotland and Germany included emotional exhaustion and problems in working practices (Aiken and Patrician 2001).

Considering the current nursing shortage is predicted to evolve into a severe global shortage, understanding the factors that influence nurses' job satisfaction should be viewed as a pressing priority. Even though nurses in Europe comprise the largest group of health care professionals, accounting for over 1.7 million nurses, there are acute problems with professional status in most parts of Europe (Kearney and Molassiotis 2003). The differences in nursing educational preparation across Europe exacerbate an already complex situation. The recent introduction of core competencies for nurses working in palliative care within Europe (see Chapter 30) is a welcome step in the right direction as the extension of the European Union (EU) has led to a more flexible employment market, with less restrictions on crossing borders.

A priority for the EU is to facilitate this standardization in the progress towards more universal education programmes for other health care disciplines. Progress over the next decade will require collaboration internationally and a close commitment by nursing education, research and practice. There is an increasing need for standard knowledge assessment measures, as well as means for evaluating clinical skills, decision-making, and a broad range of physical, psychosocial and spiritual skills necessary in palliative care (Ferrell and Coyle 2006). New teaching methodologies such as those described by Ingleton and Seymour in the Overview chapter to Part Four and new technologies to support learning (see Chapter 31) will be important resources for educators.

## Equity in palliative and end-of-life care

In some parts of the world palliative care can be regarded as a success story. As Chapter 2 illustrates, the ideas underpinning palliative care have spread around the world in a relatively short time. But even in well-resourced regions such as the UK, there remain marked equalities in access (Ahmed *et al.* 2004). In our view, one of the major challenges for the future is to improve equity of access to good quality care during the end-of-life period. It is likely that advances in medicine and health technologies will mean that greater numbers of people will survive for longer with complex health and social care needs. Formerly acute diseases may become chronic diseases. This is likely to be combined with people experiencing greater numbers of co-morbidities, especially older people. The science of palliative medicine and palliative care nursing is going to be challenged by the management of highly complex symptomatology of multiple diseases. This may mean a different type of workforce is required in specialist palliative care. For example, one scenario might be that specialist professionals become advisors and consultants (on pain and symptom control) to generalists who actually deliver care in their usual health care environments. Greater prominence might be given to other team members such as counsellors, therapists, spiritual experts, nutritionists and psychologists, as their skills become better recognized and are more often demanded by patients and their families who wish to have a 'total package' of end-of-life care. From a public health perspective, it is no longer acceptable that access to palliative care services are linked to diagnostic categories, instead they should be allocated on the basis of need (Skilbeck and Payne 2005). This may mean a breakdown in existing specialisms and greater partnership working.

We believe that consumerism and the blurring of knowledge boundaries between professionals and the public who now have greater access to information, such as via the internet, may influence issues of access and demands for improvement in end-of-life care. However, this is likely in our view to differentially advantage those with the knowledge, education and power to demand access to specialist palliative care. There are concerns that this will create greater divergence between those who have the skills to use health and social care systems and those who remain socially excluded. There is a danger that disease category, culture, ethnicity, social class and geographical location will remain the key drivers determining access rather than burden of illness. Nurses could have an important role in ensuring greater equity of access to end-of-life care, but they will have to be prepared to become more politically and socially assertive than they have generally been in the past. Whatever the configuration of services or the diversity of diseases, people will die and nurses are likely to have a central role in caring for them. As nurses, we are privileged to witness part of our common humanity – death. Palliative care belongs to everyone and, arguably, is a basic right for all those in need.

## References

Addington-Hall, J., McDonald, L.D., Anderson, H.R., Chamberlain, J., Freeling, P., Bland, J.H. and Raferty, G. (1992) Randomized Controlled Trial of Effects of Coordination Care for Terminally Ill Cancer Patients. *British Medical Journal*, 305: 1317–1322.

Addington-Hall, J., Shipman, C., Burt, J., Ream, E., Beynon, T. and Richardson A. (2006) *Evaluation of the education and support programme for district and community nurses in the principles and practice of palliative care.* London: Department of Health.

Ahmed, N., Bestall, J., Ahmedzai, S., Payne, S., Clark, D. and Noble, B. (2004) Systematic review of the problems and issues of accessing specialist palliative care by patients, carers and health and social care professionals, *Palliative Medicine*, 18(6): 525–42.

Aiken, L.H. and Patrician, P.A. (2001) Measuring organisational traits of hospitals: the revised working index. *Nursing Research*, 49(3): 145–53.

Campion, M., Papper, E. and Wedsker, G. (1996) Relations between work team characteristics and effectiveness: a replication and extension. *Personnel Psychology*, 49: 429–52.

Cartwright, C. (2007) Advance care planning in Australia: challenges of a federal legislative system. *Progress in Palliative Care*, 15(3): 113–17.

Centeno, C., Clark, D., Lynch, T., Rocafort, J., Flores, L.A., Greenwood, A., Brasch, S., Praill, D., Giordano, A., and de Lima, L. (2007) *EAPC Atlas of Palliative Care in Europe*. Milan: European Association for Palliative Care.

Christakis, N. (1999) *Death Foretold: Prophecy and Prognosis in Medical Care*. Chicago, IL: University of Chicago Press.

Corner, J. (2003) Nursing management in palliative care. *European Journal of Oncology Nursing*, 7(2): 83–90.

Ferrell, B. and Coyle, N. (2006) *Textbook of Palliative Nursing*, 2nd edn. Oxford: Oxford University Press.

Field, D. and Johnson, I. (1993) Satisfaction and change: a survey of volunteers in a hospice organisation. *Social Science and Medicine*, 36(12): 1625–33.

Field, D., Ingleton, C. and Clark, D. (1997) The costs of unpaid labour: the use of voluntary staff in the King's Mill Hospice. *Health and Social Care in the Community*, 5(3): 198–208.

Foley, K.M. (2003) How much palliative care do we need? *European Journal of Palliative Care*, 10(2): 5–7.

Gott, M., Seymour, J.E., Bellamy, G., Clark, D. and Ahmedzai, S.H. (2004) Older people's views about home as a place of care at the end of life. *Palliative Medicine*, 18(15): 460–7.

Graham, F. and Clark, D. (2005a) The syringe driver and the subcutaneous route in palliative care: the inventor, the history and the implications. *Journal of Pain and Symptom Management*, 29(1): 32–40.

Graham, F. and Clark, D. (2005b) Addressing the basics of palliative care. *International Journal of Palliative Nursing*, 11(1): 36–9.

Harding, R. and Higginson, I. (2003) What is the best way to help caregivers in cancer and palliative care? A systematic literature review of interventions and their effectiveness. *Palliative Medicine*, 17(1): 63–74.

Huntington, J. (1981) *Social Work and General Medical Practice*. London: George Allen & Unwin.

Huntington, J. (1986) The proper contributions of social workers in health practice. *Social Science and Medicine*, 22: 1151–60.

Jaramillo, I. de (2003) Death in Colombia. In: J.D. Morgan and P. Laungani (eds) *Death and Bereavement Around the World. Volume 2: Death and Bereavement in the Americas*. Amityville, New York: Baywood Publishing Company.

Kearney, M. (2000) *A Place of Healing: Working with Suffering in Living and Dying*. Oxford: Oxford University Press.

Kearney, N. and Molassiotis, A. (2003) I have a dream . . . cancer nursing leadership. *European Journal of Oncology Nursing*, 7(4): 227–90.

Kellehear, A (2005) *Compassionate cities: Public health and end of life care*. London: Routledge.

Kwaka, J. (2006) The hospice model in Sierra Leone. *International Journal of Palliative Nursing*, 12(4): 157.

Loxley, A. (1997) *Collaboration in Health and Welfare*. London: Jessica Kingsley.

Lunney, J.R., Lynn, J. and Hogan, C. (2002) Profiles of Older Medicare Decedents. *Journal of the American Geriatrics Society*, 50: 1108–12.

Mount, B.M. (2003) Existential suffering and the determinants of healing. *European Journal of Palliative Care*, 10(suppl.): 40–2.

Opie, A. and Bernhofen, D.M. (1997) Thinking teams and thinking clients: issues of discourse and representation in the work of health care teams. *Sociology of Health and Illness*, 19(3): 259–80.

Payne, S. (2002) Dilemmas in the use of volunteers to provide hospice bereavement support: evidence from New Zealand. *Mortality*, 7(2): 139–54.

Payne, S., Chapman, A., Holloway, M., Seymour, J. and Chau, R. (2005) Chinese Community Views: Promoting Cultural Competence in Palliative Care, *Journal of Palliative Care*, 21(2): 111–16.

Payne, S., Kerr, C., Hawker, S., Seamark, D., Davis, C., Roberts, H., Jarrett, N. and Smith, H. (2007) Dying in old age in community hospitals in the United Kingdom: perceptions of patients, carers and bereaved carers. *Health and Social Care in the Community*, 58(3): 236–45.

Seymour, J., Payne, S., Chapman, A. and Holloway, M. (2007) End of life care: expectations and experiences of white indigenous and Chinese older people in the UK. *Sociology of Health and Illness*, Special Edition on Ethnicity and Health.

Seymour, J., Witherspoon, R., Gott, M., Ross, H. and Payne, S. (2005) *Dying in Older Age: End-of-Life Care*. Bristol: Policy Press.

Skilbeck, J. and Payne, S. (2005) End-of-Life care: a discursive analysis of specialist palliative care nursing, *Journal of Advanced Nursing*, 51(4): 325–34.

Stordeur, S., D'Hoore, W. and the NEXT study group (2006) Organisational configuration of hospitals successful in attracting and retaining nurses. *Journal of Advanced Nursing*, 57(11): 45–54.

Vandrevala, T. and Hampson, S.E (2002) Breaking the death taboo: older people's perspectives on end of life decisions. *Quality in Aging: Policy, practice and research*, 3(3): 36–46.

Vandrevala, T., Hampson, S.E, Daly, T., Arber, S. and Thomas, H. (2006) Dilemmas in decision making about resuscitation: a focus group study of older people. *Social Science and Medicine*, 62(7): 1579–94.

Volicer, L., Hurley, A.C. and Blasi, Z.V. (2003) Characteristics of dementia end of life care across care settings. *American Journal of Hospice and Palliative Care*, 20(3): 191–200.

Wright, M. and Clark, D. (2006) *Hospice and Palliative Care in Africa: a review of developments and challenges*. Oxford: Oxford University Press.

Wright, M., Wood, J., Lynch, T. and Clark, D. (in press) Mapping levels of palliative care development: a global view. *Journal of Pain and Symptom Management*.

# Index

The index entries appear in letter-by-letter alphabetical order.
Page references in italics indicate information in figures and tables.

**Related books from Open University Press**
Purchase from www.openup.co.uk or order through your local bookseller

## ORGAN AND TISSUE DONATION
AN EVIDENCE BASE FOR PRACTICE

### Magi Sque and Sheila Payne (eds)

- What is the historical and social context that shapes our attitudes towards organ and tissue donation?
- How do the bereavement experiences of organ donor families differ from other types of bereavement?
- How can health and social care professionals support bereaved families leading up to, during and after organ and tissue donation?

This ground-breaking book is a valuable addition to the end-of-life, palliative and bereavement care literature. Using original research findings relating to the social and psychological issues surrounding organ donation, this book provides a strong evidence-base and brings together contemporary research carried out in the developed world. The book is internationally applicable, especially in countries with Westernised healthcare systems and where organ donation takes place using similar practices to the UK.

Key areas covered include:

- Examination of the historical development of human dissection and how it created a context for legislation
- Analysis of how human organ and tissue donation is currently understood
- The social theories that help explain the donation event and families' and health professionals' experiences of it

*Organ and Tissue Donation: An Evidence Base for Practice* is essential reading for transplant coordinators and qualified clinical practitioners working in intensive care, accident and emergency departments, operating theatres, palliative care units and bereavement support and counselling services. It is also a core text for specialist postgraduate programmes and a useful reference book for national organisations concerned with donation and transplant services.

**Contents**
*List of contributors – Introduction – Human dissection and organ transplantation in historical context – Contemporary views of bereavement and the experience of grief – Gift of Life or Sacrifice? Key discourses for understanding decision-making by families of organ donors – A dissonant loss: The bereavement of organ donor families – Supporting families' decision-making about organ donation – Tissue donation and the attitudes of health care professionals – Facilitating the donation discussion beyond intensive care: Lessons from specialist palliative care – Decisions about living kidney donation: A family and professional perspective – Xenotransplantation and the Post Human Future – Closing thoughts and the future – Appendix 1 – Index.*

2007   192pp

978–0–335–21692–5 (Paperback)     978–0–335–21693–2 (Hardback)

# DEATH'S DOMINION
## ETHICS AT THE END OF LIFE

## Simon Woods

I enjoyed reading this book very much. It is very readable and well argued using real life cases and thought experiments as well . . . The book provides the reader with a short history of and an overview of the most important issues in modern palliative care. Various theoretical discussions are clearly set out, such as: the relationship between the hospice movement and modern palliative care, between palliative care and health care in general, between palliative sedation and euthanasia, and the question whether euthanasia can be part of palliative care. The author starts with exploring the existing debates and then develops his own arguments in a balanced and well-structured way.

*Medicine, Health Care and Philosophy*

The text of this book is accessible, the philosophical and ethical arguments are clearly articulated, and relevant ethical principles are integrated into the critique of the issues, making this a very useful book for nurses working in palliative as well as in general care.

*Nursing Ethics*

It is crucially important for any student or researcher who is seriously considering ethical and policy matters at the end of life to embrace and tackle intellectually the issues that Woods raises in this book. I would happily recommend it.

*Journal of Medical Ethics*

- What constitutes a good death?
- Is it possible to arrange a good death?
- Is killing compatible with caring?

This book looks at death and the issues and ethical dilemmas faced at the end of life. It addresses the central issues in the field such as:

- Withholding and withdrawing treatment
- Euthanasia and assisted suicide
- Terminal sedation
- The role of autonomy
- Palliative care

Drawing on a philosophical framework, the author explores end-of-life issues in order to reflect on the nature of the good death and how this may be achieved. The book considers whether it is permissible or desirable to influence the quality of dying: offering palliative sedation as a possible alternative to terminal sedation, the argument is extended to examine why some forms of assisted dying can be shown to be compatible with the ideas of palliative care.

Consideration is also given to future developments such as life extension techniques and the ethical questions that that these techniques might raise. As such, the book follows in the ongoing philosophical tradition to critique and analyse current thought on the topic of death, encouraging self-reflection in the reader and offering suggestions for practice in end-of-life care.

*Death's Dominion* is key reading for students and professionals involved in care of the dying, as well as those with an interest in the philosophical issues surrounding end-of-life care.

### Contents
*Acknowledgements – Preface – Introduction – Ethics – Good life, good death – Palliative care: History and values – Ethics in palliative care: Autonomy and respect for persons – Respect for persons: A framework for palliative care – Terminal sedation – Assisted dying – Concluding thoughts – Bibliography – Index.*

2006   192pp

978–0–335–21160–9 (Paperback)       978–0–335–21161–6 (Hardback)

# THE PRESCRIPTION DRUG GUIDE FOR NURSES

## Sue Jordan

This book is exceedingly timely. I am certain it will be invaluable to both undergraduate and post graduate student nurses, and, also act as a continuing reference source. Thoroughly recommended.

*Molly Courtenay, Reading University, UK*

Sue Jordan has combined her deep understanding of her own discipline with her long experience of teaching nurses, to produce just the right type and level of information that nurses need, in a format that they will find relevant to their practice and easy to use. This book will be an essential reference resource for every ward bookshelf.

*Professor Dame June Clark, Swansea University, UK*

This popular *Nursing Standard* prescription drug series is now available for the first time in book format! Organised by drug type and presented in an easy-to-use reference format, this book outlines the implications for practice of 20 drug groups.

Each drug group is presented in handy quick check format, and covers:

- Drug actions
- Indications
- Administration
- Adverse effects
- Practice suggestions
- Cautions/contra-indications
- Interactions

### Contents
*Preface – Using this book – Abbreviations used in the text – Introduction – Laxatives – Controlling gastric acidity – Diuretics – Beta blockers – ACE inhibitors – Vasodilators (calcium channel blockers and nitrates) – Anticoagulants – Bronchodilators: Selective beta2 adrenoreceptor agonists – Cortico-steroids – Antipsychotics – Antidepressants: Focus on SSRIs – Anti-emetics – Opioid analgesics – Anti-epileptic drugs: Focus on carbamazepine and valproate – Antibacterial drugs – Insulin – Oral anti-diabetic drugs – Thyroid and anti-thyroid drugs – Cytotoxic drugs – Non-steroidal anti-inflammatory drugs (NSAIDs) – Idiosyncratic drug reactions – Glossary – References – Bibliography/ Further reading – Index.*

March 2008   192pp

978–0–335–22547–7 (Paperback)       978–0–335–22546–0 (Hardback)

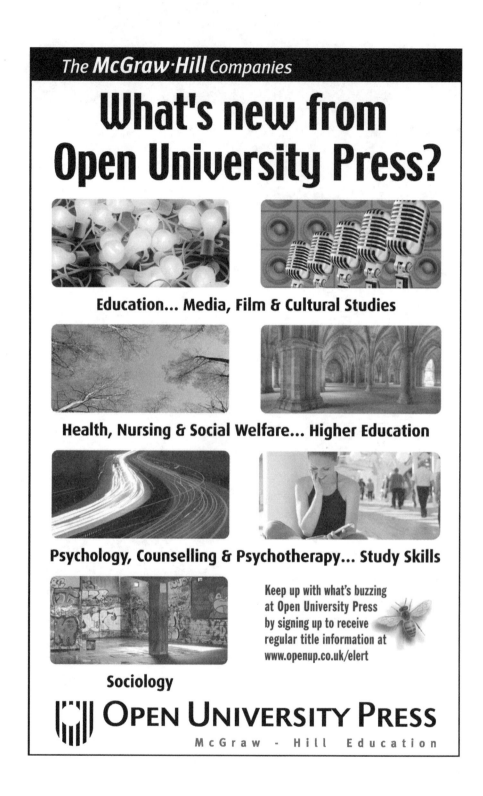